F. A. Davis Company
1915 Arch Street
Philadelphia, PA 19103
www.fadavis.com

Printed in the United States of America

Last digit indicates print number: 10 9 8 7 6 5 4 3

As new scientific information becomes available through basic and clinical research,
recommended treatments and drug therapies undergo changes. The author(s) and publisher
have done everything possible to make this book accurate, up to date, and in accord with
accepted standards at the time of publication. The author(s), editors, and publisher are not
responsible for errors or omissions or for consequences from application of the book, and make
no warranty, expressed or implied, in regard to the contents of the book. Any practice described
in this book should be applied by the reader in accordance with professional standards of care
used in regard to the unique circumstances that may apply in each situation. The reader is
advised always to check product information (package inserts) for changes and new
information regarding dose and contraindications before administering any drug.
Caution is especially urged when using new or infrequently ordered drugs.

Library of Congress Control Number: 2014960189

Foundations of Clinical Research

Applications to Practice

3rd Edition

Leslie G. Portney, DPT, PhD, FAPTA
Dean, School of Health and Rehabilitation Sciences
MGH Institute of Health Professions
Boston, Massachusetts

Mary P. Watkins, DPT, MS
Professor Emerita
MGH Institute of Health Professions
Boston, Massachusetts

F.A. Davis Company • Philadelphia

Contents

Appendices

Preface

As we approached the revision of this text for the third edition, we realized that the prevailing paradigms of clinical research in rehabilitation and medicine had continued to evolve over the past 10 years, and that we had to address several important changes in the research landscape. Probably the most notable of these changes is the emphasis on evidence-based practice (EBP) that has become central to all of health care. The World Health Organization's adoption of the *International Classification of Functioning and Disability (ICF)* has created a new vocabulary that is being integrated into research and practice across disciplines. Questions related to diagnostic accuracy and clinical decision making are prominent in research literature, and phrases like "responsiveness," "minimally important change" and "number needed to treat" are becoming essential to EBP. Attitudes about clinical research have emphasized the responsibility of every clinician to better understand how to apply evidence to patient care, and the gaps in our research knowledge have become more evident as we often search for answers that are not there.

This book has served a variety of audiences in research, professional education and clinical practice. It continues to be directed toward those in physical therapy, occupational therapy, speech therapy, nursing, medicine, exercise physiology, and public health, as well as other disciplines concerned with questions of health and health care. The book will remain a text for courses in research and critical inquiry, as well as a comprehensive reference for clinicians and researchers who are committed to evidence-based practice.

We have included varied levels of detail in design and statistics to meet the diverse needs of those who use this text. Instructors are urged to consider which portions of the text are relevant for their students, and not to expect to use it all in their courses. Students will find it user-friendly as they learn concepts and principles of research, and will keep it is a reference as they grow in their professional role. Those who are engaged in research activities or advanced education will be able to utilize the more detailed portions as they explore research questions. And clinicians will be able to apply these principles to their clinical decision making.

The application of evidence-based practice to health care requires an understanding of design and analytic methods. Our text is not going to provide the answers to clinical questions for practice—that must be left to journal articles and clinical textbooks, and to those who mentor students and clinicians, who will ask the right questions. Our contribution is to provide the foundations that are necessary for finding and interpreting research evidence. Clinicians must provide the experience and knowledge to apply the research to their practice.

Although the general organization of the book has not changed, several additions have been incorporated into this edition to provide a contemporary framework for clinical research. Part I covers the basic concepts of research, including a discussion of theory and ethical principles. In this section we introduce important contexts for research related to models of health and evidence-based practice. Part II focuses on measurement, including a comprehensive examination of reliability and validity. Part III presents the broad scope of experimental, exploratory and descriptive research approaches, including a new chapter on systematic reviews and meta-analysis.

Part IV of the text is devoted to the application of statistical procedures, from descriptive to multivariate approaches. This section now contains expanded content related to clinical decision making, including likelihood ratios, pretest and posttest probabilities, minimally important change and number needed to treat. We continue to focus on the conceptual foundations of statistics, although calculations are provided for those who desire that level of detail. We use the format for SPSS in presenting output, but with explanations that we trust will allow integration with other statistical packages.

Part V focuses on processes of research and communication, including an expanded chapter on searching the literature, development of proposals, presentation of research, and critical appraisal of published literature. Appendices provide tables of reference for statistical procedures, a newly designed algorithm for choosing statistical approaches for analysis, examples of power analysis for various designs, methods of transforming data, and a sample informed consent form.

Prentice Hall has provided a wonderful opportunity to share information related to all sections of the book on their companion website, which can be accessed at www.prenhall.com/portney. We hope you will find this a helpful addition to the text, especially for those who use it for teaching purposes.

As the health care environment evolves, we will always anticipate new directions and priorities for clinical research. Therefore, this work will always be in progress. We are proud to be part of the larger health care research and clinical communities that are clearly dedicated to the pursuit of new knowledge and the application of evidence to improve patient care. We look forward to the continued journey with all of you.

Acknowledgments

We are indebted to many friends and colleagues who have shared their thoughts and time with us as this edition has been developed. We extend our gratitude to Dale Avers, Steve Alison, Jane Baldwin, Marianne Beninato, Maura Iversen, Madhuri Kale, Kevin Kearns, Aimee Klein, Mary Knab, Virgil Mathiewitz, Ruth Purtilo, Paul Stark, Patricia Sullivan and Elise Townsend for taking the time to read, critique and provide feedback on sections of the book. Several individuals were especially helpful in providing in-depth reviews: Roy Lee Aldridge Jr, Louise Dunn, Mary Ann Holbein-Jenny, Robin Gaines Lanzi, Beth Marcoux, Keli Mu, Gerald Smith, Rebecca States, Gordon St. Michael and Frank Underwood. We thank Laurita Hack, Kay Shepherd and Kim Nixon-Cave, from Temple University, who provided significant assistance to improve the content on qualitative research, and Joy McDermid who so graciously shared her experiences with systematic reviews.

We continue to thank our students from the MGH Institute of Health Professions for their enthusiasm and generous spirit. And we are grateful to all of our colleagues who stop us at conferences and other venues to share a kind word about how the book has helped them. Those are moments of true satisfaction.

The staff at Prentice Hall has remained dedicated and understanding as we labored through this revision. We appreciate everyone's patience and will continue to be grateful to Mark Cohen for all he has done to keep this work moving. We want to thank Nicole Ragonese (Editorial Assistant), Patrick Walsh (Production Manager), and Christina Zingone (Production Liaison) for their contributions. Angela Corio has done a wonderful job writing the content for the book's Web site. Karen Berry (Production Editor) at Pine Tree Composition was wonderfully supportive through the production of the book.

As always, our families remain the foundation of our lives, and we are ever grateful for their support. Leslie's girls are out of the house, finding their way in life, and Mary's girls are married with daughters of their own. Skip and John are now doing the cooking in addition to the dishes—and we are all looking forward to the next chapters in our lives!

Reviewers

Roy Lee Aldridge Jr., PT, SCCT
Assistant Professor
Arkansas State University
State University, Arkansas

Louise Dunn, ScD, OTR/L
Assistant Professor
University of Utah
Salt Lake City, Utah

Robin Gaines Lanzi, PhD, MPH
Assistant Professor
Georgetown University
Washington, District of Columbia

Mary Ann Holbein-Jenny, PhD, DPT
Associate Professor
Slippery Rock University
Slippery Rock, Pennsylvania

Beth C. Marcoux, PT, PhD
Professor and Chair
University of Rhode Island
Kingston, Rhode Island

Keli Mu, PhD, OTR/L
Assistant Professor
Creighton University
Omaha, Nebraska

Gerald V. Smith, PT, PhD
Associate Professor and Program Director
University of Cental Florida
Orlando, Florida

Rebecca A. States, Ph.D.
Associate Professor
Long Island University
Brooklyn, New York

Gordon St. Michael, MPH, OTR/L, FAOTA
Associate Professor
Eastern Kentucky University
Richmond, Kentucky

Frank B. Underwood, PT, PhD, ECS
Professor
University of Evansville
Evansville, Indiana

PART **1**

Foundations of Clinical Research

CHAPTER 1

A Concept of Clinical Research

The ultimate purpose of a profession is to develop a knowledge base that will maximize the effectiveness of practice. To that end, health professionals have recognized the necessity for documenting and testing elements of clinical practice through rigorous and objective analysis and scientific inquiry. The concept of **evidence-based practice** represents the fundamental principle that the provision of quality care will depend on our ability to make choices that have been confirmed by sound scientific data, and that our decisions are based on the best evidence currently available. If we look at the foundations of clinical practice, however, we are faced with the reality that often compels practitioners to make intelligent, logical, best-guess decisions when scientific evidence is either incomplete or unavailable.

This situation is even more of an issue because of the economic challenges that continue to confront health care. Clinical research has, therefore, become an imperative, driving clinical judgments, the organization of practice, and reimbursement. The task of addressing the needs of the present and future is one that falls on the shoulders of all clinicians—whether we function as consumers of professional literature or scientific investigators—to collect meaningful data, to analyze outcomes, and to critically apply research findings to promote optimal clinical care. Through collaborative and interdisciplinary efforts, researchers and clinicians share a responsibility to explore the broadest implications of their work, to contribute to balanced scientific thought. The purpose of this text is to provide a frame of reference that will bring together the comprehensive skills needed to promote critical inquiry as part of the clinical decision making process.

In this chapter we develop a concept of research that can be applied to clinical practice, as a method of generating new knowledge and providing evidence to justify treatment choices. We will explore an historic perspective of clinical research, the framework of evidence-based practice, the different types of research that can be applied to clinical questions, and the process of clinical research.

DEFINING CLINICAL RESEARCH

The concept of research in health professions has evolved along with the development of techniques of practice and changes in the health care system. Traditionally, research has connoted controlled laboratory experiments, run by scientists in white lab coats using complex instrumentation; however, the maturation of a clinical profession brings with it the realization that research has a broader meaning as it is applied to the patients and situations encountered in practice. **Clinical research** is a structured process of investigating facts and theories and exploring connections. It proceeds in a systematic way to examine clinical conditions and outcomes, to establish relationships among clinical phenomena, to generate evidence for decision making and to provide the impetus for improving methods of practice.

Clinical research must be *empirical* and *critical*; that is, results must be observable, documented and examined for their validity.[1] This objective process is, however, also a dynamic and creative activity, performed in many different settings, using a variety of quantitative and qualitative measurement tools and focusing on the application of clinical theory and interventions. It is a way of satisfying one's curiosity about clinical phenomena, stimulating the intellectual pursuit of truth to understand or explain clinical events, and generating new or different ways of viewing clinical problems.

The context of clinical research is often seen within a prevailing paradigm. **Scientific paradigms** have been described as ways of looking at the world that define both the problems that can be addressed and the range of legitimate evidence that contributes to solutions.[2] We can appreciate changes in research standards and priorities in terms of three paradigm shifts that have emerged in rehabilitation and medicine through the latter half of the 20th century: the focus on outcomes research to document effectiveness, the application of models of health and disability and most recently an attention to evidence-based practice.

MEASUREMENT OF OUTCOMES

The concept of looking at outcomes as the validation of quality care is not a new one. Historically, the triad of *structure, process* and *outcomes* has been used as the barometer of healthcare quality.[3] Structure was assessed through organizational standards, and process through quality assurance programs examining details such as charges and record keeping. Outcomes of care were typically assessed in terms of morbidity, mortality, length of stay and readmissions.

In rehabilitation, outcomes were often related to improvements in impairments or pathologies, with the assumption that such changes would be linked to the ultimate outcomes of interest. Today, the concept of outcomes has been expanded to fit with the World Health Organization's definition of health, which includes physical, social and psychological well-being.[4] Looking at the effects of intervention now includes consideration of patient satisfaction, patient preferences, self-assessment of functional capacity and quality of life. Clinicians and especially patients have always considered functional outcome as the ultimate measure of the success of intervention. At this time, however, consumers and reimbursement policies have obligated health care practitioners to define and document outcomes, and to substantiate the efficiency and effectiveness of treatment.

To be meaningful the outcomes agenda must influence public policy, routine monitoring of medical care and standardized assessment of patient outcomes.[5] Clinical practice databases must be developed to include functional outcome measures and other relevant information to contribute to the evaluation of outcomes.[6] Clinical managers now use these data to support practice and organizational structure. The objective of **outcomes management** has generated a renewed understanding of the link between clinical management decisions, treatment decisions and measured documentation of effectiveness.[7–11] Outcomes management has emerged as an interdisciplinary process aimed at determining best practices and identifying opportunities for improvement of clinical quality through intermediate and long-term outcome analysis.[12]

Outcomes research refers to the study of success of interventions in clinical practice, with a focus on the end results of patient care in terms of disability and survival.[13] Such studies often use large administrative databases that include information about insurance coverage and utilization of services in addition to functional outcomes. Patients are frequently followed over time after discharge.

Outcome Measures

Outcomes can be documented in many ways. Economic indicators are traditional outcomes, interpreted within the context of cost effectiveness or cost-benefit ratio; that is, what is the relative cost in terms of success of outcomes? For example, Harp[14] demonstrated how revenue, patient outcomes, staff productivity, costs and patient satisfaction could reflect the success of a rehabilitation program for patients with back and neck problems. Fakhry and associates[15] looked at the effectiveness of using evidence-based guidelines for treating patients with traumatic brain injury (TBI), a condition they described as costing billions of dollars annually. They used a protocol based on Brain Trauma Foundation guidelines, and demonstrated that adherence to this protocol resulted in a reduction of mortality, length of stay and disability as well as financial resources.

The development of questionnaires to measure outcomes in terms of function and health status has become a major thrust of health research and has provided a mechanism for understanding how functional outcomes relate to specific elements of health care. Generic instruments that assess quality of life, and more specifically health-related quality of life (HRQOL), have provided an overarching perspective for understanding the outcomes of health care in terms of physical, psychological and social function.

Many health status scales have been developed to assess these constructs. Two of the more widely used instruments, the Medical Outcomes Study Short-Form 36 (SF-36) and the Sickness Impact Profile (SIP), have been validated in many languages[16–22] and for many different patient populations.[23–34] These scales have also been tested in abbreviated forms that demonstrate an efficiency of validity. These instruments allow for calculation of a summary score or subscale scores that are theoretically related to different dimensions of function and health status. For example, the SF-36 provides eight subscale scores that reflect physical function, physical role limitations, mental function, social function, vitality, general health, bodily pain, and emotional role limitations.[35]

Those who study HRQOL have debated the usefulness of generic measures over disease-specific (or condition or region-specific) instruments that include items focused on issues relevant to a particular disorder. For example, the Western Ontario and McMaster Osteoarthritis Index (WOMAC) is specific to arthritis.[36] The Minnesota

Living with Heart Failure Questionnaire targets individuals with heart disease.[37] Studies that compare generic and specific tools generally lead to the conclusion that specific tools are more powerful for understanding impairments and function, but both are needed to get a full picture of the individual's quality of life.[38-40]

Issues of validity for outcome measures remain paramount, as researchers and clinicians must understand the conditions and situations for which these tests are appropriate. The interpretation of outcomes based on these tests must also be made with consideration of the constructs that are being measured. Clinical decisions based on such outcomes must account for the context of the scale used and its measurement properties. Chapter 6 will focus on these issues in greater detail.

MODELS OF HEALTH AND DISABILITY

A second concept in understanding the evolution of medical research is related to the overriding framework for the delivery of health care. This was historically based on the **biomedical model**, which focuses on a linear relationship between pathology and resulting impairments. Within this model, health is viewed as the absence of disease and the assumption is made that disease and injury can be treated and cured. The biomedical model confines attention to physical aspects of health, without consideration of how the patient is affected by illness.[41] The primary outcomes of interest under this model are the traditional endpoints of cure, disease or death.[42,43] However, as health care advances and people live longer, practitioners appreciate the inadequacies of the biomedical model for dealing with the common problems of aging, chronic disease and disability, which do not fall within the rubric of "treat and cure," and the consequent need to look differently at the assessment of "successful" interventions.

An expansion of this model has been applied to a broader perspective in rehabilitation. The **disablement model** (see Figure 1.1A) has provided a framework for assessing the effect of acute and chronic conditions by emphasizing functional consequences and social role. This model demonstrates the relationships among pathology, impairments, functional limitations and disability.[44,45] Although variants of this model have been proposed with different terminology, they have all included the basic elements of pathology, organ system dysfunction, restrictions in activities of daily living (ADL) and limitations of role performance as a member of society.[46] Accordingly, this model provides a conceptual basis for looking at outcomes within the broader context of health, including psychological and social domains, general health status and quality of life.[42,47-49]

The International Classification of Functioning, Disability and Health

In 2001 the World Health Organization (WHO) published a revised model of the **International Classification of Functioning, Disability and Health (ICF)** (see Figure 1.1B).[50] The ICF is the result of an international and multidisciplinary effort to provide a common language for the classification and consequences of health conditions. Rather than focusing on disability, the intent of the ICF is to describe how people

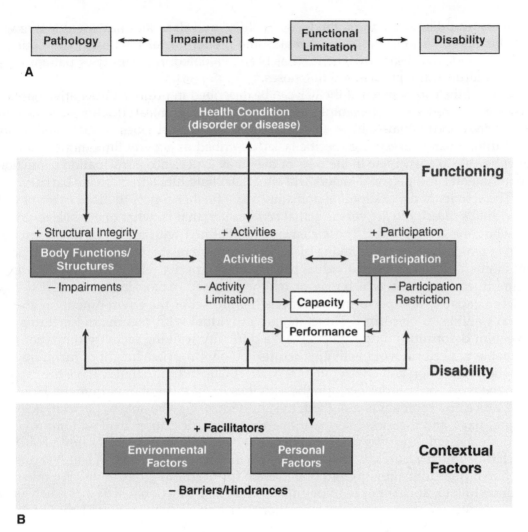

FIGURE 1.1 **A.** The model of disablement, as described by Nagi,[44] showing the relationship among pathology, impairments, functional limitations and disability. **B.** The World Health Organization International Classification of Functioning, Disability and Health (ICF).[50] Each component of the ICF can be expressed in positive or negative terms, as shown. Capacity and performance are two elements of the Activity and Participation domains.

live with their health condition. It is a comprehensive representation of health and health-related domains based on the relationships among health conditions, body functions and structures, activities and participation. The domains are classified from body, individual and societal perspectives. Since an individual's functioning and disability occur in a context, the ICF also includes specific reference to environmental and personal factors that can affect function.[51]

The ICF holds a parallel to the disablement model. Health conditions correspond to pathology; body functions/structures correspond to impairments; activity corresponds to functional limitation; and participation corresponds to disability. The ICF may be more useful, however, to understand and measure health outcomes, looking beyond mortality and disease. It shifts the focus to "life," and describes how people live with their health condition. This context makes the model useful for health promotion as well as illness and disability. The ICF has been evaluated in a variety of patient populations, cultures, age groups and diagnoses.[52-58]

Each of the components of the ICF can be described in positive or negative terms, as shown in Figure 1.1B.[59] For example, body systems or anatomical structures will be intact or impaired. Individuals will be able to perform specific activities or they will demonstrate difficulties in executing specific tasks, described as activity limitations. They will either be able to participate in life roles or they may experience participation restrictions. Environmental and personal factors will either facilitate function or create barriers.

The activity and participation domains can be further conceptualized in terms of an individual's *capacity* to act versus actual *performance;* that is, what one is *able* to do versus what one actually *does.* These elements are defined with reference to the environment in which assessment is taking place. Performance relates to the "current" or actual environment in which the individual participates. Capacity relates to a "standardized" optimum environment, which may be real or assumed. According to the ICF, the gap between capacity and performance reflects the impact of the environment on an individual's ability to perform.[59] Therefore, an individual with rheumatoid arthritis may have joint deformities (impairments), have difficulty walking (activity limitation) and be unable to perform work activities because of inappropriate height of furniture (participation restriction and environmental barrier). The individual may have the capacity to do the work, but cannot perform the activities in the current environment. However, if the office environment is modified, this individual may be able to perform activities without pain, and therefore, her performance and participation level will improve.

Both the ICF and the disablement model provide a framework for identifying which outcome measures are relevant for specific clients or patients. Health status and functional questionnaires present one avenue for examining outcomes. We must also continue to look at changes in impairments and basic functional activities, such as gait or the performance of a particular functional or occupational task, to provide a complete picture of improvement. Data on psychological and social aspects of health must also be collected, including the impact of the environment. As we become more involved in the documentation of outcomes it is imperative that we understand the measurement properties of the tools we use so they can be applied and interpreted properly (see Chapters 4–6).

EVIDENCE-BASED PRACTICE

Stressing the importance of objective documentation in clinical research does not mean that practice can be reduced to a finite science. There is no pure "scientific method" that can account for the influence of experience, intuition and creativity in clinical judgment. Making clinical decisions in the face of uncertainty and variability is part of the "art" of clinical practice. We cannot, however, dissociate the art from the science that supports it. The framework of **evidence-based practice (EBP)** helps to put this in perspective.

Sackett and colleagues[60] have provided a popular definition of evidence-based practice as the "conscientious, explicit and judicious use of current best evidence in making decisions about the care of individual patients." EBP is also described as the "integration of best research evidence with our clinical expertise and our patient's unique values and circumstances."[61] Embedded in this definition is an important concept, that evidence is applied in a process of clinical decision making within the context of a patient or clinical scenario. It emphasizes that research literature provides one, but not the only, source of information for decision making. Perhaps more aptly called *evidence-based decision making*, this process requires considering all relevant information and then making choices that provide the best opportunity for a successful outcome given the patient-care environment and available resources.

The process of EBP starts by asking a relevant clinical question. The question provides a direction for decision making related to a patient's diagnosis, prognosis or intervention. Questions may also relate to etiology of the patient's problem, the validity of clinical guidelines, safety or cost-effectiveness of care. It should not be surprising that the ability to formulate a good question is essential to finding a relevant answer! It is not a general question, but one that focuses specifically on the characteristics of the patient and issues related to his or her management. The acronym **PICO** has been used to represent the components of a good clinical question: **P**atients, **I**ntervention, **C**omparison, **O**utcome (see Box 1.1).

The question leads to a search for the best evidence that can contribute to a decision about the patient's care. The terms defined within the PICO format can be used as keywords in a search for literature. The concept of "best evidence" is important, as it refers to the availability of valid and relevant research information. Clinicians must be able to search and access literature (see Chapter 31), critically appraise studies to determine if they meet validity standards, and then determine if and how research results apply to a given clinical situation. A working knowledge of research design and statistics is important for clinicians to use this information wisely. For instance, in describing the Hypothesis-Oriented Algorithm for Clinicians II (HOAC II), Rothstein et al.[62] have made the assessment of evidence a clearly identifiable part of the decision making process.

This assessment, however, must be made by a clinician who then integrates his or her own clinical judgment and experience with the patient's needs and unique characteristics to make a decision about the patient's care (see Figure 1.2). This decision will also take into account the current circumstances of care, including available equipment, space, time, the patient's comorbidities and the clinical setting. Even Sackett acknowledges that

> . . . without clinical experience, practice risks being tyrannized by evidence, for even excellent external advice may be inapplicable to or inappropriate for an individual patient.[63] (p.vi)

There are many useful journal articles,* books[61] and websites[64-68] that describe the concepts related to EBP, including interpretation of statistical outcomes. We will include

---

*See the series of articles published by the Evidence-Based Medicine Working Group in the *Journal of the American Medical Association* from 1992 to 2001. These papers can also be found at <http://www.cche.net/usersguides/life.asp> Accessed January 15, 2006. See also articles in *Evidence-Based Medicine Reviews*, including the *Cochrane Database of Systematic Reviews*, the ACP Journal Club and the Database of Abstracts of Reviews and Effects (DARE).

BOX 1.1   Background and Foreground Questions for Evidence-Based Practice

Developing a good clinical question is the essential first step in evidence-based practice. It is important to draw a distinction between this type of question and questions that are used to guide research endeavors. The purpose of a research question is to identify and define variables that will be studied using specific design strategies, typically addressing issues of concern for populations with certain disorders. For evidence-based practice, however, we develop a clinical question that focuses on the management of a particular patient. That question will guide the search for research to support clinical decision making.

Consider the following case: Mrs. Jones is a 75-year old woman who suffered a right CVA 2 months ago. She is being seen by physical, occupational, and speech therapists in an inpatient rehabilitation setting. She is able to walk short distances with a cane with moderate assistance, and exhibits poor balance. One of your colleagues suggests that you consider training the patient on a treadmill with partial body-weight support, but you have not tried this approach before.

How one asks a question to guide practice will depend on what one needs to know. As obvious as that seems, it is useful to consider what Straus et al[61] have termed background and foreground questions. A **background question** refers to general knowledge about a disorder or intervention, often relating to etiology, pathophysiology, or prognosis. For example, in the case of Mrs. Jones we might be interested in learning more about the causes of balance disorders in stroke, or the prognosis of balance and gait in stroke survivors.

A **foreground question** relates to specific information that will guide management of the patient, typically addressing diagnosis or intervention. Such questions will have four components.

The acronym **PICO** helps us focus on the appropriate pieces of information.

P   What is the target **population?** What are the characteristics of the **patient** or **problem** that should be considered?

I   What is the **intervention** that is being considered? This component may also be a prognostic factor or diagnostic test.

C   What **comparison** or **control** condition is being considered? This component is most appropriate when comparing the effectiveness of two interventions or when comparing the accuracy of two or more diagnostic tests. It will not be relevant for a question of prognosis or when examining only one intervention or diagnostic test.

O   What are the **outcomes** of interest? What measurements will be relevant to understanding the effectiveness of an intervention, the importance of a prognostic factor, or the accuracy of a diagnostic test?

We may ask Mrs. Jones the following foreground question:

In an elderly patient two-months post stroke **(P)**, is partial body weight-supported treadmill training **(I)** more effective than traditional gait training with full weight-bearing **(C)** for improving walking speed, endurance and balance **(O)**?

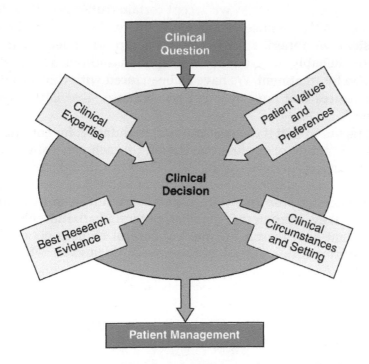

FIGURE 1.2   The components of evidence-based practice as a framework for clinical decision making.

many of these concepts throughout this text as we discuss research designs, statistical analyses and the use of published material for clinical decision making. The success of evidence-based practice will continue to be assessed as we examine outcomes based on use of published guidelines and treatment effects.

SOURCES OF KNOWLEDGE

The information that is used to make clinical decisions and to support clinical research can be acquired in many different ways. As one participates in the pursuit of knowledge, it is interesting to reflect on the sources of information that guide our thinking and decision making. How do we decide which test to perform, which intervention will be most successful, which patients have the best chance of responding positively to a given treatment? Oftentimes clinical problems can be solved on the basis of scientific evidence, but in many situations such evidence does not exist or is not directly applicable. It is important, then, to consider how we come to "know" things, and how we can appropriately integrate what we know with available evidence as we are faced with clinical problems (see Figure 1.3).

Tradition

As members of an organized culture, we accept certain truths as givens. Something is thought to be true simply because people have always known it to be true. Within such a belief system, we inherit knowledge and accept precedent, without need for external validation. Rehabilitation science is steeped in tradition as a guide to practice and as a foundation for treatment. We have all been faced with clinical, administrative or educational practices that are continued just because "that is the way they have always been done."

Tradition is useful in that it offers a common foundation for communication and interaction within a society or profession. Therefore, each generation is not responsible for reformulating an understanding of the world through the development of new concepts. Nevertheless, tradition as a source of knowledge poses a serious problem in clinical science because many traditions have not been evaluated for their validity, nor have they been tested against potentially better alternatives. Sole reliance on precedent as a reason for making clinical choices generally stifles the search for new information, and may perpetuate an idea even when contrary evidence is available.

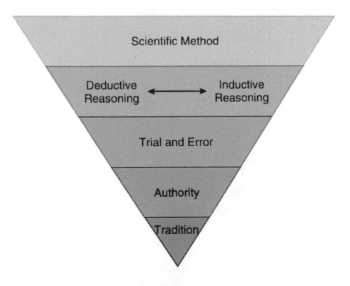

FIGURE 1.3   Ways of knowing.

Authority

We frequently find ourselves turning to specialized sources of **authority** for answers to questions. If we have a problem with finances, we seek the services of an accountant. If we need legal advice for purchasing a home, we hire a real estate lawyer. In the medical profession we regularly pursue the expertise of specialists for specific medical problems. Given the rapid accumulation of knowledge and technical advances and the need to make decisions in situations where we are not expert, it is most reasonable and natural to place our trust in those who are authoritative on an issue by virtue of specialized training or experience.

Authorities often become known as expert sources of information based on their success, experience or reputation. When an authority states that something is true, we accept it. As new techniques are developed, we often jump to use them without demanding evidence of their scientific merit, ignoring potential limitations, even when the underlying theoretical rationale is unclear.[69,70] Too often we find ourselves committed to one approach over others, perhaps based on what we were taught, because the technique is empirically useful. This is a necessary approach in situations where scientific evidence is unavailable; however, we jeopardize our professional responsibility if these techniques are not critically analyzed and if their effects are not scientifically documented.

The danger of uncritical reliance on authoritative canon is well illustrated by the unyielding belief in the medical tenets of Galen (A.D. 138–201), whose teachings were accepted without challenge in the Western world for 16 centuries. When physicians in the 16th and 17th centuries began dissecting human organs, they were not always able to validate Galen's statements. His defenders, in strict loyalty and unwilling to doubt the authority, wrote that if the new findings did not agree with Galen's teachings, the discrepancy should be attributed to the fact that nature had changed![71]

Trial and Error

The **trial and error** method of data gathering was probably the earliest approach to solving a problem. The individual faced with a problem attempts one solution and evaluates its effects. If the effects are reasonably satisfactory, the solution is generally adopted. If not, another solution is tried. We use this method when we have no other basis for making a decision. We have all used trial and error at one time or another in our personal lives and in professional practice. Trial and error incorporates the use of intuition and creativity in selecting alternatives when one approach does not work.

The major disadvantage of trial and error is its haphazard and unsystematic nature and the fact that knowledge obtained in this way is usually not shared, making it inaccessible to others facing similar problems. In situations where a good response is not obtained, a continuous stream of different solutions may be tried, with no basis for sorting out why they are not working.

Trial and error is by nature extremely time consuming and limiting in scope, for although several possible solutions may be proposed for a single problem, the process generally ends once a "satisfactory" response is obtained. Experience is often based on these solutions, and when similar situations arise, a better solution, as yet untried, may never be tested. Therefore, a clinician using this method should never conclude that the "best" solution has been found.

Logical Reasoning

Many clinical problems are solved through the use of logical thought processes. Logical reasoning as a method of knowing combines personal experience, intellectual faculties, and formal systems of thought. It is a systematic process that has been used throughout history as a way of answering questions and acquiring new knowledge. Two distinctive types of reasoning are used as a means of understanding and organizing phenomena: deductive and inductive reasoning (see Figure 1.4).

Deductive Reasoning

Deductive reasoning is characterized by the acceptance of a general proposition, or premise, and the subsequent inferences that can be drawn in specific cases. The ancient Greek philosophers introduced this systematic method for drawing conclusions by using a series of three interrelated statements, called a *syllogism*, containing (1) a major premise, (2) a minor premise and (3) a conclusion. A classic syllogism will serve as an example:

1. All living things must die.   [major premise]
2. Man is a living thing.   [minor premise]
3. Therefore, all men must die.   [conclusion]

In deductive reasoning, if the premises are true, then it follows that the conclusion must be true. Scientists use deductive logic by beginning with known scientific principles or generalizations, and deducing specific assertions that are relevant to a specific question. The observed facts will cause the scientist to confirm, to reject or to modify the conclusion. The greater the accuracy of the premise, the greater the accuracy of the conclusion.

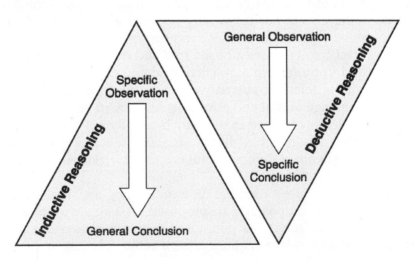

FIGURE 1.4   The relationship between deductive and inductive reasoning.

For example, we might reason that exercise will be an effective intervention to prevent falls in the elderly in the following way:

1. Impaired postural stability results in falls.
2. Exercise improves postural stability.
3. Therefore, exercise will decrease the risk of falls.

This system of deductive reasoning produces a testable hypothesis: If we develop an exercise program for individuals who have impaired stability, we should see a decrease in the number of falls. This has been the basis for a number of studies. For example, Wolf and colleagues[72] used this logic as the theoretical premise for their study comparing balance training and tai chi exercise to improve postural stability in a sample of older, inactive adults. Carter and coworkers[73] designed an exercise program aimed at modifying risk factors for falls in elderly women with osteoporosis. Similarly, Barnett et al.[74] studied the effect of participation in a weekly group exercise program over one year on the rate of falling in community dwelling older people. All three studies found that the exercise groups either had a lower incidence of falls or delayed onset of falls, supporting the premise from which the treatment was deduced.

Of course, deductive reasoning does have limitations. Its usefulness is totally dependent on the truth of its premises. In many situations, the theoretical assumptions on which a study is based may be faulty or unsubstantiated, so that the study and its conclusions have questionable validity. In addition, we must recognize that deductive conclusions are only elaborations on previously existing knowledge. Deductive reasoning can organize what is already known and can suggest new relationships, but it cannot be a source of new knowledge. Scientific inquiry cannot be conducted on the basis of deductive reasoning alone because of the difficulty involved in establishing the universal truth of many statements dealing with scientific phenomena.

Inductive Reasoning

Inductive reasoning reflects the reverse type of logic, developing generalizations from specific observations. It begins with experience and results in conclusions or generalizations that are probably true. This approach to knowing was advanced in the late 16th century by Francis Bacon, who called for an end to reliance on authority as absolute truth. He proposed that the discovery of new knowledge required direct observation of nature, without prejudice or preconceived notions.[75] Facts gathered on a sample of events could lead to inferences about the whole. This reasoning gave birth to the scientific approach to problem solving, and often acts as the basis for common sense. For example, we might observe that those patients who exercise do not fall, and that those who do not exercise fall more often. We might then conclude, through induction, that exercise will improve postural stability.

Inductive reasoning has its limitations as well. The quality of the knowledge derived from inductive reasoning is dependent on the representativeness of the specific observations used as the basis for generalizations. To be absolutely certain of an inductive conclusion, the researcher would have to observe all possible examples of the event. This is feasible only in the rare situations where the set of events in question is very small, and we therefore find ourselves relying mostly on imperfect induction based on incomplete observations. In the preceding example, if we observe the effects of exercise on a sample of elderly persons, and if balance and exercise responses are related to aging, our conclusion may not be a valid one for younger individuals.

Even with these limitations, the process of logical reasoning, both deductive and inductive, is an essential component of scientific inquiry and clinical problem solving. Both forms of reasoning are used to design research studies and interpret research data. Introductory statements in research articles often illustrate deductive logic, as the author explains how a research hypothesis was developed from an existing theory of general body of knowledge. Inductive reasoning is used in the discussion section of a research report, where generalizations or conclusions are proposed from the data obtained in the study. Even though imperfect induction does not allow us to reach infallible conclusions, it is the clinical scientist's responsibility to evaluate critically the validity of the information and to draw reasonable conclusions (see Box 1.2). These conclusions must then be verified through further empirical testing.

The following statement, attributed to Galen, illustrates the potential for the abuse of logic:

> All who drink of this remedy recover in a short time, except those whom it does not help, who all die. Therefore, it is obvious that it fails only in incurable cases.[71]

The Scientific Method

The **scientific method** is the most rigorous process for acquiring new knowledge, incorporating elements of deduction and induction in a systematic and controlled analysis of phenomena. The scientific approach to inquiry is based on two assumptions related to the nature of reality. First, we assume that nature is orderly and regular and that events are, to some extent, consistent and predictable. Second, we assume that events or conditions are not random or accidental and, therefore, have one or more causes that can be discovered. These assumptions allow us to direct clinical thinking toward establishing cause-and-effect relationships so that we can develop rational solutions to clinical problems.

The scientific approach has been defined as a *systematic, empirical, controlled and critical examination of hypothetical propositions about the associations among natural phenomena.*[1] The *systematic* nature of research implies a sense of order and discipline that will ensure an acceptable level of reliability. It suggests a logical sequence that leads from identification of a problem, through the organized collection and objective analysis of data, to the interpretation of findings. The *empirical* component of scientific research refers to the necessity for documenting objective data through direct observation. Findings are thereby grounded in reality rather than in personal bias or subjective belief of the researcher.

The element of *control*, however, is the most important characteristic that sets the scientific method apart from the other sources of knowledge. To understand how one phenomenon relates to another, the scientist practitioner must attempt to control factors that are not directly related to the variables in question. Clinical problems such as pain, functional disability, cognitive dysfunction, deformity, cardiopulmonary insufficiency or motor control concern highly complex phenomena and often involve the effects of

BOX 1.2 **The Logic of the Frog**

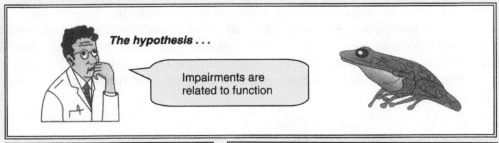

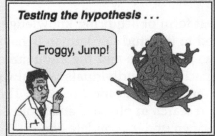

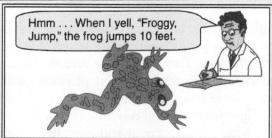

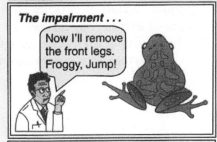

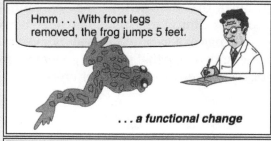

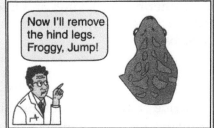

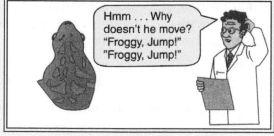

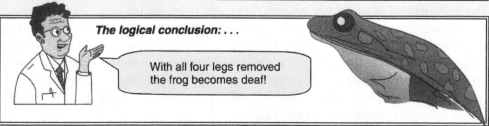

No animals were harmed in the making of this picture!

many interacting factors. Investigators must be able to control extraneous influences to have critical confidence in research outcomes. This important concept is explored in greater detail in Chapter 9.

A commitment to *critical examination* means that the researcher must subject findings to empirical testing and to the scrutiny of other scientists. Scientific investigation is thereby characterized by a capacity for self-correction based on objective validation of data from primary sources of information. This minimizes the influence of bias, and makes the researcher responsible for logical and defensible interpretation of outcomes.

Limitations of the Scientific Method

Although scientific research is considered the highest form of acquiring knowledge, it is by no means perfect, especially when it is applied to the study of human behavior and performance. The complexity and variability within nature and the environment and the unique psychosocial and physiological capacities of individuals will always introduce some uncertainty into the interpretation and generalization of data. These issues differentiate clinical research from laboratory research in physical and biological sciences, where environment and even heredity are often under complete control. This does not mean that the scientific method cannot be applied to human studies, but it does mean that clinical researchers must be acutely aware of extraneous influences to interpret findings in a meaningful way. Some clinical findings may actually be strengthened by the knowledge that patients generally improve with certain treatments despite physiological and environmental differences.

TYPES OF RESEARCH

The research process delineates a general strategy for gathering, analyzing, and interpreting data to answer a question. A variety of schema have been used to classify research strategies according to their purpose and objectives.

Quantitative and Qualitative Research

In categorizing clinical research, researchers often describe studies by distinguishing between quantitative and qualitative methods. Quantitative methods may be used all along the continuum of research approaches, whereas qualitative data are generally applied to descriptive or exploratory research. **Quantitative research** involves measurement of outcomes using numerical data under standardized conditions. The advantage of the quantitative approach is the ability to summarize scales and to subject data to statistical analysis. Quantitative information may be obtained using formal instruments which address physical or physiological parameters, or by putting subjective information into an objective numerical scale.

Qualitative research is more concerned with a deep understanding of a phenomenon through narrative description, which typically is obtained under less structured conditions. In qualitative methodology, "measurement" is based on open-ended questions, interviews and observations, as the researcher attempts to capture the context of the data, to better understand how phenomena are experienced by individuals. The purpose of the research may be to simply describe the state of conditions, or it may be to explore associations, formulate theory, or generate hypotheses.

Basic and Applied Research

One system of classification is based on the objective of the research, or the degree of utility of the findings. **Basic research** is done to obtain empirical data that can be used to develop, refine, or test theory. Basic research is directed toward the acquisition of new knowledge for its own sake, motivated by intellectual curiosity, without reference to the potential practical use of results. Typically done in a laboratory, basic research is often called "bench research." Researchers who study how blood cells function or who examine the structure and function of parts of the brain are doing basic research. Of course, basic studies may eventually lead to numerous practical applications, such as developing a treatment for leukemia or grafting brain cells to treat Parkinson's disease. But these are not the direct goals of the basic scientist.

In contrast, **applied research** is directed toward solving immediate practical problems with functional applications and testing the theories that direct practice. It is usually carried out under actual practice conditions on subjects who represent the group to which the results will be applied. Most clinical research falls into this category. When therapists study the effect of electrical stimulation for reducing muscle spasm or compare the effectiveness of eccentric and concentric exercises for increasing strength, they are doing applied research.

Although the distinction between basic and applied research appears to create a dichotomy, in reality a continuum exists between the two extremes. We recognize that rehabilitation and health care are applied sciences, but that many of the theories that guide practice are founded on basic science principles. Today, clinical research is often a hybrid, combining elements of both basic and applied science. Many studies provide clinical application as well as new knowledge that contributes to a theoretical understanding of behavior.

Translational Research

The term **translational research** refers to the application of basic scientific findings to clinically relevant issues, and simultaneously, the generation of scientific questions based on clinical dilemmas.[76] It is often described as taking knowledge from "bench to bedside," or more practically from "bedside to bench and back to bedside."[77] Although certainly not a new concept, the medical community has experienced a renewed emphasis on the application of laboratory-based findings to clinically important problems. The *NIH Roadmap*, proposed in 2002, has called for a new paradigm of research to assure that "basic research discoveries are quickly transformed into drugs, treatments, or methods for prevention."[78] Questions related to understanding the mechanisms of disease or therapies, molecular changes or different responses of normal or abnormal tissues are examples of how fundamental work at the bench can eventually benefit patients directly.[79]

All too often, the successes of scientific breakthroughs in the laboratory or in animal models have not translated into major changes in medical care for humans. The success of the Human Genome Project is an example of where important scientific discoveries have not yet realized their full potential.[80] Although markers for specific genetic defects can be identified, these do not exist in isolation from other physical and physiological conditions, and so the complexity of the human organism creates a challenge to apply these discoveries to patient outcomes. Other examples of promising translational research include the study of regeneration in spinal cord injury,[81] and new interventions to optimize treatment of diabetes.[82] Research aimed at developing therapies for inhibiting angiogenesis in tumors has also sparked questions related to their use in nononcological diseases, such as rheumatoid arthritis, psoriasis and diabetic retinopathy.[83] As these examples illustrate, the success of translational research will lie in the close collaboration among laboratory researchers who understand the basic science, clinicians who understand human behavior and response to disease, and patient communities.[78,84] It will include reflection on challenging clinical problems, rigorous investigation with basic science techniques, insights into clinical innovations, and consideration of new directions for future research.[77]

Experimental and Nonexperimental Research

Another common classification defines research as either experimental or nonexperimental. **Experimental research** refers to investigations where the researcher manipulates and controls one or more variables and observes the resultant variation in other variables. The major purpose of an experiment is to compare conditions or intervention groups, to suggest cause-and-effect relationships. **Nonexperimental research** refers to investigations that are generally more descriptive or exploratory in nature and that do not exhibit direct control over the studied variables. This latter type of research is often referred to as **observational research**, to reflect the idea that phenomena are observed rather than manipulated.

A Continuum of Research

In a more practical scheme, research can be viewed along a continuum that reflects the type of question the research is intended to answer. Within this continuum, illustrated in Figure 1.5, research methods can be classified as descriptive, exploratory, or experimental. These classifications reflect different purposes of research, and within each one various types of research can be used. As a continuum suggests, however, different types of research can overlap in their purpose and may incorporate elements of more than one classification.

While many view this continuum as a hierarchy, with experimental designs at the top (suggesting a relative value for these research approaches), each type of research fulfills a particular purpose and need. Each brings specific strengths to an investigation of clinical phenomena. The appropriate use of various designs will depend on the research question and the available data, with questions related to intervention, diagnosis and prognosis requiring different approaches.

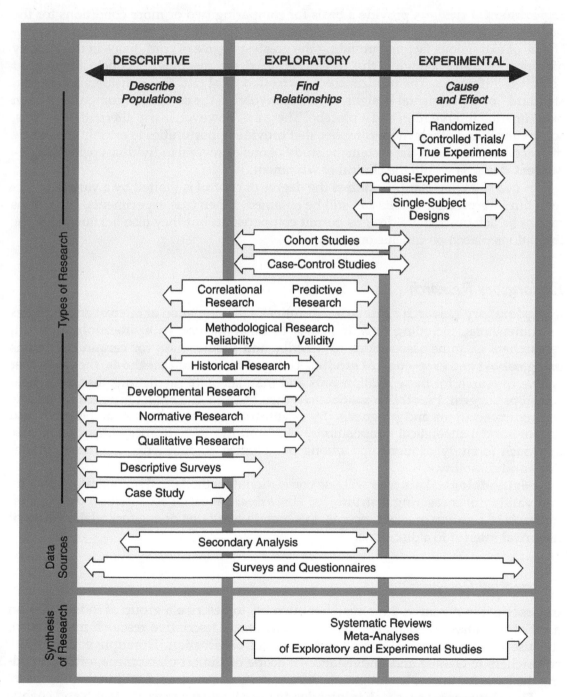

FIGURE 1.5   A continuum of research across descriptive, exploratory and experimental categories, showing types of research, relevant data sources and synthesis of literature.

Experimental Research

Experimental designs provide a basis for comparing two or more conditions for the purpose of determining cause and effect relationships. They control or account for the effects of extraneous factors, providing the greatest degree of confidence in the validity of outcomes, and allowing the researcher to draw meaningful conclusions about observed differences. The **randomized controlled trial (RCT)** is considered the "gold standard" of experimental designs, typically involving the controlled comparison of an experimental intervention and a placebo. There are, however, many alternative models, some simple and others more complex, that provide opportunities to examine the cause of outcomes, including the systematic study of one or several individuals using **single-subject designs** within the clinical environment.

In **quasi-experimental studies** the degree of control is limited by a variety of factors, but interpretable results can still be obtained. When true experimental conditions cannot be achieved, these designs permit comparisons, but they also acknowledge the limitations placed on conclusions.

Exploratory Research

In **exploratory research** a researcher examines a phenomenon of interest and explores its dimensions, including how it relates to other factors. In **epidemiology** health researchers examine associations to describe and predict risks for certain conditions using **cohort** and **case-control studies**. Using **correlational methods**, the researcher is able to search for these relationships and may generate predictions that these relationships suggest. **Predictive models** can then be used as a basis for decision making, setting expectations and prognosis. By establishing associations, researchers can also test or model theoretical propositions. Many efforts in outcomes research use this approach to study relationships among pathologies, impairments, functional limitations and disability.

Methodological studies will use correlational methods to demonstrate reliability and validity of measuring instruments. **Historical research** reconstructs the past, on the basis of archives or other records, to generate questions or suggest relationships of historical interest to a discipline.

Descriptive Research

In **descriptive research** the researcher attempts to describe a group of individuals on a set of variables, to document their characteristics. Descriptive research may involve the use of questionnaires, interviews or direct observation. Descriptive data allow researchers to classify and understand the scope of clinical phenomena, often providing the basis for further investigation. Several designs can be used within this approach.

Developmental research is intended to investigate patterns of growth and change over time within selected segments of a population, or it may chronicle the natural history of a disease or disability. **Normative studies** focus on establishing normal values for specific variables, to serve as guidelines for diagnosis and treatment planning. **Qualitative research** involves collection of data through interview and observation, in an effort to characterize human experience as it occurs naturally, and to generate hypotheses about human behavior. A **case study** or **case series** may consist of a description of one or several patients, to document unusual conditions or the effect of innovative interventions.

Sources of Data

In designing research studies, investigators will describe the methods used for collecting data. Most research involves direct data collection based on the performance of subjects, according to the investigator's defined protocol. **Surveys** or **questionnaires** are often used to collect data on subject characteristics or opinions, as part of descriptive, exploratory or experimental studies. As large databases begin to develop, researchers often use **secondary analysis** as a mechanism for exploring relationships. This approach typically involves the use of data that were collected for another purpose, or it may be based on data from ongoing surveys.

Synthesis of Literature

As bodies of evidence continue to grow through publication of research, clinicians face the challenge of aggregating information to adequately answer a clinical question. **Systematic reviews** present a comprehensive analysis of the full range of literature on a particular topic, typically an intervention, diagnostic test or prognostic factors. **Meta-analysis** is a process of statistically combining the findings from several studies to obtain a summary analysis. These forms of review, when done well, provide the clinician with a critical analysis of current research that can be used for clinical decision making. They also allow the clinician to recognize the scope of research and knowledge in a particular content area, and to appreciate a balance in the interpretation of information.

THE RESEARCH PROCESS

Clinical research involves a systematic process of sequential steps that guide thinking, planning and analysis. Whether one is collecting quantitative or qualitative data, the research process assures that there is a reasonable and logical framework for a study's design and conclusions. We conceptualize research as a series of nine sequential steps shown in Figure 1.6, recognizing that the order may vary and the steps may overlap in different research models. These steps can be grouped into five major categories.

Step 1: Identify the Research Question

The first step of the research process involves delimiting the area of research and formulating a specific research question that provides an opportunity for scientific testing (see Chapter 7). During this stage, the researcher must define the type of individual to whom the results will be generalized. Through a review of scientific literature, the researcher should be able to provide a rationale for the study, a justification of the need to investigate the problem, and a theoretical framework for interpreting results. Research hypotheses are proposed to predict how response variables and treatment variables will

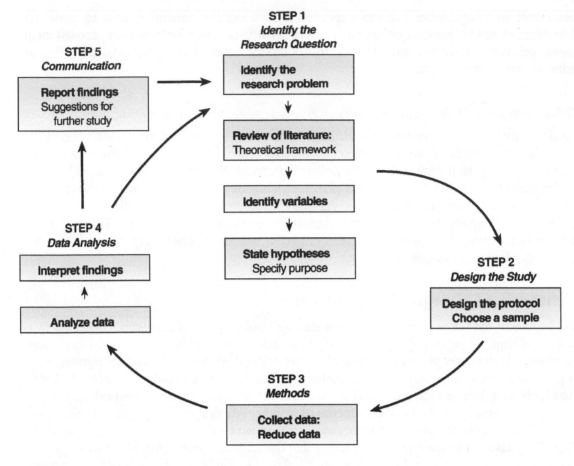

FIGURE 1.6   A model of the research process.

be related and to predict clinically relevant outcomes. In descriptive or qualitative studies, guiding questions may be proposed that form the framework for the study.

Step 2: Design the Study

In step 2, the researcher designs the study and plans methods of subject selection, testing, and measurement so that all procedures are clearly mapped out (see Chapters 5–16). The choice of research method reflects how the researcher conceptualizes the research question. Many alternative approaches are available, depending on the nature of the data and the type of subjects. The researcher must carefully define all measurements and interventions so that the methods for data analysis are clear. The completion of the first two steps of planning results in the formulation of a *research proposal* (see Chapter 32).

Step 3. Methods

During the third step of the research process, the researcher implements the plans designed in steps 1 and 2. *Data collection* is typically the most time consuming part of the research process. After data are collected and recorded, the researcher must reduce and collate the information into a useful form for analysis. Forms or tables are created for compiling the "raw data." Just as much attention to precision must be given during data reduction as during data collection (see Chapter 30).

Step 4: Data Analysis

The fourth step of the research process involves analyzing, interpreting, and drawing valid *conclusions* about the obtained data. It is the pulling together of all the materials relevant to the study, to apply them to a generalized or theoretical framework. Statistical procedures are applied to summarize quantitative information in a meaningful way, usually with the assistance of a computer (see Chapters 17–29). It is at this stage that the research hypothesis will be either supported or rejected. In qualitative studies, the researcher will look for themes that characterize the data. Through the analysis of results, the study should also lead to new questions that will stimulate further study.

Step 5: Communication

Research done in a vacuum is of little use to anyone. Researchers have a responsibility to share their findings with the appropriate audience so that others can apply the information either to clinical practice or to further research. Research reports can take many forms including journal articles, abstracts, oral presentations, and poster presentations. Students may be required to report their work in the lengthier form of a thesis or dissertation (see Chapter 33).

Finally, no research project is a dead end. Results of one study always lead to new questions. Researchers contribute to the advancement of their own work by offering suggestions for further study and recommending what kinds of additional studies would be useful for contributing to the theoretical foundations addressed in the current study.

UNDERSTANDING METHOD, CONTENT AND PHILOSOPHY

The focus of a text such as this one is naturally on the methods and procedures of conducting research, on the mechanisms of how research is done: how phenomena are observed and measured; how different types of research fit varied research questions; how to design conditions so that relationships can be examined; and how to control and manipulate variables to demonstrate cause-and-effect relationships. By understanding the processes, definitions and analytic procedures of research, the clinician has the building blocks to structure an investigation or interpret the work of others.

Methodology is only part of research, however. Research designs and statistical techniques cannot lead us to a research question, nor can they specify the technical procedures needed for studying that question. Designs cannot tell us what to investigate, nor do they assign meaning to the way clinical phenomena behave. Two other aspects are equally important to the concept of research: knowledge of the subject matter that will be studied and the research philosophy of the clinical discipline.

A thorough knowledge of content related to a research question is necessary to determine relevant applications of the methods for answering the question. The researcher must be able both to determine which instruments are appropriate for measuring different variables and to apply measurement tools properly. The scientific bases for observed responses must be thoroughly understood to design a study and interpret results. Without a complete background in the relevant content, the researcher may make serious errors in data collection and analysis.

The philosophy of a discipline concerns itself with the way the subject matter is conceptualized, the overall significance of the knowledge generated by research, and what scientific approaches will contribute to an understanding of practice. How one conceives of a discipline's objectives and the scope of practice will influence the kinds of questions one will ask. We must recognize the influence of professional values on these applications. These values reflect the researcher's inclinations to consider treatment alternatives, to search for new knowledge to substantiate certain types of clinical decisions, or to investigate particular types of questions with particular methods. For instance, different paradigms will direct some clinical investigators to study behavior at the level of impairments versus outcomes, or to use qualitative versus quantitative methods.

There is no right or wrong in these contrasts. As we explore the variety of research approaches and the context of evidence-based practice, we urge the reader to continually apply his or her own framework for applying these methods. Our emphasis on clinical examples throughout the book is a limited attempt to demonstrate these connections. It is also relevant to consider the interdisciplinary clinical associations inherent in health care, the team approach to patient care, and the shared research agendas that might emerge from such associations. The framework that supports a research question will likely be broader than any one discipline's objectives and might be well served by a team of professionals.

COMMENTARY

Research and Evidence-Based Practice: Investigation vs. Clinical Decision Making

As we discuss the clinical research process and its contribution to evidence-based practice, it is useful to recognize the analogy that can be drawn between research and clinical decision making. Decisions usually begin with the definition of specific clinical problems, which are understood within the context of a theoretical framework. The clinician then applies literature, professional judgment and patient considerations to generate a list of alternative solutions and selects one reasonable course of action. The process continues with the design of a plan of care, implementation of that plan and the evaluation of change. It is easy to see the commonalities of this process to the design and analysis of a research question, as presented in Figure 1.6.

Two major differences distinguish clinical decision making from clinical research, however. One is the purpose for which each process is used. Decision making is used to determine solutions to particular clinical problems. Research concerns broader questions about recurrent phenomena, and is used to obtain knowledge that is generalizable beyond individual situations. In clinical decision making, the process usually ends with a solution. In research, outcomes generate more questions. The outcomes of clinical decisions may be shared with colleagues, but as a rule, the decisions are not intended to contribute to an overall understanding of the clinical problem beyond the immediate situation. In contrast, the goal of clinical research is to contribute to a scientific understanding of clinical phenomena, to predict outcomes and strengthen the theoretical foundations of treatment and evaluation.

The other difference between these processes concerns the degree of control that is required. Clinical decision making is a process used within the clinical environment, and deals with events and variations within that environment as they occur naturally. In contrast, the researcher attempts to control or at least account for the environment. When asking questions about intervention, the researcher wants to have confidence that observed differences are due to the imposed intervention and not due to extraneous environmental influences.

The experienced clinician will also recognize that information is not always available to justify clinical decisions. Therefore, research questions often develop out of clinical practice. In this way, decision making and clinical research become interdependent. Research provides information on which to base clinical decisions, and problem solving contributes to the development of research questions. Both processes involve the application of orderly and systematic procedures to guide the interpretation of outcomes.

In this text, we emphasize the elements of and approaches to clinical research and the development of clinical theory. We also focus on the idea that research and practice are inseparable components of clinical science, recognizing that clinicians are uniquely qualified to study, analyze and integrate evidence into clinical practice.

REFERENCES

1. Kerlinger FN. *Foundations of Behavioral Research.* New York: Holt, Rinehart & Winston, 1973.
2. Kuhn TS. *The Structure of Scientific Revolutions.* Chicago: University of Chicago Press, 1970.
3. Donabedian A. *Explorations in Quality Assessment and Monitoring.* Ann Arbor, MI: Health Administration Press, 1980.
4. World Health Organization. Constitution. *WHO Chronicle* 1947;1:29.
5. Ware JE. Conceptualizing and measuring generic health outcomes. *Cancer* 1991;67:774–779.
6. Shields RK, Leo KC, Miller B, Dostal WF, Barr R. An acute care physical therapy clinical practice data base for outcomes research. *Phys Ther* 1994;74:463–470.
7. Urden LD. Decision support systems to manage outcomes. *Outcomes Manag* 2003; 7:141–143.
8. Urden LD. Leading and succeeding in outcomes management. *Outcomes Manag* 2004;8:2–4.
9. Ellwood PM. Outcomes management: A technology of patient experience. *N Engl J Med* 1988;318:549–556.
10. Hart DL, Geril AC, Pfohl RL. Outcomes process in daily practice. *PT Magazine* 1997; 5(9):68–77.
11. Nemeth LS. Implementing change for effective outcomes. *Outcomes Manag* 2003; 7:134–139.
12. Wojner AW. Outcomes management: An interdisciplinary search for best practice. *AACN Clin Issues* 1996;7:133–145.
13. Geyman JP, Deyo RA, Ramsey SD. *Evidence-Based Clinical Practice: Concepts and Approaches.* Boston: Butterworth Heinemann, 2000.

14. Harp SS. The measurement of performance in a physical therapy clinical program: A ROI approach. *Health Care Manag* 2004;23:110–119.

15. Fakhry SM, Trask AL, Waller MA, Watts DD. Management of brain-injured patients by an evidence-based medicine protocol improves outcomes and decreases hospital charges. *J Trauma* 2004;56:492–499; discussion 499–500.

16. Li L, Wang HM, Shen Y. Chinese SF-36 Health Survey: Translation, cultural adaptation, validation, and normalisation. *J Epidemiol Community Health* 2003;57:259–263.

17. Micciolo R, Valagussa P, Marubini E. The use of historical controls in breast cancer. An assessment in three consecutive trials. *Control Clin Trials* 1985;6:259–270.

18. Aaronson NK, Muller M, Cohen PD, Essink-Bot ML, Fekkes M, Sanderman R, et al. Translation, validation, and norming of the Dutch language version of the SF-36 Health Survey in community and chronic disease populations. *J Clin Epidemiol* 1998; 51:1055–1068.

19. Fukuhara S, Bito S, Green J, Hsiao A, Kurokawa K. Translation, adaptation, and validation of the SF-36 Health Survey for use in Japan. *J Clin Epidemiol* 1998;51:1037–1044.

20. Apolone G, Mosconi P. The Italian SF-36 Health Survey: Translation, validation and norming. *J Clin Epidemiol* 1998;51:1025–1036.

21. Arocho R, McMillan CA, Sutton-Wallace P. Construct validation of the USA-Spanish version of the SF-36 health survey in a Cuban-American population with benign prostatic hyperplasia. *Qual Life Res* 1998;7:121–126.

22. Perneger TV, Leplege A, Etter JF, Rougemont A. Validation of a French-language version of the MOS 36-Item Short Form Health Survey (SF-36) in young healthy adults. *J Clin Epidemiol* 1995;48:1051–1060.

23. Hunskaar S, Vinsnes A. The quality of life in women with urinary incontinence as measured by the sickness impact profile. *J Am Geriatr Soc* 1991;39:378–382.

24. Davis GL, Balart LA, Schiff ER, Lindsay K, Bodenheimer HC, Jr., Perrillo RP, et al. Assessing health-related quality of life in chronic hepatitis C using the Sickness Impact Profile. *Clin Ther* 1994;16:334–343.

25. Jensen MP, Strom SE, Turner JA, Romano JM. Validity of the Sickness Impact Profile Roland scale as a measure of dysfunction in chronic pain patients. *Pain* 1992;50:157–162.

26. Gerety MB, Cornell JE, Mulrow CD, Tuley M, Hazuda HP, Lichtenstein M, et al. The Sickness Impact Profile for nursing homes (SIP-NH). *J Gerontol* 1994;49:M2–8.

27. Post MW, Gerritsen J, Diederikst JP, DeWittet LP. Measuring health status of people who are wheelchair-dependent: Validity of the Sickness Impact Profile 68 and the Nottingham Health Profile. *Disabil Rehabil* 2001;23:245–253.

28. Streppel KR, de Vries J, van Harten WH. Functional status and prosthesis use in amputees, measured with the Prosthetic Profile of the Amputee (PPA) and the short version of the Sickness Impact Profile (SIP68). *Int J Rehabil Res* 2001;24:251–256.

29. Van de Port IG, Ketelaar M, Schepers VP, Van den Bos GA, Lindeman E. Monitoring the functional health status of stroke patients: The value of the Stroke-Adapted Sickness Impact Profile-30. *Disabil Rehabil* 2004;26:635–640.

30. Gee L, Abbott J, Conway SP, Etherington C, Webb AK. Validation of the SF-36 for the assessment of quality of life in adolescents and adults with cystic fibrosis. *J Cyst Fibros* 2002;1:137–145.

31. Bourke SC, McColl E, Shaw PJ, Gibson GJ. Validation of quality of life instruments in ALS. *Amyotroph Lateral Scler Other Motor Neuron Disord* 2004;5:55–60.

32. Thumboo J, Feng PH, Boey ML, Soh CH, Thio S, Fong KY. Validation of the Chinese SF-36 for quality of life assessment in patients with systemic lupus erythematosus. *Lupus* 2000;9:708–712.

33. Bensoussan A, Chang SW, Menzies RG, Talley NJ. Application of the general health status questionnaire SF36 to patients with gastrointestinal dysfunction: Initial validation and validation as a measure of change. *Aust N Z J Public Health* 2001;25:71–77.

34. Anderson C, Laubscher S, Burns R. Validation of the Short Form 36 (SF-36) health survey questionnaire among stroke patients. *Stroke* 1996;27:1812–1816.

35. Ware JE, Sherbourne CD. The MOS 36-item Short Form Health Survey (SF-36). I. Conceptual framework and item selection. *Med Care* 1992;30:473–483.

36. Bellamy N, Buchanan WW, Goldsmith CH, Campbell J, Stitt LW. Validation study of WOMAC: A health status instrument for measuring clinically important patient relevant outcomes to antirheumatic drug therapy in patients with osteoarthritis of the hip or knee. *J Rheumatol* 1988;15:1833–1840.

37. Rector TS, Kubo SH, Cohn JN. Validity of the Minnesota Living with Heart Failure questionnaire as a measure of therapeutic response to enalapril or placebo. *Am J Cardiol* 1993;71:1106–1107.

38. Bombardier C, Melfi CA, Paul J, Green R, Hawker G, Wright J, et al. Comparison of a generic and a disease-specific measure of pain and physical function after knee replacement surgery. *Med Care* 1995;33:AS131–144.

39. Davies GM, Watson DJ, Bellamy N. Comparison of the responsiveness and relative effect size of the western Ontario and McMaster Universities Osteoarthritis Index and the short-form Medical Outcomes Study Survey in a randomized, clinical trial of osteoarthritis patients. *Arthritis Care Res* 1999;12:172–179.

40. Ni H, Toy W, Burgess D, Wise K, Nauman DJ, Crispell K, et al. Comparative responsiveness of Short-Form 12 and Minnesota Living with Heart Failure Questionnaire in patients with heart failure. *J Card Fail* 2000;6:83–91.

41. Minaire P. Disease, illness and health: Theoretical models of the disablement process. *Bull World Health Org* 1992;70:373–379.

42. Bergner M. Quality of life, health status and clinical research. *Med Care* 1989;27: S148–S156.

43. Wilkins EG, Lowery JC, Smith Jr DJ. Outcomes research: A primer for plastic surgeons. *Ann Plast Surg* 1996;37:1–11.

44. Nagi SZ. Disability concepts revisited: Implications for prevention. In AM Pope, AR Tarlov (Eds.), *Disability in America: Toward a National Agenda for Prevention*. Washington, DC: Division of Health Promotion and Disease Prevention, Institute of Medicine, National Academy Press, 1991.

45. Verbrugge LM, Jette AM. The disablement process. *Soc Sci Med* 1994;38:1–14.

46. Whiteneck GG, Fongeyrollas P, Gerhart KA. Elaborating the model of disablement. In MJ Fuhrer (Ed.), *Assessing Medical Rehabilitation Practices: The Promise of Outcomes Research*. Baltimore: Brookes Publishing, 1997.

47. Jette AM. Physical disablement concepts for physical therapy research and practice. *Phys Ther* 1994;74:380–386.

48. Patrick DL, Bergner M. Measurement of health status in the 1990s. *Ann Rev Public Health* 1990;11:165–183.

49. Pope AM, Tarlov AR (Eds.). *Disability in America: Toward a National Agenda for Prevention*. Washington, DC: Division of Health Promotion and Disease Prevention, Institute of Medicine, National Academy Press, 1991.

50. World Health Organization. International classification of functioning, disability and health. Available at: <http://www3.who.int/icf/icftemplate.cfm> Accessed November 7, 2004.

51. Reed GM, Brandt DE, Harwood KJ. ICF clinical manual. Presentation at Physical Therapy 2004 Annual Conference and Exposition. Chicago, July 1, 2004.

52. Bilbao A, Kennedy C, Chatterji S, Ustun B, Barquero JL, Barth JT. The ICF: Applications of the WHO model of functioning, disability and health to brain injury rehabilitation. *NeuroRehabilitation* 2003;18:239–250.

53. Worral L, McCooey R, Davidson B, Larkins B, Hickson L. The validity of functional assessments of communication and the Activity/Participation components of the ICIDH-2: Do they reflect what really happens in real life? *J Commun Disord* 2002;35:107–137.

54. Kennedy C. Functioning and disability associated with mental disorders: The evolution since ICIDH. *Disabil Rehabil* 2003;25:611–619.

55. Geyh S, Kurt T, Brockow T, Cieza A, Ewert T, Omar Z, et al. Identifying the concepts contained in outcome measures of clinical trials on stroke using the International Classification of Functioning, Disability and Health as a reference. *J Rehabil Med* 2004:56–62.

56. Stucki G, Ewert T. How to assess the impact of arthritis on the individual patient: The WHO ICF. *Ann Rheum Dis* 2005;64:664–668.

57. Brockow T, Duddeck K, Geyh S, Schwarzkopf S, Weigl M, Franke T, et al. Identifying the concepts contained in outcome measures of clinical trials on breast cancer using the International Classification of Functioning, Disability and Health as a reference. *J Rehabil Med* 2004:43–48.

58. Crews JE, Campbell VA. Vision impairment and hearing loss among community-dwelling older Americans: Implications for health and functioning. *Am J Public Health* 2004;94:823–829.

59. World Health Organization. *International Classification of Functioning, Disability and Health.* Geneva: World Health Organization, 2001.

60. Sackett DL, Rosenberg WM, Gray JA, Haynes RB, Richardson WS. Evidence based medicine: What it is and what it isn't. *BMJ* 1996;312:71–72.

61. Straus SE, Richardson WS, Glasziou P, Haynes RB. *Evidence-based Medicine: How to Practice and Teach EBM* (3rd ed.). Edinburgh: Churchill Livingstone, 2005.

62. Rothstein JM, Echternach JL, Riddle DL. The Hypothesis-Oriented Algorithm for Clinicians II (HOAC II): A guide for patient management. *Phys Ther* 2003;83:455–470.

63. Sackett DL. Foreword. In RA Dixon, JF Muno, PB Silcocks (Eds.). *The Evidence Based Medicine Workbook: Critical Appraisal for Evaluating Clinical Problem Solving.* Oxford: Butterworth Heinemann, 1997:vii–viii.

64. Center for Evidence-based Physiotherapy. Physiotherapy Evidence Database. Available at: <http://www.pedro.fhs.usyd.edu.au/index.html> Accessed October 17, 2004.

65. American Physical Therapy Association. Hooked on Evidence. Available at: <http://www.apta.org/hookedonevidence/index.cfm> Accessed October 17, 2004.

66. Center for Evidence-Based Medicine. Available at: <http://www.cebm.utoronto.ca/practise/formulate/eduprescript.htm> Accessed October 17, 2004.

67. University of Michigan Department of Pediatrics. Available at: <http://www.med.umich.edu/pediatrics/ebm/Cat.htm> Accessed October 17, 2004.

68. University of North Carolina. Available at: <http://www.med.unc.edu/medicine/edursrc/!catlist.htm> Accessed October 17, 2004.

69. Harris SR. How should treatments be critiqued for scientific merit? *Phys Ther* 1996;76:175–181.

70. Rothstein JM. Editors note: Say it ain't so. *Phys Ther* 1994;74:175–181.

71. Silverman WA. *Human Experimentation: A Guided Step into the Unknown.* New York: Oxford University Press, 1985.

72. Wolf SL, Barnhart HX, Ellison GL, Coogler CE. The effect of Tai Chi Quan and computerized balance training on postural stability in older subjects. *Phys Ther* 1997;77:371–381.

73. Carter ND, Khan KM, McKay HA, Petit MA, Waterman C, Heinonen A, et al. Community-based exercise program reduces risk factors for falls in 65- to 75-year-old women with osteoporosis: Randomized controlled trial. *CMAJ* 2002;167:997–1004.

74. Barnett A, Smith B, Lord SR, Williams M, Baumand A. Community-based group exercise improves balance and reduces falls in at-risk older people: A randomised controlled trial. *Age Ageing* 2003;32:407–414.

75. Gould SJ. Bacon, brought home—Philosophy of Francis Bacon about natural world. *Natural History* June, 1999.

76. Rustgi AK. Translational research: What is it? *Gastroenterology* 1999;116:1285.

77. Fontanarosa PB, DeAngelis CD. Translational medical research. *JAMA* 2003;289:2133.

78. National Institutes of Health. Overview of the NIH roadmap. Available at: <http://nihroadmap.nih.gov/overview.asp> Accessed January 30, 2005.

79. Dische S, Saunders M. Translational Research—A new entity? *Acta Oncol* 2001;40: 995–999.

80. Mayer L. The real meaning of translational research. *Gastroenterology* 2002;123:665.

81. Kleitman N. Keeping promises: Translating basic research into new spinal cord injury therapies. *J Spinal Cord Med* 2004;27:311–318.

82. Narayan KM, Benjamin E, Gregg EW, Norris SL, Engelgau MM. Diabetes translation research: Where are we and where do we want to be? *Ann Intern Med* 2004;140:958–963.

83. Augustin HG. Translating angiogenesis research into the clinic: The challenges ahead. *Br J Radiol* 2003;76 Spec No 1:S3–10.

84. Marincola FM. Translational Medicine: A two-way road. *J Transl Med* 2003;1:1.

CHAPTER 2

The Role of Theory in Clinical Research

Clinical research is a systematic method for evaluating the effectiveness of treatment and for establishing a basis for inductive generalizations about intervention. The ultimate goal is to further intellectual progress by contributing to the scientific base of practice through the development of **theory**. Theories are created out of a need to organize and give meaning to a complex collection of individual facts and observations.

Methods are the means by which we conduct investigations in a reliable and valid way so that we can understand clinical phenomena. But it is theory that lets us speculate on the questions of why and how treatment works, accounting for what we observe. Theories provide the explanations for findings within the context of what is already known from the successes and failures of previous investigations. As we continue to examine observations, we try to create theoretical generalizations to form a basis for predicting future outcomes. Without such explanations we risk having to reinvent the wheel each time we are faced with a clinical problem.

A theory is a set of interrelated concepts, definitions, or propositions that specifies relationships among variables and represents a systematic view of specific phenomena.[1] Theories have always been a part of human cultures, although not all theories have been scientific. Philosophy and religion historically have played a significant part in the acceptance of theory. The medieval view that the world was flat was born out of the theory that angels held up the four corners of the earth. Naturally, the men of the day were justified in believing that if one sailed toward the horizon, eventually one would fall off the edge of the earth. Such theories went untested because of a lack of instrumentation and because it was not considered necessary to test that which was already known to be true.

In contrast, scientific theory deals with the empirical world of observation and experience, and requires constant verification. We use theory to generalize beyond a specific situation and to make predictions about what *should* happen in other similar situations. The validity of these predictions can be tested through research. The purpose of this chapter is to define the elements of theory and to describe mechanisms for developing and testing clinical theories.

PURPOSES OF THEORIES

Theories can serve several purposes in science and clinical practice, depending on how we choose to use them. Theories *summarize* existing knowledge, giving meaning to isolated empirical findings. They provide a framework for interpretation of observations.

For example, theories of motor learning bring together the results of many separate studies that have examined schedules of practice, types of skills, psychomotor components of performance, and other elements of the learning process. Theories are also used to *explain* observable events by showing how variables are related. For instance, a theory of motor learning would explain the relationship between feedback and feedforward mechanisms in the learning, performance, and refinement of a motor skill.

Theories allow us to *predict* what should occur, given a set of specific circumstances. For example, one theory of motor learning states that greater changes take place during stages of initial learning than during later stages, as illustrated by a decelerating learning curve. On the basis of this theory, we could anticipate that a patient using an exercise device for the first time will experience a spurt of improvement in force output during early trials as a result of practice that will not necessarily be related to strength increases.[2]

Theories can also provide a basis for predicting phenomena that cannot be empirically verified. For instance, through deductions from mathematical theories, Newton was able to predict the motion of planets around the sun long before technology was available to confirm their orbits. The element of prediction also affords us a measure of control. This is illustrated by analysis of the germ theory of disease, which explains how organisms in the environment cause disease states. The theory allows us to predict how changes in the environment will affect the incidence of disease. This, in turn, suggests mechanisms to control disease, such as the use of drugs, vaccines, or attention to hygiene.

Theories also help to stimulate the *development of new knowledge* by providing motivation and guidance for asking significant clinical questions. On the basis of a theoretical premise, a clinician can use the process of deduction to formulate a hypothesis which can then be tested, providing evidence to support, reject, or modify the theory. For instance, based on the theory that reinforcement will facilitate learning, a clinician might deduce that verbal encouragement will decrease the time required for a patient to learn a program of home exercises. This hypothesis can be tested by comparing patients who do and do not receive reinforcement, and, if supported, the hypothesis will lend credence to the original theory. A wide variety of hypotheses can be deduced from this same theory. For instance, a clinician may hypothesize that reinforcement will improve learning for spinal cord injured patients working to master the use of a hand splint. The results of testing each hypothesis will provide additional affirmation of the theory or demonstrate specific situations where the theory is not substantiated.

Theory provides the basis for asking a question in applied research. Sometimes there will be sufficient background in the literature to build this framework; other times the researcher must build an argument based on what is known from basic science. In descriptive or exploratory research, the study's findings may contribute to the development of theory. The researcher uses a theoretical premise to project how the variables being studied should be related and what outcomes are expected. The theoretical framework is usually discussed within the introduction or discussion section of a paper. Without a theoretical framework a researcher will be unable to understand the implications of his findings, and observations will not have a context.

COMPONENTS OF THEORIES

Concepts and Constructs

The role that theory plays in clinical practice and research is best described by examining the structure of a theory. Figure 2.1 shows the basic organization of scientific thought, building from observation of facts to laws of nature.

The essential building blocks of a theory are **concepts**. Concepts are abstractions that allow us to classify natural phenomena and empirical observations. From birth we begin to structure empirical impressions of the world around us in the form of concepts, such as "mother," "father," "play," or "food," each of which implies a complex set of recognitions and expectations. We develop these concepts within the context of experience and feelings, so that they meet with our perception of reality. We supply labels to sets of behaviors, objects, or processes that allow us to identify them and discuss them.

We use concepts in professional communication in the same way. Even something as basic as a "wheelchair" is a concept from which we distinguish chairs of different types, styles, and functions. Almost every term we incorporate into our understanding of human and environmental characteristics and behaviors is a conceptual entity. When concepts can be assigned values, they can be manipulated as **variables**, so that their relationships can be examined. In this context, variables become the concepts used for building theories and planning research. Variables must be operationally defined, that is, the methods for measuring or evaluating them must be clearly delineated.

Some concepts are observable and easily distinguishable from others. For instance, a wheelchair will not be confused with an office chair. But other concepts are less tangible, and can be defined only by inference. Concepts that represent nonobservable behaviors or events are called **constructs**. Constructs are invented names for abstract

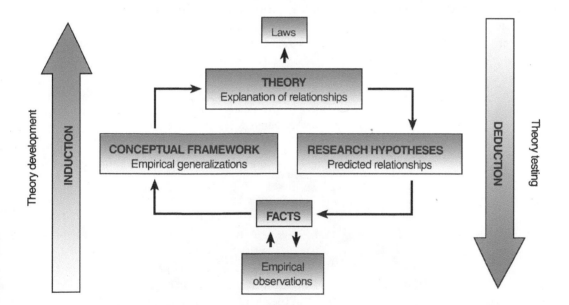

FIGURE 2.1   A model of scientific thought, showing the circular relationship between facts and theory and the integration of inductive and deductive reasoning.

variables that cannot be seen directly, but are inferred by measuring relevant or correlated behaviors that are observable. The construct of intelligence, for example, is one that we cannot see, and yet we give it very clear meaning. We evaluate a person's intelligence by observing his behavior, the things he says, what he "knows." We can also measure a person's intelligence using standardized tests and use a number to signify intelligence. An IQ score of 125 tells us something about that individual, but the number by itself has no empirical value. We cannot observe 125 intelligence "points" like we can 125 degrees of shoulder joint motion. Constructs are often manipulated as variables in psychosocial and behavioral research.

Propositions

Once the concepts that relate to a theory are delineated, they are formed into a generalization, or **proposition**. Propositions state the relationship between variables, which can be described in several ways. For example, a *hierarchical* proposition shows a vertical relationship, establishing ordered levels of concepts. Maslow's theory of the relationship of human needs to motivation demonstrates this principle.[3] He described five levels, beginning at the bottom with basic physiological needs, moving up to safety, social needs, esteem, and finally ending at the top with self-actualization, or the fulfillment of one's self (see Figure 2.2).

A *quantitative* proposition is based on the frequency or duration of a specific behavior. For example, theories of fatigue are based partly on the concept of repetitions of exercise and how that relates to muscular endurance.[4] A *temporal* proposition orders concepts in time and states a sequence of events. For instance, the transtheoretical model explains behavior change as a process along a continuum of motivational readiness, with five stages: precontemplation, contemplation, preparation, action, and maintenance.[5] Rather than seeing change as a unidimensional act, such as simply quitting

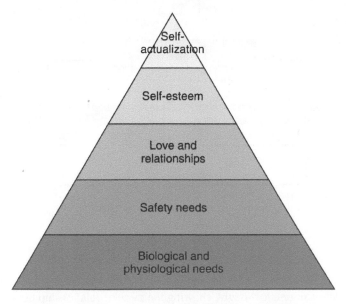

FIGURE 2.2   Maslow's hierarchy of human needs; example of a hierarchical proposition.[3]

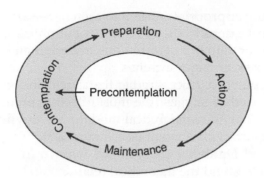

FIGURE 2.3   The transtheoretical model of behavior change; example of a temporal proposition.[5]

smoking or starting to exercise, this model suggests that individuals progress through a series of stages in recognizing the need to change and finally engaging in a new behavior (see Figure 2.3). The model also clarifies the importance of identifying the stage an individual is in before a successful intervention can be implemented.

Models

Many of the concepts we deal with in professional practice are so infinitely complex that we cannot truly comprehend their real nature. In an effort to understand them we try to simplify them within the context of a **model** that serves as an analogy for the real phenomenon. To understand the concept of an "atom," for example, it was helpful for scientists to delineate a conceptual model that is likened to a solar system. The intricacies of genetic processes were clarified by the development of a helical model of DNA. Function of the neuromuscular system is often taught using a model of the muscle spindle. These models are considered simplified approximations of reality. The model leaves out much of the detail, but describes the conceptual structure closely enough to give us a better understanding of the phenomenon. Models are symbolic representations of the elements within a system. Where a theory is an explanation of phenomena, a model is a structural representation of the concepts that comprise the theory.

Some physical models are used to demonstrate how the real behavior might occur. For example, engineers study models of bridges to examine the stresses on cables and the effects of different loading conditions. The benefit of such models is that they obey the same laws as the original, but can be controlled and manipulated to examine the effects of various conditions in ways that would not otherwise be possible. Rehabilitation engineers develop prototypes of prostheses or motor-driven wheelchairs, to evaluate their performance and to perfect their design. Scientists also use animal models to mimic specific anatomical or physiological deficits in the human to examine the effects of pathology, trauma and intervention.

Sometimes a model is a schematic representation, such as an architect's plans or a map. Therapists might use this type of model when evaluating a client's home for architectural barriers, by drawing a diagram of rooms and doorways and plotting out the spatial requirements for use of a wheelchair. Such a model provides opportunities for considering the implications of different approaches without physically carrying them out, and facilitates making appropriate changes when necessary. Computer simulations are the most recent contributions to the development of physical models. Scientists can experiment with an infinite number of variations in design and can analyze the implications of each without risk or major expense.

A model can also represent a process rather than a real object. For example, decision-making models can be used to suggest the most effective progression of intervention with specific disorders.[6] The transtheoretical model provides a framework for understanding the process of behavior change (see Figure 2.3).[5] The International Classification of Functioning and Disability (ICF) model (shown in Figure 1.1 in Chapter 1) creates a structure to understand the theoretical relationship between impairments and functional activities, and can be used to offer explanations as to why specific impairments might lead to certain types of disability.[7]

Quantitative models are used to describe the relationship among variables by using symbols to represent them. Models in physical science allow for accurate prediction of quantities, such as the summary of the relationship between force, mass, and acceleration ($F = m \times a$). In the behavioral sciences, however, quantitative models are less precise, usually containing some degree of error resulting from the variability of human behavior and physical characteristics. For instance, a clinician might want to determine the level of strength a patient could be expected to achieve following a period of training. A model that demonstrates the influence of a person's height, weight, and age on muscle strength would be useful in making this determination.[8-10] This type of quantitative model can serve as a guide for setting long-term goals and for predicting functional outcomes. Research studies provide the basis for testing these models and estimating their degree of accuracy for making such predictions.

DEVELOPMENT OF THEORIES

As the previous examples illustrate, theories are not discovered, they are created. A set of observable facts may exist, but they do not become a theory unless someone has the insight to understand the relevance of the observed information and pulls the facts together to make sense of them. Certainly, many people observed apples falling from trees before Newton was stimulated to consider the force of gravity. Theories can be developed using inductive or deductive processes.

Inductive Theories

Inductive theories are data based and evolve through a process of inductive reasoning, beginning with empirically verifiable observations. Through multiple investigations and observations, researchers determine those variables that are related to a specific phenomenon and those that are not. The patterns that emerge from these studies are developed into a systematic conceptual framework, which forms the basis for generalizations. This process involves a degree of abstraction and imagination, as ideas are manipulated and concepts reorganized, until some structural pattern is evident in their relationship.

For instance, this process was used by Skinner in the formulation of his theories of learning and behavior, based on previous work and his own observations of human behavior.[11] Through the examination and clarification of the interrelationships between stimuli and responses, he formulated a systematic explanation for the observed behaviors. Glaser and Strauss[12] used the term "grounded theory" to describe the development of theory by reflecting on individual experiences in qualitative research. As an example, Resnik and Jensen[13] used this method to describe characteristics of therapists who were classified as "expert" or "average" based on the outcomes of their patients. Building on their observations, they theorized that the meaning of "expert" was not based on years of experience, but on academic and work experience, utilization of colleagues, use of reflection, a patient-centered approach to care, and collaborative clinical reasoning.

Deductive Theories

The alternative approach to theory building is the intuitive approach, whereby a theory is developed on the basis of great insight and intuitive understanding of an event and the variables most likely to impact on that event. This type of theory, called a **hypothetical-deductive theory**, is developed with few or no prior observations, and often requires the generation of new concepts to provide adequate explanation. Freud's theory of personality fits this definition.[14] It required that he create concepts such as "id," "ego" and "superego" to explain psychological interactions and motivations. Because they are not developed from existing facts, hypothetical-deductive theories must be continually tested in the "real world" to develop a database that will support them. Einstein's theory of relativity is an excellent example of this type of theory; it was first advanced in 1905 and is still being tested and refined through research today.

Most theories are formulated using a combination of both inductive and hypothetical-deductive processes. Observations initiate the theoretical premise, and then hypotheses derived from the theory are tested. As researchers go back and forth in the process of building and testing the theory, concepts are redefined and restructured. This process occurs along a circular continuum between fact and theory, whereby a theory can be built on facts, but must also be tested by them (see Figure 2.1).

CHARACTERISTICS OF THEORIES

As we explore the many uses of theories in clinical research, we should also consider criteria that can be used to evaluate the utility of a theory. First and foremost, a theory should provide a thorough and *rational explanation* of observed facts. It should provide a basis for classifying relevant variables and predicting their relationships. A theory should also provide a means for its own verification; that is, it should be sufficiently developed and clear enough to permit deductions that form testable hypotheses.

A Good Theory Is *Economical*.   It should be the most efficient explanation of the phenomenon, using only those concepts that are truly relevant and necessary to the explanation offered by the theory. Complex theories are difficult to interpret and less likely to provide meaningful direction to practice or research. Theories are also most useful when they apply to a broad range of situations, not one specific segment of a discipline.

A Theory Should Be *Important*.   It should reflect that which is judged significant by those who will use it. In this sense, theories become the mirror of a profession's values and identity. When we examine the theories that are adopted by clinicians in the course of their practice, their intellectual investments become clear. For example, many therapists rely on neurophysiological theory as a basis for choosing therapeutic exercise techniques that use diagonal and rotational patterns of motion, as opposed to the traditional use of anatomical theory as a basis for exercises in straight planes. This suggests that research is needed to test hypotheses that predict the superiority of multiple-plane movement over single-plane exercise for given purposes.

Acceptance of Theory Can Change. Theories must be consistent with observed facts and the already established body of knowledge. Therefore, our acceptance of a particular theory will reflect the present state of knowledge and must adapt to changes in that knowledge as technology and scientific evidence improve. Therefore, a theory is only a tentative explanation of phenomena. It should be reasonable according to what has been observed, but may not be the only explanation. Many theories that are accepted today will be discarded tomorrow (see Box 2.1). Some will be "disproved" by new evidence, and others may be superseded by new theories that integrate the older ones. For example, Gardner's theory of multiple intelligences challenged long-held assumptions about general intelligence and the ability to measure it with a single score, such as an IQ test.[15] He proposes eight distinct intelligences and suggests that different cultures will perceive these differently.

Theory recognition also evolves with social change. For instance, the *disengagement theory of aging* was originally proposed to account for observations of age-related decreases in social interaction.[16] The explanation this theory offered was that older individuals withdrew from social involvements in anticipation of death. As sociological theory progressed, however, new perspectives emerged, such as *exchange theory,* which suggested that interactions in old age become limited because the old have fewer resources to offer, therefore bringing less to a relationship.[17] In a further generation of exchange theory, *socioemotional selectivity theory* tried to explain reduced social exchange of older persons as a function of increasing selectivity in interactions.[18] This theory suggests that older persons decide to reduce emotional closeness with some people while they increase closeness with others; that is, interactions reflect the rewards of specific emotional support with a selective group of individuals. The most recent progression of this theory is *gerotranscendence,* which looks at human development as a process that extends into old age. The theory proposes that aging, from childhood through old age, is a process that can be obstructed or accelerated by life crises, culture and support systems. Old age is yet another phase in development. When optimized, the process ends in a new and qualitatively different perspective on life.[19]

This evolution of theory illustrates how the explanations of an observed psychosocial phenomenon have continued to change as our understanding and perceptions of social interaction have grown. It also demonstrates how caregivers and health professionals may change their perspective on how to support and interact with aging individuals, depending on how they view the psychological focus of the aging process.

THEORY AND RESEARCH

Every theory serves, in part, as a research directive. The empirical outcomes of research can be organized and ordered to build theories using inductive reasoning. Conversely, theories must be tested by subjecting deductive hypotheses to scientific scrutiny. The

BOX 2.1 Ancient Medical Theory: The Four Humours

Originating in the work of Aristotle and Hippocrates, traditional medical theory from Greco-Roman times through the Middle Ages was based on the belief that the body was made up of four elemental liquids: blood, yellow bile, black bile and phlegm. Physical and mental health depended on a balance of these humours, called *eucrasia*. An imbalance of humours, or *dyscrasia*, was believed to be the cause of all diseases.

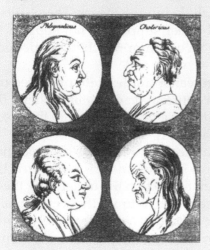

Image of a woodcut from an 18th-century text by Johann Kaspar Lavater.

Each humour corresponded to one of the four elements, specific seasons, qualities and personalities. Blood was associated with air, spring, hot and moist, and a sanguine temperament—amorous, happy, generous, and optimistic. Black bile was associated with earth, autumn, cold and dry, and a melancholic personality—introspective, sentimental and lazy. Yellow bile was paired with fire, summer, hot and dry, and a choleric disposition—vengeful, violent and easily angered. And phlegm was linked to water, winter, cold and moist, and a phlegmatic temperament—calm, unemotional and dull.

This theoretical context was used as the basis for diagnosis and treatment, geared toward identifying and pushing out a harmful surplus of a humour. For example, if someone had a fever, they were thought to have too much blood in their body, which was therefore treated by blood letting. Sweating from a fever was considered hot and wet, and foods were given that were associated with cold and dry. The baby with "cholic" was thought to be constantly angry. Epilepsy was believed to be due to phlegm blocking the airways that caused the body to thrash about to free itself. Manic behavior was due to bile boiling in the brain. Black bile was associated with melancholy.

In every era, our theories grow to meet the state of knowledge and science. The humours replaced the theory that health could be explained by divine intervention. Many of the practices associated with the four humours were still part of mainstream medicine in the late 1800s. You can undoubtedly see the connections between the four personalities and many words we use today to describe physical and mental states.

Sources: Four humours. Wikipedia. <http://en.widipedia.org/wiki/Four_bodily_humours>; The Four Humours. Kheper website. <http://www.kheper.net/topics/typology/four_humours.html>; Warren P. The Roots of Scientific Medicine. Hippocrates on the Web. http://www.umanitoba.ca/faculties/medicine/units/history/notes/roots/index.html> Accessed May 15, 2007.

processes of theory development and theory testing are represented in the model shown in Figure 2.1. It integrates the concepts of inductive and deductive reasoning as they relate to the elements of theory design.

Theory Testing

When we speak of testing a theory, we should realize that a theory itself is not testable. The validity of a theory is derived through the empirical testing of hypotheses that are deduced from it and from observation of the phenomenon the theory describes. The hypotheses predict the relationships of variables included in the theory. The results of research will demonstrate certain facts, which will either support or not support the hypothesis. If the hypothesis is supported, then the theory from which it was deduced is also supported.

When we compare the outcomes of individual research studies with predicted outcomes, we are always aware of the potential for disconfirmation of the underlying theory. In essence, the more that research does *not disconfirm* a theory, the more the theory is supported. This may sound backwards, but in actuality we can never "prove" or "confirm" a theory. We can only demonstrate that a theoretical premise does not hold true in a specific situation. When a research hypothesis is tested and it is *not rejected*, that is, the study turns out the way we expected, we cannot state that the underlying theory is definitely true. To make such a statement, we would have to verify every possible application of the theory and demonstrate that the outcomes were absolutely consistent. As this is not feasible, we can only interpret individual hypotheses and conclude that a theory has not been disproved.

Utilization of Theory in Research and Practice

Clinicians are actually engaged in theory testing on a regular basis in practice. Theories guide us in making clinical decisions. Specific therapeutic modalities are chosen for treatment because of expected outcomes that are based on theoretical assumptions. Treatments are modified according to the presence of risk factors, based on theoretical relationships. Therefore, the theory is tested each time the clinician evaluates treatment outcomes. When a theory is used as the basis for a treatment, the clinician is, in effect, hypothesizing that the treatment will be successful. If results are as expected, the theory has been supported. When evidence is obtained that does not support a theory, or that cannot be explained by the theory, alternative explanations must be considered. There may be reason to question how measurements were taken and how concepts were defined, to determine if these were truly consistent with the theory's intent. The validity of the theory may be questioned, or the application of the theory to the specific problem being studied may need to be re-evaluated. It may also be necessary to re-examine the theory and modify it, so that it does explain the observed outcome. If this is not practical, a new theory may need to be considered that will encompass this and all previous observations.

As an example of the application of theory to clinical decision making, Mueller and Maluf[20] have described *physical stress theory,* which states that changes in levels of physical stress cause a predictable adaptive response in all biological tissue. According to this premise, stresses less than normal will result in decreased tolerance of tissues to subsequent stresses, and stresses greater than normal will result in increased tolerance. If we accept this premise, we can assume that when muscle is not sufficiently stressed (not exercised), we would predict decreased tension and power (weakness), which would limit the muscle's future tolerance to outside forces. When muscle is challenged at high stresses (as through exercise), we will see increases in contractile strength. Stresses at either extreme will cause the tissue to fail. When stresses are absent, the muscle will atrophy; when stresses are excessive, the muscle will be strained.

We can use this theory to help with decision making when an individual's muscle performance does not fall within normal limits. As shown in Figure 2.4, for a condition of weakness, due to prolonged low stress levels, the threshold for adaptation will decrease. Therefore, a patient who has a weakened muscle is likely to suffer an injury at a lower force threshold than someone who is stronger. Similarly, a weakened muscle will increase in strength with a lower level of exercise than a stronger muscle would require. This theory goes beyond this specific example, to demonstrate how intrinsic and extrinsic factors can modify the adaptive responses of various tissues. The authors clearly illustrate how continued testing of the theory and its relationships is needed to contribute to the foundations of practice.[20]

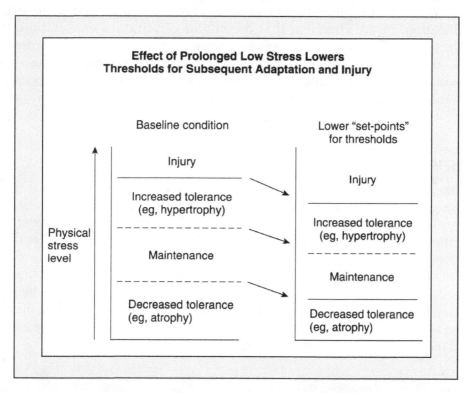

FIGURE 2.4 Representation of the physical stress theory, illustrating the effect of prolonged low stress on biological tissue. Low stress results in a lower threshold for subsequent adaptation and injury. Although relative thresholds remain the same, the absolute magnitude of physical stress is lower for each threshold. Injury (and all other adaptations) occurs at a lower level of physical stress than required previously. (From Mueller MJ, Maluf KS. Tissue adaptation to physical stress: A proposed "Physical Stress Theory" to guide physical therapist practice, education, and research. *Phys Ther* 2002;82:383–403, Figure 2, p. 387. Reprinted with permission of the American Physical Therapy Association.)

Theory as a Foundation for Understanding Research

Understanding clinical phenomena cannot be achieved in a single study. It is a process within a community of researchers involving discussion, criticism and intellectual exchange to analyze the connection between new and previous findings and explanations. This type of exchange allows the inconsistencies to surface, to identify findings that cannot be explained by current theories. This process can serve as a catalyst for a *paradigm shift*, or a change in the basic framework that governs the way knowledge is pursued.[21] For instance, the focus on outcomes in research represents a paradigm shift in rehabilitation science, as constructs such as disability and quality of life become a major focus, rather than the traditional emphasis on changes in physical impairments.[22] The ICF is another example, allowing interactions with theories of self-efficacy and health behaviors, and incorporating environmental factors as influences on performance.[23] By looking at outcomes in this way, researchers recognize that questions and their underlying theories will take a different direction than in the past.

The importance of theory for understanding research findings is often misunderstood. Whenever a research question is formulated, there is an implicit theory base that suggests how the variables of interest are related. Unfortunately, many authors do not make this foundation explicit. Empirical results are often described with only a general explanation, or an admission that the author can find no explanation. It is the author's responsibility, however, to consider what is known, to examine potential relationships, and help the reader understand the context within which the results can be understood. It is incumbent upon all researchers to project their expectations into the realm of theory, to offer an interpretation of findings, and thereby contribute to the growth of knowledge.[24]

THEORY AND LAW

When a theory does reach the level of absolute consistency in outcomes, it is called a **law**. Laws generally have a wider scope than theories, and allow precise predictions. For example, Newton made many mathematical observations that were used to describe the motion of the planets around the sun. These motions can be described with great precision, allowing great accuracy of prediction. What started as a theoretical observation eventually came to be accepted as a universal law. Generally, laws are not established in the applied sciences as they are in the physical sciences. The nature of human beings and their interactions with the environment does not allow our theories to become so precise in their prediction. We are left, therefore, with the necessity of continuing the quest for affirmation of our theories.

COMMENTARY

Applying Theory

History documents many dramatic changes in society's acceptance of theories, such as the belief that the world was round not flat and that the sun was the center of our solar system. In medicine we are aware of significant modifications to our understanding of the human body, as evidenced in the shift from Galen's view of "pores" in the heart to Harvey's theory of circulation. We have also witnessed major changes in cultural values that have influenced the acceptance of some theories, such as the effect of the feminist movement on theories of social interaction and management.

The concept of **metatheory** has been used to reflect theories that attempt to reconcile several theoretical perspectives in the explanation of sociological, psychological and physiological phenomena. A metatheory places specific research questions within a broader framework and encourages the integration of theorizing for a range of potentially disparate ideas.[25] For example, metatheories have been proposed to explain the complex nature of depression,[26] adaptation to chronic illness[27] and compensatory phenomena observed in studies of early brain damage.[28] Openness to synthesizing various concepts provides the impetus for continually posing new research questions.

The fact that scientists are constantly adapting or developing theories to accommodate new information is, of course, healthy and of critical importance to clinical science if we expect our treatments to reflect the most up-to-date scientific information available. Evidence-based practice requires that we consider the latest research in the context of our own clinical judgment and experience. We cannot ignore the possibility that any theory will need to be modified or discarded. At any given time a particular theory will be accepted by some scientists for some purposes, and not by others. Theories need to be tested in different ways in a variety of contexts. Research is, therefore, essential to the continued refinement of the theoretical basis for treatment.

Much of clinical practice is based on empirical successes which clinicians have attempted to explain using theories that are currently accepted. As new knowledge is advanced, these theories may be dismissed or changed. This does not mean that the treatment does not work. It just suggests that the theory was incorrectly applied to that situation and that we do not yet fully understand why the treatment is successful. We must continue to test theories in an effort to refine them in the context of human behavior, and eventually reformulate them to reflect more precisely what we actually observe in practice.

REFERENCES

1. Kerlinger FN. *Foundations of Behavioral Research.* New York: Holt, Rinehart & Winston, 1973.
2. Mawdsley RH, Knapik JJ. Comparison of isokinetic measurements with test repetitions. *Phys Ther* 1982;62:169–172.
3. Maslow AH. *Motivation and Personality* (2nd ed.). New York: Harper & Row, 1970.
4. Maughan RJ, Harmon M, Leiper JB, Sale D, Delman A. Endurance capacity of untrained males and females in isometric and dynamic muscular contractions. *Eur J Appl Physiol* 1986;55:395–400.
5. Prochaska JO, Velicer WF. The transtheoretical model of health behavior change. *Am J Health Promot* 1997;12:38–48.
6. Allen KR, Hazelett SE, Palmer RR, Jarjoura DG, Wickstrom GC, Weinhardt JA, et al. Developing a stroke unit using the acute care for elders intervention and model of care. *J Am Geriatr Soc* 2003;51:1660–1667.
7. Verbrugge LM, Jette AM. The disablement process. *Soc Sci Med* 1994;38:1–14.

8. Hamzat TK. Physical characteristics as predictors of quadriceps muscle isometric strength: A pilot study. *Afr J Med Med Sci* 2001;30:179–181.

9. Neder JA, Nery LE, Shinzato GT, Andrade MS, Peres C, Silva AC. Reference values for concentric knee isokinetic strength and power in nonathletic men and women from 20 to 80 years old. *J Orthop Sports Phys Ther* 1999;29:116–126.

10. Hanten WP, Chen WY, Austin AA, Brooks RE, Carter HC, Law CA, et al. Maximum grip strength in normal subjects from 20 to 64 years of age. *J Hand Ther* 1999;12:193–200.

11. Gewirtz JL, Pelaez-Nogueras M. B. F. Skinner's legacy to human infant behavior and development. *Am Psychol* 1992;47:1411–1422.

12. Glaser BG, Strauss AI. *The Discovery of Grounded Theory: Strategies for Qualitative Research.* New York: Aldine, 1967.

13. Resnik L, Jensen GM. Using clinical outcomes to explore the theory of expert practice in physical therapy. *Phys Ther* 2003;83:1090–1106.

14. von Keutz P. The character concept of Sigmund Freud. *Schweiz Arch Neurol Neurochir Psychiatr* 1971;109:343–365.

15. Gardner H. *Intelligence Reframed: Multiple Intelligences for the 21st Century.* New York: Basic, 2000.

16. Cummings E, Henry WE. *Growing Old: The Process of Disengagement.* New York: Basic Books, 1961.

17. Bengtson VL, Dowd JJ. Sociological functionalism, exchange theory and life-cycle analysis: A call for more explicit theoretical bridges. *Int J Aging Hum Develop* 1981;12:55–73.

18. Carstensen LL. Social and emotional patterns in adulthood: Support for socioemotional selectivity theory. *Psychol Aging* 1992;7:331–338.

19. Wadensten B, Carlsson M. Theory-driven guidelines for practical care of older people, based on the theory of gerotranscendence. *J Adv Nurs* 2003;41:462–470.

20. Mueller MJ, Maluf KS. Tissue adaptation to physical stress: A proposed "Physical Stress Theory" to guide physical therapist practice, education, and research. *Phys Ther* 2002;82:383–403.

21. Kuhn T. *The Structure of Scientific Revolutions.* New York: Norton, 1962.

22. Jette AM. Outcomes research: Shifting the dominant research paradigm in physical therapy. *Phys Ther* 1995;75:865–970.

23. van der Ploeg HP, van der Beek AJ, van der Woude LH, van Mechelen W. Physical activity for people with a disability: A conceptual model. *Sports Med* 2004;34:639–649.

24. Royce JR. Pebble picking versus boulder building. *Psychol Rep* 1965;16:447–450.

25. Abrams D, Hogg MA. Metatheory: Lessons from social identity research. *Pers Soc Psychol Rev* 2004;8:98–106.

26. Karasu TB. Developmentalist metatheory of depression and psychotherapy. *Am J Psychother* 1992;46:37–49.

27. Paterson BL. The shifting perspectives model of chronic illness. *J Nurs Scholarsh* 2001; 33:21–26.

28. Gottlieb G. The relevance of developmental-psychobiological metatheory to developmental neuropsychology. *Dev Neuropsychol* 2001;19:1–9.

CHAPTER 3
Ethical Issues in Clinical Research

We will complete our conceptual framework of clinical research by discussing ethical issues related to the conduct of human studies. We ask people to participate as subjects in studies for the purpose of gaining new knowledge that may or may not have an impact on their lives. Clinical research is conducted because we have questions and do not have the answers; therefore, participation in research may come with some risk to the health and well-being of the subjects. In this society, we recognize a responsibility to research subjects for assuring their rights as individuals. Since the middle of the 20th century, the rules of conducting research have been and continue to be discussed, legislated and codified.

The purpose of this chapter is to present the principles and practices that have become standards in the planning and implementation of research involving human subjects. These principles elucidate the ethical obligation of researchers to engage in meaningful research and to acknowledge the participation of not only the subjects under study but also professional colleagues who contribute substantially to a research project. We will cite the major documents that define public policy.

INTEGRITY OF THE RESEARCHER

Researchers have a responsibility for honesty and integrity in all phases of the research process, beginning with choice of a research question. Researchers who are health professionals must set priorities and pursue questions that are relevant to important health care issues. Today, for example, we see an emphasis on research to examine the outcomes of emerging health care strategies. Changes in the population profile, public health problems and scientific or technological advances have stimulated research in specific areas, such as geriatrics, acquired immune deficiency syndrome (AIDS) and stem cell research. External forces such as the priorities of private and governmental funding agencies affect the research direction of most clinical scientists. These complex factors influence the selection of ongoing research efforts.

Researchers also have an ethical responsibility to do clinical research that is meaningful. We should be able to justify a project based on the potential scientific value of its results. This implies an obligation to base our research on rational theoretical principles and to carry it out according to a sound research design with an appropriate sample. It also suggests that research should be conducted by competent investigators who have the expertise to do reliable and valid work. It is not ethical to involve patients in a study, with potential risks to them, when the study has little chance of making a scientific contribution.

During data collection researchers must be careful to minimize the effect of personal bias in measurement. Rosenthal[1] has described several types of experimenter bias that can have significant effects on experimental outcomes. These include unconscious or purposeful inaccuracies in measurement that will tend to support the research hypothesis and influential interactions between researcher and subject that alter the subject's behavior. Bias cannot be eliminated entirely simply because of human nature, but it should be recognized and controlled as much as possible.

Unfortunately, there have been several instances of misconduct in the medical research community such as falsification or misrepresentation of data that serve only to hinder the pursuit of truth and progress.[2] Statistical procedures should be appropriate, and should not be used to manipulate data for the sole purpose of obtaining a significant result. All data should be included in an analysis, and true differences or the lack of true differences should be reported. Researchers should be aware of potential conflicts of interest that may lead to misconduct. It is not unusual today to find research funded by government or private agencies or equipment manufacturers. The researcher should know who would control the dissemination of information. That agent may want to suppress results that do not conform to expectations. The researcher should be clear on who owns the data and who has access to it once the project is completed.

A researcher has an obligation to publish findings and to be thorough and honest in reporting results. In the 2004 update of the Uniform Requirements for Manuscripts Submitted to Biomedical Journals, the International Committee of Medical Journal Editors has included a section on the obligation to publish negative results.[3] The Uniform Requirements are accepted by over 500 journal editorial boards.

Credit of authorship is an issue for research publications. Authors should have made major contributions to a project,[3] although many research directors are routinely listed as a formality. Some journals now require a description of the role of each contributor. The order in which authors are listed in the byline is usually determined according to each individual's contribution. Agreements about authorship should be made early in the course of a project to avoid later conflicts. Most research involves the input of many contributors, and researchers should not hesitate to give authorship credit where it is due. Authors should also give credit to those who helped during the project, but who might not merit authorship, through an acknowledgment.

THE PROTECTION OF HUMAN RIGHTS IN CLINICAL RESEARCH

Our primary professional purpose in conducting clinical research is to document the effectiveness and efficiency of treatment intervention. Our patients or normal subjects are, therefore, the *sine qua non* of our research activities. Commitment to the protection of their rights and dignity must be inherent in the design and conduct of any clinical research project.

Guiding Principles

Research with human subjects requires adherence to three basic principles: autonomy of each individual, beneficence, and justice. Personal **autonomy** refers to self-determination and the capacity of individuals to make decisions affecting their lives and to act on those decisions. Beauchamp and Childress[4] describe autonomous action as intentional, carried out with understanding and without controlling influence. It is essential that researchers demonstrate all due respect for the elements of autonomy. Some individuals who may be appropriate subjects for research, such as children or patients with cognitive problems, may be unable to understand adequately. In these cases, the researcher is obliged to assure that an authorized surrogate decision maker is available, has the ability to make a reasoned decision and is committed to the well-being of the compromised individual.

Beneficence refers to the obligation to attend to the well-being of individuals. All who engage in clinical research are bound to "maximize possible benefits and minimize possible harm."[5] The balance between risks and benefits must be weighed as a part of the decision to go forward with a specific project. Risks may be physical, economic, social or psychological. Potential benefits may include new knowledge that can be applied to future subjects or patients, or that may have a direct impact on study participants, such as improved health status. The point is that the "risks to the subjects [must be] reasonable in relation to anticipated benefits."[6] The analysis of the *risk-benefit* relationship measures the probability and magnitude of benefit against the probability of anticipated harm or discomfort. For example, if a new powerful chemotherapeutic agent with known serious side effects requires testing, the selection of normal subjects would be unacceptable; whereas testing on subjects who are terminally ill, and for whom the drug has the potential to effect a positive change, might be acceptable.

Justice refers to fairness in the research process, or the equitable distribution of the benefits and burdens.[4] This principle speaks to the fair selection of subjects who are appropriate for a given study, drawn from a defined population that is most likely to benefit from the research findings. The selection of subjects should not be discriminatory on some irrelevant criterion, but based on reasons directly related to the problem being studied.[5] The principle of justice also has meaning in multigroup studies where subjects have an equal chance of being assigned to an experimental or control (or alternative) group. Current practices are followed to ensure consideration of and adherence to these three basic principles.

Use of Control Groups

A historical dilemma for medical researchers has been the need for a **control group**, or placebo group, as a basis for experimental comparison. Randomized controlled trials (RCTs) have become an accepted way to determine whether an intervention has a significant effect on subjects who receive the treatment compared to those who receive no treatment or a sham treatment. The RCT is preferred for this purpose over observation or retrospective analysis of data. Through the process of random assignment of subjects to the treatment or control group, researchers are best able to control confounding variables that could affect the outcome of the study.

A dilemma may arise when the researcher is also the clinician responsible for the care of the patient who might be a research subject. Rothman and Michels[7] reported several examples of this problem in drug studies where a placebo condition was employed when, in fact, effective therapeutic methods existed. The current *Declaration of Helsinki* addresses this issue, stating that: "The benefits, risks, burdens and effectiveness of a new method should be tested against those of the best current prophylactic, diagnostic, and therapeutic methods" (principle 29).[8] In this case, the research goal is to determine which of the alternative treatments is more effective. This allows us to say that one treatment is different from another, but it does not establish if treatment conditions are more effective than no intervention at all (see Chapter 10).

The researcher can support the concept of a placebo control group from several perspectives. First, there may be some clinical conditions for which no treatments have been effective.[8] In that case it is necessary to compare a new treatment with a no-treatment condition. It is also necessary to make such a comparison when the purpose of the research is to determine whether a particular treatment approach is not effective. In situations where the efficacy of a treatment is being questioned because current knowledge is inadequate, it may actually be more ethical to take the time to make appropriate controlled comparisons than to continue clinical practice using potentially ineffective techniques. The researcher is obliged to inform the potential participants when a study is planned that includes a control group. Subjects should know that there is a chance that they will receive the treatment being studied and a chance that they will not receive the treatment. According to the 2002 edition of the *Declaration of Helsinki*, as a form of compensation, the experimental treatment may be offered to the control group patients after data collection is complete, if results indicate that treatment is beneficial (principle 30).[8] As clinician-researchers, we are obliged to discuss alternative treatments that would be appropriate for each patient-subject if such alternatives are employed in clinical practice. This is an important element of the informed consent process that will be discussed later in this chapter.

Evolution of Regulations for the Conduct of Research Involving Human Subjects

Establishment of formal guidelines delineating rights of research subjects and obligations of professional investigators became a societal necessity as clear abuses of experimentation came to light. In the United States, many unconscionable studies have been identified over the years.[9] In one case, elderly patients were injected with live malignant cancer cells without their knowledge.[10] Another much publicized study, begun in the 1930s, withheld treatment from men with syphilis to observe the natural course of the disease.[11] This study continued until the early 1970s, long after penicillin had been identified as an effective cure.

The first formal guidelines document defining ethical human research practices was the *Nuremberg Code of 1949*. This document was developed in concert with the Nuremberg trials of Nazi physicians who conducted criminal experimentation on captive victims during World War II. The code clearly emphasized that every individual should voluntarily consent to participate as a research subject. Consent should be given only after the subject has sufficient knowledge of the purposes, procedures, inconveniences, and potential hazards of the experiment. This principle underlies the current practice of obtaining informed consent prior to initiation of clinical research or therapeutic intervention. The Nuremberg Code also addresses the competence of the investigator, stating that research "should be conducted only by scientifically qualified persons."

The World Medical Association originally adopted the *Declaration of Helsinki* in 1964. This document addressed for the first time the concept of independent review of research protocols by a committee of individuals who are not associated with the proposed project (Principle 13 in the current edition of the Declaration).[8] These and other essential principles set forth in this document have been incorporated into the U.S. Department of Health and Human Services (DHHS) Rules and Regulations.[6] The *Declaration of Helsinki* also declares that reports of research that has not been conducted according to stated principles should not be accepted for publication (Principle 27).[8] This principle has led to an editorial challenge to professional journals to obtain assurance that submitted reports of human studies do indeed reflect proper attention to ethical conduct. DeBakey[12] suggests that all reports should contain information on the procedures used for obtaining informed consent and ethical review. Most journals now require acknowledgment that informed consent was obtained from subjects used in any research project.

Based on the ethical principles guiding biomedical research and the rules and regulations promulgated pursuant to the 1974 National Research Act (PL-93-348), procedures to ensure protection of human subjects in research have been delineated and are now considered "standard" throughout the United States. There must be a fully developed research proposal that identifies the problem or question to be studied and provides the rationale of, need for, and importance of the study. The research design must be clearly stated and deemed appropriate to answer the question. Informed consent must be obtained from individuals or their legally authorized representatives. This is usually accomplished by signature affixed to a written informed consent document. Both the written proposal and the informed consent form are submitted to an Institutional Review Board for approval.

The National Research Act (1976) established the National Commission for the Protection of Human Subjects of Biomedical and Behavioral Research. The deliberations and recommendations of this commission resulted in the Belmont Report (1979) that delineates the guiding principles discussed previously in this chapter and the manner in which these principles apply to human research studies.[5] Based on that report, both the Department of Health and Human Services (DHHS) and the Food and Drug Administration (FDA) established the rules and regulations that govern the conduct of research in the United States today. The Office for Human Research Protection (OHPR) is the administrative arm of the DHHS that is responsible for implementing the regulations and providing guidance to those who conduct human studies.

The Health Insurance Portability and Accountability Act of 1996 (HIPAA) and the resultant regulations (the *Privacy Rule*) issued by the DHHS, Office of Civil Rights have added a new dimension to the process of protecting research subjects[13,14] The DHHS regulations (45 CFR 46),[6] known as the *Common Rule*, and the FDA regulations (21 CFR, parts 50 and 56)[15] have always included rules for protecting individual confidentiality.

THE INSTITUTIONAL REVIEW BOARD

According to federal regulations, an **Institutional Review Board (IRB)** must review research proposals prior to implementation to ensure that the rights of research subjects are protected.[6] The IRB must be composed of at least five members. It may not consist of all males, or all females or all members of one professional group, although the IRB must be able to competently review the scientific details of proposed research. At least one member must be concerned primarily with nonscientific issues and may be a lawyer, clergyman or ethicist. One member, a "public" member, must not be otherwise affiliated with the institution where the research is to be conducted. One of the responsibilities of the OHRP is to approve IRB documents that assure compliance with ethical principles and regulations.

Review of Proposals

The responsibility of the IRB is to review research proposals at convened meetings. The decision to approve, require modifications in, defer or deny approval of a proposal must be that of a majority. In arriving at a decision, the IRB considers the scientific merit of the project, the competence of the investigators, the risk to subjects, and the feasibility based on identified resources. If the project is not scientifically sound or practical, there can be no benefit; therefore, no risk to subjects is justified. Reviewers will consider the evidence that the risks and discomforts to the subject have been minimized and are sufficiently outweighed by the potential benefits of the proposed study. This is the **risk-benefit ratio**. The Board also studies the procedures for selecting subjects, ensuring voluntary informed consent based on complete and understandable descriptions and conforming to the applicable elements of the Privacy Rule. The majority of proposals submitted to an IRB are reviewed in this detailed manner.

Expedited or Exempt Review

Some categories of research activity, however, may qualify for an expedited review or may be exempted from the review process. A project may qualify for **expedited review** in circumstances such as "recording data from subjects 18 years of age or older using noninvasive procedures routinely employed in clinical practice" and "moderate exercise by healthy volunteers."[6] In the case of an expedited review, the chairman and at least one designated member of the IRB conduct the review. The advantage of expedited review is that it is usually completed in less time than that required for a full Board review.

Projects may be **exempted** from committee review if they are surveys, interviews, or studies of existing records, provided that the data are collected in such a way that subjects cannot be identified. Surveys or interviews will only be given exempt status if they do not deal with sensitive issues, such as drug abuse, sexual behavior or criminal activity. Secondary analysis of existing data from databases ("limited data sets") where subject information is appropriately de-identified may be exempt. On the other hand, when actual patient clinic records are used, IRB approval is required.[16] Researchers must describe methods of coding data to assure patient confidentiality. Given the advent of the HIPAA Privacy Rule, some institutions have eliminated the exempt review category.

All proposals for studies involving human subjects must be submitted to the IRB, which then determines whether a project qualifies for full review, expedited review or is exempt.

Institutional Guidelines

Each institution establishes its own guidelines for review in accordance with federal and state regulations. Clinicians should, therefore, become familiar with the requirements in their own institutions. Clinicians should also be aware that the process could take several weeks, depending on the IRB's schedule and whether or not the proposal needs revision. This review process should be included in the timetable for any research project. No research on human subjects should be done without prior review and approval of a designated review committee.

ELEMENTS OF INFORMED CONSENT

Perhaps the most important ethical tenet in human studies is the individual's ability to agree to participate with full understanding of what will happen to him. The **informed consent** process and all of its elements address the basic principles of autonomy, beneficence and justice. The components of the process consist of **information elements**, including disclosure of information and the subject's comprehension of that information, **consent elements**, ensuring the voluntary nature of participation and the subject's competence to consent and **authorization** to use data in a manner specified in the protocol.[15,17]

Information Elements

Subjects Must Be Fully Informed

The informed consent process begins with an invitation to participate. A statement of the purpose of the study permits potential subjects to decide whether they believe in or agree with the worth and importance of the research. The process then requires that the researcher provide, in writing, a fair explanation of the procedures to be used and how they will be applied. This explanation must be complete, with no deception by virtue of commission or omission. Subjects should know what will be done to them, how long it will take, what they will feel, what side effects can be expected, and what types of questions they may be asked. If subjects cannot read the informed consent document, it should be read to them. Children should be informed to whatever extent is reasonable for their age. Subjects should also know why they have been selected to participate in terms of inclusion criteria for the study, such as clinical condition or age. If the subjects are patients, they should understand the distinction between procedures that are experimental and procedures, if any, that are proposed to serve their personal needs.

An ethical dilemma occurs when complete disclosure of procedures might hinder the outcomes of a study by biasing the subjects so that they do not respond in a typical way. When the risks are not great, review boards may allow researchers to pursue a deceptive course, but subjects must be told that information is being withheld and that they will be informed of all procedures after completion of data collection. For example, when the research design includes a control or placebo group, subjects will not know what treatment they are receiving. They should know that they will be told their group assignment at the completion of the study.

An important aspect of informed consent is the description of all reasonable foreseeable risks or discomforts to which the patient will be subjected, directly or indirectly, as part of the study. **Risk** refers to physical, psychological or social harm that goes beyond expected experiences in daily life. The researcher should detail the steps that will be taken to protect against these risks and the treatments that are available for potential side effects. For example, if a patient is likely to become fatigued as a result of performing maximal physical exercise, the researcher may include rest periods during the experimental trial. If a patient were receiving electrical stimulation, the researcher would explain the risk of shock and how that risk is minimized by proper grounding and by regular inspection of the equipment. The subject should be advised against such behaviors as taking certain medications or driving a car, which could be hazardous during or after the experimental period. A statement should be included whereby subjects agree to exercise appropriate caution. They are not bound by this, but they should understand the potential harm of not honoring the agreement. If the research involves more than a minimal risk, a statement should be included concerning the availability of medical care and whether compensation will be provided. Subjects should also be informed of new information, such as the identification of previously unknown risks that becomes available during the course of the study. This may affect their willingness to continue participation.

The researcher also delineates the potential **benefits** of participation. Some studies may result in a beneficial reduction of symptoms. For example, subjects who participate in a study to test the effectiveness of treatment for migraine headache may find their pain relieved by the experimental treatment. The subject should be advised that such a benefit is possible but is not guaranteed. Studies that are geared more toward theory testing may provide no direct benefits. The researcher should explain the potential application of theoretical findings and how the findings will contribute to future research or future patient care.

When a study involves a form of therapeutic intervention, subjects must be informed that alternative treatments are available and that they have the right to choose among them instead of accepting the experimental intervention. Patients must also be told if "standard" treatments to which they are entitled are being withheld as part of the study. This information is essential if a patient is to make an informed decision about accepting the experimental conditions.

Subject Information Should Be Confidential and Anonymous

Research subjects should be told what steps are being taken to ensure confidentiality of all information, including descriptive and experimental data. Whenever possible, a subject's anonymity should be protected. This becomes an issue with surveys, for example, when respondents wish to remain unidentified. In experimental situations anonymity is often not feasible, but the researcher can code the data without using names. Identifying codes can be kept separate from the rest of the data. Researchers should also be aware of this responsibility when disseminating results. Researchers also have a responsibility to know the requirements of the Privacy Rule[15,17] and the procedures established by their Institutional Review Boards.

If the subject is to be videotaped or photographed during the study, this should be disclosed in the consent form. The subject should know who will have access to tapes or photographs, who will keep them, and how they will be used. Subjects retain the right to review such material and to withdraw permission for its use at any time. Subjects should also be informed if one-way windows will be used and who the observers will be.

The Informed Consent Form Must Be Written in Lay Language

Informed consent is more than telling subjects about the research; the process implies that they understand what they are being told and what they are reading. The language must be clear and basic so that the average reasonable individual can follow it. Professional jargon is unacceptable. Instead of "perform a maximal isometric contraction," the subject should be told to "pull up as hard as you can without moving." This is the language that clinicians use routinely in patient education. As a rule of thumb, language should be written for the lowest educational level that would be expected for subjects.

The Researcher Must Offer to Answer Questions at Any Time

The researcher is responsible for ensuring that the subject understands all relevant information. A verbal description is almost always a part of the process, so that the researcher can "personalize" the information for each subject. The subjects should have sufficient time to assimilate the details of the proposed project, prior to making their decision to participate. They should feel free to question the procedures at any time during the course of the study, and should be provided with the name and telephone number of an appropriate contact person.

Consent Elements

Consent Must Be Voluntary

Subjects should participate in a research project of their own free will. Patients are usually quite motivated to help, but they must be informed that there is no penalty to them if they refuse. Some studies may involve monetary compensation for participation. It should be clear if such compensation will be received whether or not the subject completes the study.

Special Consideration Must Be Given to Subjects Who Are Particularly "Vulnerable"

Some individuals cannot give informed consent because they may not be able to understand the information. In cases of mental illness, developmental disability, or diminished mental capacity, the ability of the subject to consent must be evaluated by the researcher and others who know the subject well. If the subject is not competent, consent must be provided by a legal guardian or advocate.[6]

The regulations regarding children as research subjects require that parents or guardians give permission for participation. Furthermore, if a child is considered competent to understand, regardless of age, his or her assent, that is, his or her affirmative agreement to participate must be obtained and documented. Researchers should be particularly cautious about influencing subjects who are considered "captive."[7] For example, there are specific regulations regarding research involving prisoners.[9] More subtle circumstances exist with the use of students or nursing home residents. In both cases, the sense of pleasing those in authority may affect the subjects' decisions.

Subjects Must Be Free to Withdraw Consent at Any Time

The informed consent document must indicate that the subject is free to discontinue participation for any reason at any time without prejudice; that is, the subject should be assured that no steps will be taken against him, and, if he is a patient, that the quality of his care will not diminish. This can occur before or during an experiment, or even after data collection when a subject might request that his data be discarded. It should also be clear that the researcher would discontinue the experiment at any time if necessary for the subject's safety or comfort.

The Informed Consent Form

All subjects must give informed consent prior to participating in a project. This is done by providing a written informed consent form that is signed and dated by the subject, researcher and a witness. Subjects should receive a copy of this form and the researcher must retain a signed copy. Although it is a general contractual agreement, the informed consent form is not binding on subjects. Subjects never waive their rights to redress if their participation should cause them harm. The form should not contain language that appears to release the researcher from liability. The required elements of an informed consent form are listed in Table 3.1. A sample informed consent form can be found in Appendix E. The format of this sample informed consent form is used in many institutions. It specifically identifies and acknowledges all of the elements of informed consent. Of special note, the signature page should not stand alone, but must contain some of the text of the document to show that the signatures are applied in the context of the larger document.

Although written consent is preferable, some agencies allow oral consent in selected circumstances. In this case, a written "short form" can be used that describes the information presented orally to the subject or his or her legally authorized representative.[6] This short form is submitted to the review committee for approval.

Informed Consent and Usual Care

Clinical research projects are often designed to test specific treatment protocols that are accepted as standard care, and subjects are recruited from those who would receive such treatments. Therapists often ask if informed consent is necessary for a research

---

TABLE 3.1   ELEMENTS OF INFORMED CONSENT

---

1. Purpose of the research project
  • A clear explanation of the reason for doing the study and why it is important
  • Reason for selecting this particular individual

2. Procedures
  • A clear detailed explanation of what will be done to or by the individual

3. Risks and discomforts
  • Truthful and inclusive statements of risks that may result and discomforts that can be expected

4. Benefits
  • A description of potential benefits of the individual participant, to the general knowledge, or to future administration of health care

5. Alternatives to participation
  • A description of reasonable alternative procedures that might be used in the treatment of this individual when a treatment intervention is being studied

6. Confidentiality
  • Statements of the procedures used to ensure the anonymity of the individual in collecting, storing, and reporting information and who (persons or agencies) will have access to the information
  • Specific authorization
  • What information may be used?
  • Who may use the information?
  • For what purpose? (May be referred to the description of the study)
  • Is there an expiration date? Is so, what is it?
  • This authorization must be signed as part of the informed consent document or as a separate document.

7. Request for more information
  • A statement that the individual may ask questions about or discuss participation in the study at any time, naming an individual to contact

8. Refusal or withdrawal
  • A statement that the individual may refuse to participate or discontinue participation at any time without prejudice

9. Injury statement
  • A description of measures to be taken if injury occurs as a direct result of the research activity

10. Consent statement
  • A confirmation that the individual consents to participate in the research project

11. Signatures
  • Participant
  • Parent or guardian (for the care of minors)
  • Assent of minors over age 7
  • Witness

---

project when the procedures would have been used anyway. The answer is yes! Even where treatment is viewed as usual care, patients are entitled to understand alternatives that are available to them. Patients must always be informed of the use of the data that are collected during their treatments, and they should have sufficient information to decide to participate or not, regardless of whether treatment is viewed as experimental or accepted clinical practice.

COMMENTARY

A Patient Care Perspective

The concepts of informed consent for human research have also been applied to medical practice.[18,19] Patients entering hospitals are asked to sign standard consent forms that indicate agreement to routine medical care and tests. Additional forms are signed for surgery or special tests. This practice has not been applied as readily to clinical situations in allied health, although the concepts of disclosure and voluntary participation are becoming more important to the protection of patients' rights. Although the idea of explaining treatments to patients is by no means unusual, the structure and formal requirements of informed consent have important implications for the patient–provider relationship. The clinician can give the patient a description of the planned treatment and available alternatives and explain inherent risks, consequences, advantages and disadvantages. Clinicians recognize the possibilities of inflicting harm on patients through thermal modalities, resistive exercise, or mobilization and should identify these potential effects prior to treatment. It is not necessary for the average patient to understand the physiological rationale for treatment, but clinicians should be able to explain things in reasonable detail and within the scope of the patient's understanding. With sufficient information, the patient can participate in the setting of treatment goals, consider whether or not he or she wants to be treated, and express a preference for particular types of treatment. In this manner, patients, like research subjects, can assume an appropriate role in making decisions about the activities that affect their lives.

REFERENCES

1. Rosenthal R. *Experimenter Effects in Behavioral Research.* New York: Appleton-Century-Crofts, 1966.
2. Department of Health and Human Services, Office of Research Integrity. Available at: <http://ori.dhhs.gov> Accessed on April 7, 2005.
3. International Committee of Medical Journal Editors. Uniform requirements for manuscripts submitted to biomedical journals. Available at: <http://www.icmje.org/#obligation> Accessed March 25, 2005.
4. Beauchamp TL, Childress JF. *Principles of Biomedical Ethics* (5th ed.). New York: Oxford University Press, 2001.
5. The National Commission for the Protection of Human Subjects of Biomedical and Behavioral Research. *The Belmont Report: Ethical Principles and Guidelines for the Protection of Human Subjects of Research.* Washington, DC: National Institutes of Health. Office of Human Subject Research. Available at: <http://www.hhs.gov/ohrp/humansubjects/guidance/belmont.htm> Accessed March 25, 2005.
6. Title 45 Code of Federal Regulations. Part 46: Protection of human subjects (HHS). Washington, DC: National Institutes of Health. Office of Human Subject Research. Available at: <http://www.hhs.gov/ohrp/humansubjects/guidance/belmont.htm> Accessed March 25, 2005.

7. Rothman KJ, Michels KB. The continuing unethical use of placebo controls. *N Engl J Med* 1994;331:394–398.
8. World Medical Association. Declaration of Helsinki. Recommendations guiding physicians in biomedical research involving human subjects. Available at: <http://www.wma.net/e/policy/b3.htm> Accessed March 25, 2005.
9. Beecher HK. Ethics and clinical research. *N Engl J Med* 1966;274:1354–1360.
10. Langer E. Human experimentation: New York verdict affirms human rights. *Science* 1966;151:663.
11. *Final Report of the Tuskegee Syphilis Study Ad Hoc Advisory Panel.* Washington, DC: United States Public Health Service, 1973.
12. DeBakey L. *The Scientific Journal: Editorial Policies and Practicies.* St. Louis: CV Mosby, 1976.
13. U.S. Department of Health and Human Services, National Institutes of Health. Protecting Personal Health Information in Research: Understanding the HIPAA Privacy Rule. Available at: <http://privacyruleandresearch.nih.gov/pr_02.asp> Accessed March 25, 2005.
14. Woods GW. Impact of the HIPAA privacy rule on academic research. <http://www.acenet.edu>, Accessed March 25, 2005.
15. U.S. Food and Drug Administration. Guidance for Institutional Review Boards and Clinical Investigators. Washington, DC. Available at: <http://www.fda.gov/oc/ohrt/irbs/appendixb.html> Accessed March 25, 2005.
16. Huston P, Naylor CD. Health services research: Reporting on studies using secondary data sources [editorial]. *CMAJ* 1996;155:1697–1709.
17. Woods GW: Impact of the HIPAA Privacy Rule on Academic Research. Available at: <http://www.acenet.edu> Accessed March 25, 2005.

PART **II**

Concepts of Measurement

CHAPTER 4

Principles of Measurement

Scientists and clinicians use measurement as a way of understanding, evaluating and differentiating characteristics of people and objects. Measurement provides a mechanism for achieving a degree of precision in this understanding, so that we can describe physical or behavioral characteristics according to their quantity, degree, capacity or quality.[1] We can document that a patient's shoulder can flex to 75 degrees, rather than say motion is "limited," or indicate that the air temperature is 95° F, rather than just "hot." This ability helps us communicate information in objective terms, giving us a common sense of "how much" or "how little" without ambiguous interpretation. Principles of measurement, therefore, are basic to our ability to describe phenomena, demonstrate change or relationship, and to communicate this information to others.

Measurement is used as a basis for making decisions or drawing conclusions in several ways. At its most basic, measurement is used to describe the quality or quantity of an existing variable, such as the measurement of intelligence, attitude, range of motion or muscle strength. We can also use measurement to make absolute decisions based on a criterion or standard of performance, such as the requirement that a student achieve at least a grade of C to pass a course or that a certain degree of spinal curvature be present to indicate a diagnosis of scoliosis. We use measurement as a basis for choosing between two courses of action. In this sense a clinician might decide to implement one treatment approach over another based on the results of a comparative research study. Clinicians use measurement as a means of evaluating a patient's condition and response to treatment; that is, we measure change or progress. We also use measurements to compare and discriminate between individuals or groups. For instance, a test can be used to distinguish between children who do and do not have learning disabilities or between different types of learning disabilities. Finally, measurement allows us to draw conclusions about the predictive relationship between variables. We might use grades on a college entrance examination to predict a student's ability to succeed in an academic program. We can measure the functional status of an elderly patient to determine the level of assistance that will be required when the patient returns home. There are virtually no decisions or clinical actions that are independent of some type of measurement.

Measurement has been defined as the *process of assigning numerals to variables to represent quantities of characteristics according to certain rules.*[2] The purpose of this chapter is to explore this definition as it is applied to clinical research. In doing so, we consider several aspects of measurement theory and discuss how these relate to measurement, analysis and interpretation of clinical variables.

QUANTIFICATION AND MEASUREMENT

The first part of the definition of measurement emphasizes the process of *assigning numerals to variables.* A numeral is a symbol or label in the form of a number. A variable is a property that can differentiate individuals or objects. It represents an attribute that can have more than one value. Value can denote quantity, such as age or blood pressure, or quality, such as gender or geographic region. Numerals are used to represent qualitative values, with no quantitative meaning. Therefore, we can assign numerals to football players, or code data on a questionnaire using a "0" to represent Male and a "1" to represent Female. A numeral becomes a mathematical number only when it represents a known quantity.

A number reflects how much of an attribute or variable is present. A **continuous variable** can theoretically take on any value along a continuum within a defined range. Between any two values an indefinitely large number of fractional values can occur. In reality, continuous values can never be measured exactly, but are limited by the precision of the measuring instrument. For instance, joint range could be measured as 50 degrees, 50.5 degrees or even 50.3 degrees, depending on the gradations on the goniometer and skill of the measurer. Strength, distance, weight, and chronological time are other examples of continuous variables.

Other variables can be described only in whole units, and are considered **discrete variables.** Heart rate, for example, is measured in beats per minute, not in fractions of a beat. Variables such as the number of trials needed to learn a motor task or the number of children in a family are also examples of discrete variables. Qualitative variables represent discrete categories, such as male/female. When qualitative variables, such as gender, can take on only two values, they are called **dichotomous variables.**

Precision refers to the exactness of a measure. For statistical purposes, this term is usually used to indicate the number of decimal places to which a number is taken. Therefore, 1.473826 is a number of greater precision than 1.47. The degree of precision in a measurement is a function of the sensitivity of the measuring instrument and data analysis system as well as the variable itself. It is not useful, for example, to record blood pressure in anything less than integer units (whole numbers with no decimal places). It may, however, be meaningful to record strength to a tenth or hundredth of a kilogram. Computer programs will often record values with four or more decimal places by default. It is generally not informative, however, to report results to so many places. How important is it to know that a mean age is 84.5 years as opposed to 84.5283 years? Cohen[3] suggests that such values create statistical "clutter" and are not meaningful for understanding data.

THE INDIRECT NATURE OF MEASUREMENT

The definition of measurement also indicates that measured values *represent quantities of characteristics.* Most measurement is a form of abstraction or conceptualization; that is, very few variables are measured directly. Range of motion and length are among the few examples of measures that involve direct observation of a physical property. We can actually see how far a limb rotates or how tall a person is, and we can compare angles and heights between people. Most characteristics are not directly observable, however, and we can measure only a correlate of the actual property. Therefore, most behavioral variables are actually indirect measures of these characteristics. For example, we do not observe temperature, but only the height of a column of mercury in a thermometer; we are not capable of visualizing the electrical activity of a heartbeat or muscle contraction, although we can evaluate the associated recording of an electrocardiogram (EKG) or electromyogram (EMG); force is observable only as the reading on a dynamometer, not as movement of the contractile elements of muscle. For most variables, then, we use some form of direct observation to *infer* a value for a phenomenon.

Constructs

The ability to measure a variable, no matter how indirectly, is dependent on one's ability to define it. Unless we know what a term means we cannot show that it exists. This is not difficult for variables such as temperature, weight, and heart rate, which can be defined by direct physical or physiological methods, but is much harder for abstract terms such as intelligence, health, strength, or pain. Any explanation of what these variables mean will undoubtedly involve descriptions of behaviors or outcomes that indicate if someone is "intelligent," "healthy," "strong," or "in pain"; however, there is no logical, unidimensional definition that will satisfy these terms. For instance, intelligence cannot be assessed as a single estimate of either verbal performance, memory, or quantitative skill, but is conceptualized as a complex, combined measure of IQ. Different aspects of strength may be assessed by dynamometry, strain gauges, lifting weights, or manual resistance, with specific reference to type of contraction, joint position, speed of movement, and type of resistance. No one measurement can be interpreted as an absolute measure of a person's "strength."

These types of abstract variables are called **constructs** (see Chapter 2). Measurement of a construct is based on expectations of how a person who possesses the specified trait would behave, look or feel in certain situations. Therefore, a construct is associated with some value or values that are assumed to represent the original variable. Some constructs are derived from one or more quantities of other variables.[4] For instance, velocity is calculated by first determining values for distance and time. Work is derived from the product of force and distance. These constructs have no inherent meaning except as a function of other constructs.

Most constructs must be defined as a function of many interrelated concepts or multiple dimensions. For example, we each have a conceptual understanding of the clinical term "disability," but researchers still struggle to develop meaningful ways to measure it. How might a physical therapist look at disability as compared with an occupational therapist, nurse, psychologist, neurologist, orthopedist, or social worker? Can we devise a scale so that one sum or average number is indicative of a patient's level of disability? Many such scales exist. But can we make the inferential leap from this number to an assessment of the psychological, social, physical, and physiological manifestations of disability? To do so we must be able to define the construct of disability in terms of specific and limited properties of behavior that are relevant to our own frame of reference. It is important to appreciate this difficulty in operationally defining construct measures as a basis for interpretation of clinical variables.

RULES OF MEASUREMENT

The last element of the definition of measurement concerns the need for establishing purposeful and precise *rules* for assigning values to objects. These rules designate how numbers are to be assigned, reflecting both amount and units of measurement. In some cases the rules are obvious and easily learned, as in the use of a yardstick (inches), scale (pounds), goniometer (degrees), or dynamometer (pounds of force). This is not the case for many clinical variables, for which the rules of measurement must be invented. Concepts such as sensation, quality of life, muscle tone, manual resistance, gait, function, and developmental age have been operationally defined by researchers who have developed instruments with complex rules of measurement that are by no means intuitive or obvious. Often, these rules require rigorous training and practice for the instruments to be applied effectively.

The criteria for assigning values and units to these types of variables must be systematically defined so that levels of the behavior can be objectively differentiated; that is, rules of assignment stipulate certain relationships among numbers or numerals. For example, we assume that relationships are consistent within a specific measurement system, so that objects or attributes can be equated or differentiated. For instance, we assume that either A equals B, or A does not equal B, but both cannot be true. We also assume that if A equals B, and B equals C, then A should also equal C (see Box 4.1).

Numbers are also used to denote relative order among variables. If A is greater than B, and B is greater than C, it should also be true that A is greater than C. We can readily see how this rule can be applied to a direct variable such as height. Similarly, we might assume that if A is stronger than B, and B is stronger than C, then A is also stronger than C. As logical as this may seem, however, there are measurement scales that do not fit within this structure. For example, if patient A receives a 4+ grade on a manual muscle test, and patient B receives a 4 grade, we cannot assume that A is stronger than B. The "rules" for manual muscle testing define a system of order that is valid *within* an individual, but not *across* individuals. A similar system is employed with a visual analogue scale for evaluating pain. Two patients may mark a point at 6.5 cm, but there is no way to establish that their levels of pain are equal. If, after a period of treatment, each patient marks a point at 2.0 cm, we know that their pain has decreased, but we still do not know if one patient has more pain than the other. Therefore, a researcher must understand the conceptual basis of a particular measurement to appreciate how the rules for that measurement can logically be applied and interpreted.

Rules of measurement also apply to the acceptable operations with which numerals can be manipulated. For instance, not all types of data can be subjected to arithmetic operations such as division and multiplication. Some values are more appropriately analyzed using proportions or frequency counts. The nature of the attribute being measured will determine the rules that can be applied to its measurement. To clarify this process, four **scales** or **levels of measurement** have been identified—nominal, ordinal, interval, and ratio—each with a special set of rules for manipulating and inter-

BOX 4.1 **When Does "A" Not Equal "B"?**

If you ever doubt the "far-reaching" consequences of not specifying well-defined terms, consider this. On December 11, 1998, the National Aeronautics and Space Administration (NASA) launched the Mars Climate Orbiter,

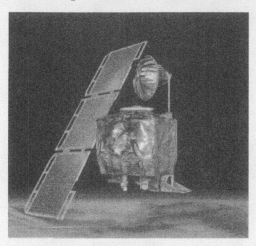

designed to be the world's first complete weather satellite orbiting another planet, with a price tag of $125 million.

On September 23, 1999, the orbiter crashed into the red planet, disintegrating on contact. After a 415 million mile journey over nine months, the orbiter came within 36 miles of the planet's surface, lower than the lowest orbit the craft was designed to survive.

After several days of investigation, NASA officials admitted to an embarrassingly simple mistake. The project team of engineers at Lockheed Martin in Colorado, who had built the spacecraft, transmitted the orbiter's final course and velocity to Mission Control in Pasadena using units of *pounds per second* of force. The navigation team at Mission Control, however, used the metric system in their calculations, which is generally the accepted practice in science and engineering. Their computers sent final commands to the spacecraft in *grams per second* of force (a measure of newtons). As a result, the ship just flew too close to the planet's surface, and was destroyed by atmospheric stresses.

www.googleimages.com

Oops!

Sources: http://www4.cnn.com/TECH/space/9909/24/mars.folo.03/index.html; http://www.sfgate.com; http://nssdc.gsfc.nasa.gov/nmc/tmp/1998-073A.html.

preting numerical data.[5] The characteristics of these four scales are summarized in Figure 4.1.

Nominal Scale

The lowest level of measurement is the **nominal scale**, also referred to as the *classificatory scale*. Objects or people are assigned to categories according to some criterion. Categories may be coded by name, number, letter or symbol, although none of these have any quantitative value. They are used purely as labels for identification. Blood type, handedness, type of mental illness, side of hemiplegic involvement, and

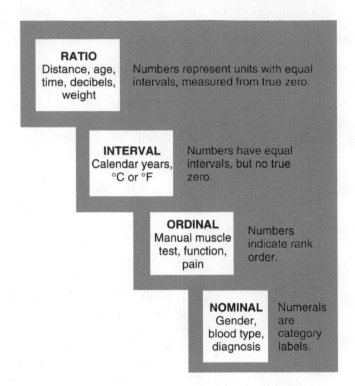

FIGURE 4.1   Summary of characteristics of scales of measurement.

area code are examples of nominal variables. Questionnaires often code nominal data as numerals for responses such as (0) no and (1) yes, (0) male and (1) female, or (0) disagree and (1) agree.

Based on the assumption that relationships are consistent within a measurement system, nominal categories are *mutually exclusive,* so that no object or person can logically be assigned to more than one. This means that the members within a category must be equivalent on the property being scaled, but different from those in other categories. We also assume that the rules for classifying a set of attributes are *exhaustive;* that is, every subject can be accurately assigned to one category. Classifying sex as male–female would follow these rules. Classifying hair color as only blonde or brunette would not.

The numbers or symbols used to designate groups on a nominal scale can be altered without changing the values or characteristics they identify. The categories cannot, therefore, be ordered on the basis of their assigned numerals. The only permissible mathematical operation is *counting* the number of subjects within each category, such as 35 males and 65 females. Statements can then be made concerning the frequency of occurrence of a particular characteristic or the proportions of a total group that fall within each category.

Ordinal Scale

Measurement on an **ordinal scale** requires that categories be rank ordered on the basis of an operationally defined characteristic or property. Data are organized into adjacent categories exhibiting a "greater than–less than" relationship. Many clinical measurements are based on this scale, such as sensation (normal > impaired > absent), spasticity (none < minimal < moderate < severe), and balance (good > fair > poor). Most clinical tests of constructs such as function, strength and development are also based on ranked scores. Surveys often create ordinal scales to describe attitudes or preferences (strongly agree > agree).

The intervals between ranks on an ordinal scale may not be consistent and, indeed, may not be known. This means that although the objects assigned to one rank are considered equivalent on the rank criterion, they may not actually be of equal value along the continuum that underlies the scale. Therefore, ordinal scales often record ties even when true values are unequal. For example, manual muscle test grades are defined according to ranks of 5 > 4 > 3 > 2 > 1 > zero. Although 4 is always stronger than 3, this scale is not sensitive enough to tell us what this difference is. Therefore, the interval between grades 4 and 3 on one subject will not necessarily be the same as on another subject, and one 4 muscle may not be equal in strength to another 4 muscle.

Ordinal scales can be distinguished on the basis of whether or not they contain a natural origin, or true zero point. For instance, military rank is ordinal, but has no zero rank. Manual muscle testing grades do have a true zero, which represents no palpable muscle contraction. In some cases, an ordinal scale can incorporate a natural origin within the series of categories, so that ranked scores can occur in either direction away from the origin (+ and –). This type of scale is often constructed to assess attitude or opinion, such as agree–neutral–disagree. For construct variables, it may be impossible to locate a true zero. For example, what is zero function? A category labeled "zero" may simply refer to performance below a certain criterion or at a theoretical level of dependence.

Limitations for interpretation are evident when using an ordinal scale. Perhaps most important is the lack of arithmetic properties for ordinal "numbers." Because ranks are assigned according to discrete categories, ordinal scores are essentially labels, similar to nominal values; that is, an ordinal value does not represent quantity, but only relative *position* within a distribution. For example, manual muscle test grades have no arithmetic meaning. No matter how one chooses to label categories, the ranks do not change. Any scheme can be used to assign values, as long as the numbers get bigger with successive categories. Therefore, we know a manual muscle test grade of 4 is greater than 2, but it does not mean twice as much strength. We know that the distance from 2 to 3 is not equal to the distance from 3 to 4, even within one individual. This means that the difference between two ordinal scores will be difficult to interpret.

This concern is relevant to the use of ordinal scales in clinical evaluation, especially those that incorporate a sum. For instance, the Functional Independence Measure (FIM) uses the sum of 18 items, each scored 1-7, to reflect the degree of assistance needed in functional tasks.[6] The Oswestry Low Back Pain Disability Questionnaire is scored as the total of 10 items, each scored on 0–5 scale, with higher scores representing greater disability.[7] The sums are used to describe a patient's functional level, but their interpretation for research purposes must acknowledge that these numbers are not true quantities, and therefore, have no coherent meaning.[8] Therefore, ordinal scores are generally considered appropriate for descriptive analysis only. Although ordinal numbers can be subjected to arithmetic operations, such as calculating an average rank for a group of subjects or subtracting to document change over time, such scores are not meaningful as true quantities. Issues related to interpreting ordinal scores are discussed further in Chapter 6 (see also the Commentary in this chapter).

Interval Scale

An **interval scale** possesses the rank-order characteristics of an ordinal scale, but also demonstrates known and equal distances or intervals between the units of measurement. Therefore, relative difference and equivalence within a scale can be determined. What is not supplied by an interval scale is the absolute magnitude of an attribute because interval measures are not related to a true zero (similar to an ordinal scale without a natural origin). This means that negative values may represent lesser amounts of an attribute. Thus, the standard numbering of calendar years (B.C. and A.D.) is an interval scale. The year 1 was an arbitrary historical designation, not the beginning of time. Measures of temperature using Fahrenheit and Celsius scales are also at the interval level. Both have artificial zero points that do not represent a total absence of heat and can indicate temperature in negative degrees. Within each temperature scale we can identify that the numerical difference between 10° and 20° is equal to the numerical difference between 70° and 80° (in each case 10°); however, these differences are based on the numerical values on the scale, not on the true nature of the variable itself. Therefore, the actual difference in amount of heat or molecular motion generated between 10° and 20° is not necessarily the same as the difference between 70° and 80°.

Because of the nature of the interval scale, we must consider the practical implications for interpreting measured differences. Interval values can be added and subtracted, but these operations cannot be used to interpret actual quantities. The interval scale of temperature best illustrates this point, as shown in Figure 4.2. We know that the freezing point on the Celsius scale is 0°, while on the Fahrenheit scale it is 32°. This is so because the zero point on each scale is arbitrary. A temperature of 50° Fahrenheit corresponds to 10° Celsius. Therefore, while each scale maintains the integrity of its intervals, measurement of the same quantities will yield different scores. Although the relative position of each quantity is the same, the actual values of each measurement are quite different. Therefore, it is not reasonable to develop a ratio based on interval data because the numbers cannot be logically measured against true zero.

Because the actual values within any two interval scales are not equivalent, one interval scale cannot be directly transformed to another. For instance, the designation

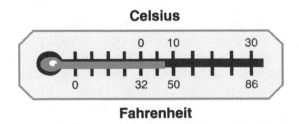

FIGURE 4.2   Temperature as an interval scale, showing quantities expressed with two different zero points on Celsius and Fahrenheit scales.

of 100 °C cannot be compared with 100 °F; however, because the actual values are irrelevant, it is the ordinal positions of points or the equality of intervals that must be maintained in any mathematical operation. Therefore, we can transform scales by multiplying or adding a constant, which will not change the relative position of any single value within the scale. After the transformation is made, intervals separating units will be in the same proportion as they were in the original scale. This is classically illustrated by the transformation of Fahrenheit to Celsius by subtracting 32 and multiplying by 5/9.

Ratio Scale

The highest level of measurement is achieved by the **ratio scale**, which is an interval scale with an absolute zero point that has empirical, rather than arbitrary, meaning. A score of zero at the ratio level represents a total absence of whatever property is being measured. Therefore, negative values are not possible. Range of motion, height, weight and force are all examples of ratio scales. Although a zero on such scales is actually theoretical (it could not be measured), it is nonetheless unambiguous. Numbers on this scale reflect actual amounts of the variable being measured. It makes sense, then, to say that one person is twice as heavy as another, or that one is half as tall as another. Ratio data can also be directly transformed from one scale to another, so that 1 in. = 2.54 cm, and 1 pound = 2.2 kg. All mathematical and statistical operations are permissible with ratio level data.

Identifying Measurement Scales

As shown in Figure 4.1, the four scales of measurement constitute a hierarchy based on the relative precision of assigned values, with nominal measurement at the bottom and ratio measurement at the top. Although most variables will be optimally measured at one level of measurement, it is always possible to operationally define a variable at lower levels. Suppose we were interested in measuring step length in a sample of four children. We could use a tape measure with graduated centimeter markings to measure the distance from heelstrike to heelstrike. This would constitute a ratio scale because we have a true zero point on a centimeter scale and clearly equal intervals. Our measurements would allow us to determine the actual length of each child's step, as well as which children took longer steps than others. Hypothetical data for such measures are presented in Table 4.1.

TABLE 4.1   **HYPOTHETICAL DATA FOR STEP LENGTH MEASURED ON DIFFERENT SCALES**

Subject	Ratio Measure	Interval Measure	Ordinal Measure	Nominal Measure
A	23	4	2	Long
B	24	5	3	Long
C	19	0	1	Short
D	28	9	4	Long

We could convert these ratio measures to an interval scale by arbitrarily assigning a score of zero to the lowest value and adjusting the intervals accordingly. We would still know which children took longer steps, and we would have a relative idea of how much longer they were, but we would no longer know what the actual step length was. We would also no longer be able to determine that Subject D takes a step 1.5 times as great as Subject C. In fact, using interval data, it erroneously appears as if Subject D takes a step 9 times the length of Subject C.

An ordinal measure can be achieved by simply ranking the children's step lengths. With this scale we no longer have any indication of the magnitude of the differences. On the basis of ordinal data we could not establish that Subjects A and B were more alike than any others. We can eventually reduce our measurement to a nominal scale by setting criteria for "long" versus "short" steps and classifying each child accordingly. With this measurement we have no way of distinguishing any differences in performance between Subjects A, B and D.

Clearly, we have lost significant amounts of information with each successive reduction in scale. It will always be to the researcher's advantage, therefore, to achieve the highest possible level of measurement. Data can always be manipulated to use a lower scale, but not vice versa. In reality, clinical researchers usually have access to a limited variety of measurement tools, and the choice is often dictated by the instrumentation available and the therapist's preference or skill. We have measured step length using four different scales, although the true nature of the variable remains unchanged. Therefore, we must distinguish between the underlying nature of a variable and the scale used to measure it.

COMMENTARY

Do I Really Care about the Level of Measurement?

Identifying the level of measurement for a particular variable is not always as simple as it seems. The underlying properties of many behavioral variables do not fit neatly into one scale or another.[9] Consider the use of a visual analog scale to evaluate the intensity of pain. A patient makes a mark along a 10 cm line to indicate his level of pain, on a continuum from "no pain" to "pain as bad as it could be." The mark can be measured in precise millimeters from the left anchor. When the patient makes a second mark, however, to show a change in pain level, can we interpret the distance on a ratio scale, or does it actually represent a ranked or ordinal measurement? Is the patient able to equate the exact difference in millimeters with his change in pain? How different is this from asking the patient to rate his level of pain on an ordinal scale of 1–10? Researchers have shown that these questions are not simple, and can be affected by many factors, such as instructions given to subjects, the length of the line and the words used at the anchors.[10–12] These considerations bear out the multidimensional influences on measurement properties.

An understanding of the scales of measurement is more than an academic exercise. The importance of determining the measurement scale for a variable lies in the determination of which mathematical operations are appropriate and which inter-

of 100 °C cannot be compared with 100 °F; however, because the actual values are irrelevant, it is the ordinal positions of points or the equality of intervals that must be maintained in any mathematical operation. Therefore, we can transform scales by multiplying or adding a constant, which will not change the relative position of any single value within the scale. After the transformation is made, intervals separating units will be in the same proportion as they were in the original scale. This is classically illustrated by the transformation of Fahrenheit to Celsius by subtracting 32 and multiplying by 5/9.

Ratio Scale

The highest level of measurement is achieved by the **ratio scale**, which is an interval scale with an absolute zero point that has empirical, rather than arbitrary, meaning. A score of zero at the ratio level represents a total absence of whatever property is being measured. Therefore, negative values are not possible. Range of motion, height, weight and force are all examples of ratio scales. Although a zero on such scales is actually theoretical (it could not be measured), it is nonetheless unambiguous. Numbers on this scale reflect actual amounts of the variable being measured. It makes sense, then, to say that one person is twice as heavy as another, or that one is half as tall as another. Ratio data can also be directly transformed from one scale to another, so that 1 in. = 2.54 cm, and 1 pound = 2.2 kg. All mathematical and statistical operations are permissible with ratio level data.

Identifying Measurement Scales

As shown in Figure 4.1, the four scales of measurement constitute a hierarchy based on the relative precision of assigned values, with nominal measurement at the bottom and ratio measurement at the top. Although most variables will be optimally measured at one level of measurement, it is always possible to operationally define a variable at lower levels. Suppose we were interested in measuring step length in a sample of four children. We could use a tape measure with graduated centimeter markings to measure the distance from heelstrike to heelstrike. This would constitute a ratio scale because we have a true zero point on a centimeter scale and clearly equal intervals. Our measurements would allow us to determine the actual length of each child's step, as well as which children took longer steps than others. Hypothetical data for such measures are presented in Table 4.1.

TABLE 4.1   HYPOTHETICAL DATA FOR STEP LENGTH MEASURED ON DIFFERENT SCALES

Subject	Ratio Measure	Interval Measure	Ordinal Measure	Nominal Measure
A	23	4	2	Long
B	24	5	3	Long
C	19	0	1	Short
D	28	9	4	Long

14. Wang ST, Yu ML, Wang CJ, Huang CC. Bridging the gap between the pros and cons in treating ordinal scales as interval scales from an analysis point of view. *Nurs Res* 1999;48:226–229.
15. Cohen ME. Analysis of ordinal dental data: Evaluation of conflicting recommendations. *J Dent Res* 2001;80:309–313.
16. Gaito J. Measurement scales and statistics: Resurgence of an old misconception. *Psychol Bull* 1980;87:564–567.
17. Velleman PF, Wilkinson L. Nominal, ordinal, interval and ratio typologies are misleading. *Am Statistician* 1993;47:65–72.
18. Kerlinger FN. *Foundations of Behavioral Research* (3rd ed.). New York: Holt, Rinehart & Winston, 1985.
19. White LJ, Velozo CA. The use of Rasch measurement to improve the Oswestry classification scheme. *Arch Phys Med Rehabil* 2002;83:822–831.
20. Decruynaere C, Thonnard JL, Plaghki L. Measure of experimental pain using Rasch analysis. *Eur J Pain* 2007;11:469–474.
21. Jacobusse G, van Buuren S, Verkerk PH. An interval scale for development of children aged 0–2 years. *Stat Med* 2006;25:2272–2283.
22. Wright BD, Linacre JM. Observations are always ordinal; measurements, however, must be interval. *Arch Phys Med Rehabil* 1989;70:857–860.
23. Wright BD, Linacre JM, Smith RM, Heinemann AW, Granger CV. FIM measurement properties and Rasch model details. *Scand J Rehabil Med* 1997;29:267–272.
24. Andres PL, Skerry LM, Thornell B, Portney LG, Finison LJ, Munsat TL. A comparison of three measures of disease progression in ALS. *J Neurol Sci* 1996;139 Suppl:64–70.
25. Stevens SS. On the theory of scales of measurement. *Science* 1946;103:677–680.
26. Lord FM. On the statistical treatment of football numbers. *Am Psychol* 1953;8:750–751.
27. Rothstein JM, Echternach JL. *Primer on Measurement: An Introductory Guide to Measurement Issues*. Alexandria, VA: American Physical Therapy Association, 1993.

CHAPTER 5

Reliability of Measurements

The usefulness of measurement in clinical research and decision making depends on the extent to which clinicians can rely on data as accurate and meaningful indicators of a behavior or attribute. The first prerequisite, at the heart of measurement, is **reliability,** or the extent to which a measurement is consistent and free from error. Reliability can be conceptualized as reproducibility or dependability. If a patient's behavior is reliable, we can expect consistent responses under given conditions. A reliable examiner is one who will be able to measure repeated outcomes with consistent scores. Similarly, a reliable instrument is one that will perform with predictable consistency under set conditions. Reliability is fundamental to all aspects of measurement, because without it we cannot have confidence in the data we collect, nor can we draw rational conclusions from those data.

The second prerequisite is **validity**, which assures that a test is measuring what it is intended to measure. Validity is necessary for drawing inferences from data, and determining how the results of a test can be used. Both reliability and validity are essential considerations as we explore ways in which measurement is used in both clinical practice and research. We will address issues of validity in depth in the next chapter.

The purpose of this chapter is to present the conceptual basis of reliability and to describe different approaches for testing the reliability of clinical measurements. Statistical procedures for reliability testing are presented in Chapter 26.

MEASUREMENT ERROR

The nature of reality is such that measurements are rarely perfectly reliable. All instruments are fallible to some extent, and all humans respond with some inconsistency. Consider the simple process of measuring an individual's height with a tape measure. If measurements are taken on three separate occasions, either by one tester or three different testers, we can expect to find some differences in results from trial to trial, even when the individual's true height has not changed. If we assume all the measurements were made using the same exact procedures and with equal concern for accuracy, then we cannot determine which, if any, of these three values is a true representation of the subject's height, that is, we do not know how much error is included in these measurements.

Theoretically, then, it is reasonable to look at any *observed score* (*X*) as a function of two components: a *true score* (*T*) and an *error component* (*E*). This relationship is summarized by the equation

$$X = T \pm E \tag{5.1}$$

This expression suggests that for any given measurement (*X*), a hypothetically true or fixed value exists (*T*), from which the observed score will differ by some unknown amount (*E*). The true component is the score the subject would have gotten had the measurement been taken by a perfect measuring instrument under ideal conditions. The difference between the true value and the observed value is **measurement error**, or "noise" that gets in the way of our finding the true score. For example, if we measure a height of 65 in., when the true height is 65.5 in., our assessment will be too short; that is, our measurement error is –0.5 in. On a second assessment, if we measure 66 in., our measurement error will be +0.5 in. In reality, we cannot calculate these error components because we do not know what the true score really is. Therefore, we must come up with some way of *estimating* how much of our measurement is attributable to error and how much represents an accurate reading. That estimate is reliability.

Systematic and Random Error

To understand reliability, we must distinguish between two types of measurement errors. **Systematic errors** are predictable errors of measurement. They occur in one direction, consistently overestimating or underestimating the true score. Such error is constant and biased. Therefore, if a systematic error is detected, it is usually a simple matter either to correct it by recalibrating the system or to adjust for it by adding or subtracting the appropriate constant. For example, if the end of a tape measure is incorrectly marked, so that markings actually begin 0.25 in. from the end, measurements of height will consistently record values that are too long by 0.25 in. We can correct this error by cutting off the extra length at the end of the tape or by subtracting 0.25 in. from all measurements. By definition, systematic errors are constant and, therefore, do not present a problem for reliability. Systematic errors are primarily a concern of validity, because, although they are consistent, test values are not true representations of the quantity being measured.

   Random errors of measurement are due to chance and can affect a subject's score in an unpredictable way from trial to trial. They are as likely to increase the observed score as to decrease it. Random errors occur from unpredictable factors such as fatigue, inattention, mechanical inaccuracy or simple mistakes. If the patient moves slightly while his height is being measured or does not stand fully erect each time measurements are taken, scores will be inconsistent. The tester might observe markings at an angle and read them incorrectly, or the tape measure might be stretched out more on one occasion than another. Reliability focuses on the degree of random error that is present within a measurement system. As random errors diminish, the observed score moves closer to the true score, and the measurement is more reliable. The assumption is made that random error is not related to the magnitude of the true score, and that if enough measurements were taken, random errors would eventually cancel each other out, making the average score a good estimate of the true score.

Sources of Measurement Error

The development or testing of a measuring instrument typically involves specification of a protocol that maximizes the reliability of the instrument; that is, procedures are detailed to ensure consistent application and scoring. In developing such a protocol, researchers have to address known or expected sources of error that could limit the reliability of the test. Once these errors are identified, they can often be controlled or eliminated to some extent. Generally, measurement errors can be attributed to three components of the measurement system: (1) the individual taking the measurements (often called the tester or *rater*), (2) the measuring instrument and (3) variability of the characteristic being measured. Many sources of error can be minimized through careful planning, training, clear operational definitions and inspection of equipment. Therefore, a testing protocol should thoroughly describe the method of measurement, which must be uniformly performed across trials. Isolating and defining each element of the measure reduces the potential for error, thereby improving reliability.

Even when the anticipated sources of error are controlled, a researcher is still faced with the unpredictability of the environment and the human response as a normal and inevitable part of measurement. Many instruments, especially mechanical ones, will always be subject to some level of background noise and random fluctuation of performance. Responses of raters and subjects will be influenced by variable personal characteristics, such as motivation, cooperation, or fatigue, and environmental factors such as noise and temperature. These contributions to error may not be controllable. We assume that these factors are random and, therefore, their effect will be canceled out in the long run.

The most difficult challenge to reliability testing is faced when the response being measured is inherently unstable. For instance, if we measure blood pressure, we might expect a natural fluctuation from session to session. When a response is very unstable, no one measurement can be considered an accurate representation of it, and it is virtually impossible to estimate the reliability of the instrument used to measure it. It is important, therefore, for researchers to understand the theoretical and practical nature of response variables, so that sources of error in reliability testing can be interpreted properly.

Regression toward the Mean

When we examine the effect of measurement error on reliability, we must also consider the extremeness of observed scores; that is, very high scores may reflect substantial positive error, and very low scores may reflect substantial negative error. Cook and Campbell[1] use the example of students taking academic exams to illustrate this concept. Everyone has, at one time or another, done worse than they expected on a test, with any number of possible "excuses," such as getting a poor night's sleep, being distracted, or accidentally marking the wrong space on the answer sheet. If we think of these factors as random sources of error, then the low grade is not an accurate assessment of the student's knowledge or ability; that is, the student's true score is confounded by negative error. On a subsequent test this student's grade is likely to be higher because, all things being equal, these negative "errors" would probably not be operating to the same extent. Conversely, if a student obtained an unusually high score on the first test, we might suspect that favorable conditions were operating (positive error), such as several good guesses on questions for which the student did not really know the answer. On a second test, this student is just as likely to score lower, because these favorable conditions would not necessarily exist.

This phenomenon is called **regression toward the mean**. It means that extreme scores on a pretest are expected to move closer, or regress, toward the group average (the mean) on a second test; that is, the error component of an extreme pretest score is likely to be less extreme on a posttest (see Figure 5.1). Therefore, using our student example, higher test scores will decrease and lower test scores will increase, moving closer to the class average—even though the students' actual degree of knowledge does not change. The reliability of the test will have an impact on the extent to which this effect will be present. As a more reliable score contains less error, a reliable test should produce a score close to the true score. Therefore, there is less chance for regression to occur. If the tests are not reliable, the error component within each test will be large, and therefore, the chances of observing a regression effect are considerably higher.

Regression toward the mean is potentially most serious in situations where subjects are specifically assigned to groups on the basis of their extreme scores (see Box 5.1). For instance, we might be interested in the differential effect of a particular teaching technique on different levels of students. Suppose we give a class a pretest to determine their initial ability and find that the average score is 80. Then we distinguish two experimental groups on the basis of these pretest scores, one composed of those scoring above 90 and the other of those scoring below 70. According to regression theory, we would expect to see both groups respond with scores closer to 80 (the total group mean)

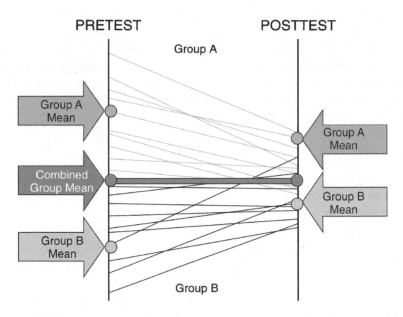

FIGURE 5.1   Illustration of regression toward the mean. Each line represents an individual's score from pretest to posttest. Test scores have tended to decrease on the posttest for Group A, and increase for Group B, both coming closer to the original group mean. If we treated these groups differently, and then compared their posttests, we could not be sure if the intervention made a difference, as we could expect to see these changes just by chance.

BOX 5.1 **The Regression Fallacy**

The impact of regression toward the mean can be illustrated by a practical example of standardized testing. The Commonwealth of Massachusetts has implemented a statewide mandatory student testing program, called the

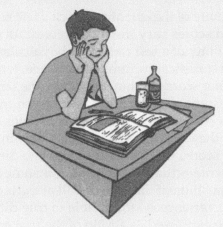

Massachusetts Comprehensive Assessment System (MCAS). Students in the 4th, 8th and 10th grades are tested and must eventually pass the exam to graduate high school. School districts are being evaluated based on average student MCAS scores. In 1998 districts were ranked in one of six categories from very high to critically low, based on their MCAS ratings. The next year, schools were given improvement targets based on these 1998 scores. The schools in the highest categories were expected to increase scores by 1 to 2 points, while schools in the lowest categories were expected to improve by 4 to 7 points.

Results for 1999 and 2000 indicated that many lower ranked schools had indeed met or exceeded their goals. However, many higher ranking schools failed to meet their target scores, even those with higher SAT scores and one high school with 18 National Merit Scholars! The interpretation, of course, was that the weaker schools had improved while the stronger schools did not. As expected, some superintendents were boastful, and others were irate.

These findings prompted much controversy among educators and statisticians, given the extensive funding and efforts attached to the standardized tests, and rewards for school districts based on their scores. Many have argued that these results are a case of regression toward the mean: Those who started at a higher point were likely to decrease their scores, and those who started at a lower point were likely to improve—just by chance! Therefore, drawing conclusions about the success or failure of teachers and students based on these numbers is likely an example of the "regression fallacy."

Source: A Vaishnav. Some top-scoring schools faulted. Many question MCAS assessment. *Boston Globe,* January 10, 2001.

on a second test, even if the teaching technique had no effect. The effect can be minimized, however, if we can improve the reliability of the test as a measure of the students' ability.

RELIABILITY COEFFICIENTS

Reliability can be conceptually defined as an estimate of the extent to which a test score is free from error; that is, to what extent observed scores vary from true scores. As it is not possible to know the true score, the true reliability of a test can never be calculated; however, we can estimate reliability based on the statistical concept of **variance**, which is a measure of the variability or differences among scores within a sample. The larger the variance, the greater the dispersion of scores; the smaller the variance, the more homogeneous the scores. If we were to measure a patient's blood pressure 10 times, we do not expect the scores to be identical; that is, they will exhibit a certain amount of variance. Some of this total variance in observed scores will be the result of true differences among the scores (the patient's blood pressure actually changed), and some can be attributed to random sources of error, such as position of the arm or skill of the tester. Reliability is a measure of how much of this total variance is attributable to true differences between scores. Therefore, reliability can be expressed as a ratio of the true score variance to the total variance, or

$$\frac{\text{True score variance}}{\text{True score variance} + \text{Error variance}} = \frac{T}{T + E} \tag{5.2}$$

This ratio yields a value called the **reliability coefficient**. From this ratio, we can see that reliability increases as the observed score approaches the true score ($T + E \Rightarrow T$). With maximum reliability (zero error), this ratio will produce a coefficient of 1.00; that is, the observed score *is* the true score. As error increases ($T + E \Rightarrow E$), the ratio approaches zero. The reliability coefficient can range between 0.00 and 1.00, with 0.00 indicating no reliability and 1.00 indicating perfect reliability. There are actually many reliability coefficients, each applied under different design conditions and with different types of data.

What Is Acceptable Reliability?

Reliability cannot be interpreted as an all-or-none condition. It is a property of a measurement system that is attained to varying degrees. Because reliability is hardly ever perfect, reliability coefficients of 1.00 are rare. Most researchers establish limits that define "acceptable" levels of reliability. Although such limits are essentially arbitrary, as a general guideline coefficients below .50 represent poor reliability, coefficients from .50 to .75 suggest moderate reliability, and values above .75 indicate good reliability. *We hasten to add, however, that these limits must be based on the precision of the measured variable and how the results of the reliability test will be applied.*

We hesitate to even suggest these guidelines, as they are often inappropriately applied as standards. They are intended only as a starting point to judge acceptable standards for any specific measurement. The level of acceptable reliability must be put in context. How much error is tolerable depends on the criteria for the measurement.

For instance, we generally accept a 5 degree error for goniometric measurements. But does it matter if we are assessing range of motion of the shoulder or the distal phalanx of the finger? If we performed a 6 minute walk test, how precise must we be in measuring distance walked? If we were off by 6 inches, would that change how we used that value? But what if we were measuring leg length? A difference of millimeters could change how we manage the patient. When is it okay to be "close enough"? Wainner[2] uses the examples of a baseball pitch in the strike zone, or a field goal in football passing through the uprights. A certain margin of error is built into the criteria for success. How this translates into acceptable clinical measurement is not so obvious.

Researchers may be able to tolerate lower reliability for measurements that are used for description, whereas those used for decision making or diagnosis need to be higher, perhaps at least .90 to ensure valid interpretations of findings. When only one form of measurement exists for a particular variable, researchers are often faced with the choice of using a less reliable test or no test at all. The validity of the test will also make a difference (see Chapters 6 and 27), especially when using measurement for diagnosis. For some purposes, even a test with moderate reliability can add sufficient information to justify its use, especially when used in conjunction with other tests. "Acceptable reliability" is a judgment call by the researcher or clinician who understands the nature of the measured variable and whether the measurements are precise enough to be used meaningfully. In a reliability study, it is the researcher's obligation to justify the level of acceptable reliability based on the purpose of the measurement.

Correlation and Agreement

Many reliability coefficients are based on measures of correlation. Although we discuss the concept of correlation in detail in Chapter 23, it is necessary to provide a brief introduction here, to understand how reliability coefficients can be interpreted. **Correlation** reflects the degree of *association* between two sets of data, or the consistency of position within the two distributions. For example, if we were to measure height and shoe size on a sample of adult men, we would probably find a correlation between the two variables; that is, those with bigger feet tend to be taller, and those with smaller feet tend to be shorter.

Reliability can be interpreted in a similar way. For instance, if we measured height on two separate occasions, we would expect that the tallest man on Test 1 would also be the tallest on Test 2; the shortest man on Test 1 would also be measured as the shortest on Test 2. If the relative position of each subject remains the same from test to test, we would obtain a high measure of correlation. We assume that any variations in observed measurements are due to random error. If systematic errors occur, the correlation would be unaffected because each subject's relative position will not change. This means that systematic errors of measurement will not have any effect on the size of the reliability coefficient.

Consider the two sets of scores shown in Figure 5.2. In both sets the scores are *directly proportional* for X and Y; hence, their relationship is depicted on a straight line. The relative positions of the scores are also consistent; that is, the highest score in X is paired with the highest score in Y, and so on. The scores in graph A also show direct **agreement** for each pair of scores. This is not the case in graph B, where all pairs

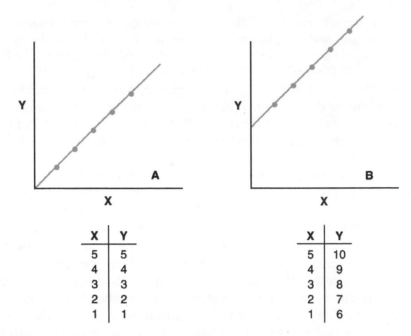

X	Y
5	5
4	4
3	3
2	2
1	1

X	Y
5	10
4	9
3	8
2	7
1	6

FIGURE 5.2   Examples of the association between X and Y in two sets of scores. In **A** the graph shows a *line of identity,* where each measure on X and Y is equal, resulting in perfect correlation as well as agreement, indicating excellent reliability. In **B** there is still perfect correlation, but no agreement, illustrating poor reliability.

disagree. But both graphs show perfect correlation. Therefore, while correlation tells us how the scores vary together, it cannot tell us the extent of agreement between the two sets of measurements. For most research and clinical applications, however, the essence of reliability is agreement between the two tests; that is, we want to know that the actual values obtained by two measurements are the same, not just proportional to each other. For example, range of motion measurements are used to evaluate joint dysfunction on the basis of actual, not relative, limitations. We need to know the true value of the limitation, not just that one patient is more limited than another. It would not be enough to know that repeated measurements were proportionally consistent; it would be necessary to establish that repeated tests resulted in the same angular measurements. Therefore, the correlation coefficient is not effective as a measure of reliability. Because of this, statistical approaches to reliability testing should include estimates of agreement that can be used in conjunction with correlation.

TYPES OF RELIABILITY

Estimates of reliability vary depending on the type of reliability being analyzed. We discuss four general approaches to reliability testing: test–retest reliability, rater reliability, alternate forms reliability, and internal consistency. For each approach we will identify the most commonly used reliability coefficients. These statistical indices are described in detail in Chapter 26.

Test–Retest Reliability

One basic premise of reliability is the stability of the measuring instrument; that is, a reliable instrument will obtain the same results with repeated administrations of the test. **Test–retest reliability** assessment is used to establish that an instrument is capable of measuring a variable with consistency. In a test–retest study, one sample of individuals is subjected to the identical test on two separate occasions, keeping all testing conditions as constant as possible. The coefficient derived from this type of analysis is called a *test–retest reliability coefficient*. This estimate can be obtained for a variety of testing tools, and is generally indicative of reliability in situations where raters are not involved, such as self-report survey instruments and physical and physiological measures with mechanical or digital readouts. If the test is reliable, the subject's score should be similar on multiple trials. In terms of reliability theory, the extent to which the scores vary is interpreted as measurement error.

Because variation in measurement must be considered within the context of the total measurement system, errors may actually be attributed to many sources. Therefore, to assess the reliability of an instrument, the researcher must be able to assume stability in the response variable. Unfortunately, many variables *do* change over time. For example, a patient's self-assessment of pain may change between two testing sessions. We must also consider the inconsistency with which many clinical variables naturally respond over time. When responses are labile, test–retest reliability may be impossible to assess.

Test–Retest Intervals

Because the stability of a response variable is such a significant factor, the time interval between tests must be considered carefully. Intervals should be far enough apart to avoid fatigue, learning, or memory effects, but close enough to avoid genuine changes in the measured variable. The primary criteria for choosing an appropriate interval are the stability of the response variable and the test's intended purpose. For example, if we were interested in the reproducibility of electromyographic measurements, it might be reasonable to test the patient on two occasions within one week. Range of motion measurements can often be repeated within one day or even within a single session. Measures of infant development might need to be taken over a short period, to avoid the natural changes that rapidly occur at early ages. If, however, we are interested in establishing the ability of an IQ test to provide a stable assessment of intelligence over time, it might be more meaningful to test a child using intervals of one year. The researcher must be able to justify the stability of the response variable to interpret test–retest comparisons.

Carryover and Testing Effects

With two or more measures, reliability can be influenced by the effect of the first test on the outcome of the second test. For example, practice or carryover effects can occur with repeated measurements, changing performance on subsequent trials. A test of dexterity may improve because of motor learning. Strength measurements can improve following warm-up trials. Sometimes subjects are given a series of pretest trials to neutralize this effect, and data are collected only after performance has stabilized. A retest score can also be influenced by a subject's effort to improve on the first score. This is especially relevant for variables such as strength, where motivation plays an important role. Researchers may not let subjects know their first score to control for this effect.

It is also possible for the characteristic being measured to be changed by the first test. A strength test might cause pain in the involved joint and alter responses on the second trial. Range of motion testing can stretch soft tissue structures around a joint, increasing the arc of motion on subsequent testing. When the test itself is responsible for observed changes in a measured variable, the change is considered a **testing effect**. Oftentimes, such effects will be manifested as systematic error, creating consistent changes across all subjects. Such an effect will not necessarily affect reliability coefficients, for reasons we have already discussed.

Reliability Coefficients for Test–Retest Reliability

Test–retest reliability has traditionally been analyzed using the Pearson product-moment coefficient of correlation (for interval-ratio data) or the Spearman rho (for ordinal data). As correlation coefficients, however, they are limited as estimates of reliability. The intraclass correlation coefficient (ICC) has become the preferred index, as it reflects both correlation and agreement. With nominal data, percent agreement can be determined and the kappa statistic applied. In situations where the stability of a response is questioned, the standard error of measurement (SEM) can be applied.

Rater Reliability

Many clinical measurements require that a human observer, or *rater*, be part of the measurement system. In some cases, the rater is the actual measuring instrument, such as in a manual muscle test or joint mobility assessment. In other situations, the rater must observe performance and apply operational criteria to subjective observations, as in a gait analysis or functional assessment. Sometimes a test necessitates the physical application of a tool, and the rater becomes part of the instrument, as in the use of a goniometer or taking of blood pressure. Raters may also be required simply to read or interpret the output from another instrument, such as an electromyogram, or force recordings on a dynamometer. However the measurements are taken, the individual performing the ratings must be consistent in the application of criteria for scoring responses.

This aspect of reliability is of major importance to the validity of any research study involving testers, whether one individual does all the testing or several testers are involved. Data cannot be interpreted with confidence unless those who collect, record and reduce the data are reliable. In many studies, raters undergo a period of training, so that techniques are standardized. This is especially important when measuring devices are new or unfamiliar, or when subjective observations are used. Even when raters are experienced, however, rater reliability should be documented as part of the research protocol.

To establish rater reliability the instrument and the response variable are considered stable, so that any differences between scores are attributed to rater error. In many situations, this may be a large assumption, and the researcher must understand the nature of the test variables and the instrumentation to establish that the rater is the true source of observed error.

Intrarater Reliability

Intrarater reliability refers to the stability of data recorded by one individual across two or more trials. When carryover or practice effects are not an issue, intrarater reliability is usually assessed using trials that follow each other with short intervals. Reliability is best established with multiple trials (more than two), although the number of trials needed is dependent on the expected variability in the response. In a test–retest situation, when a rater's skill is relevant to the accuracy of the test, intrarater reliability and test–retest reliability are essentially the same estimate. The effects of rater and the test cannot be separated out.

Researchers may assume that intrarater reliability is achieved simply by having one experienced individual perform all measurements; however, the objective nature of scientific inquiry demands that even under expert conditions, rater reliability should be evaluated. Expertise by clinical standards may not always match the level of precision needed for research documentation. By establishing statistical reliability, those who critique research cannot question the measurement accuracy of data, and research conclusions will be strengthened.

Rater Bias. We must also consider the possibility for bias when one rater takes two measurements. Raters can be influenced by their memory of the first score. This is most relevant in cases where human observers use subjective criteria to rate responses, but can operate in any situation where a tester must read a score from an instrument. The most effective way to control for this type of error is to blind the tester in some way, so that the first score remains unknown until after the second trial is completed; however, as most clinical measurements are observational, such a technique is often unreasonable. For instance, we could not blind a clinician to measures of balance, function, muscle testing or gait where the tester is an integral part of the measurement system. The major protections against tester bias are to develop grading criteria that are as objective as possible, to train the testers in the use of the instrument, and to document reliability across raters.

Interrater Reliability

Interrater reliability concerns variation between two or more raters who measure the same group of subjects. Even with detailed operational definitions and equal skill, different raters are not always in agreement about the quality or quantity of the variable being assessed. Intrarater reliability should be established for each individual rater before comparing raters to each other.

Interrater reliability is best assessed when all raters are able to measure a response during a single trial, where they can observe a subject simultaneously and independently. This eliminates true differences in scores as a source of measurement error when comparing raters' scores. Videotapes of patients performing activities have proved useful for allowing multiple raters to observe the exact same performance.[3-5] Simultaneous scoring is not possible, however, for many variables that require interaction of the tester and subject. For example, range of motion and manual muscle testing could not be tested simultaneously by two clinicians. With these types of measures, rater reliability may be affected if the true response changes from trial to trial. For instance, actual range of motion may change if the joint tissues are stretched from the first trial. Muscle force can decrease if the muscle is fatigued from the first trial.

Researchers will often decide to use one rater in a study, to avoid the necessity of establishing interrater reliability. Although this is useful for attempting consistency within the study, it does not strengthen the generalizability of the research outcomes. If interrater reliability of measurement has not been established, we cannot assume that other raters would have obtained similar results. This, in turn, limits the application of the findings to other people and situations. Interrater reliability allows the researcher to assume that the measurements obtained by one rater are likely to be representative of the subject's true score, and therefore, the results can be interpreted and applied with greater confidence.

Reliability Coefficients for Rater Reliability

The intraclass correlation coefficient (ICC) should be used to evaluate rater reliability. For interrater reliability, ICC model 2 or 3 can be used, depending on whether the raters are representative of other similar raters (model 2) or no generalization is intended (model 3). For intrarater reliability, model 3 should be used (see Chapter 26).

Alternate Forms

Many measuring instruments exist in two or more versions, called equivalent, parallel or alternate forms. Interchange of these alternate forms can be supported only by establishing their parallel reliability. **Alternate forms reliability** testing is often used as an alternative to test-retest reliability with paper-and-pencil tests, when the nature of the test is such that subjects are likely to recall their responses to test items. For example, we are all familiar with standardized tests such as the Scholastic Aptitude Test (SAT) and the Graduate Record Examination (GRE), professional licensing exams or intelligence tests, which are given several times a year, each time in a different form. These different versions of the tests are considered reliable alternatives based on their statistical equivalence. This type of reliability is established by administering two alternate forms of a test to the same group, usually in one sitting, and correlating paired observations. Because the tests are ostensibly different, they can be given at relatively the same time without fear of bias from one to the other. Although the idea of alternate forms has been applied mostly to educational and psychological testing, there are many examples in clinical practice. For example, clinicians use parallel forms of gait evaluations, tests of motor development, strength tests, functional evaluations, and range of motion tests. Many of these have not been tested for alternate forms reliability.

The importance of testing alternate forms reliability has been illustrated in studies of hand dynamometers. Several models are available, each with slightly different design features. Because these tools are often used to take serial measurements, patients might appear to be stronger or weaker simply because of error if different instruments were used. Studies comparing various models have shown that some instruments generate significantly different strength scores,[6] while others have shown comparable values.[7] Establishing this method comparison is necessary if absolute values are to be compared or equated across tests, and to generalize findings from one study to another or from research to practice.

Reliability Coefficients for Alternate Forms Reliability

Correlation coefficients have been used most often to examine alternative forms reliability. The determination of *limits of agreement* has been proposed as a useful estimate of the range of error expected when using two different versions of an instrument. This estimate is based on the standard deviation of difference scores between the two instruments (see Chapter 26).

Internal Consistency

Software instruments, such as questionnaires, written examinations and interviews are ideally composed of a set of questions or items designed to measure particular knowledge or attributes. **Internal consistency,** or **homogeneity,** reflects the extent to which items measure various aspects of the same characteristic and nothing else. For example, if a professor gives an exam to assess students' knowledge of research design, the items should reflect a summary of that knowledge; the test should not include items on anthropology or health policy. If we assess a patient's ability to perform daily tasks using a physical function scale, then the items on the scale should relate to aspects of physical function only. If some items evaluated psychological or social characteristics, then the items would not be considered homogeneous. The scale should, therefore, be grounded in theory that defines the dimension of physical function, thereby distinguishing it from other dimensions of function.

The most common approach to testing internal consistency involves looking at the correlation among all items in a scale. For most instruments, it is desirable to see some relationship among items, to reflect measurement of the same attribute, especially if the scale score is summed. Therefore, for inventories that are intended to be multidimensional, researchers generally establish subscales that are homogenous on a particular trait (even though items are often mixed when the test is administered). For example, the Short-Form 36-item (SF-36) health status measure is composed of eight subscales, including physical function, limitations in physical role, pain, social function, mental health, limitations in emotional role, vitality and general health perception.[8] Each of these subscales has been evaluated separately for internal consistency.[9]

Split-Half Reliability

If we wanted to establish the reliability of a questionnaire, it would be necessary to administer the instrument on two separate occasions, essentially a test–retest situation. Oftentimes, the interval between testing is relatively brief, to avoid the possibility for true change. Recall of responses, then, becomes a potential threat, as it might influence the second score, making it impossible to get a true assessment of reliability. One solution to this problem is the use of parallel forms, but this shifts the measure of reliability to a comparison of instruments, rather than reliability of a single instrument.

A simpler approach combines the two sets of items into one longer instrument, with half the items being redundant of the other half. One group of subjects takes the test at a single session. The items are then divided into two comparable halves for scoring, creating two separate scores for each subject. Typically, questions are divided according to odd and even items. This is considered preferable to comparing the first half of the test with the second half, as motivation, fatigue and other psychological elements can influence performance over time, especially with a long test. Reliability is then assessed by correlating results of two halves of the test. If each subject's half-test scores are highly correlated, the whole test is considered reliable. This is called **split-half reliability.** This value will generally be an underestimate of the true reliability of the scale, since the reliability is proportional to the total number of items in the scale. Therefore, because the subscales are each half the length of the full test, the reliability coefficient is too low.

The obvious problem with the split-half approach is the need to determine that the two halves of the test are actually measuring the same thing. In essence, the two halves can be considered alternate forms of the same test; however, the split-half method is considered superior to test–retest and alternate forms procedures because there is no time lag between tests, and the same physical, mental and environmental influences will affect the subjects as they take both sections of the test.

Reliability Coefficients for Internal Consistency

The statistic most often used for internal consistency is **Cronbach's coefficient alpha (α).**[10] This statistic can be used with items that are dichotomous or that have multiple choices.* Conceptually, coefficient α is the average of all possible split-half reliabilities for the scale. This statistic evaluates the items in a scale to determine if they are measuring the same construct or if they are redundant, suggesting which items could be discarded to improve the homogeneity of the scale. Cronbach's α will be affected by the number of items in a scale. The longer the scale, the more homogeneous it will appear, simply because there are more items.

For split-half reliability, the *Spearman-Brown prophecy* statistic is used as an estimate of the correlation of the two halves of the test.

We can also assess internal consistency by conducting an **item-to-total correlation;** that is, we can examine how each item on the test relates to the instrument as a whole. To perform an item-to-total correlation, each individual item is correlated with the total score, omitting that item from the total. If an instrument is homogeneous, we would expect these correlations to be high. With this approach it is not necessary to create a doubly long test. The *Pearson product-moment correlation coefficient* is appropriate for this analysis (see Chapter 23).

---

*When items are dichotomous, Cronbach's alpha is identical to a statistic called KR-20 (Kuder-Richardson formula 20).

GENERALIZABILITY

Measurement in clinical research or practice is never used as an end unto itself. Measurements are used as information for decision making, evaluation or prediction. The score we obtain from a test is given a meaning beyond the specific situation in which it was taken; that is, we make generalizations about performance or behavior based on measurements. In many ways, reliability provides the foundation for making such generalizations, as we must have confidence in the dependability of measurements if they are to be applied in different situations or used to make decisions for future action.

On this basis, Cronbach and his colleagues[11] introduced the idea that reliability theory should be more accurately conceptualized in terms of **generalizability theory**. They suggested that every individual score can be thought of as a sample from a universe of possible scores that might have been obtained under the same testing conditions. These specific testing conditions define the universe to which measures of reliability can be generalized. For example, we can test the grip strength of a patient with rheumatoid arthritis using a hand dynamometer. A single measured score of 15 pounds would be one of a universe of possible scores that might have been obtained under the same testing conditions, using the same dynamometer, at the same time of day, and by the same examiner. Because most research involves taking small samples of measurements, we assume that our observations are representative of this infinite distribution of possible scores. A single measurement then becomes the *best estimate* of a true score under those testing conditions. Reliability is essentially a measure of how good an estimate that measurement is.

According to classical reliability theory, an individual's observed score can be partitioned into a true component and an error component. The true score is assumed to be a fixed value that exists independently of any other conditions of measurement. Therefore, any differences between the observed score and the true score are due to random error (see Figure 5.3A). This theory also assumes that the error component is undifferentiated; that is, it comes from many different sources in an unbiased form. If we accept this premise, then we should be comfortable applying a given reliability estimate to any other situation where the same measurement is taken, because the error in each situation should be equally random.

In generalizability theory, however, the conditions of testing are not considered independent factors; that is, the true score is a function of an underlying theoretical component *only as it exists under specific conditions*. This means that not all variations from trial to trial should be attributed solely to random error. If we can identify relevant testing conditions that influence test scores, then we should be able to explain and predict more of the variance in a set of scores, effectively leaving less variance unexplained as error.

Facets of Reliability

The concept of generalizability, therefore, forces us to interpret reliability within a multidimensional context, that is, in relation to a set of specific testing conditions. Each condition that defines this context is called a **facet.** A particular combination of facets characterizes the universe to which reliability can be generalized. The researcher determines

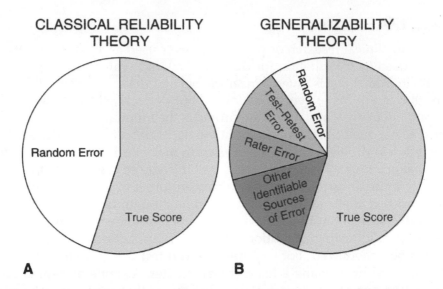

FIGURE 5.3 **A.** Circle A illustrates classical reliability theory, where the actual score is made up of the true score and unexplained random error. **B.** Circle B illustrates generalizability theory, which accounts for specific sources of error in addition to random error. These identified sources of error may be accounted for by evaluating their effects statistically.

which facets are relevant to the measurement of a particular variable. By specifying those facets of greatest relevance, it is possible to statistically determine how much of the variance in observed scores can be attributed to each facet (see Figure 5.3B).

For instance, suppose we set up a test–retest situation for goniometric measurements of elbow flexion. In one scenario, we obtain two sets of ratings taken by one rater on a sample of 10 patients. By comparing these two sets of scores, we can establish the reliability of data across two occasions. Therefore, "occasion" becomes a facet of reliability. These occasions may be trials within one session or over two separate days. How these occasions are defined determines how the results can be generalized. Similarly, if we collect data from four clinicians' ratings within a single session, we can establish the reliability of data across four raters. Therefore, "rater" becomes a facet of reliability. In this case, we would have to establish the criteria that would characterize these raters, such as their years of experience or special training. Then results can be generalized to other raters with similar training.

The concept of generalizability is a clinically useful one, especially in terms of the development and standardization of measurement tools, because it provides a frame of reference for interpretation of reliability coefficients and suggests areas of improvement of protocols. Because we cannot expect to verify the reliability of every instrument on every patient for every rater, we must be able to document those characteristics that are relevant to generalizing measurement consistency. Generalizability theory also emphasizes that reliability is not an inherent quality of an instrument, but exists only within the context in which it was tested. Accordingly, we cannot automatically assume that estimates of reliability from one study can be applied to other raters, environments, testing conditions, or types of patients, unless we specifically address these factors in our analysis. Most reliability studies look at rater as the most important single facet.

The essence of generalizability theory suggests, however, that other facets must be examined before an instrument's reliability can be fully understood.

In effect, then, there is no one coefficient that provides a complete estimate of reliability for a given test or measurement. Separate coefficients that address different facets can be obtained and applied to relevant situations. Without such documentation, it is not possible to make reasonable claims of general reliability for any instrument. Statistical and design considerations that are appropriate for generalizability studies are discussed further in Chapter 26.

Minimal Detectable Difference

Measurement error is of special interest in the assessment of change. When we take two measurements of the same variable at different times, we are usually doing so to determine if there is a difference in value, perhaps due to a specific intervention or the passage of time. When we observe a difference in the measurement, we want to assume that it represents a change in the true score—the variable really did change. But because all measurements are subject to some degree of error, the accuracy of this assumption will depend on the reliability of the measurement.

We can appreciate, then, that when we measure a difference between two scores, some portion of that change may be error, and some portion may be real. The concept of a **minimal detectable difference (MDD)** has been used to define that amount of change in a variable that must be achieved to reflect a true difference.[†] This is the smallest amount of difference that passes the threshold of error for a specific instrument and application.[12] It is the smallest amount of change an instrument can accurately measure.[‡] The greater the reliability of the measurement, the smaller the MDD. The precision and level of measurement will also affect this detectable difference.

Methodological studies that focus on an instrument's ability to measure change will report the MDD as an important characteristic of the measurement tool. By knowing the MDD, clinicians can generalize the information from such a report to their specific clinical situation. To illustrate this concept, van der Esch et al.[13] studied measurement of knee joint laxity in healthy subjects using an instrumented system. Based on test–retest measures, they determined that the MDD was 3.73 degrees, with a 95% confidence interval of 2.66–6.37. This means that we can be 95% confident that measurements outside of this range would represent true change. They also found that the mean score for knee joint laxity was approximately 6 degrees. Therefore, the researchers concluded that it would be difficult to interpret measurement of change since the observed change and the expected error were in the same range. It would not be possible to distinguish error from true joint change using their instrument. Statistical application of the MDD is discussed in Chapters 26 and 27.

[†]The minimal detectable difference (MDD) may also be called the minimal detectable change (MDC).

[‡]The minimal detectable difference (MDD) is not the same as the minimal clinically important difference (MCID), which is an estimate of the amount of change that is meaningful. Depending on the nature of the variable being measured and the use of the measurement for decision making, the MDD will typically be smaller than the MCID. See Chapter 26 for further discussion of MDD and Chapters 6 and 27 for discussion of the MCID.

Population-Specific Reliability

The concept of generalizability also emphasizes the need to consider characteristics of those involved in establishing reliability. This includes the patients or subjects being tested and the raters who do the testing. Reliability that is established on subjects from one population cannot automatically be attributed to other populations. This has been termed **population-specific reliability**. Clearly, factors such as pain, deformity, weakness, anxiety, and spasticity can alter the way a patient responds to a measurement and the consistency with which a clinician can take those measurements. Doing a manual muscle test on a patient with shoulder pain may be a different experience from doing the test on someone with limited range of motion. Range of motion measurements may be difficult to standardize among patients with joint deformities, joint pain or tenderness, or severe limitations of movement. Similarly, rater reliability must take into account the skill, experience and training of the individual performing the test. Therefore, reliability of measurement must be documented according to the characteristics of a specific group of individuals who will be part of the measurement.

PILOT TESTING

When choosing an instrument for clinical or research measurement, it would certainly make sense to use a tool for which reliability has already been demonstrated. Even then, however, there is no guarantee that the same degree of reliability will be achieved in every situation. Therefore, researchers often perform pilot studies to establish reliability prior to the start of actual data collection. This should be a routine part of the research process, especially when observational measurements are used. It allows the researcher to determine if raters are adequately trained to obtain valid measurements. It may be important to consider, however, that specific characteristics of the pilot test situation may be quite different from those that will be encountered during data collection. At the least, raters are often much more careful when they know the scores will be examined for reliability. Mitchell suggests that actual data collection should include multiple trials of each measurement, and that these trials should be assessed for reliability as part of the study's data analysis.[14] Although training and testing prior to data collection are essential for developing measurement accuracy, the validity of an experiment will be well served by documenting the error rate of measurement within the actual data used for analysis. For generalization of findings, it is probably more meaningful to report the reliability of these data than those obtained during pilot testing.

COMMENTARY

What Is the True Score?

It is hard to imagine any measurement system that is free from error. The concept of reliability is based on the premise that we can expect some deviation from the "true score" in every measurement we take. This presents an interesting dilemma when quantitative performance data are collected. If we take measures of range of motion or strength, for example, how do we determine which scores are useful for analysis? What strategies can we apply in data collection procedures to ensure the most reliable outcome? In addition to test–retest and rater reliability studies, most researchers recognize the need for taking more than one measurement of a behavior or characteristic whenever possible. But then we must ask, Out of these several trials, which value best represents the individual's true score?

Most investigators will not use the first score alone as the test value. The initial trial is often confounded by a warm-up or learning effect that will be evident as performance improves on subsequent trials. Some researchers use the final score in a series. They rationalize that the last repetition in a set of trials will be stabilized following warm-up or practice effects; however, depending on the number of trials, the final score may also be influenced by fatigue and, therefore, will not necessarily represent the subject's true effort.

A more common approach is to take the "best" score. Many researchers prefer using the subject's best effort as a reflection of what the subject is maximally capable of doing. If we consider reliability theory, however, this is not necessarily the most accurate representation because random error can contribute both positive and negative components to an observed score. Therefore, any observed score may be an overestimate or an underestimate of the true score. It is possible that the subject's maximal score in a set of two or three trials may actually be a function of positive error. Using the maximal score for data analysis may lend a positive bias to the outcome that would not be seen if the study were repeated on another sample.

Theoretically, then, the most representational score should be achieved through the mean or average score, because the sum of the error components over an infinite number of trials would be zero. Thus, the true score can be thought of as the average of the observed scores for a large number of trials, with the error components canceled out. Of course, there is room for argument in this rationale, because this theory operates in the "long run"; that is, we can expect a canceling of error components over an infinite number of trials. With only a few trials, this may be an unrealistic assumption; however, several studies have shown that taking a mean value provides a more reliable measurement than any single value in a series of trials.[15,16]

Which score should be used? There is no easy answer to this question. Researchers grapple with this decision for every study, based on the types of variables being measured and the precision those measurements achieve. It is often useful to take a series of measurements and estimate reliability using both single scores and average scores, to determine which approach provides the most reliable basis for data analysis. Generally, reliability of measurements that are less stable can be improved if averages are used. Reliability is also an important issue in statistical inference, as greater error (low reliability) will reduce the chances of finding statistically significant differences between groups. Therefore, the researcher always tries to make measurements as reliable as possible. This issue does reinforce, however, the constant need to confirm reliability as part of every study.

REFERENCES

1. Cook TD, Campbell DT. *Quasi-experimentation: Design and Analysis Issues for Field Settings.* Boston: Houghton Mifflin, 1979.
2. Wainner RS. Reliability of the clinical examination: How close is "close enough"? *J Orthop Sports Phys Ther* 2003;33:488–490.
3. Cusick A, Vasquez M, Knowles L, Wallen M. Effect of rater training on reliability of Melbourne Assessment of Unilateral Upper Limb Function scores. *Dev Med Child Neurol* 2005;47:39–45.
4. McConvey J, Bennett SE. Reliability of the Dynamic Gait Index in individuals with multiple sclerosis. *Arch Phys Med Rehabil* 2005;86:130–133.
5. Baer GD, Smith MT, Rowe PJ, Masterton L. Establishing the reliability of Mobility Milestones as an outcome measure for stroke. *Arch Phys Med Rehabil* 2003;84:977–981.
6. Flood-Joy M, Mathiowetz V. Grip strength measurement: A comparison of three Jamar dynamometers. *Occup Ther J Res* 1987;7:235–243.
7. Bohannon RW. Parallel comparison of grip strength measures obtained with a MicroFET 4 and a Jamar dynamometer. *Percept Mot Skills* 2005;100:795–798.
8. Ware JE, Sherbourne CD. The MOS 36-item Short Form Health Survey (SF-36). I. Conceptual framework and item selection. *Med Care* 1992;30:473–483.
9. McHorney CA, Ware JE, Jr., Lu JF, Sherbourne CD. The MOS 36-item Short Form Health Survey (SF-36): III. Tests of data quality, scaling assumptions, and reliability across diverse patient groups. *Med Care* 1994;32:40–66.
10. Cronbach LJ. *Essentials of Psychological Testing* (5th ed.). New York: Harper & Row, 1990.
11. Cronbach LJ, Gleser GC, Nanda H, Rajaratnam N. *The Dependability of Behavioral Measurements: Theory of Generalizability for Scores and Profiles.* New York: Wiley, 1972.
12. Beaton DE, Bombardier C, Katz JN, Wright JG, Wells G, Boers M, et al. Looking for important change/differences in studies of responsiveness. OMERACT MCID Working Group. Outcome Measures in Rheumatology. Minimal Clinically Important Difference. *J Rheumatol* 2001;28:400–405.
13. van der Esch M, Steultjens M, Ostelo RW, Harlaar J, Dekker J. Reproducibility of instrumented knee joint laxity measurement in healthy subjects. *Rheumatology (Oxford)* 2006;45:595–599.
14. Mitchell SK. Interobserver agreement, reliability, and generalizability of data collected in observational studies. *Psychol Bull* 1979;36:376–390.
15. Beattie P, Isaacson K, Riddle DL, Rothstein JM. Validity of derived measurements of leg-length differences obtained by use of a tape measure. *Phys Ther* 1990;70:150–157.
16. Mathiowetz V, Weber K, Volland G, Kashman N. Reliability and validity of grip and pinch strength evaluations. *J Hand Surg [Am]* 1984;9:222–226.

CHAPTER 6
Validity of Measurements

Measurement validity concerns the extent to which an instrument measures what it is intended to measure. Validity places an emphasis on the objectives of a test and the ability to make inferences from test scores or measurements. For instance, a goniometer is considered a valid instrument for testing range of motion because we can assess joint range from angular measurements. A ruler is considered a valid instrument for calibrating length, because we can judge how long an object is by measuring inches or centimeters. We would, however, question the validity of assessing low back pain by measuring leg length because we cannot make reasonable inferences about back pain based on that measurement.

Therefore, validity addresses what we are able to do with test results. Tests are usually devised for purposes of discrimination, evaluation, or prediction. For instance, we may ask, Is the test capable of *discriminating* among individuals with and without certain traits? Can it *evaluate* change in the magnitude or quality of a variable from one time to another? Can we make useful and accurate *predictions* or diagnoses about a patient's potential function based on the outcome of the test? These are all questions of test validity.

The determination of validity for any test instrument can be made in a variety of contexts, depending on how the instrument will be used, the type of data it will generate, and the precision of the response variables. The purpose of this chapter is to define different types of validity and to describe the application of validity testing for clinical measurements. Discussion of statistical procedures related to validity will be covered in Chapter 27.

VALIDITY AND RELIABILITY

Validity implies that a measurement is relatively free from error; that is, a valid test is also reliable. An instrument that is inconsistent cannot produce meaningful measurements. If we use a goniometer with a loose axis that alters alignment, our results will no longer be valid indicators of joint range. Random measurement error will make it difficult to determine a true reading.

An invalid test can be reliable, however. For instance, we could obtain reliable measures of leg length time after time, but those measurements would still not tell us anything about back pain. Similarly, we might be able to establish that the reliability of leg length measurements is greater than the reliability of scores on a less objective test, such as a graphic pain scale, but this fact could not be used to support the validity of leg length as a measure of back pain. In addition we must consider the effect of systematic error or bias in the recording of data. If a tape measure is incorrectly marked, so that

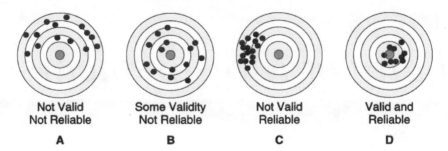

Not Valid	Some Validity	Not Valid	Valid and
Not Reliable	Not Reliable	Reliable	Reliable
A	**B**	**C**	**D**

FIGURE 6.1   Illustration of the relationship between reliability and validity, using a target analogy. The center of the target represents the true score. **A.** Scores are neither reliable nor valid, demonstrating random error. **B.** Scores are somewhat valid, demonstrating a useful average score, but not reliable **C.** Scores are quite reliable, but not valid. **D.** Scores are both reliable and valid.

readings are consistently one inch more than the actual length, we may see strong reliability, but we will not have a valid measure of length.

These examples illustrate the importance of separating out issues of reliability and validity when evaluating a test (see Fig. 6.1). Although reliability is a prerequisite to validity, this relationship is unidirectional; that is, reliability sets the limits of validity, but it is no guarantee of it. Low reliability is automatic evidence of low validity, whereas strong reliability does not automatically suggest strong validity.

VALIDITY OF INFERENCES

In Chapter 4 we discussed the indirect nature of clinical measurement. We explained that most clinical variables are assessed by taking a correlate of the actual property being measured; that is, we make inferences about the magnitude of a particular variable based on a relevant observable behavior or response. Validity is basic to establishing these inferences. We must be able to document that the values assigned to a variable are representative of that response. We can verify that a thermometer is a valid instrument for measuring temperature because mercury expands and contracts in proportion to changes in heat. A dynamometer is valid for measuring strength because the transducer responds with a signal proportional to the exerted force. Similarly, it is logical to assess the level of serum creatinine in the body as an indicator of renal disease, since the kidneys regulate the level of creatinine in the body. Unfortunately, for the measurement of more abstract variables, such as intelligence, function and perception, measurement scales are not so obviously related to the variable of interest, and validity is harder to verify.

We also draw inferences from tests that go beyond the simple values assigned to a variable. When we measure a patient's muscle strength or range of motion, it is not the muscle grade or joint angle that is of interest for its own sake, but what those values mean in terms of the integrity of the patient's musculoskeletal system. We use those values to infer something about the cause of that person's symptoms, the degree of disability, or the level of improvement following treatment. If we were told that the scores were not related to any other characteristics or future performance, we would wonder why anyone bothered to measure them.

Measurements are important, therefore, insofar as they allow us to make generalizations beyond a specific score. For example, clinical trials in Duchenne muscular dystrophy have examined the effects of various drug interventions by documenting changes in manual muscle test grades, range of motion, pulmonary function, and functional status.[1] These assessments can be considered valid for the measurement of the effectiveness of drug intervention only if we can make inferences about the state of the disease or disease progression based on their values.

Specificity of Validity

At issue here is the specificity of validity. Just like reliability, validity is not inherent to an instrument, but must be evaluated within the context of the test's intended use. The question of validity should not be: "Is an instrument valid?" It is more accurately: "How valid is it for a given purpose?" For instance, manual muscle testing, which was first developed to evaluate patterns of denervation in patients with poliomyelitis, may not be valid for use on patients who exhibit upper motor neuron involvement because grading criteria do not account for the interference of abnormal muscle tone. Similarly, an instrument designed to assess function in patients who have had a stroke may not be valid for patients with Alzheimer's disease. In another context, an instrument designed to describe the health status of a specific population may not be appropriate for assessing change in an individual's function. Therefore, validity is not a universal characteristic of an instrument.

Because measurement inferences are difficult to verify, establishing validity is not as straightforward as establishing reliability. For many variables there are no obvious rules or formulas for judging that a test is indeed measuring the critical property of interest. Like reliability, we do not think of validity in an all-or-none sense, but rather as a characteristic that an instrument has to some degree or other. It is often a source of frustration to clinical scientists that, when dealing with abstract constructs, the documentation of test validity remains ongoing.

Types of Measurement Validity

Validation procedures are based on the types of evidence that can be offered in support of a test's validity. We can think of validation as a process of hypothesis testing, determining if scores on a test are related to specific behaviors, characteristics or level of performance. Evidence to support hypotheses is generally defined according to four types of measurement validity: face validity, content validity, criterion-related validity, and construct validity (see Table 6.1).

FACE VALIDITY

The least rigorous method for documenting a test's validity is face validation. **Face validity** indicates that an instrument *appears* to test what it is supposed to and that it is a plausible method for doing so. To establish face validity, one must be clear about the

TABLE 6.1   TYPES OF MEASUREMENT VALIDITY

Face validity	Indicates that an instrument appears to test what it is supposed to; the weakest form of measurement validity.
Content validity	Indicates that the items that make up an instrument adequately sample the universe of content that defines the variable being measured. Most useful with questionnaires and inventories.
Criterion-related validity	Indicates that the outcomes of one instrument, the target test, can be used as a substitute measure for an established reference standard criterion test. Can be tested as concurrent or predictive validity.
Concurrent validity	Establishes validity when two measures are taken at relatively the same time. Most often used when the target test is considered more efficient than the gold standard and, therefore, can be used instead of the gold standard.
Predictive validity	Establishes that the outcome of the target test can be used to predict a future criterion score or outcome.
Construct validity	Establishes the ability of an instrument to measure an abstract construct and the degree to which the instrument reflects the theoretical components of the construct.

definition of the concept that is being measured. For some instruments, face validity is easily established because the instrument measures the property of interest through some form of direct observation. Therefore, face validity is generally attributed to tests of range of motion, length, strength, tactile discrimination, sensation, gait, and balance. The separate items on a functional status scale, such as eating, dressing, and transferring, would have face validity. Some instruments do not have obvious face validity, and must be validated in some other way to document their usefulness. For instance, the measurement of temperature using a mercury thermometer does not have face validity; however, physicists can show how mercury reacts to changes in molecular motion and heat to provide validation.

For scientific purposes, face validity should not be considered sufficient documentation of a test's validity because there is no standard for judging it or determining "how much" of it an instrument has. Essentially, face validity is assessed as all or none. Therefore, assessments of face validity are considered subjective and scientifically weak. There will be times, however, when no other form of validation is possible, when an instrument is one of a kind, and no other instrument or test can be used for comparison. In that case, the investigator may be forced to rely on face validity to support an instrument's use. The disadvantage of relying on face validation as the only justification for a test is that it provides no clout against potential challenges because it is based solely on the opinion of the investigator. Goldsmith[2] suggests that one way to evaluate face validity is to determine who the stakeholders are, such as patients, physicians, physical therapists, occupational therapists or social workers, and then to describe a simple percentage of how many consider the test credible.

Face validity does serve an important purpose, however, in that an instrument lacking in face validity may not be acceptable to those who administer it, those who are tested by it, or those who will use the results. For example, respondents on a questionnaire may not answer questions with honesty or motivation if they do not see the relevance of the questions. Patients may not be compliant with repeated testing if they do not understand how a test relates to their difficulty. Consumers of research reports may not accept results if they feel the test is irrelevant. Therefore, although face validity should not be considered sufficient, it is a useful property of a test.

CONTENT VALIDITY

Most behavioral and educational variables have a theoretical domain or universe of content that consists of all the behaviors, characteristics, or information that could possibly be observed about that variable. **Content validity** refers to the adequacy with which this universe is sampled by a test. Because the content universe is theoretical, it must be defined by representative parts of the whole. An instrument is said to have content validity if it covers all parts of the universe of content and reflects the relative importance of each part. Content validity is an especially important characteristic of questionnaires, examinations, inventories, and interviews that attempt to evaluate a range of information by selected test items or questions.

Content validity demands that a test is free from the influence of factors that are irrelevant to the purpose of the measurement. For instance, a test of gross motor skills should not contain items that assess language skills, nor should it be influenced by the patient's anxiety level or ability to read. If these factors influence the patient's score, the test would be measuring something other than what it was intended to measure and would not be a valid reflection of gross motor skill. Perhaps more important, content validity means that the test does contain all the elements that reflect the variable being studied. For example, an evaluation of pain using a visual analogue scale (VAS) that assesses the intensity of an individual's pain reflects only one element of the experience of pain. A tool such as the McGill Pain Questionnaire may have greater content validity because it includes a comprehensive assessment of many elements of pain such as location, quality, duration and intensity.[3]

The determination of content validity is essentially a subjective process. There are no statistical indices that can assess content validity. Claims for content validation are made by a panel of "experts" who review the instrument and determine if the questions satisfy the content domain. This process often requires several revisions of the test. When all agree that the content domain has been sampled adequately, content validity is supported.

Content validity is specific to the content universe as it is defined by the researcher. For some content areas this will be fairly obvious. For instance, an instructor preparing a final examination can determine if the questions address each unit covered during the semester and if the requested information was included in course materials. Other content universes are less obvious. Consider the following: What range of activities are representative of "function"? Should a functional status questionnaire include questions related to physical, cognitive, social and emotional function? How important are each of these domains to the assessment of function of a patient with a stroke, a patient with spinal cord injury, or a well elderly person? If we are interested in dressing skills, how many different tasks must be sampled to make a valid judgment? Will physical thera-pists define this universe differently from occupational therapists or nurses?

These types of questions must be answered by the researcher before the validity of the test can be determined. The answers will depend on the rationale for the test, the operational definitions of the test variable, and the specific objectives of the test instru-ment. The content universe should be described in sufficient detail so that the domain of interest is clearly identified for all who use the instrument.

CRITERION-RELATED VALIDITY

Criterion-related validity is the most practical and objective approach to validity test-ing. It is based on the ability of one test to predict results obtained on an external crite-rion. The test to be validated, called the *target test*, is compared with a **gold standard**, or criterion measure that is already established or assumed to be valid. When both tests are administered to one group of subjects, the scores on the target test are correlated with those achieved by the criterion measure. If the correlation is high (the correlation coefficient is close to 1.00), the target test is considered a valid predictor of the criterion score. For instance, we can investigate the validity of heart rate (the target test) as an indicator of energy cost during exercise by correlating it with values obtained in stan-dardized oxygen consumption studies (the criterion measure). We could establish the validity of observational gait analysis (the target test) by comparing results with those obtained with computerized motion analysis systems (the criterion measure). In each case, the criterion measure is known or assumed to be a valid indicator of the variable of interest, and therefore, comparable results achieved with the target test are support-ive of that test's validity.

Validity of the Criterion

The most crucial element of criterion validation is the ability to demonstrate validity of the criterion measure. If the criterion is not valid, it is plainly useless as a standard. Sev-eral characteristics can be used to judge the utility of a criterion measure. First, it is nec-essary to demonstrate its *reliability* in a test–retest situation, so that the instrument's stability is confirmed. Second, the criterion and target ratings should be *independent* and *free from bias*. For instance, if we use a supervisor's ratings as the criterion to validate a new scale of clinical competence for evaluating staff performance, we want to be sure that the supervisor's relationship with the staff does not influence the rating. We also want to blind the supervisor to the staff person's scores on the clinical scale to avoid the temptation of giving higher ratings to those who achieved higher clinical scores. It is often helpful to have different raters perform the target and criterion tests.

A third, and probably the most important, characteristic of a good criterion is its rel-evance to the behavior being measured by the target test. We must be able to establish that the criterion is a valid measure of the variable being addressed by the target test; that is, the *criterion and the target test must be measuring the same thing*. For instance, some studies have used measures of range of motion to document changes in joint pain. One might believe that active movement in a joint will be proportional to the amount of pain experienced during movement. Others might argue, however, that range of motion measures do not assess pain and would be inappropriate as a criterion for validation of other pain scales. This issue is of obvious importance to the interpretation of correlations between tests.

In many areas of physical and physiological science, standard criteria are readily available for validating clinical tools. For example, to validate methods of measuring physical activity levels, we can use oxygen consumption data;[4] to validate methods of measuring finger range of motion, we can refer to radiographic images.[5] Unfortunately, the choice of a gold standard for more abstract constructs is not always as obvious. If we want to establish the validity of a functional status questionnaire, with what referent should it be compared? What standard can be used to validate a scale designed to assess perceptions of quality of life in a nursing home population? How can we establish an external criterion to judge a person's degree of pain? Sometimes the best one can do is use another instrument that has already achieved a degree of validation or acceptance. For abstract variables such as these, criterion validation may be based on a **reference standard** that may not be a true "gold standard," but is considered an acceptable criterion. A more complex approach, construct validation, is often necessary to validate the measurement of more abstract variables. This process is discussed in the next section.

Criterion-related validity is often separated into two components: concurrent validity and predictive validity. These approaches are differentiated on the basis of the time frame within which predictions are made.

Concurrent Validity

Concurrent validity is studied when the measurement to be validated and the criterion measure are taken at relatively the same time (concurrently), so that they both reflect the same incident of behavior. This approach is often used to establish the validity of diagnostic or screening tests for determining the presence or absence of diseases or conditions. For example, the Autism Screening Questionnaire was developed to distinguish children with autism and pervasive development disorders, based on parental interview as the reference standard.[6]

Concurrent validity is also useful in situations where a new or untested tool is potentially more efficient, easier to administer, more practical, or safer than another more established method, and is being proposed as an alternative. For instance, the distinction between stress and urge incontinence requires an extensive and time consuming clinical examination by a urologist. Brown et al.[7] demonstrated the validity of a 3-item questionnaire to make this distinction, using the clinical evaluation as the reference standard. As another example, Perkins and associates[8] studied the characteristics of four simple sensory screening maneuvers compared with standardized electrophysiological tests in the diagnosis of diabetic polyneuropathy. They demonstrated that monofilament sensory examination, superficial pain sensation, and vibration testing, all requiring only minutes to administer, were able to identify those with likely neuropathy.

Predictive Validity

Predictive validity attempts to establish that a measure will be a valid predictor of some future criterion score. A test with good predictive validity helps an investigator make successful decisions by providing a basis for predicting outcomes or future behaviors. To assess predictive validity, a target test is given at one session and is followed by a period of time after which the criterion score is obtained. The interval between these two tests is dependent on the time needed to achieve the criterion, and may be as long as several years. The relationship between the target and criterion scores is examined to determine if the target test score is a valid predictor of the outcome on the criterion measure. A classic example is the use of college admissions criteria, such as the Scholastic Aptitude Test (SAT) or grade point average (GPA), based on their presumed ability to predict future academic success.

Predictive validity is an essential concept in screening procedures to assess future risk (see Chapter 27). For instance, we may use an instrument like the Berg Balance Scale[9] or the Timed Up and Go test[10] as a screen to predict risk for falls in elderly individuals. Salaffi[11] developed an algorithm based on age, weight, history of previous low impact fracture, early menopause and corticosteroid therapy to identify women at increased risk of low bone mineral density. Prediction of cognitive impairment following stroke has been shown to be related to side and type of stroke, gender, and the presence of aphasia.[12] The results of screening tests allow clinicians to initiate appropriate preventive strategies.

Prediction is also used for prognosis and setting long-term goals. We engage in prediction when we examine the relationship between impairments and activity limitations or disability. For example, Cress and Meyer[13] were able to show that maximal voluntary muscle force and performance in daily activities could predict the ability to live independently without self-reported functional limitation in elderly individuals. Lombardino et al.[14] tested 149 kindergarteners using the Early Reading Screening Instrument (ERSI) and followed the children for one year. They demonstrated a strong correlation between first grade reading skills and the ERSI score, with the strongest relationship for reading comprehension. By knowing the ERSI score, then, intervention can be started early to prevent or diminish future risk for reading failure.

We also estimate the potential for rehabilitation or change on the basis of a patient's initial status. For instance, Katz and co-workers[15] studied a sample of 105 patients who underwent arthroscopic partial meniscectomy, to identify factors that were predictive of poor outcomes. They examined demographic factors, medical history, preoperative impairments and functional status, and operative variables to determine their relationship to postoperative function, as measured by the SF-36 physical activity scale. Through multivariate statistical analyses, they found that the extent of cartilage damage, worker's compensation and preoperative functional status were most predictive of a poor outcome. The authors suggested that these findings should be routinely measured and incorporated into prognostic data, to provide a basis for discussing the advantages and disadvantages of the procedure with patients.

A practical limitation exists, however, when trying to assess the predictive validity of screening procedures. One must be able to follow subjects who *do* and *do not* have positive initial findings, so that follow-up measures can distinguish between them. For instance, in setting academic admissions criteria, presumably, we only admit the most qualified students. Therefore, when examining the outcome of academic success we are not able to determine if those with lesser scores would have also succeeded. They were never given the chance. This makes it difficult to truly determine if the admissions criteria have predictive validity.

CONSTRUCT VALIDITY

Construct validity reflects the ability of an instrument to measure an abstract concept, or construct. The process of construct validation presents a considerable challenge to the researcher because constructs are not "real"; that is, they are not directly observable, and exist only as concepts that are constructed to represent an abstract trait. Because constructs are typically multidimensional, it is not easy to determine if an instrument is actually measuring the variable of interest.

For example, everyone agrees that "health" is an important clinical construct, but because of its complexity, clinicians are generally unable to agree on how it should be defined or measured. Therefore, the definition of a construct like "health status" can be determined only by the instrument used to measure it. A test that focuses on physical activity alone will suggest a very different definition than a more global test that also incorporates cognitive, social and psychological elements. Similarly, a scale that looks at activities of daily living (ADL) according to categories of self-care, transfers and dressing will provide a different perception of function than one that also evaluates locomotion, housekeeping and recreation skills. An instrument that evaluates ADL according to an individual's perception of the *difficulty* performing given tasks will produce a measurement that is interpreted differently than one which focuses on the *time* needed to perform, the *assistance* required, or another that assesses the level of *pain* associated with specific tasks. Each of these provides a different theoretical foundation for defining the construct of function.

Part of construct validity, therefore, is based on content validity; that is, one must be able to define the content universe that represents that construct to develop a test to measure it. Beyond content, however, constructs must also be defined according to their underlying *theoretical context*. Thus, the "meaning" of a construct is based on assumptions about how an individual with that trait would behave under given conditions and how the various dimensions that form the construct interrelate. One can generate hypotheses regarding the overt behaviors of individuals with high and low scores on the test. An instrument is said to be a valid measure of a construct when its measurements support these theoretical assumptions.

For example, pain is a difficult construct to define, as it represents a subjective phenomenon rather than a performance behavior. However, we may also question whether "pain" is a stimulus, a perception, a response or a behavior. Looking at the construct of pain, then, requires that we conceptualize what is actually being evaluated. For instance, Sim and Waterfield[16] discuss the *experience of pain* as a subjective outcome that varies from individual to individual. They describe the pain experience as having sensory, affective, evaluative, cognitive and behavioral dimensions, with sensory, emotional and physiological outcomes (Figure 6.2). Further analysis suggests the need to look at memory, cultural factors, social networks, sex and age, personality and other

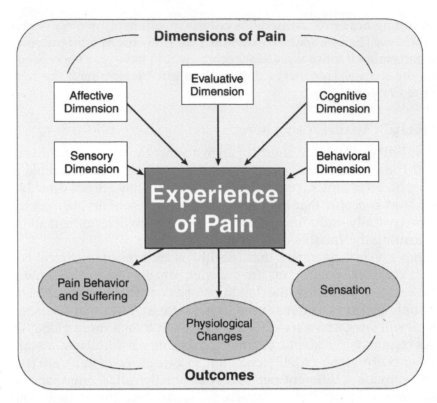

FIGURE 6.2 Theoretical model of the multidimensional nature of the experience of pain, illustrating how the construct of pain may be conceptualized. Several dimensions contribute to the individual nature of the experience, as well as how the outcomes of the pain experience are perceived. (Adapted from Sim J, Waterfield J. Validity, reliability and responsiveness in the assessment of pain. *Physiother Theory Pract* 1997; 13:23–37.)

elements that contribute to the individual perception of pain. The differentiation between chronic and acute pain is more than just the time over which the pain occurs. Then there are characteristics of pain, such as intensity, quality, location, and duration.

How one chooses to "measure" pain, therefore, will affect how the outcome will be interpreted. For instance, a study of patients in cancer trials looked at several outcome measures to evaluate pain treatment.[17] A visual analog scale (VAS) using the anchors of "no pain" to "pain as bad as it could be" focused solely on intensity. A Pain Relief Scale assessed complete relief to worsening of pain. A Patient Satisfaction Scale rated how satisfied patients were with their treatment, and pain management scales were based on medication use. The authors showed that the adequacy of treatment for pain varied from 16% to 91%, depending on the type of outcome measure used. The construct is defined, therefore, by the instrument used to measure it. Different elements may be important, depending on the clinical or research situation.

Methods of Construct Validation

Construct validation provides evidence to support or refute the theoretical framework behind the construct. Construct validation is an ongoing process, wherein we are continually learning more about the construct and testing its predictions. This evidence can be gathered by a variety of methods. Some of the more commonly used procedures include the known groups method, convergence and discrimination, factor analysis, hypothesis testing and criterion validation.

Known Groups Method

The most general type of evidence in support of construct validity is provided when a test can discriminate between individuals who are known to have the trait and those that do not. Using the **known groups method**, a criterion is chosen that can identify the presence or absence of a particular characteristic, and the theoretical context behind the construct is used to predict how different groups are expected to behave. Therefore, the validity of a particular test is supported if the test's results document these known differences. For example, Megens and associates[18] examined the construct validity of the Harris Infant Neuromotor Test (HINT), a screening tool to identify neuromotor or cognitive/behavioral problems in infants who are healthy or at risk within the first year of life. They studied 412 low-risk infants and 54 infants who were identified as high risk based on preterm birth weight or exposure to drugs or alcohol *in utero*. The researchers found that the HINT distinguished between the two groups of infants in their mean scores, supporting the construct validity of the tool.

Convergence and Discrimination

Campbell and Fiske[19] have suggested that the construct validity of a test can be evaluated in terms of how its measures relate to other tests of the same and different constructs. In other words, it is important to determine what a test does measure as well as what it does not measure. This determination is based on the concepts of convergence and discrimination.

Convergent validity indicates that two measures believed to reflect the same underlying phenomenon will yield similar results or will correlate highly. For instance, if two health status scales are valid methods for measuring quality of life, they should produce correlated scores. Convergence also implies that the theoretical context behind the construct will be supported when the test is administered to different groups in different places at different times. Convergence is not a sufficient criterion for construct validity, however. It is also necessary to show that a construct can be differentiated from other constructs.

Discriminant validity indicates that different results, or low correlations, are expected from measures that are believed to assess different characteristics. Therefore, the results of an intelligence test should not be expected to correlate with results of a test of gross motor skill. To illustrate these concepts, the Sickness Impact Profile (SIP) has been compared to several other measures of function in an effort to establish its construct validity. The SIP is a health status measure which indicates the changes in a person's behavior due to sickness, scored on the total scale as well as on separate physical and psychosocial subscales.[20] Convergent validity has been supported by a high correlation between the physical dimensions of the SIP scale and the SF-36 health survey questionnaire.[21] Discriminant validity is illustrated by a lower correlation between the physical SIP scale and the Carroll Rating Scale for Depression.[22]

Campbell and Fiske[19] also suggest that validity of a test should be evaluated in terms of both the characteristic being measured and the method used to measure it. They call this a *trait-method unit;* that is, a trait cannot be assessed independently of some method. Therefore, the validity of the assessment must take both elements into account. On the basis of this concept, a validation process was proposed that incorporates an analysis of two or more traits measured by two or more methods. The intercorrelations of variables within and between methods are arranged in a matrix called a **multitrait-multimethod matrix** (see Figure 6.3). By arranging scores in this way, we can verify that tests measuring the same trait produce high correlations, demonstrating convergent validity, and those that measure different traits produce low correlations, demonstrating discriminant validity.

Factor Analysis

Another common approach to construct validation is the use of a statistical procedure called **factor analysis**. The concept of factor analysis is based on the idea that a construct contains one or more underlying dimensions, or different theoretical components. For example, Wessel and associates[23] used the Western Ontario Rotator Cuff (WORC) Index to study the quality of life of individuals with that disorder. The index is composed of 21 items that were originally designed to reflect five dimensions: (1) pain and physical symptoms, (2) sports and recreation, (3) work, (4) lifestyle, and (5) emotions. Using a factor analysis, the researchers were able to recombine these variables as three *factors:* Emotions and Symptoms, Disability–Strength Activities, and Disability–Daily Activities. These separate groupings of correlated variables represent subsets of test items or behaviors that are related to each other, but are not related to items in other factors; that is, each factor represents a unique combination of items that reflects a different theoretical component of the construct. The statistical basis for this

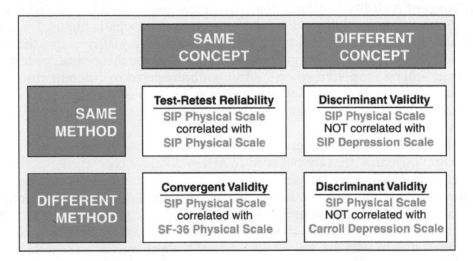

FIGURE 6.3   A multitrait-multimethod matrix, showing the relationship between reliability and validity, and the concepts of convergent and discriminant validity. The physical scale of the Sickness Impact Profile (SIP) shows high correlations (convergent validity) with the physical scale of the SF-36 Health Status Questionnaire, but low correlations (discriminant validity) with different measures of depression.

process is quite complex and beyond our current discussion, but we will devote considerable attention to it in Chapter 29.

Hypothesis Testing

Because constructs have a theoretical basis, an instrument's validity can also be assessed by using it to test specific hypotheses that support the theory. For instance, the construct validity of the Functional Independence Measure (FIM) was assessed by Dodds et al.,[24] based on the assumption that the instrument should be able to distinguish functional differences between people with varied clinical conditions. The construct of function that forms the foundation for the FIM relates to the burden of care, or the degree of assistance needed for a patient to fulfill activities in ADL, mobility and cognitive domains. Using this theoretical premise, the authors proposed three hypotheses: (1) that FIM scores should decrease with increasing age and comorbidities, (2) that the score would be related to a patient's discharge destination according to the level of care provided in that setting (such as home or skilled nursing facility), and (3) that there would be a relationship between FIM scores and degree of severity for patients with amputations, spinal cord injury and stroke. Using data collected on more than 11,000 patients, their results supported some hypotheses better than others, demonstrating a strong relationship between FIM scores and discharge destination, and severity of spinal cord injury and stroke. This type of analysis provides distinct evidence of construct validity for the instrument, but it leaves unanswered many theoretical questions regarding its use over the broad range of rehabilitation situations. Therefore, it also points to the need for continued testing to determine how the FIM score relates to various diagnoses and clinical findings.

Criterion Validation

Construct validity can also be supported by comparison of test results with those of relevant criterion tests. This approach is not used as often as other approaches, because it is typically difficult to find a suitable criterion. In most cases, when a new instrument is developed to measure a construct, it is because no other acceptable instruments are available. Therefore, no standard can be applied to test it; however, it is often possible to find criterion tests that can be applied to subparts of the overall instrument. For example, Podsiadlo and Richardson[10] used the Berg Balance Scale, gait speed and an ADL scale as criterion values to establish the construct validity of the timed "Up and Go" test. These individual criterion tests were assumed to represent components of the overall construct of functional mobility that the "Up and Go" test was intended to measure. Through a series of correlations the authors were able to demonstrate that each criterion test was related to the outcome variable, and although these were not perfect correlations, taken together they supported the overall concept that was being evaluated.

MEASURING CHANGE

As clinicians and researchers, we could reasonably argue that a primary goal of treatment is to effect a positive change in a patient's status. The difference between the outcome and the initial score is called a **change score** or **difference score**. The use of change scores as the basis for analysis of treatment outcomes is pervasive throughout clinical research. This practice is actually quite complex, however, in terms of statistical and practical interpretation. Perhaps the most important consideration is the purpose of measuring change. We measure change to determine if an individual's performance or condition has gotten better. The amount of change will indicate a strong versus weak response. We also look at differences between individuals in the amount of change, to distinguish those who changed a lot from those who changed a little and to draw inferences about treatment effects.

Issues Affecting Validity of Change

Four measurement issues have the potential to influence the validity of change scores.[25]

Level of Measurement

The use of nominal, ordinal, interval or ratio data is an important consideration in the calculation of change scores. Nominal scores, of course, cannot be subtracted, and therefore, cannot demonstrate change. At the other end of the continuum, true change can only be measured using ratio scores, because all measures are known quantities. Interval level data present a problem for evaluating change (refer to Figure 4.2 in Chapter 4), because although we can determine the *distance* of change, we may not know the true *amount* of change.

The risk of misinference is greatest, however, with ordinal measures because the distance between intervals is not known and may not be equal. For instance, Andres and co-workers[26] examined changes in strength in patients with amyotrophic lateral sclerosis using manual muscle test grades (ordinal scale) and isometric force measures with a strain gauge (ratio scale). They found that early changes in strength were evident with the ratio scale measure, which were not evident using the ordinal measure. Significant declines in functional strength occurred within a single manual muscle test grade. During later stages, strength decrements were more dramatic and were clear with both measures. The choice of tool, therefore, could make a distinct difference in evaluative decisions early in the disease.

This creates a potentially troublesome situation for clinicians and researchers, as so many tools used to measure impairments, function and quality of life are based on ordinal scores. Assessment of change with such tools must take into account their limitations for interpretation. To illustrate, consider again the Functional Independence Measure (FIM) which is used extensively in rehabilitation settings.[27] This instrument includes 18 items related to independence in physical and cognitive domains. Each item is scored on a 1–7 ordinal scale, with lower scores representing the need for more assistance. We would have to question an assumption, however, that would equate a one-point improvement from 1 to 2 with the same "amount" of improvement from 6 to 7. Similarly, a change from 1 to 2 on a manual muscle test could not be validly equated with a change from 3 to 4. Therefore, efforts to show improvement in individual patients or groups through change scores can be ambiguous.

This measurement issue is a concern for interpretation of scores. For instance, most functional scales present a total score, derived by summing item scores. This process could be considered meaningless if the "numbers" that are used to create the sum have no inherent mathematical relationship; that is, an ordinal number is nothing more than a categorical label, and has no arithmetic properties. Therefore, the sum and its derived change score may be uninterpretable. See the Commentary in Chapter 4 for further discussion of this question.

Reliability

A second important issue in evaluating the validity of change concerns the reliability of the factor being measured. This consideration refers back to the concepts of measurement error and minimal detectable difference (see Chapter 5). Suppose we take a pretest measurement and a subsequent posttest, but the true value does not change. The score will probably be different on the posttest because of random measurement error. Now we subtract the pretest from the posttest to obtain a change score. Assuming that the *true score* has not changed, measurement theory suggests that the difference will cancel out the true score, essentially leaving nothing but error in the change score. Therefore, even with true change, reliability is a necessary precondition for the application of change scores. Streiner and Norman[28] suggest that one should only use change scores when the reliability of a measure exceeds 0.50, although for many clinical variables reliability should probably be higher. Perhaps more relevant, the minimal detectable change will provide a useful reference to determine how much change can be reasonably interpreted as real. It is important to remember that being reliable does not automatically imply that a measure will be able to detect change.

Stability

In addition to the reliability of the measurement system, we must also consider the stability of the variable being measured. If we are working with a variable that is labile, it may be difficult to determine if change is a function of improvement in a therapeutic element, or if it is a reflection of an unstable behavior. For instance, measurement of blood pressure may vary from trial to trial with no true change in physiological status, whereas measures of function should be fairly stable even though precise performance may vary from time to time. Establishing stability may require that several measurements be taken at both baseline and outcome to demonstrate that the performance is reliable.

Baseline Scores

A fourth concern in the interpretation of improvement or decline is the status of patients at baseline. Sometimes the extent to which a variable changes will depend on its starting point. For example, a patient with poor health status may not demonstrate deterioration if the baseline score on a quality of life scale is already at the lowest point (a **floor effect**). Conversely, a patient who is functioning well in basic activities of daily living (ADL) may show no improvement in function if a functional scale is not able to assess high level instrumental ADLs (a **ceiling effect**).

Therefore, when describing the effectiveness of a therapeutic program, information should be included about gains as a function of initial scores. It would be useful to know if the likelihood of improvement is similar across all levels of baseline scores. Patterns may become evident when the starting point is examined. If some patients do not improve as much as others, it would be helpful to understand if their status upon admission was different. Those with greater impairments may need to be treated differently.

Responsiveness to Change

If we are interested in documenting change, one of the first choices we must make is which measuring instrument we will use. For some variables this decision is rather straightforward. When we want to measure ROM or strength, for instance, we have a fairly traditional set of tools to employ. For more abstract variables, however, researchers have generated a vast set of instruments that can be applied in different situations. Much of the research in the development of these tools has focused on construct validity, determining if the instrument is able to reflect a person's status at a given point in time. However, if we intend to use an instrument for evaluation, we must extend our concern for validity beyond the construct itself to a discussion of the **responsiveness** of the instrument, or its ability to detect minimal change over time.[29] Responsiveness is an important quality if a test is to be used to assess the effectiveness of intervention; that is, the score must change in proportion to the patient's status change, and must remain stable when the patient is unchanged. This change must be large enough to be statistically significant for research purposes and precise enough to reflect increments of meaningful change in an external criterion for clinical application.

Minimal Clinically Important Difference

An important question, then, relates to just how much change can be considered clinically meaningful. From a research standpoint, we often find ourselves referring to statistical significance as a way of defining important differences. But this may not reflect a difference that has clinical significance. Decisions about the effectiveness of interventions must be made on the basis of clinical importance and relevant change.

The concept of the **minimal clinically important difference (MCID)** has become central to assessing change. The MCID is the smallest difference in a measured variable that signifies an important rather than trivial difference in the patient's condition.[30] It has also been defined as the smallest difference a patient would perceive as beneficial, and that would result in a change in the management of the patient, assuming an absence of excessive side effects or cost.[31,32] The determination of the MCID is critical for judging the benefit of intervention.[33] Only when we know if treatment has resulted in meaningful change can we truly compare the effectiveness of treatments.

The MCID is usually based on an "anchor" or external criterion that indicates when change has occurred. This is typically associated with the patient's perception that he is "better," by the clinician's judgment of the patient's improvement, or an external health status measure. The minimal clinically important difference has been determined for several instruments. For example, Kocks et al.[34] studied the Clinical COPD Questionnaire, and found that a change of 0.44 points on the 0–10 scale was related to the patient's perception that he was "somewhat better." A change of 0.39 points was established as the MCID based on a criterion reference of hospital readmission. Iyer et al.[35]

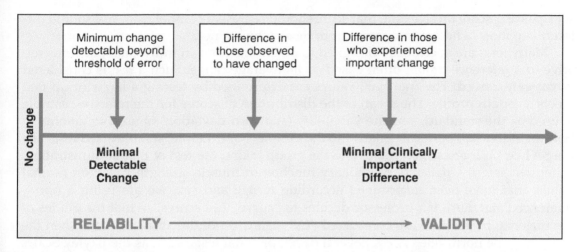

FIGURE 6.4 Continuum of reliability to validity, related to the measurement of important clinical changes.

studied the Pediatric Evaluation of Disability Inventory (PEDI) and found that an 11 point change (0–100 scale) was meaningful based on ratings from physical therapists, occupational therapists and speech and language pathologists. Quintana et al.[36] showed that a change of 20–40 points on the Physical Function scale of the SF-36 was important to patients six months following hip replacement surgery.

Interpretation of the MCID must be made within the context of a given study, with specific reference to the outcome measures used, the population and setting, and the design of the study. It must also be interpreted with reference to the minimal detectable difference (MDD) to determine how much change is potentially attributable to error (see Chapter 5). Although change may be observed beyond the MDD, clinicians must determine if the values reported will be useful in understanding when an individual patient has had an important improvement (see Figure 6.4). Further discussion of MCID and methods for calculating it are provided in Chapter 27.

CRITERION REFERENCING AND NORM REFERENCING

The validity of a measurement is also related to how one makes judgments from the test results. Tests may be developed to assess performance based on an absolute criterion. The results of a **criterion-referenced test** are interpreted relative to a fixed standard that represents an acceptable model or level of performance. If we know that a patient with a total knee replacement needs at least 90 degrees of knee flexion to negotiate stairs, then we will establish 90 degrees as an acceptable outcome. A functional test will establish how much assistance a patient needs to perform certain tasks using specific definitions of dependence and independence. In educational programs, a grade of 70 on a test might be used to specify competence for the material being tested. This absolute standard will indicate passing, and everyone could pass or everyone could fail. Each student's grade is independent of how the rest of the group performs. The validity of a criterion-referenced score, of course, depends on the validity of the criterion. So if we set a passing score on an exam, that score should represent competence, and should differentiate those who are competent from those who are not.

Many tests are specifically designed to determine how an individual performs relative to a reference group, often based on an average range. Such a test is considered **norm-referenced**. The "normal" values are determined by testing a large group that meets a certain profile. The mean of the distribution of scores for the reference sample is used as the standard, and the variability (standard deviation) is used to determine how an individual performs relative to the sample. For example, standardized tests like the SAT or GRE are scored relative to the group taking the test at that administration. When we assess a patient's pulmonary function or muscle strength based on normal values that have been determined according to age and sex, we are using a norm-referenced standard. If a professor decides to "curve" test scores, so that the grades of the majority of the class are considered "C," regardless of the absolute score, then the test would be norm referenced. Several developmental tests, such as the Bayley Scales of Infant Development[37] or the Gesell development scales,[38] are based on data collected on children within specified age groups. These standardized tests allow the clinician to determine if a child's developmental status falls within the range of the majority of children in that age group. The validity of a norm-referenced test will depend on the validity of the sample that was used to provide the normal values.

The distinction between criterion-referenced and norm-referenced scores is an important one, and should be understood by those who administer and interpret tests. The relative utility of these scores will depend on the purpose of the test and the action that will be taken based on the results. Norm-referenced tests are usually used to establish placement or for diagnosis, as in standardized college board exams or developmental tests. A criterion-referenced test is used to examine the proficiency of performance along a continuum of skill, and does not depend on the performance of others. Criterion-based scores are generally more useful for establishing treatment goals and measuring change, as they tend to be based on an analysis of the tasks that are required for successful performance. Both types of tests should demonstrate reliability and validity.

CROSS-VALIDATION

The purpose of validation studies is to document that a test can be used effectively for a particular purpose. When we deal with predictive tests or screening procedures, we collect data on an experimental sample and use these data to create predictive equations or cutoff scores that will be applied to the larger population. For example, if we want to determine the appropriate criteria for screening scoliosis patients, we would look at results obtained on a particular sample and then apply the most effective cutoff score to other samples.

Unfortunately, the data obtained on an experimental sample are often different from those that would be obtained on a sample of different subjects. Therefore, the error components within predictive equations or cutoff scores will usually be greater for subsequent samples than they were for the original sample. This means that the test's accuracy will not necessarily be as great as it was on the original sample.

The predictive models or cutoff scores obtained from validation studies should, therefore, always be cross-validated on a second sample, to determine if the test criteria can be generalized across samples. **Cross-validation** is accomplished by trying out a previously developed test on a new group with characteristics as close as possible to those of the original. Of course, we assume that the original and test groups are both good representatives of the population for which the test will be used. It is also possible to cross-validate the test on a sample with different characteristics that may be appropriate for the test. For instance, certain perceptual tests may be used for different age groups and could be validated across groups of children and adults. If cross-validation is not documented, a substantial reduction in the validity of a test on subsequent applications can be anticipated.

COMMENTARY

The Ongoing Pursuit of Validity

The process of developing a measuring instrument involves several stages of planning, test construction, reliability testing, and validation. In the planning stages, the purpose of the test must be stipulated, including specification of the relevant content universe or the theoretical construct and the target population for which the instrument will be used. A literature review is usually necessary, to determine that an appropriate instrument does not already exist and to formulate operational definitions of the construct to be measured. For educational or physical tests, these operational definitions will refer to specific content that the subject is expected to know or perform. For physiological or behavioral tests, operational definitions must specify how the construct theory will be manifested in a person's actions or responses. The literature will often help identify the types of test items that are likely to best evaluate the construct of interest.

When mechanical instruments are developed for measurement of physical or physiological variables, the construction phase of development involves the actual building of the device, usually starting with the development of a prototype. The instrument is field tested on a variety of subjects to see if it reacts properly and if the resulting scores represent the construct of interest. For educational and psychological tests, the construction phase is facilitated by the listing of behavioral objectives that are relevant to the test's purpose and that define the content areas that should be included. Depending on the purpose of the test, these objectives may relate to the cognitive, affective, and psychomotor domains. The number of items that address each content area will reflect the relative importance of each objective to the test's ultimate goal. Writing test items is a long process, usually incorporating contributions from many experts, and several stages of review to support content validity.

Validation is almost never a complete process, nor is it ever accomplished with only one study. Numerous research efforts are required to substantiate a test's validity using different testing methods. The choice of which type of evidence is required to document validity will depend on the test's purpose. For most instruments, more than one method will be used. In many instances, construct validity will subsume the other forms of evidence and require that multiple approaches to validation be used.

Choosing a sample for validation studies is an important part of the process, as the results that are obtained must be generalizable to the target population for which the test is being developed. The characteristics of the target population should be clearly defined. It is important that the test sample reflect some variance in the measured characteristics, and not just the population average. One criterion for establishing a test's validity is its ability to discriminate among individuals with different levels of the construct. If a sample is composed of a homogeneous group with similar values for the test trait, it will be impossible to determine if the test fulfills this purpose.

Concepts of validity are of vital importance in the contemporary health care environment, where outcomes and quality of life constructs are seen as relevant end points for evaluating the success of treatment and justifying continued intervention. As clinicians become more familiar with the vast number of generic and condition-specific health instruments that are being used, they must also be able to determine which instrument is appropriate under which conditions and for which patient, and they must be able to interpret the scores on these instruments with meaningful analyses. If an instrument is used to demonstrate change or improvement, but it is not sensitive enough to pick up small but clinically important changes, then the treatment will appear unsuccessful. As we attempt to use these tools to show effectiveness, we must understand the concepts of validity to make reasonable judgments and more informed choices. We must be able to evaluate validity, and we must critically scrutinize the literature to make these determinations.

Perhaps the most significant message, however, concerns how one goes about choosing an instrument. Many clinicians are ambitious in their attempt to design forms and tests for specific purposes. Unfortunately, many are unaware of the need to be accountable for the validity of the instrument, and their measurements are often not meaningful. This practice hinders communication and obstructs the ability to examine patterns, compare findings or draw generalizations regarding outcomes. It would make more sense to try to find an existing instrument that might serve the purpose. This also presents the responsibility, however, for confirming reliability and validity. Given the large number of instruments that are presently being tested, we can all contribute significantly to our understanding of their capabilities by using them with different populations in varied settings, to determine their useful measurement properties.

REFERENCES

1. Escolar DM, Scacheri CG. Pharmacologic and genetic therapy for childhood muscular dystrophies. *Curr Neurol Neurosci Rep* 2001:168–174.
2. Goldsmith CH. Commentary: Measurement validity in physical therapy research. *Phys Ther* 1993;73:113–114.
3. Melzack R, Katz J. The McGill Pain Questionnaire: Appraisal and current status. In DC Turk, R Melzack, (Eds.). *Handbook of Pain Assessment.* New York: Guilford Press, 1992.

4. Buckley JP, Sim J, Eston RG, Hession R, Fox R. Reliability and validity of measures taken during the Chester step test to predict aerobic power and to prescribe aerobic exercise. *Br J Sports Med* 2004;38:197–205.

5. Groth GN, VanDeven KM, Phillips EC, Ehretsman RL. Goniometry of the proximal and distal interphalangeal joints, Part II: Placement prefereces, interrater reliability, and concurrent validity. *J Hand Ther* 2001;14:23–29.

6. Berument SK, Rutter M, Lord C, Pickles A, Bailey A. Autism screening questionnaire: Diagnostic validity. *Br J Psychiatry* 1999;175:444–451.

7. Brown JS, Bradley CS, Subak LL, Richter HE, Kraus SR, Brubaker L, et al. The sensitivity and specificity of a simple test to distinguish between urge and stress urinary incontinence. *Ann Intern Med* 2006;144:715–723.

8. Perkins BA, Olaleye D, Zinman B, Bril V. Simple screening tests for peripheral neuropathy in the diabetes clinic. *Diabetes Care* 2001;24:250–256.

9. Berg KO, Wood-Dauphinee SL, Williams JI, Maki B. Measuring balance in the elderly: Validation of an instrument. *Can J Public Health* 1992;83 Suppl 2:S7–11.

10. Podsiadlo D, Richardson S. The timed "Up & Go": A test of basic functional mobility for frail elderly persons. *J Am Geriatr Soc* 1991;39:142–148.

11. Salaffi F, Silveri F, Stancati A, Grassi W. Development and validation of the osteoporosis prescreening risk assessment (OPERA) tool to facilitate identification of women likely to have low bone density. *Clin Rheumatol* 2005;24:203–211.

12. Hochstenbach J, Mulder T, van Limbeek J, Donders R, Schoonderwaldt H. Cognitive decline following stroke: A comprehensive study of cognitive decline following stroke. *J Clin Exp Neuropsychol* 1998;20:503–517.

13. Cress ME, Meyer M. Maximal voluntary and functional performance levels needed for independence in adults aged 65 to 97 years. *Phys Ther* 2003;83:37–48.

14. Lombardino LJ, Morris D, Mercado L, DeFillip F, Sarisky C, Montgomery A. The Early Reading Screening Instrument: A method for identifying kindergarteners at risk for learning to read. *Int J Lang Commun Disord* 1999;34:135–150.

15. Katz JN, Harris TM, Larson MG, Krushell RJ, Brown CH, Fossel AH, et al. Predictors of functional outcomes after arthroscopic partial meniscectomy. *J Rheumatol* 1992;19:1938–1942.

16. Sim J, Waterfield J. Validity, reliability and responsiveness in the assessment of pain. *Physiother Theory Pract* 1997;13:23–38.

17. de Wit R, van Dam F, Abu-Saad HH, Loonstra S, Zandbelt L, van Buuren A, et al. Empirical comparison of commonly used measures to evaluate pain treatment in cancer patients with chronic pain. *J Clin Oncol* 1999;17:1280–1287.

18. Megens AM, Harris SR, Backman CL, Hayes VE. Known-groups analysis of the Harris Infant Neuromotor test. *Phys Ther* 2007; 87:164–169.

19. Campbell DT, Fiske DW. Convergent and discriminant validation by the multitrait-multimethod matrix. *Psychol Bull* 1959;56:81–105.

20. Bergner M, Bobbitt RA, Carter WB, Gilson BS. The Sickness Impact Profile: Development and final revision of a health status measure. *Med Care* 1981;19:787–805.

21. Ho AK, Robbins AO, Walters SJ, Kaptoge S, Sahakian BJ, Barker RA. Health-related quality of life in Huntington's disease: A comparison of two generic instruments, SF-36 and SIP. *Mov Disord* 2004;19:1341–1348.

22. Brooks WB, Jordan JS, Divine GW, Smith KS, Neelon FA. The impact of psychologic factors on measurement of functional status. Assessment of the sickness impact profile [see comments]. *Med Care* 1990;28:793–804.

23. Wessel J, Razmjou H, Mewa Y, Holtby R. The factor validity of the Western Ontario Rotator Cuff Index. *BMC Musculoskelet Disord* 2005;6:22.

24. Dodds TA, Martin DP, Stolov WC, Deyo RA. A validation of the Functional Independence Measurement and its performance among rehabilitation inpatients. *Arch Phys Med Rehabil* 1993;74:531–536.
25. Johnston MV, Keith RA, Hinderer SR. Measurement standards for interdisciplinary medical rehabilitation. *Arch Phys Med Rehabil* 1992;73:S3–S23.
26. Andres PL, Skerry LM, Thornell B, Portney LG, Finison LJ, Munsat TL. A comparison of three measures of disease progression in ALS. *J Neurol Sci* 1996;139 Suppl:64–70.
27. Liang MH, Fossel AH, Larson MG. Comparisons of five health status instruments for orthopedic evaluation. *Med Care* 1990;28:632–642.
28. Streiner DL, Normal GR. *Health Measurement Scales: A Practical Guide to Their Development and Use* (3rd ed.). New York: Oxford University Press, 2003.
29. Patrick DL, Chiang YP. Measurement of health outcomes in treatment effectiveness evaluations: Conceptual and methodological challenges. *Med Care* 2000;38:II14–25.
30. Redelmeier DA, Guyatt GH, Goldstein RS. Assessing the minimal important difference in symptoms: A comparison of two techniques. *J Clin Epidemiol* 1996;49:1215–1219.
31. Jaeschke R, Singer J, Guyatt GH. Measurement of health status. Ascertaining the minimal clinically important difference. *Control Clin Trials* 1989;10:407–415.
32. Wells G, Beaton D, Shea B, Boers M, Simon L, Strand V, et al. Minimal clinically important differences: Review of methods. *J Rheumatol* 2001;28:406–412.
33. Wright JG. The minimal important difference: Who's to say what is important? *J Clin Epidemiol* 1996;49:1221–1222.
34. Kocks JW, Tuinenga MG, Uil SM, Van Den Berg JW, Stahl E, Van Der Molen T. Health status measurement in COPD: The minimal clinically important difference of the Clinical COPD Questionnaire. *Respir Res* 2006;7:62.
35. Iyer LV, Haley SM, Watkins MP, Dumas HM. Establishing minimal clinically important differences for scores on the pediatric evaluation of disability inventory for inpatient rehabilitation. *Phys Ther* 2003;83:888–898.
36. Quintana JM, Escobar A, Bilbao A, Arostegui I, Lafuente I, Vidaurreta I. Responsiveness and clinically important differences for the WOMAC and SF-36 after hip joint replacement. *Osteoarthritis Cartilage* 2005;13:1076–1083.
37. Bayley N. *The Bayley Scales of Infant Development.* New York: The Psychological Corporation, 1969.
38. Knobloch H, Stevens F, Malone AF. *Manual of Developmental Diagnosis: The Administration and Interpretation of the Revised Gesell and Amtruda Developmental and Neurological Examination.* Hagerstown, MD: Harper & Row, 1980.

PART III

Designing Clinical Research

CHAPTER 7
Asking the Research Question

The first step in any research effort is identification of the specific question that will be investigated. This is the most important and often most difficult part of the research process, because it controls the direction of all subsequent planning and analysis. The delineation of a precise question is an analytic and evolutionary process, requiring a thorough search through the literature to determine what information is already available on the topic. Throughout the search the researcher re-examines and redefines the purpose of the research, honing it and clarifying it until, finally, an important "researchable" question is asked.

The overall process for identifying a research question starts with the selection of a research *topic* that sparks some interest, and the subsequent exploration of that topic by examining issues in clinical practice and theory, and reading the professional literature. This information leads to the identification of a *research problem*, a broad statement that begins to focus the direction of study. The problem is then refined to a *research question*, which is specific and defined. The "question" may actually be in the form of a statement or an interrogatory; in either case, it delimits the purpose of the study. Several components will shape the question, including an evaluation of its *importance and feasibility*, specification of the *population* to be studied, development of a *research rationale* to support the question, and a description of the specific *variables* to be studied. Throughout this process, the researcher relies on a comprehensive *review of the literature* to provide the background necessary for decision making. The research question is then translated into a statement that reflects the expected outcomes of the study, clarifying the *research objectives* in the form of *hypotheses* or a *statement of purpose* for the study.

The development of a question as the basis for a research study must be distinguished from the process for development of a clinical question in evidence-based practice. In the latter instance, the clinician formulates a question to guide a literature search that will address a particular decision regarding a patient's intervention, diagnosis or prognosis (see Chapter 1).

The purpose of this chapter is to clarify the framework for developing and refining a feasible research question, to define the different types of variables that form the basis for the question, to describe how research objectives guide a study, and to discuss how the review of literature contributes to this process.

SELECTING A TOPIC

The research process begins when a researcher identifies a specific **topic** of interest (see Figure 7 1). Many beginning researchers approach the initial phase of the research process by "looking for a question." Students may be required to generate a question for a project to meet academic requirements. Certainly, there is no paucity of clinical problems that need to be investigated, however, developing a research question should not be merely a fishing expedition. The intellectual and problem solving processes that are part of all clinical or academic endeavors will generate questions of interest. Questions grow out of these experiences because the clinician or researcher feels a need to know something that is not already known, to resolve a conflict, or to clarify some piece of information that is not sufficiently documented. Even in situations where the research task is an academic exercise, the investigator's intellectual curiosity is bound to uncover some uncertainty or special interest that can be translated into a research question. Researchers are usually able to identify that they are interested in studying a certain patient population, a specific type of intervention, a clinical theory, or a fundamental policy issue in the profession.

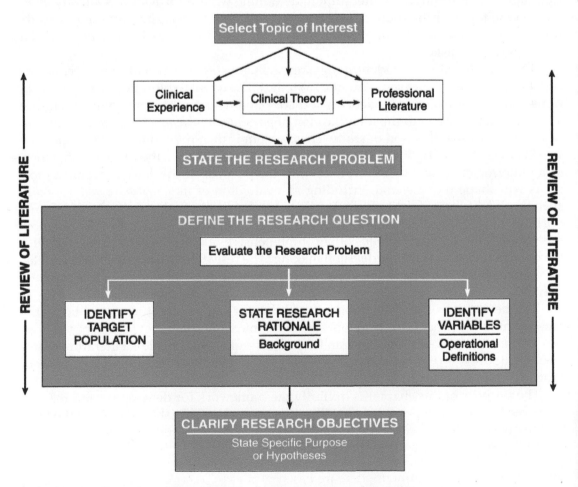

FIGURE 7 1   Illustration of the process for developing a research question.

THE RESEARCH PROBLEM

Once a topic is identified, the process of clarifying a research problem begins by sorting through ideas, facts and theories based on clinical experience and professional literature to determine what we know, what we don't know, and what we need to find out. The application of this information will lead to identification of a **research problem** that will provide the foundation for delineating a specific **research question** that can be answered within a single study (see Figure 7.1). Typically, research problems start out broad, concerned with general clinical problems or theoretical issues. They must be manipulated and modified several times before they become narrowed sufficiently to propose a specific question. Reading the literature and discussing ideas with colleagues are invaluable as one works toward crystallizing a research question. For instance, a researcher might be interested in exploring issues related to wound care. The topic then has to be made more explicit, perhaps specifically, "How can we effectively treat pressure ulcers?" This problem could then be addressed in many ways, leading to several different types of studies. For example, a researcher might look at the effects of ultrasound, electrical stimulation, negative pressure therapy or surgical intervention to promote healing. Another might be concerned with the timing or duration of intervention. Another might address co-morbidities that affect healing. Questions may relate to location or size of the ulcer, debridement techniques, influences of age or gender, or the best ways to measure healing. Many other approaches could be taken to address the same general problem. Each one will contribute to the overall knowledge base that helps us understand the problem. Beginning researchers are often unprepared for the amount of time and thought required to formulate a precise question that is testable. It is sometimes frustrating to accept that only one small facet of a problem can be addressed in a single study.

Clinical Experience

Research problems often emerge from some aspect of practice that presents a dilemma. A clinician's knowledge, experience and curiosity will influence the types of questions that are of interest. We often ask why a particular intervention is successful for some patients but not for others. Are new treatments more effective than established ones? What outcomes can be expected following a particular intervention? Would a particular treatment be more or less effective if we changed the technique of application or combined it with other treatments?

For example, neuromuscular electrical stimulation (NMES) has been shown to be an effective adjunct treatment for quadriceps strengthening following anterior cruciate ligament (ACL) repair when performed against isometric resistance using a dynamometer with the knee positioned in flexion. Fitzgerald et al.[1] had found that some patients had difficulty tolerating that protocol and many clinics did not have instrumented dynamometers. They developed a modified version of the published NMES procedures and then studied the effectiveness of their adapted protocol.

Often, through trial and error, clinicians find interesting solutions to clinical problems. These present a challenge to objectively document effects of treatment on specific patient populations. Treatments that are based in tradition or authority should also be examined, to test their underlying assumptions in the effort to support evidence-based practice. For instance, research has been unable to substantiate the effects of craniosacral therapy as a technique to assess pain and dysfunction.[2-4] In many cases, our empirical observations suggest that a treatment works and we do not feel a need to pursue documentation further; however, evidence-based practice requires systematic study of traditional treatment biases and a critical analysis of treatment alternatives.

Research problems may reflect a need to describe patterns of normal behaviors or the natural history of clinical phenomena. What values can we use to judge the degree of dysfunction we find in our patients? Does one clinical problem consistently accompany others? What is the natural progression of physical disability following a specific injury or onset of disease?

Questions about methodology are also of interest. How can we measure change? What tools are needed to document and diagnose patient problems? Many new instruments have been developed in recent years for measuring physical, physiological, and psychological performance. These need to be analyzed for reliability and validity under varied clinical conditions and on different patient groups.

Clinical Theory

Clinicians will often examine the theories that govern their practice as a source of research questions. Theories allow us to explain relationships and to predict outcomes based on given information (see Chapter 2); however, theories are applicable only to the extent that they can be empirically confirmed. For example, the validity and scope of theories that address motor control, motor learning, cognitive and physical development, neuromuscular function, language acquisition, personal interaction or compliance can be tested in clinical situations. To formulate a specific research question, a clinician must first examine the principles behind a theory and then determine what clinical outcomes would support or not support the theory. The answers will be the basis for a research question.

The International Classification of Functioning and Disability (ICF) is an example of a model that lends itself to important research questions.[5,6] Among the theoretical constructs that support the model, we can look at the relationship between positive (functioning) and negative (disability) aspects of activity and participation (see Chapter 1). For instance, researchers have focused on the relationships between measures of personal characteristics, impairment and activity/participation levels in patients with ankylosing spondylitis.[7] Results showed that impairment variables explained only a small portion of the activity and participation restrictions perceived by patients. Therefore, the researchers concluded that further research should identify how social, structural and attitudinal barriers (contextual factors) influence activity and participation in these patients.

Several researchers have begun to examine how specific instruments reflect the components of the ICF in the measurement of quality of life and function.[7-12] These studies have examined the theoretical construct of function, and have found that many instruments reflect all the dimensions of the ICF, while others do so in only a limited way. As clinicians and researchers select measuring tools, they must be aware of the components that are addressed in these instruments, and the potential areas that are not covered at all.[13] Once we understand the theoretical scope of our measurements, we can begin to ask questions that will verify how changes in body functions and structure (impairments) will directly or indirectly impact functional activities.

Professional Literature

Reference to professional literature plays an essential role in the delineation of a research problem and ultimately in deriving the specific research question. In the initial phases, the literature will help the researcher determine the issues of importance. Using this information, an initially broad or vague problem can begin to take a more structured and concise form. This initial review of the literature is preliminary and not necessarily extensive. The researcher will explore a variety of references on a particular subject and examine a breadth of materials to become oriented to practical and theoretical issues, as well as the kinds of variables or clinical problems that others have addressed.

Finding Gaps and Conflicts in the Literature

Professional literature provides the basis for developing a research problem in several ways. First, it will clarify holes in professional knowledge, areas where we do not have sufficient information for making clinical decisions. For example, Ingham and co-workers[14] were interested in the possible association between stuttering and speech effort, but they were not able to find studies that addressed this relationship. They did find, however, several studies that showed successful treatment for stuttering through prolonged speech, such as chorus reading. This led them to an investigation of the effect of chorus reading on self-rated speech effort in adult stuttering speakers and normally fluent control participants.

Another common source of ideas derives from conflicts in the literature, when studies present contradictory findings. For instance, many researchers have looked at the effect of patellar taping for reduction of pain associated with patellofemoral syndromes. However, studies have variously shown significant effects, short-lived effects, or no change in patellar alignment. Whittingham and colleagues[15] addressed this inconsistent evidence by designing a randomized trial to investigate the effect of exercise and taping on pain and function in patients with knee pain.

Professional literature may also identify disagreements due to differences or flaws in study design or measurement methods. For example, a systematic review of the efficacy and safety of common interventions for tears of the rotator cuff in adults showed little evidence to support or refute the superiority of conservative or surgical interventions.[16] This supports the need for well designed clinical trials that incorporate consistent methods for defining interventions and validated outcome measures.

Research questions may also arise out of data from descriptive studies, which document trends, patterns or characteristics that can subsequently be examined more thoroughly using alternative research approaches. For example, several descriptive studies have documented characteristics of individuals who have suffered spinal cord injuries. These studies have provided the foundation for testing new devices to improve function.[17]

Replication

In many instances, replication of a study is a useful strategy to correct for design limitations or to examine outcomes with different populations or in different settings. A study may be repeated using the same variables and methods or slight variations of them. Replication is an extremely important process in research, because one study is never sufficient to confirm a theory or to verify the success or failure of a treatment. We are often unable to generalize findings of one study to a larger population because of the limitations of small sample size in clinical studies. Therefore, the more studies we find that support a particular outcome, the more confidence we can have in the validity of those findings. As an example, Miltner and co-workers[18] studied the effects of constraint-induced movement therapy in patients with chronic stroke. They cited previous research in American laboratories showing success of this intervention to improve use of the affected upper extremity. They were able to replicate these results in Germany, where the health care system and context of therapy is different than in the United States.

Although many authors conclude research papers with a recommendation for further study, researchers do not often take up that challenge.[19] Because we recognize the uncertainty and variation that can be part of each study, it is necessary to demonstrate consistency of findings across settings and samples, to confirm an intervention's effectiveness or a test's diagnostic validity. Replication is essential for adding strength to our efforts for evidence-based practice.

That said, it is also important to consider the limits of replication as a useful strategy. There will come a point when the question must move on, to further knowledge, not just repeat it. Fergusson and co-workers[20] provide an illustration of this point in their discussion of the use of aprotinin to reduce perioperative blood loss. Through meta-analysis, they showed that 64 trials on the drug's effectiveness were published between 1987 and 2002, although the effectiveness had been thoroughly documented by 1992 after 12 trials. They suggested that the following 52 trials were unnecessary, wasteful and even unethical, and that authors "were not adequately citing previous research, resulting in a large number of RCTs being conducted to address efficacy questions that prior trials had already definitively answered."[20] Replication is a reasonable approach when prior research has not yet arrived at that threshold.

IMPORTANCE AND FEASIBILITY OF THE RESEARCH QUESTION

Throughout the process of identifying and refining a research question, three general criteria should be considered to determine that it is worth pursuing: The question should be important, answerable and feasible for study.

The Question Should Be Important: The "So What?" Test

Clinical research should have potential impact on treatment, on theoretical foundations, or on policies related to practice. Basic research should address questions that contribute to scientific knowledge and theory. Because of the commitment of time and resources required for research, a researcher should believe that the effort is worthy of investigation, that is, it should generate new information that will further the profession's knowledge base. Although it is important to keep a project simple and direct, it should not be so trivial as to make no difference to anyone. Researchers should consider if the outcomes of the study will resolve inconsistencies in previous research, or if they will contribute to explanations of clinical theory. It may be relevant to ask how often this clinical problem occurs in practice. Will the findings provide useful information for clinical decision making or be generalizable to other clinical situations?

Statements that support the importance of the research question are often considered the *justification* for a study. We often say that the research question must be able to pass the "so what?" test; that is, the results should be meaningful and useful. Researchers should look at trends in practice and health care to identify those problems that have clinical or professional significance for contributing to evidence-based practice.

The Question Should Be Answerable

Not all questions can be studied scientifically. For instance, questions involving judgments or philosophical issues are often difficult to study. We should not consider asking, "Are all patients entitled to treatment regardless of their ability to pay for services?" If this issue is of interest, however, related questions can be investigated: "What is the extent of health insurance coverage for different age groups or socioeconomic groups?" "What types of treatments are being denied reimbursement by various insurers?" These questions are not the same as the original question, but they would provide related information that can be used by clinicians in considering the ethical and moral consequences of the issue.

Questions that begin with "why" are also difficult to answer using clinical research methods. Why does one treatment approach work better than another for reducing spasticity? The answer to such a question goes beyond the capability of clinical tools. Rather than asking why a patient responds a certain way to a treatment, we can document that a treatment does or does not change the level of response and examine whether that response supports a particular theory of spasticity. Similarly, it is not the function of science to judge if one or another treatment is "preferable." Such judgments reflect personal values but are not based on research evidence.

The research problem should also incorporate variables that can be defined and measured. Consider the question, "How can we improve a patient's motivation to exercise?" How can we define the term "motivation"? What criteria can be established to assess that a person is motivated? How will those who are motivated be distinguished from those who are not? Motivation becomes a construct for which some relevant measure must be identified. If a variable cannot be adequately defined, it cannot be studied.

The Study Should Be Feasible

Many factors influence the feasibility of a research study. The researcher must have the necessary skill, background and resources to be able to complete the project properly. In many cases, consultants and advisors will be needed for technical and statistical assistance. Can a realistic timetable be developed? Pilot studies are helpful for estimating the time requirements of a study. Are sufficient numbers of subjects available, and can they be counted on to participate? Problems often occur when patients are discharged or develop medical complications that prevent their participation. What type of space is needed to carry out the project, and when will it be available? Can the necessary equipment be obtained? Does the project have the necessary administrative or budgetary support? Lastly, are the rights of subjects being protected? The researcher must determine risks and benefits, and be able to justify the demands placed on the subject during data collection (see Chapter 3). These considerations must be addressed prior to continuing with plans for a study. Many questions will be refocused by the practicalities of the process.

TARGET POPULATION

As we proceed with the development of a research question, we must identify *who* we want to study. The **target population** refers to the group of individuals to which the results of the study will apply. It represents the totality of all members of this group who conform to a designated set of specifications. For example, suppose we are interested in studying the effectiveness of electrical stimulation for increasing muscle strength. We could designate a healthy population of "normal" subjects as our population, or we could select patients with total knee replacements or ACL reconstruction. But further restriction may be necessary to make this designation clear. Once again, the literature is a consistent source of information for decision making. Should the subjects be within a certain age range? Will we include males and females? Should we specify a time since onset of pain or surgery? Is the cause of the knee surgery a relevant factor? Does it matter if symptoms are unilateral or bilateral? Other considerations may be based on availability of patients. For instance, the age range of the population may be dictated by the age range of patients at the researcher's facility. We might specify a general target population of otherwise healthy males between 20 and 40 years of age with no prior history of orthopedic or neuromuscular dysfunction, who have had an ACL repair within the last 6 months. The definition of the target population should be sufficiently clear and complete that it will be obvious who will and who will not be considered a member (see Chapter 8).

THE RESEARCH RATIONALE

Once the research problem has been defined, a full review of literature will establish the background for the research question. This foundation will clarify the **research rationale** that will support the research question, guide decisions in designing the study, and most importantly, provide the basis for interpreting results. The rationale presents a logical argument that shows how and why the question was developed. It provides a **theoretical framework** by explaining the constructs and mechanisms behind the question. It helps us understand why the question makes sense. The research rationale includes references to previous research as well as logical assumptions that can be made from current theory. Without a strong rationale, the results of a study will be hard to interpret.

For example, many researchers have looked at the effectiveness of electrical stimulation for increasing muscle strength in healthy and patient populations. Some studies have looked at the comparison of neuromuscular electrical stimulation (NMES) and voluntary exercise. The research rationale for these studies focuses on the suggested mechanisms for this effect.[21] Why should electrical stimulation be expected to produce strength gains? One explanation proposes that training with NMES is similar to strengthening with voluntary exercise in terms of muscle physiology. If this is true, then we should be able to observe comparable strength gains with each technique, and the protocol for strengthening with NMES should follow currently accepted guidelines for voluntary exercise, including number of repetitions and load. Another mechanism suggests that NMES selectively recruits high force muscle fibers, thereby increasing muscle strength. Researchers have used this rationale as the basis for comparing the recruitment order of fast and slow twitch muscle fibers during NMES and voluntary exercise. The study rationale, therefore, incorporates current knowledge of muscle physiology, theories related to how muscle increases functional strength, the physiological properties of neuromuscular electrical stimulation and an understanding of what other studies have been able to demonstrate. These concepts form a logical foundation for the research question.

VARIABLES

Now we must specify *what* we want to test. **Variables** are the building blocks of the research question. A variable is a property that can differentiate members of a group or set. It represents a concept, or **factor,** that can have more than one *value*. By definition, variables are characteristics that can vary. A factor becomes a variable by virtue of how it is used in a study. For instance, if we wanted to compare levels of back pain between men and women, then pain and gender are the variables of interest. Pain can take on a range of values, depending on how we measure it, and gender can take on two "values" (male and female). If, however, in another study, we compare the effects of two different treatments for decreasing back pain in men, then gender is no longer a variable. It has only one "value" (male) and is, therefore, a constant. In this latter example, type of treatment and pain are the variables of interest.

Research is performed to examine the relationship among variables or describe how variables exist in nature. In descriptive and correlational studies, variables represent the phenomena being examined, and their measurement may take many forms. The investigator looks at these characteristics one at a time, describes their values and their interrelationships. In exploratory and experimental studies the investigator examines relationships among two or more variables to predict outcomes or to establish that one variable influences another. For these types of studies, research variables are generally classified as independent or dependent, according to how they are used.

Independent and Dependent Variables

A predictor variable is an **independent variable**. It is a condition, intervention or characteristic that will predict or cause a given outcome. The outcome variable is called the **dependent variable**, which is a response or effect that is presumed to vary depending on the independent variable.

In exploratory studies, independent and dependent variables are usually measured together, to determine if they have a predictive relationship. For example, researchers have studied the relationship between back pain and age, gender, cognitive status, ambulatory status, analgesic use, osteoporosis and osteoarthritis in a long-term care population.[22] The dependent variable (the outcome variable) was the presence of back pain and the independent variables (predictor variables) were the characteristics of age, gender, cognitive status and so on. These types of studies often involve several independent variables, as the researcher tries to establish how different factors interrelate to explain the outcome variable.

Experimental studies involve comparison of different conditions to investigate causal relationships, where the independent variable is controlled and the dependent variable is measured. For instance, researchers have compared the effect of a back class versus usual medical care to determine if the back class was an effective program for reducing pain in those with acute low back pain.[23] Outcomes included changes in a disability score and a pain scale rating. In this example the independent variable is the back class (intervention), and the two dependent variables are the disability and pain scores (response). A change in the dependent variables is presumed to be caused by the "value" of the independent variable; that is, the dependent variable is a function of the condition of the independent variable.

Comparative studies can be designed with more than one independent variable. We could look at the patients' gender in addition to intervention, for instance, to determine if effectiveness of a back class is different for males and females. We would then have two independent variables: type of intervention and gender. A study can also have more than one dependent variable. In the previously mentioned study, researchers measured both disability rating and pain.

Levels of the Independent Variable

In comparative studies, independent variables are given "values" called **levels**. The levels represent groups or conditions that will be compared. Every independent variable will have at least two levels. Dependent variables are not described as having levels.

For example, in the study comparing a back class and usual care, the independent variable of "intervention" has two levels: back class and usual care. If the study had included additional interventions, such as physical therapy or bed rest, it would have changed the number of *levels* of the intervention variable, not the number of variables.

Operational Definitions

Once the variables of interest have been identified, the researcher still faces some major decisions. Exactly what procedures will be used? If we are interested in studying the effects of different interventions on back pain, exactly what will the interventions be? How will they be applied? How will we measure a change in back pain? Are we interested in pain at the time that treatment begins or when it ends? On the same day or later in the week? What aspect of pain should we measure? As the research question continues to be refined we continually refer to the literature and our clinical experience to make these judgments. How often will subjects be treated? In what position will the subjects be tested? How often will they be tested? These questions must be answered before adequate definitions of variables are developed.

Variables must be defined in terms that explain how they will be used in the study. For research purposes, we distinguish between conceptual definitions and operational definitions. A *conceptual definition* is the dictionary definition, one that describes the variable in general terms, without specific reference to its methodological use in a study. For instance, "back pain" can be defined as the degree of discomfort in the back. This definition is useless, however, for research purposes because it does not tell us what measure of discomfort is used or how we could interpret discomfort.

In contrast, an **operational definition** defines a variable according to its unique meaning within a study (see Box 7.1). The operational definition should be sufficiently detailed that another researcher could replicate the procedure or condition. Independent variables are operationalized according to how they are manipulated by the investigator. For example, in the study comparing a back class and usual care, an operational

BOX 7.1 **The Relevance of Operational Definitions**

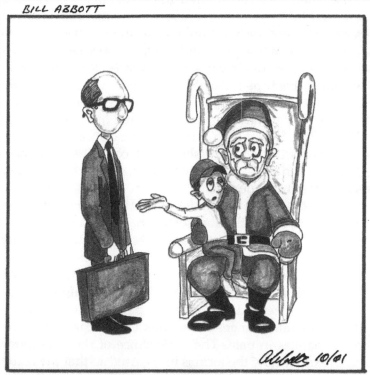

BILL ABBOTT

"and this is Mort, my attorney, who will help us to accurately define naughty"

Source: www.CartoonStock.com

definition for the independent variable "back class" should include the number of sessions, the type of training and materials, expectations of compliance, who will teach the class and so on. The subjects' activities and other treatment specifications should be included. We also need to describe the control group's activities of usual care. Operational definitions for independent variables must differentiate the various levels of the variable.

Dependent variables are operationally defined by describing the method of measurement, including delineation of tools and procedures used to obtain measurements. A variable like "low back pain" could be defined operationally as the score on a visual analog scale (VAS), reflecting the magnitude of pain at a particular time of day under specific activity conditions. An individual reading this definition should be able to know precisely how the variable "pain" could be interpreted in this study.

Some variables do not require substantial operational definitions. The application of the term *age*, for example, is readily understood, as is the identification of male and female. It is usually sufficient to define variables such as height and weight simply by specifying units of measurement and the type of measuring instrument. Some variables can be defined according to standardized criteria, such as manual muscle tests and intelligence; however, many variables whose definitions appear self-evident still present sufficient possibilities for variation that they require explanation. Consider the concept of hand preference. We often take for granted the designation of right-handed or left-handed. But when used in a study that concerns laterality, this may not be sufficient. Some researchers might accept the hand used for writing as the preferred hand. Others may want to include mixed handedness, and use a standardized test for dominance.

There are many examples of concepts for which multiple measurements may be acceptable. For example, back pain can be measured using a VAS, the McGill Pain Questionnaire, or the Oswestry Disability Rating Scale. The results of studies using these different tools would be analyzed and interpreted quite differently because of the different information provided by each form. The measurement properties, feasibility of use and sensitivity of an instrument should be considered in choosing the most appropriate dependent variable. A comparison of measurement methods can also become the basis for a research question.

There may be instances when the reader of a research report does not agree with the validity of an operational definition set forth by an investigator. For example, researchers have examined changes in pain as a function of decreased usage of medication;[24] others have considered greater active joint range of motion a useful indicator.[25] These investigators have made certain assumptions about the relationship between pain and intake of medication or mobility. Some clinicians might argue, however, that these measures could be influenced by a subject's pain tolerance and that a more stoic individual might demonstrate changes in the measured variable that are not necessarily representative of changes in pain. The importance of the operational definition is that it communicates exactly how the term is being used so that the reader understands the researcher's conceptualization of the variable and the implications of the findings. Whatever measure is chosen will reflect only certain characteristics of the construct, and thereby influence our interpretation of changes. It is the researcher's responsibility to justify the operational definition in terms of the purpose of the research.

RESEARCH OBJECTIVES

The final step in delineating a researchable question is to clarify the objective of the study. This is the culmination of all the reasoning and reading that has gone before to determine the target population, describe the research rationale and define the research variables. The objectives may be presented as **hypotheses**, **specific aims**, the **purpose** of the research or the **research objectives**. The terms used will vary among researchers, journals and disciplines. Most important, however, this statement must specifically and concisely delineate what the study is expected to accomplish.

There are four general types of research objectives:

1. The intent of the study may be *descriptive,* in an effort to characterize clinical phenomena or existing conditions in a particular population.

2. Many research problems stem from the lack of appropriate *measuring instruments* to document outcomes. Studies may involve the investigation of reliability and validity in measuring tools to determine how different instruments can be used meaningfully for clinical decision making. Sometimes the problem will address different uses of a known tool, and other times it will suggest the need for a new instrument.

3. A third type of research objective is the *exploration of relationships* to determine how clinical phenomena interact. By determining these relationships, studies can suggest risk factors that contribute to impaired function and provide ideas for prevention and treatment options.

4. The study may be based on a *comparison*, in an attempt to define a cause-and-effect relationship using an experimental model. This type of study evaluates differences between groups or the effectiveness of interventions.

The choice of one of these approaches will frame the research design, the types of data collection that will be appropriate, and the applicable data analysis procedures. Each of these approaches is examined in detail in subsequent chapters.

Specific Aims

Descriptive studies will usually be based on **specific aims** or **guiding questions** that describe the study's purpose. For instance, researchers may specify that they want to describe attitudes about a particular issue, the demographic profile of a given patient group, or the natural progression of a disease. Survey researchers will design a set of questions to organize a questionnaire. Because descriptive studies have no fixed design, it is important to put structure into place. Setting specific aims or guiding questions allows the researcher to organize data and discuss findings in a meaningful way.

Hypotheses

For experimental investigations and many exploratory studies involving the examination of relationships, the researcher must be more precise in setting expectations. This requires that the researcher propose an educated guess about the outcome of the study. This guess is presented as a statement called a **hypothesis:** a declarative statement that predicts the relationship between the independent and dependent variables, specifying the population that will be studied. The purpose of the study is to test the hypothesis and, ultimately, to provide evidence so that the researcher can accept or reject it. The researcher generally formulates a **research hypothesis** following identification of the problem, a review of relevant literature and final conceptualization of the research variables. A research question might ask: Is knee range of motion improved by the addition of continuous passive motion (CPM) to a postoperative rehabilitation program following total knee replacement?[26] The clinical researcher may then hypothesize that "Knee range of motion in flexion and extension at time of discharge will be greater for patients who receive CPM following total knee replacement than for those who do not receive CPM." Hypotheses are developed at the outset to provide a definitive structure for the investigation by assisting the researcher in planning the design and methods and in determining the data analysis procedures. Hypotheses also provide the reader of a research report with an understanding of what the researcher was expecting to find.

Characteristics of Hypotheses

Useful hypotheses can be evaluated according to several criteria. Consider the statement:

> Patients with total knee replacements who receive CPM following surgery will have fewer postoperative complications.

This statement includes a reference to a target population, but is not complete because it contains only one variable, the number of postoperative complications. CPM treatment is not a variable in this statement because only one condition is presented. We can modify the statement to express a relationship and thereby make it a complete hypothesis:

> Patients with total knee replacements who receive CPM following surgery will have fewer postoperative complications than patients who do not receive CPM.

Now CPM is an independent variable, with two levels. We will be able to distinguish the responses of those patients who receive CPM from those who do not. Hypotheses usually incorporate phrases such as "greater than," "less than," "different from" or "related to" as a way of indicating the type of relationship that is being examined.

An acceptable hypothesis must be testable and should be based on a sound rationale. This implies that a body of knowledge exists that will support the hypothesis. A researcher does not propose a hypothesis purely on the basis of speculation. Hypotheses can be derived from theory or suggested from previous research, clinical experience, or observation. **Deductive hypotheses** are based on a theoretical premise, allowing the clinician to predict what outcomes would be expected under a given set of conditions. When contradictions exist in the literature researchers must examine these variances to draw relevant parallels with their own research questions. **Inductive hypotheses** are based on trends, regularities, patterns, or relationships that are observed in clinical practice. Clinicians can also use other sources of knowledge, such as authority, tradition, and trial and error, as a basis for formulating a hypothesis. When a new area is being addressed, the researcher's own experiences and logical reasoning may be the only foundation available.

Stating the Hypothesis

A **research hypothesis** states the researcher's true expectation of results, guiding the interpretation of outcomes and conclusions. Analysis of data is based on testing a statistical hypothesis, which differs from the research hypothesis in that it will always express no difference or no relationship between the independent and dependent variables. The statistical hypothesis is called the **null hypothesis** (see Chapter 18).

Researchers use a great deal of flexibility in the phrasing of research hypotheses. The same research problem can be translated into a hypothesis in different ways. Some research hypotheses predict *no difference* between variables:

1. There is no difference in perceived learning between students enrolled in online classes and those enrolled in on-campus courses.[27]

More often, research hypotheses propose a relationship in terms of a difference:

2. There will be a difference in expressive language scores at 6 and 12 months in preschool children with language delay who receive routine speech and language therapy as compared to those who are managed with a strategy of watchful waiting.[28]

Hypotheses 1 and 2 are considered **nondirectional hypotheses** because they do not predict a direction of change. In other cases, a researcher will have a definite idea about the expected direction of outcomes. Consider the following hypotheses:

3. Children with cerebral palsy who receive botulinum toxin A injections in combination with serial casting will have significantly faster resolution of contracture, greater reduction of spasticity, and greater improvement in gross motor function when compared with children who receive casting alone.[29]

4. Patients with chronic plantar fasciitis who are managed with a structure-specific plantar fascia-stretching program for eight weeks have a better functional outcome than do patients managed with a standard Achilles tendon-stretching protocol.[30]

These are examples of **directional hypotheses**. They not only describe the relationship between variables in terms of a difference, but they also assign a direction to that difference.

Hypotheses can also be phrased to predict a *relationship,* between variables, rather than a *difference,* as illustrated by the following:

5. There is an association between decreased length of stay and reduced functional status at follow-up for patients receiving inpatient rehabilitation.[31]

6. Improvements in exercise capacity following training programs for patients with chronic obstructive pulmonary disorders are related to changes in body composition.[32]

Hypothesis 5 is considered directional because the authors predict the presence of a relationship between two variables and the direction of that relationship. We can expect that patients with a shorter length of stay will tend to have poorer function. Hypothesis 6 does not tell us the expected direction of the proposed relationship.

Research hypotheses can be phrased in simple or complex forms. A **simple hypothesis** includes one independent variable and one dependent variable. For example, Hypotheses 1, 4, 5 and 6 are simple hypotheses. A **complex hypothesis** contains more than one independent or dependent variable. Hypotheses 2 and 3 contain several dependent variables. Complex hypotheses are often nondirectional because of the potential difficulty in clarifying multiple relationships. Complex hypotheses are efficient for expressing expected research outcomes in a research report, but they cannot be tested. Therefore, for analysis purposes, such statements must be broken down into several simple hypotheses. Several hypotheses can be addressed within a single study.

REVIEWING THE LITERATURE

Every research question can be considered an extension of all the thinking and investigation that has gone before it. The results of each study contribute to that accumulated knowledge and thereby stimulate further research. For this process to work, researchers must be able to identify prior relevant research and theory. This is accomplished through the **review of literature.** The review of literature is usually conducted in two phases. The initial review is a preliminary one, intended to achieve a general understanding of the state of knowledge in the area of interest. Once the research problem has been clearly formulated, however, the researcher begins a full and extensive review. This will provide a detailed and complete understanding of the relevant background to assist in formulating the research question.

A review of literature provides the foundation for a research study. It helps us understand what is already known, what has already been done (successfully or unsuccessfully) and how we can contribute further to the current state of knowledge. Conducting a thorough and successful search for relevant references is an essential first step in this process. Strategies for carrying out a literature search are described in Chapter 31.

The review of literature is not the same as a systematic review, which is a critical analysis of a set of studies focused on a particular clinical issue for use in evidence-based decision-making. Systematic reviews, however, may be part of a review of literature. Systematic reviews will be covered in detail in Chapter 16.

Scope of the Review of Literature

Clinicians and students are often faced with a dilemma in starting a review of literature in terms of how extensive a review is necessary. How does a researcher know when a sufficient amount of material has been read? There is no magic formula to determine that 20, 50 or 100 articles will provide the necessary background for a project. The number of references needed for a review depends first on the researcher's familiarity with the topic. A beginning researcher may have limited knowledge and experience, and might have to cover a wider range of materials to feel comfortable with the information.

In addition, the scope of the review will depend on how much research has been done in the area, and how many relevant references are available. Obviously, when a topic is new and has been studied only minimally, fewer materials will exist. In that situation, it is necessary to look at studies that support the theoretical framework for a question. When a topic has been researched extensively, the researcher need only choose a representative sample of articles to provide sufficient background. The important consideration is the relevancy of the literature, not the quantity. Researchers will always read more than they will finally report in the written review of literature.

The review of literature should focus on several aspects of the study. As we have already discussed, the researcher tries to establish a theoretical framework for the study based on generalizations from other studies. It is often necessary to review material on the patient population, to understand the underlying pathology that is being studied. Researchers should also look for information on methods, including equipment used and operational definitions of variables. Often it is helpful to replicate procedures from previous studies so that results have a basis for comparison. It may be helpful to see what statistical techniques have been used by others for the same reason.

Literature also provides the basis for validating assumptions. **Assumptions** are concepts or principles that are assumed to be true, based on documented evidence of accepted theoretical premises. Assumptions allow us to go on with our research without having to document every aspect of our procedures. For instance, if a study involves strength testing over several trials, the research protocol might call for a 2-minute rest between trials, based on the assumption that this time interval will be sufficient to avoid fatigue effects. This assumption can be validated by reviewing the literature on fatigue and recovery rates, rather than testing it on every subject.

The review of literature should be as up-to-date as possible, but should include some classical works as well. It is generally practical, however, to limit the review of older studies, so as not to review every historic document in the field. The review should cover all relevant studies, even if findings are contradictory to the study's objectives. It is helpful to check the reference lists at the end of recent articles. As more and more is read, the researcher will begin to find the same references cited again and again, and will have an indication that most relevant sources have been obtained.

Primary and Secondary Sources

It is important to differentiate the roles of primary and secondary sources in a review of literature. A **primary source** is a report or document provided directly by the person who authored it. Most research articles in professional journals are primary sources, as are oral presentations of direct research results, diaries, interviews and eyewitness accounts. A **secondary source** is a description or review of one or more studies presented by someone other than the original author. Review articles and most textbooks are secondary sources, as are newspaper accounts and biographies.*

Both primary and secondary references are important to the literature review; however, secondary references should not be considered substitutes for primary sources. They are most useful for providing bibliographical information on relevant primary sources. Beginning researchers should try to avoid the temptation to rely solely on secondary sources just because they conveniently summarize many studies. Secondary references often provide insufficient, inaccurate or biased information about other studies. Researchers are often amazed when they go back to a primary source to discover how different their own interpretation of results can be from those that are provided in review articles.

---

*Systematic reviews and meta-analyses, which include critical analyses of published works, are technically secondary references. They do become primary sources, however, as a form of research in generating new knowledge through the synthesis of previous research.

As another consideration in choosing references, researchers should know whether a journal is refereed. This means that articles are reviewed by content experts before being accepted for publication. Refereed journals generally require several levels of review and revision prior to publication, although this is no guarantee of validity. Papers in nonrefereed journals do not undergo this scrutiny.

Organizing the Review of Literature

Because the review of literature can be extensive, researchers usually find it helpful to establish a process for organizing and notating references as they read them. The first step is to identify the relevant information from each reference. The research question, key elements of the method, findings and conclusions should be summarized. If a reference is being used for a specific purpose, such as a description of a particular outcome instrument, this should be indicated. The researcher should critique each article for validity of design and measurement, and record critical comments. The summary should include how data were analyzed and a description of the pertinent results.

The researcher should take note of how each article is related to the research study and to other articles. This information will be invaluable when writing a review of literature for an article or thesis. It will allow the researcher to look through reference summaries and find those studies that present similar or conflicting information (see Chapter 33). Some people keep these records on index cards for each article. More recently, researchers have begun to take advantage of bibliographic management programs such as RefWorks® or EndNote® that provide a structure for cataloging references by author, title or keywords.[†] These tools allow the researcher to develop a personal database of references in one or more electronic libraries. They are designed to be compatible with most word processing programs. They store many types of information, can insert citations and generate and format bibliographies or reference lists in a written report. Most of these programs allow the researcher to download and import full references, including abstracts, from electronic databases.

COMMENTARY

Putting the Horse Before the Cart

Research is about answering questions. But before we can get to the answers, we must be able to ask the right question. What we ask will depend on our goal. If we are looking for information to direct a clinical decision for a particular patient problem, we must ask a question that allows us to focus a literature search on relevant evidence. If we are asking a question to structure a research study, we must determine appropriate variables, designs and methods. In either case, we will use our clinical judgment in concert with the literature to guide this process. We must be careful to distinguish these two types of questions, however. The research question, the focus of this chapter, creates a framework for a study based on a perceived gap

---

[†]For RefWorks® go to <http://www.refworks.com>; for information on Endnote® Thomson Corporation, go to http://www.endnote.com.

in knowledge, whereas an evidence-based question concerns information relevant to a specific clinical situation or patient. Asking a good evidence-based question is essential to good clinical decision making.

From a research standpoint, it is no exaggeration to speak of the extreme importance of the development of the right question. Albert Einstein[33] once wrote:

> The formation of a problem is far more often essential than its solution . . . to raise new questions, new possibilities, to regard old problems from a new angle, requires creative imagination and marks real advance in science.

This process is often arduous and painstaking; however, it forms the foundation for all that will follow and crystallizes the researcher's expectations for results. The research question is developed in detail in a research proposal, which provides a specific and comprehensive outline of the entire research project, including the delineation of variables and operational definitions, and a review of literature that forms the background for the study and the hypotheses (see Chapter 32). A strong research study addresses questions that are spelled out clearly and that lead to conclusions within the limits of the research design. If the question is too vague, it cannot guide the development of data collection or analytic methods.

In the process of doing research, novice researchers will often jump to a methodology and design, eager to collect data and analyze it. It is an unfortunate situation, that has occurred all too often in our experience, when a researcher has invested hours of work and has obtained reams of data, and cannot figure out what to do with the information. There is nothing more frustrating than a statistical consultant trying to figure out what analysis to perform, and asking the researcher, "What is the question you are trying to answer?" The frustrating part is when the researcher realizes that the question cannot be answered with the data that were collected. Beginning researchers often "spin their wheels" as they search for what to measure, rather than starting their search with the delineation of a specific and relevant question. It doesn't matter how complex or simple the design, it is not as important to know how to answer the question as it is to know how to ask the question.[34]

REFERENCES

1. Fitzgerald GK, Piva SR, Irrgang JJ. A modified neuromuscular electrical stimulation protocol for quadriceps strength training following anterior cruciate ligament reconstruction. *J Orthop Sports Phys Ther* 2003;33:492–501.
2. Moran RW, Gibbons P. Intraexaminer and interexaminer reliability for palpation of the cranial rhythmic impulse at the head and sacrum. *J Manipulative Physiol Ther* 2001;24: 183–190.
3. Green C, Martin CW, Bassett K, Kazanjian A. A systematic review of craniosacral therapy: Biological plausibility, assessment reliability and clinical effectiveness. *Complement Ther Med* 1999;7:201–207.
4. Rogers JS, Witt PL, Gross MT, Hacke JD, Genova PA. Simultaneous palpation of the craniosacral rate at the head and feet: intrarater and interrater reliability and rate comparisons. *Phys Ther* 1998;78:1175–1185.

5. World Health Organization. *International Classification of Functioning, Disability and Health.* Geneva: World Health Organization, 2001.
6. Stucki G. International Classification of Functioning, Disability and Health (ICF): A promising framework and classification for rehabilitation medicine. *Am J Phys Med Rehabil* 2005;84:733–740.
7. Dagfinrud H, Kjeken I, Mowinckel P, Hagen KB, Kvien TK. Impact of functional impairment in ankylosing spondylitis: Impairment, activity limitation, and participation restrictions. *J Rheumatol* 2005;32:516–523.
8. Brockow T, Duddeck K, Geyh S, Schwarzkopf S, Weigl M, Franke T, et al. Identifying the concepts contained in outcome measures of clinical trials on breast cancer using the International Classification of Functioning, Disability and Health as a reference. *J Rehabil Med* 2004:43–48.
9. Geyh S, Kurt T, Brockow T, Cieza A, Ewert T, Omar Z, et al. Identifying the concepts contained in outcome measures of clinical trials on stroke using the International Classification of Functioning, Disability and Health as a reference. *J Rehabil Med* 2004:56–62.
10. Jette AM, Haley SM, Kooyoomjian JT. Are the ICF Activity and Participation dimensions distinct? *J Rehabil Med* 2003;35:145–149.
11. Mayo NE, Poissant L, Ahmed S, Finch L, Higgins J, Salbach NM, et al. Incorporating the International Classification of Functioning, Disability, and Health (ICF) into an electronic health record to create indicators of function: Proof of concept using the SF-12. *J Am Med Inform Assoc* 2004;11:514–522.
12. Salter K, Jutai JW, Teasell R, Foley NC, Bitensky J, Bayley M. Issues for selection of outcome measures in stroke rehabilitation: ICF activity. *Disabil Rehabil* 2005;27:315–340.
13. Stamm TA, Cieza A, Machold KP, Smolen JS, Stucki G. Content comparison of occupation-based instruments in adult rheumatology and musculoskeletal rehabilitation based on the International Classification of Functioning, Disability and Health. *Arthritis Rheum* 2004;51:917–924.
14. Ingham RJ, Warner A, Byrd A, Cotton J. Speech effort measurement and stuttering: Investigating the chorus reading effect. *J Speech Hearing Disorders* 2006;49:660–670.
15. Whittingham M, Palmer S, Macmillan F. Effects of taping on pain and function in patellofemoral pain syndrome: A randomized controlled trial. *J Orthop Sports Phys Ther* 2004;34:504–510.
16. Ejnisman B, Andreoli CV, Soares BG, Fallopa F, Peccin MS, Abdalla RJ, et al. Interventions for tears of the rotator cuff in adults. *Cochrane Database Syst Rev* 2004:CD002758.
17. Mulcahey MJ, Betz RR, Smith BT, Weiss AA, Davis SE. Implanted functional electrical stimulation hand system in adolescents with spinal injuries: An evaluation. *Arch Phys Med Rehabil* 1997;78:597–607.
18. Miltner WH, Bauder H, Sommer M, Dettmers C, Taub E. Effects of constraint-induced movement therapy on patients with chronic motor deficits after stroke: A replication. *Stroke* 1999;30:586–592.
19. Klein JG, Brown GT, Lysyk M. Replication research: a purposeful occupation worth repeating. *Can J Occup Ther* 2000;67:155–161.
20. Fergusson D, Glass K, Hutton B, Shapiro S. Randomized controlled trials of aprotinin in cardiac surgery: Could clinical equipoise have stopped the bleeding? *Clin Trials* 2005;2:218–232.
21. Requena Sanchez B, Padial Puche P, Gonzalez-Badillo JJ. Percutaneous electrical stimulation in strength training: An update. *J Strength Cond Res* 2005;19:438–448.
22. D'Astolfo CJ, Humphreys BK. A record review of reported musculoskeletal pain in an Ontario long term care facility. *BMC Geriatr* 2006;6:5.

23. Underwood MR, Morgan J. The use of a back class teaching extension exercises in the treatment of acute low back pain in primary care. *Fam Pract* 1998;15:9–15.

24. Hollinger JL. Transcutaneous electrical nerve stimulation after cesarean birth. *Phys Ther* 1986;66:36–38.

25. Inaba MK, Piorkowski M. Ultrasound in treatment of painful shoulders in patients with hemiplegia. *Phys Ther* 1972;52:737–742.

26. Bennett LA, Brearley SC, Hart JA, Bailey MJ. A comparison of two continuous passive motion protocols after total knee arthroplasty: A controlled and randomized study. *J Arthroplasty* 2005;20:225–233.

27. Business communication: High-touch (on campus) vs. high tech (online) learning in Silicon Valley. Association for Business Communication Annual Convention, 2003, Albuquerque, NM. Association for Business Communication.

28. Glogowska M, Roulstone S, Enderby P, Peters TJ. Randomised controlled trial of community based speech and language therapy in preschool children. *BMJ* 2000;321:923–926.

29. Kay RM, Rethlefsen SA, Fern-Buneo A, Wren TA, Skaggs DL. Botulinum toxin as an adjunct to serial casting treatment in children with cerebral palsy. *J Bone Joint Surg Am* 2004;86-A:2377–2384.

30. DiGiovanni BF, Nawoczenski DA, Lintal ME, Moore EA, Murray JC, Wilding GE, et al. Tissue-specific plantar fascia-stretching exercise enhances outcomes in patients with chronic heel pain. A prospective, randomized study. *J Bone Joint Surg Am* 2003;85-A: 1270–1277.

31. Ottenbacher KJ, Smith PM, Illig SB, Linn RT, Ostir GV, Granger CV. Trends in length of stay, living setting, functional outcome, and mortality following medical rehabilitation. *JAMA* 2004;292:1687–1695.

32. Franssen FM, Broekhuizen R, Janssen PP, Wouters EF, Schols AM. Effects of whole-body exercise training on body composition and functional capacity in normal-weight patients with COPD. *Chest* 2004;125:2021–2028.

33. Einstein A, Infield L. *The Evolution of Physics*. New York: Simon and Schuster, 1938.

34. Findley TW. Research in physical medicine and rehabilitation. I. How to ask the question. *Am J Phys Med Rehabil* 1991;70 (Suppl):S11–S16.

CHAPTER 8
Sampling

In the process of defining a research question, the researcher must also decide who will be studied. The goal, of course, will be to make generalizations beyond the individuals studied to others with similar conditions or characteristics. Generalization is basic to all types of research, where scientists continually draw conclusions about human behavior and the environment based on limited experiences and measurements. The purpose of this chapter is to describe how the responses of a small representative group can be used with confidence to make predictions about the larger world.

POPULATIONS AND SAMPLES

The larger group to which research results are generalized is called the **population**. A population is a defined aggregate of persons, objects or events that meet a specified set of criteria. For instance, if we were interested in studying the effects of various treatments for osteoarthritis, the population of interest would be all people in the world who have osteoarthritis; however, it is not reasonable to test every person who has osteoarthritis. Working with smaller groups is generally more economical, more time efficient, and potentially more accurate than working with large groups because it affords better control of measurement. Therefore, through a process of *sampling*, a researcher chooses a subgroup of the population, called a **sample**. This sample serves as the reference group for estimating characteristics of or drawing conclusions about the population.

Populations are not necessarily restricted to human subjects. Researchers may be interested in studying characteristics of institutions or geographical areas, and these may be the units that define the population. In test–retest reliability studies, the population will consist of an infinite series of measurements. The sample would be the actual measurements taken. An epidemiological study may focus on blood samples. Industrial quality control studies use samples of items from the entire inventory of a particular manufacturing lot. Surveys often sample households from a population of housing units. A population can include people, places, organizations, objects, animals, days or any other unit of interest.

Sampling Bias

To make generalizations, the researcher must be able to assume that the responses of sample members will be representative of how the population members would respond in similar circumstances. Human populations are, by nature, heterogeneous, and the variations that exist in behavioral, psychological or physical attributes should also be present in a sample. Theoretically, a good sample reflects the relevant characteristics and variations of the population in the same proportions as they exist in the population.

Although there is no way to guarantee that a sample will be representative of a population, sampling procedures can minimize the degree of bias or error in choosing a sample. It is not so much the size of a sample that is of concern. A small representative sample of 50 may be preferable to an unrepresentative sample of 1,000. For example, in 1968 the Gallup and Harris polls predicted that Richard Nixon would receive 43% and 41% of the popular vote, respectively, based on samples of only 2,000 voters. Nixon actually received 42.9%.[1] In contrast, a 1936 Literary Digest poll predicted that Alf Landon would win the presidential election based on the preference of over 2 million voters, chosen from lists of automobile owners and telephone directories. Although 57% of the respondents indicated they would vote for Alf Landon, Franklin Roosevelt was elected by the largest margin in history up to that time. Roosevelt's support came primarily from lower income voters, most of whom did not own automobiles or telephones. This historical polling blunder has served as a classic example of a *biased* sample.

Sampling bias occurs when the individuals selected for a sample overrepresent or underrepresent certain population attributes that are related to the phenomenon under study. Such biases can be conscious or unconscious. Conscious biases occur when a sample is selected purposefully. For example, a clinician might choose only patients with minimal dysfunction to demonstrate a treatment's effectiveness, eliminating those subjects who were not likely to improve. Unconscious biases might occur if an interviewer interested in studying attitudes of the public toward the disabled, stands on a busy street corner in a downtown area and interviews people "at random," or haphazardly. The interviewer may unconsciously choose to approach only those who look cooperative, on the basis of appearance, gender, or some other characteristics. Persons who do not work or shop in that area will not be represented. The conclusions drawn from such a sample cannot be useful for describing attitudes of the "general public." The validity of generalizations made from a sample to the population depend on the method of selecting subjects. Therefore, some impartial mechanism is needed to make unbiased selections.

Target Populations and Accessible Populations

The first step in planning a study is to identify the overall group of people to which the researcher intends to generalize findings. This universe of interest is the **target population**, or **reference population**. The target population for a study of motor skills could be defined as all children with learning disabilities in the United States today. Because it is not possible to gain access to every child with a learning disability, some portion of the target population that has a chance to be selected must be identified. This is the **accessible population**. For example, an accessible population might include all children identified as having a learning disability in a given city's school system. The units within this population are the individual children. The study sample will be chosen from this accessible population (see Figure 8.1).

Strictly speaking, a sample can only be representative of the accessible population, not necessarily the target population. For example, some school systems may be more

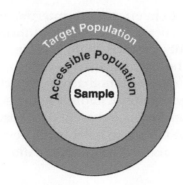

FIGURE 8.1   Levels of the sampling process.

proficient at diagnosing children with learning disabilities; others may have more advanced programs that address motor skills. Such differences can complicate generalizations to the target population. When the differences between the target and accessible populations are potentially too great, it is often appropriate to identify a more restricted target population. For example, we could designate a target population of children with learning disabilities who have participated in a comprehensive motor skills program for at least one year. The results of the study would then be applicable only to children meeting this criterion. Because the validity of the accessible population is not readily testable, researchers must exercise judgment in assessing the degree of similarity with the target population.

Inclusion and Exclusion Criteria

In defining the target population, an investigator must first specify selection criteria that will govern who will and will not be subjects. **Inclusion criteria** describe the primary traits of the target and accessible populations that will qualify someone as a subject. The researcher must consider the variety of characteristics present in the population in terms of clinical findings, demographics and geographic factors, and whether these factors are important to the question being studied. For example, consider a study to look at the effect of physical activity on cognitive performance of students with learning disabilities. The investigator may need to consider the specific type of learning disability, gender and age, or the state or city where subjects will be found. Therefore, a researcher might decide to include only students who have been identified as having dyslexia, only males, and only schools within one town in Massachusetts. The accessible population may be further defined by temporal factors, such as students who were in the school system between 1997 and 1999. It is vitally important to remember, however, that as the researcher restricts the population, and creates a more homogeneous sample, the ability to generalize research findings will also be restricted; that is, the findings will only be applicable to a population with those specific characteristics. Such a scenario may be quite artificial in terms of the patients that are typically seen in the clinic.

Exclusion criteria indicate those factors that would preclude someone from being a subject. These factors will generally be considered potentially confounding to the results; that is, they are likely to interfere with interpretation of the findings. Perhaps students who also have other types of learning disabilities or attention deficit disorders will be excluded. If tests are only given in English, subjects may be excluded if they are not fluent in that language. The researcher may want to eliminate students who have physical disabilities or some other factors that would limit their ability to participate actively in physical exercise programs. Children with asthma may be eliminated, for example. The specification of inclusion and exclusion criteria is an important early step in the research process because it helps to narrow the possibilities for seeking an accessible population. These criteria also define the population.

Subject Selection

Once an accessible population is identified, the researcher must devise a plan for subject selection, inviting members to participate. This process may involve written invitations mailed to potential subjects' homes, telephone calls or personal contacts in the clinical setting. All members of the subpopulation may be approached, or a smaller group may be selected. Not all of these invited individuals will be interested or willing to participate, and so the sample becomes further reduced to those who agree to participate. With survey questionnaires, many subjects will not respond. In an experimental study, where participants are further divided into groups, subjects may drop out before completion of data collection. In all types of studies, the researcher may have to discard the data of some subjects because of inaccuracies in procedure or missing responses. In the end, the sample used for data analysis may actually be a select subgroup of the population, and is likely to differ from nonparticipants in many ways that could affect the variables being studied.[2-4] A flowchart that details how participants pass through various stages of a study should be included in a research report.[5] Figure 8.2 shows a generic flow chart for this purpose, showing expected information about how many subjects were included or excluded at the start of the study, how many left the study (and their reasons) and finally how many completed the study.

SAMPLING TECHNIQUES

Sampling techniques can be categorized as probability or nonprobability methods. **Probability samples** are created through a process of **random selection**. Random is not the same as haphazard. It means that every unit in the population has an equal chance, or "probability," of being chosen. This also means that every unit that is chosen has an equal chance of having some of the characteristics or exposures that are present throughout the population. Therefore, the sample *should* be free of any bias and is considered representative of the population from which it was drawn. Note that we say it is *considered* representative, not that it *is* representative. Because this process involves the operation of chance, there is always the possibility that a sample's characteristics will be different from those of its parent population.

   If we summarize sample responses using averaged data, this average will most likely be somewhat different from the total population's average responses, just by chance. The difference between sample averages (called **statistics**) and population averages (called **parameters**) is **sampling error**, or sampling variation. The essence of

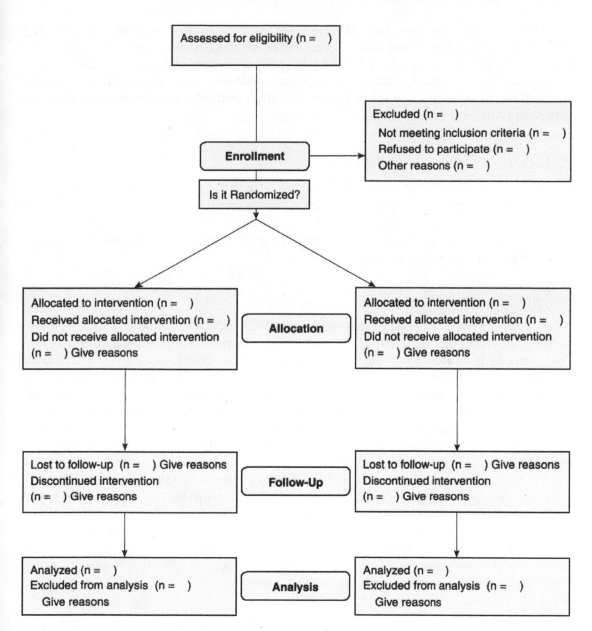

FIGURE 8.2 Flowchart for subject progression in a randomized trial, including those who withdrew or were lost to follow-up. (From http:www.consort-statement.org <http:www.consort-statement.org> Accessed May 29, 2007.)

random sampling is that these sampling differences are due to chance and are not a function of any human bias, conscious or unconscious. Because this process controls for the potential effect of bias, it provides a basis for statistically estimating the degree of sampling error (see Chapter 18). Although it is not perfect, random selection affords the greatest possible confidence in the sample's validity because, in the long run, it will produce samples that most accurately reflect the population's characteristics.

The selection of **nonprobability samples** is made by nonrandom methods. The probability of selection is not known, and therefore, the degree of sampling error cannot be estimated. This limits the ability to generalize outcomes beyond the specific sample studied. Nonprobability techniques are probably used more often in clinical research out of necessity, but we recognize that their outcomes require some caution for generalization.

PROBABILITY SAMPLING

The most basic method of probability sampling is through simple random selection, giving every member of a population an equal opportunity, or probability, of being selected; however, this technique is rarely used in practice because of practical difficulties in accessing total populations. For clinical experiments, researchers often use more efficient variations on this theme.

Simple Random Sampling

A random sample is *unbiased* in that each selection is independent, and no one member of the population has any more chance of being chosen than any other member. A random sample is drawn from the accessible population, often taken from a listing of persons, such as membership directories, or institutions, such as lists of accredited hospitals. Often, the accessible population is actually defined according to the available listings. For example, if we use a professional membership directory to create a sample of therapists, the accessible population would be defined as therapists who were members. Not all therapists belong to the association, however, and it may not be valid to generalize responses of such a sample to all practicing therapists.

Once a listing is available, a random sampling procedure can be implemented. Suppose we were interested in choosing a sample of 100 occupational therapy students to study their interest in working with the elderly after graduation. We could define the accessible population as the total number of students attending 25 programs in the Northeast. The simplest approach would be to place each student's name on a slip of paper, place these slips into a container, and blindly draw 100 slips. If the accessible population had 56 or fewer elements, we could number them 11 through 66 and choose them on the basis of the throw of two dice.

A more convenient method involves the use of a *table of random numbers*, such as the one given in Table 8.1. Tables of random numbers can be found in most statistics texts. They are generated by computers and comprise thousands of digits (0 to 9) with no systematic order or relationship. The selections made using a table of random numbers are considered unbiased, as the order of digits is completely due to chance. To use this system, the accessible population must be in numbered list form, so that every element has a unique number, or identifying code. In this example, if there were a total of 985 students, they would be numbered 001 through 985. Each identification code has the same number of digits, in this case three.

We enter Table 8.1 at random, choosing a starting point using an arbitrary method, such as blindly placing a pencil at a point on the page. For this example, we will start at the seventh digit in row 12. Note that the digits are grouped in twos, but this is just

TABLE 8.1   TABLE OF RANDOM NUMBERS

18	42	05	66	77	22	33	61	62	97	50	71	90	18	35	18	06	45	41	76
35	70	40	86	20	56	89	87	83	09	32	01	75	37	92	51	28	84	59	90
37	85	69	44	98	65	38	42	56	66	74	03	13	50	92	32	09	55	79	68
50	38	82	97	46	96	64	01	78	69	48	29	25	72	49	96	05	43	62	57
86	13	35	34	91	95	55	29	76	09	99	13	72	36	51	22	12	46	23	37
41	38	49	28	71	48	69	03	33	47	55	45	06	50	07	47	71	85	24	79
64	47	22	59	25	40	33	54	56	27	68	95	79	75	16	31	49	21	11	58
36	23	62	73	74	92	51	01	69	36	92	06	23	76	55	71	15	81	75	36
68	47	84	38	77	98	50	99	41	80	50	81	05	69	50	42	37	79	33	58
32	24	66	46	57	36	95	92	17	82	28	85	05	04	73	13	10	63	41	08
66	87	08	69	50	61	89	46	23	12	76	07	45	07	67	12	08	01	22	69
19	01	69	64	77	50	11	95	64	98	83	37	02	29	72	91	20	90	25	78
15	65	31	09	15	14	86	61	04	55	54	14	59	64	51	15	35	51	13	89
73	31	22	85	67	59	96	06	34	19	23	76	38	91	85	42	03	67	66	23
03	35	15	24	04	13	49	60	45	43	79	05	51	57	74	31	28	84	88	86
11	70	01	64	27	86	87	16	26	82	43	83	86	84	76	33	32	02	92	52
23	33	50	74	21	08	54	74	53	51	61	79	36	02	67	07	94	57	77	35
48	19	48	77	93	99	13	12	75	19	02	91	11	29	99	42	61	29	87	89
89	43	85	63	67	14	26	64	34	50	49	27	24	05	72	06	82	26	12	77
59	80	24	08	18	80	71	49	96	65	75	07	42	14	36	75	13	08	33	37
43	18	91	99	51	72	58	44	43	70	76	34	97	75	62	31	07	18	03	87
27	51	98	08	78	35	95	79	33	57	01	98	19	59	33	53	83	61	49	96
83	27	52	53	25	91	10	29	02	10	39	46	81	93	88	28	02	31	72	18
38	42	07	12	77	05	85	80	72	01	83	27	02	47	29	39	35	58	89	73
85	85	93	78	63	16	80	92	86	47	39	89	99	64	38	86	62	34	86	50
55	62	47	27	87	24	26	50	29	49	47	08	61	11	74	94	53	31	06	09
84	40	33	94	97	91	05	08	69	52	62	73	11	02	17	96	78	64	28	53
94	69	20	11	73	75	10	72	63	75	85	08	56	51	42	83	76	18	94	63
36	61	57	56	99	52	65	02	21	50	87	18	75	94	56	36	09	17	89	04
06	38	78	61	02	06	39	84	92	95	36	31	06	19	95	72	25	25	68	11
48	02	69	90	65	25	86	85	12	21	49	53	79	19	58	05	45	51	60	26
01	50	11	32	05	81	30	84	35	06	60	03	25	33	12	34	48	59	16	88
80	56	55	40	19	47	19	34	28	24	06	48	58	5	36	16	04	77	53	55
64	19	70	99	37	69	51	40	70	94	37	36	60	56	39	39	86	31	98	36
15	63	18	73	46	83	08	34	08	31	56	68	48	96	53	03	77	24	71	90
54	13	86	88	50	81	63	67	79	46	49	92	19	32	44	06	79	23	95	14
12	54	89	58	29	44	22	04	95	31	40	94	38	85	37	26	27	65	51	67
98	35	65	04	39	87	01	80	46	22	81	45	95	03	03	63	13	78	25	98
37	98	69	62	51	84	77	85	02	76	84	80	97	84	43	61	12	06	97	80
48	35	71	30	64	74	70	99	29	04	08	98	64	10	46	70	13	85	81	01
90	37	34	23	88	61	49	62	75	68	77	23	11	47	91	90	07	69	05	74
55	74	82	98	59	17	33	25	97	50	16	80	04	61	37	15	43	13	50	86
35	77	79	59	38	23	35	02	58	45	17	40	64	48	51	88	79	87	73	19
54	85	11	53	73	89	84	46	98	75	66	48	92	69	75	27	01	44	89	86

for ease of reading. Some tables group numbers differently. As we are interested in three-digit numbers, we will use the first three digits from our starting point, number 647. Therefore, the student numbered 647 is the first subject selected. We can then move up, down, or across to continue the process. If we choose to move across the row, the next student is number 750, then 119, then 564, and so on, until we choose 100 names. Note that the next number in the series will be 988, a value beyond the range of codes used. Any number that comes up out of range is simply ignored and the next three-digit number is used. Similarly, if a student's number should occur again in the list of random numbers, it is also ignored and the next random number used. This process is called **simple random sampling**, or *sampling without replacement*, as once a unit is selected it has no further chance of being selected.*

Random selections can be made by computer, using statistical packages, given a numbered list of subjects in a data set. The total data set usually will represent an accessible population. The computer can then generate a random list of any specified size to select the sample.

Systematic Sampling

Random sampling can be a laborious technique, unless the accessible population is organized as a short, prenumbered list. When lists are arranged alphabetically or in some other ordered fashion, an alternative approach can be used that simplifies this procedure, called **systematic sampling**. To use this sampling technique, the researcher divides the total number of elements in the accessible population by the number of elements to be selected. Therefore, to select a sample of 100 from a list of 1,000 students, every tenth person on the list is selected. The interval between selected elements is called the **sampling interval**, in this case 10. The starting point on the list is determined at random, often using a table of random numbers. This approach is usually the least time consuming and most convenient way to obtain a sample from an available listing of potential subjects. Systematic sampling is generally considered equivalent to random sampling, as long as no recurring pattern or particular order exists in the listing.

Stratified Random Sampling

In random and systematic sampling, the distribution of characteristics of the sample can differ from that of the population from which it was drawn just by chance because each selection is made independently of all others. It is possible, however, to modify these methods to improve a sample's representativeness (and decrease sampling error) through a process known as stratification.

Stratified random sampling involves identifying relevant population characteristics, and partitioning members of a population into homogeneous, nonoverlapping subsets, or **strata**, based on these characteristics. For example, in our study of students'

---

*Random sampling can also be performed using the technique of *sampling with replacement*, in which each unit that is selected is put back into the pool before the next selection is made. Therefore, each unit truly has an equal chance of being chosen throughout the selection procedure. This method is not used in clinical studies, because subjects cannot represent themselves more than once. Sampling with replacement is used primarily in probability and mathematical studies.

attitudes toward working with the elderly, we may be concerned about the differential effect of level of education. Those who have had more professional education may have different attitudes than those who have not yet been exposed to clinical education. Let us assume that our accessible population consists of 300 freshmen, 300 sophomores, 200 juniors, and 200 seniors. In a simple random sample drawn from the list of 1,000 students, it is possible, just by chance, that the distribution of subjects will not reflect the differential proportions of these classes in the population. To control for this, we can create a **proportional stratified sample**, by first separating the population into the four classes and then drawing random or systematic samples from each class in the proportion that exists in the population (see Figure 8.3). Therefore, to obtain a sample of 100, we would choose 30 freshmen, 30 sophomores, 20 juniors, and 20 seniors. The resulting sample would intuitively provide a better estimate of the population than simple random sampling.

Stratification increases the precision of estimates only when the stratification variable is closely related to the variables of experimental interest. It would not be of any benefit to stratify subjects on the basis of blood type, for example, in a study of attitudes toward the elderly. It might be important to use variables such as age, gender or race. National samples for surveys and polls are often stratified by geographic area so that the distribution of regional variables mirrors the population. Stratification can be done on more than one variable when this is appropriate. Sometimes, however, variables are correlated in such a way that only one variable needs to be the basis for stratification. For instance, age and college class are generally related, and therefore, stratification on class should also control for variations in age.

Although stratified sampling takes additional time, it can actually provide a more representative sample than random sampling, with no sampling error on the stratified

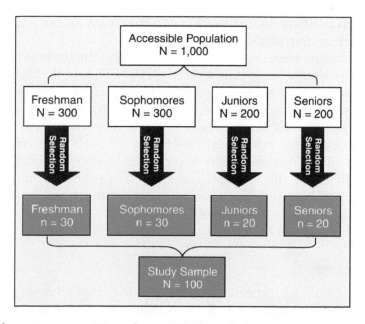

FIGURE 8.3 Schematic representation of proportional stratified sampling, drawing a random sample of 100 subjects from an accessible population of 1,000 people.

variable. Therefore, whenever relevant strata can be identified, this approach presents an opportunity to strengthen a research design.

Disproportional Sampling

The benefits of stratified sampling can be frustrated when the researcher knows in advance that strata are of greatly unequal size, creating a situation where one or more strata may provide insufficient samples for making comparisons. Suppose, for example, that we are interested in drawing a sample of 200 therapists from a professional organization with 2,000 members, including 1,700 females and 300 males. Using proportional selection, we would choose 10% of each group, 170 females and 30 males; however, such a small number of males would probably not provide adequate representation for drawing conclusions about that segment of the population.

One way of dealing with this situation is to use a simple random sample and leave the proportional representation to chance; however, unless the sample is unusually large, the differential effect of gender will probably not be controlled. Alternatively, we can adopt a **disproportional sampling** design, in which we select random samples of adequate size from each category. For example, we might select 100 females and 100 males. This sample of 200 cannot be considered random, because each male has a much greater chance (higher probability) of being chosen. This approach creates an adequate sample size, but it presents problems for data analysis, because the characteristics of one group, in this case males, will be overrepresented in the sample. We can control for this effect by weighting the data, so that females receive a proportionally larger mathematical representation in the analysis of scores than males.

To calculate *proportional weights,* we first determine the probability that any one female or male will be selected. For example, to choose 100 females, the probability of any one female being chosen is 100 of 1,700, or 1 of 17 (1/17). The probability of any one male being chosen is 100 of 300, or 1 of 3 (1/3). Therefore, each male has a probability of selection more than five times that of any female.

Next, we determine the assigned weights by taking the inverse of these probabilities.[2] Therefore, the weight for female scores is 17/1 = 17, and that for males is 3/1 = 3. This means that when data are analyzed, each female's score will be multiplied by 17 and each male's score will be multiplied by 3. In any mathematical manipulation of the data, the total of the females' scores would be larger than the total of the males' scores. Therefore, the proportional representation of each group is differentiated in the total data set. Because all subjects in a group will have the same weight, the average scores for that group will not be affected; however, the relative contribution of these scores to overall data interpretation will be controlled. This approach has been used, for example, in large surveys such as the National Health Interview Survey, to assure adequate representation of minorities in the study sample.

Cluster Sampling

In many research situations, especially those involving large dispersed populations, it is impractical or impossible to obtain a complete listing of a population. For instance, if we wanted to sample therapists in rehabilitation hospitals across the country, it is unreasonable to expect that we could easily compile such a list. We therefore need some strategy that will allow us to link members of the population to some already established grouping that can be sampled. We could start by randomly choosing 10 states, then randomly choosing 5 hospitals in each state, then randomly choosing 10 therapists from each hospital. This approach is called **cluster sampling**, or **multistage sampling**.

Cluster sampling involves successive random sampling of a series of units in the population. For example, Emery et al.[6] used this approach in their study of balance training for reducing sports injuries in adolescents, illustrated in Figure 8.4. They randomly selected 10 of 15 high schools in one city, then chose a specific physical education class in each school, then randomly chose students from that class. Schools were randomly assigned to receive either home-based exercise or a control condition.

The advantage of cluster sampling is its obvious convenience and efficiency when dealing with large populations; however, this comes at the price of increased sampling error. Because two or more samples are drawn, each is subject to sampling error, potentially compounding the inaccuracy of the final sample. This disadvantage can be minimized by choosing as large a sample as possible within each cluster and by stratifying within any stage of sampling.

Survey researchers often use multistage sampling to generate random samples of households. One technique, called **area probability sampling**, allows a population to

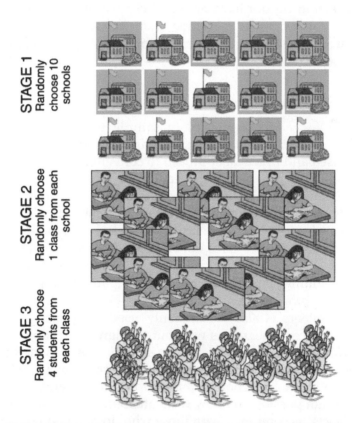

STAGE 1
Randomly choose 10 schools

STAGE 2
Randomly choose 1 class from each school

STAGE 3
Randomly choose 4 students from each class

FIGURE 8.4   Multistage cluster sampling process to select a random sample of students in one city. In Stage 1 10 schools are randomly chosen from 15 schools in the city. In Stage 2, one physical education class is chosen randomly from each school. In Stage 3, four students are randomly chosen from each class.

be sampled geographically. The total target land area is divided into mutually exclusive sections. A list is then made of housing units in each section, and a sample is drawn from these lists. The final survey may be administered to all selected housing units, or the list may be subdivided further into individuals within households.

Another survey sampling technique, called **random-digit dialing**, involves the random selection of phone numbers based on multistage sampling of area codes and telephone exchanges. Most of us have had experience with this type of survey. Many studies in marketing research use this approach. Obviously, this method presents problems in that only households with listed telephone numbers have a chance of being selected. In addition, bias may be introduced by timing. Calls made during working hours or weekdays versus weekends may alter the characteristics of sample respondents. For certain research questions, however, random-digit dialing is most useful for generating a sizable sample over a large area.

NONPROBABILITY SAMPLING

In practice, it is sometimes difficult, if not impossible, to obtain a true random sample. Clinical researchers are often forced to use **nonprobability samples,** created when samples are chosen on some basis other than random selection. Because all the elements of the population do not have an equal chance of being selected under these circumstances, we cannot readily assume that the sample represents the target population. The probability exists that some segment of the population will be disproportionately represented.

Convenience Sampling

The most common form of nonprobability sample is a **convenience sample**, or **accidental sample**. With this method, subjects are chosen on the basis of availability. Perhaps the most used and practical approach to convenience sampling is **consecutive sampling**, which involves recruiting all patients who meet the inclusion and exclusion criteria as they become available. Essentially, a consecutive sample includes the entire accessible population within the defined time period of the study. This can be problematic if the study period is too short, and a sufficient number of qualified subjects cannot be obtained, or if the time period does not allow a representative group. For example, if we were studying causes of low back pain, and we only included patients who came to the clinic in the summer months, we might miss patients whose pain is caused by shoveling snow or slipping on ice.

The use of volunteers is also a commonly used convenience sampling method because of its expedience. Researchers who put up signs in dormitories or hospitals to recruit subjects with specific characteristics are sampling by this method. Polls in magazines or on street corners and most commercial advertisements are based on samples of convenience. The major limitation of this method, however, is the potential bias of **self-selection**. It is not possible to know what attributes are present in those who offer themselves as subjects, as compared with those who do not, and it is unclear how these attributes may affect the ability to generalize experimental outcomes. Those who volunteer may be quite atypical of the target population in terms of such characteristics as age, motivation, activity level, and other correlates of health consciousness.[7,8] Although all samples, even random samples, are eventually composed of those who participate voluntarily, those who agree to be part of a random sample were not self-selected. Therefore, characteristics of subjects in a random sample can be assumed to represent the target population. This is not necessarily a safe assumption with nonrandom samples.

Quota Sampling

Nonprobability sampling can also incorporate elements of stratification. Using **quota sampling,** a researcher can control for the potential confounding effect of known characteristics of a population by guiding the sampling process so that an adequate number of subjects are obtained for each stratum. This approach requires that each stratum is represented in the same proportion as in the population. For example, using the previous example examining students' attitudes toward the elderly, we could call for volunteers to take the questionnaire and stop the call once we have achieved the proper number of subjects for each class. Although this system still faces the potential for nonprobability biases, it does improve on the process by proportionally representing each segment of the population in the sample.

Purposive Sampling

A third nonprobability approach is **purposive sampling,** in which the researcher handpicks subjects on the basis of specific criteria. The researcher may locate subjects by chart review or interview patients to determine if they fit the study. A researcher must exercise fair judgment to make this process meaningful. For instance, in a study to test the effectiveness of an exercise program, the researcher may choose patients who are likely to be compliant from among the patients seen in his clinic. In studies to establish the validity of newly developed measuring instruments, researchers may want to test a variety of subjects with specifically different degrees of limitation in the variable being measured. Purposive sampling is similar to convenience sampling, but differs in that specific choices are made, rather than simple availability. This approach has the same limitations to generalization as a convenience sample, in that it can result in a biased sample. However, in many instances, purposive sampling can yield a sample that will be representative of the population if the investigator wisely chooses individuals who represent the spectrum of population characteristics.[9] Purposive samples are commonly used in qualitative research to assure that subjects have the appropriate knowledge and will be a good informant for the study.[10]

Snowball Sampling

Snowball sampling is a method that is often used to study sensitive topics, rare traits, personal networks, and social relationships. This approach is carried out in stages. In the first stage, a few subjects who meet selection criteria are identified and tested or interviewed. In the second stage, these subjects are asked to identify others who have the requisite characteristics. This process of "chain referral" or "snowballing" is continued until an adequate sample is obtained. The researcher must be able to verify the eligibility of each respondent to ensure a representative group.[11,12] Snowball sampling is used extensively, for example, in studies involving homeless persons and drug abusers.[13–15] In a study of postpartum depression, researchers used snowball sampling through a hospital network to identify appropriate subjects.[16] As these examples illustrate, snowball sampling is most useful when the population of interest is rare, unevenly distributed, hidden, or hard to reach.

RECRUITMENT

The practicalities of clinical research demand that we consider feasibility issues in initial stages of planning a study. One of the most serious of these considerations is how to recruit the sample. Once the inclusion and exclusion criteria have been defined, the researcher begins the process of finding appropriate subjects in sufficient numbers.

Where subjects come from will depend on the research question. Community studies will often involve the use of advertisements, newspapers or mailings. Large studies may be based on samples derived from telephone listings or membership directories. Health clubs, schools and day care centers may be helpful. For clinical studies, subjects are often recruited from the patient population in the researcher's facility. Investigators must be aware of the ethical concerns that arise when using their own patients as subjects, including fair descriptions of the study in an effort to gain their trust and secure their participation (see Chapter 3). Subjects may also be recruited from other facilities or agencies, usually through the cooperation of colleagues at those institutions. In this case, the researcher should obtain written endorsements from the appropriate administrative officials to confirm their cooperation and to include with applications for funding. Researchers should be prepared to give administrative officials a copy of the study proposal, often in abbreviated form. When subjects are patients, researchers must contact the physician in charge of the patient's care. Sometimes it is efficient to work with a particular physician or practice group to recruit patients on an ongoing basis through the practice. Once the physician's approval has been obtained, the researcher can then contact individual patients to secure their participation. This may be done in person or by letter, explaining the purpose of the study, and assurance that their treatment will not be affected whether or not they participate. The consent form will be given to the patients to read and to discuss with the researcher, with a contact number if they have further questions.

Many of the individuals who are contacted will consent to participate in the study, and many others will not. To obtain a sample of sufficient size, it is often necessary to contact a large number of prospective individuals. The researcher should report the number of subjects who were screened for eligibility, the number who were determined to be eligible, and the number of those who finally enrolled in the study. It is also potentially useful to understand the characteristics of those who refuse to participate.[17] This information is important to the reader of a research report, to assess the extent to which the subjects represent the overall population or a select subgroup.[18]

A question about the number of subjects needed is often the first to be raised. The issue of sample size is an essential one, as it directly affects the statistical power of the study. **Power** is the ability to find significant differences when they exist.[†] With a small

---

[†]Statistical implications of sample size and power are discussed in Chapter 18 and Appendix C.

sample, power tends to be low, and a study may not succeed in demonstrating the desired effects. As the researcher explores the availability of subjects, we can generally be sure that fewer subjects will agree to enter the study than originally projected (see Figure 8.2). Every investigator should have a contingency plan in mind, such as recruiting subjects from different sites or expanding inclusion criteria, when the sample size falls substantially short of expectations. For studies that involve the use of questionnaires, sample size is a function of response rate, and should be a factor in deciding how many questionnaires to send out.

Once the study is completed, it is also appropriate to offer to send a summary of the findings to physicians, agencies and subjects. The results may have an impact on the patient's care or future clinical decisions. Maintaining such contact will often encourage colleagues to be part of future studies as well.

COMMENTARY

Sampling, Like Life, Is a Compromise

Nonprobability samples are used more often than probability samples in clinical research because of the difficulties in obtaining true access to populations. We frequently encounter statements such as "Subjects were selected from the patient population at Hospital X between 2000 and 2002," and "Subjects were volunteers from the senior class at University Y." Most clinical situations require that samples of convenience be used. Patients are often recruited as they become available, making true random selection impossible. Inclusion and exclusion criteria may be made sufficiently broad so that a sample of sufficient size can be obtained within a reasonable amount of time. Recruiting subjects from more than one site can also increase generalizability of findings.

Generalizations of data collected from nonrandom samples must be made with caution; however, this is not to say that studies with nonrandom samples are invalid. The data collected are still meaningful within the confines of the defined group being tested. The researcher must determine if the characteristics of the sample are an adequate representation of the target population. When using convenience samples, the researcher has an added responsibility to identify important extraneous variables that might influence the dependent variable. It is important to decide if a restricted sample, with homogeneous subjects, would be more useful, or if the full variation in the population should be represented. The risk of interpretative error can be reduced by comparing sample characteristics to other groups from the population that may be described in the literature, and by replicating studies to show that subjects chosen nonrandomly from different sources respond in a similar way.[17] Sample size is also an important consideration. In qualitative studies, samples may be quite small, as compared to quantitative studies that will require statistical comparisons. Researchers must consider the effect of sample size on their analytic process. Sometimes the restrictions set for inclusion and exclusion criteria must be modified to obtain a large enough sample, and the implications of this process must be considered.

Keppel suggests that researchers can distinguish between statistical and nonstatistical generalizations.[19] Statistical inferences theoretically require random sampling and are based on the validity of representativeness. Strictly speaking, it is inappropriate to apply many inferential statistical procedures to data that were obtained from nonprobability samples, although most researchers are willing to make assumptions about the representativeness of their sample so that the statistical analysis can be carried out. Generalizations from nonprobability samples can be justified on the basis of knowledge of the research topic, experience, the logic of the study, and consistency in replicated outcomes. Often, one can conclude that a convenience sample will provide data that, for all practical purposes, are as "random" as those obtained with a probability sample, especially with relatively small samples.[9] It is important, however, that this determination is critically assessed, not simply assumed, based on the specific circumstances of the study. Researchers must be aware of the limitations inherent in any sampling method and should try to incorporate elements of random sampling whenever possible.

From an evidence-based practice perspective, we must decide if results obtained in a research study can be applied to an individual patient. The clinician must determine if the study subjects are sufficiently similar to the patient to allow generalizations of findings. When the study sample clearly matches the patient's characteristics, the decision may be simple. However, quite often researchers have specified exclusion criteria in an effort to decrease variability, and this may decrease generalizability. The age ranges may not be exactly the same as the patient. Perhaps the setting or geographic region is markedly different. We must be able to weigh the impact of these differences and use the study's results with as much relevance as possible. An exact match between a study sample and a patient is not likely, but are the similarities sufficient that the results could be useful? If the study sample ranges in age from 40 to 60 years old, and my patient is 70, can I assume that physiological processes causing the outcome might still apply? Or does my patient's age totally preclude the application of the findings? This is a cautionary reminder that we must use our judgment to decide how we want to use the information. Evidence comes in all sizes and forms, and we must evaluate it within the context of our experience and our patients to determine how it can be best applied.

REFERENCES

1. Babbie ER. *Survey Research Methods*. Belmont, CA: Wadsworth, 1973.
2. Friedman LM, Furberg CD, DeMets DL. *Fundamentals of Clinical Trials*. Littleton, MA: PSG, 1985.
3. Wilhelmsen L, Ljungberg S, Wedel H, et al. A comparison between participants and non-participants in a primary preventive trial. *J Chron Dis* 1976;29:331–339.
4. Fetter MS, Feetham SL, D'Apolito K, Chaze BA, Fink A, Frink BB, et al. Randomized clinical trials: Issues for researchers. *Nurs Res* 1989;38:117–120.
5. The Standards of Reporting Trials Group. A proposal for structured reporting of randomized controlled trials. *JAMA* 1994;272:1926–1931.

6. Emery CA, Cassidy JD, Klassen TP, Rosychuk RJ, Rowe BH. Effectiveness of a home–based balance–training program in reducing sports–related injuries among healthy adolescents: A cluster randomized controlled trial. *CMAJ* 2005; 172: 749–754.

7. Hennekens CH, Buring JE. *Epidemiology in Medicine.* Boston: Little Brown, 1987.

8. Ganguli M, Lytle ME, Reynolds MD, Dodge HH. Random versus volunteer selection for a community-based study. *J Gerontol* 1998;53A:M39-M46.

9. Hahn GJ, Meeker WQ. Assumptions for statistical inference. *Am Statistician* 1993; 47:1–11.

10. Morse JM. Strategies for sampling. In JM Morse (Ed.) *Qualitative Nursing Research: A Contemporary Dialogue.* Rockville, MD: Aspen, 1989:117–131.

11. Biernacki P, Waldorf D. Snowball sampling: Problems and techniques of chain referral sampling. *Sociol Methods Res* 1981;10:141–163.

12. Lopes CS, Rodriguez LC, Sichieri R. The lack of selection bias in a snowball sampled case-control study on drug abuse. *Int J Epidemiol* 1996;25:1267–1270.

13. Boys A, Marsden J, Strang J. Understanding reasons for drug use amongst young people: A functional perspective. *Health Educ Res* 2001;16:457–469.

14. Heimer R, Clair S, Grau LE, Bluthenthal RN, Marshall PA, Singer M. Hepatitis-associated knowledge is low and risks are high among HIV-aware injection drug users in three US cities. *Addiction* 2002;97:1277–1287.

15. Willems JC, Iguchi MY, Lidz V, Bux DAJ. Change in drug-using networks of injecting drug users during methadone treatment: A pilot study using snowball recruitment and intensive interviews. *Subst Use Misuse* 1997;32:1539–1554.

16. Ugarriza DN. Postpartum depressed women's explanation of depression. *J Nurs Scholarsh* 2002;34:227–233.

17. Halpern SD. Reporting enrollment in clinical trials [Letter to the Editor]. *Ann Int Med* 2002;137:1007.

18. Gross CP, Mallory R, Heiat A, Krumholz HM. Reporting the recruitment process in clinical trials: Who are these patients and how did they get there? *Ann Intern Med* 2002;137:10–16.

19. Keppel G. *Design and Analysis: A Researcher's Handbook* (4th ed.). Englewood Cliffs, NJ: Prentice Hall, 2004.

CHAPTER 9
Validity in Experimental Design

The most rigorous form of scientific investigation for testing hypotheses is the **experiment.** Experiments are based on a logical structure, or design, within which the investigator systematically introduces changes into natural phenomena and then observes the consequences of those changes. The purpose of an experiment is to support a **cause-and-effect relationship** between a particular action or condition (the independent variable) and an observed response (the dependent variable).

The essence of an experiment lies in the researcher's ability to manipulate and control variables and measurements, so that rival hypotheses are ruled out as possible explanations for the observed response. These rival hypotheses concern the potential influence of unrelated factors, called **extraneous variables** (also called nuisance variables or intervening variables). An extraneous variable is any factor that is not directly related to the purpose of the study, but that may affect the dependent variable. Extraneous variables can be extrinsic factors that emerge from the environment and the experimental situation or intrinsic factors that represent personal characteristics of the subjects of the study.

When extraneous variables are not controlled, they exert a **confounding** influence on the independent variable, that is, they contaminate the independent variable in such a way that their separate effects are obscured. For example, if we wanted to examine the effect of cryotherapy for relieving shoulder pain, and our subjects were on pain medication, the medication would be a confounding factor. If we observe a decrease in pain following treatment, we could not determine if the effect was due to the treatment, the medication, or some combination of the two. Other extraneous factors that could interfere with conclusions could be spontaneous healing or other treatments the patient is receiving. Experiments are designed to **control** for this type of confounding.

In reality, of course, clinical experiments seldom have the ability to completely eliminate confounding effects; however, even though causality can never be demonstrated with complete certainty, the experimental method provides the most convincing evidence of the effect one variable has on another. The purpose of this chapter is to examine issues of experimental control that must be addressed if the researcher is to have confidence in the validity of experimental outcomes.

CHARACTERISTICS OF EXPERIMENTS

To be considered a true experiment, a study must have three essential characteristics: The independent variable must be manipulated by the experimenter, the subjects must be randomly assigned to groups and a control or comparison group must be incorporated within the design.

Manipulation of Variables

Manipulation of variables refers to a deliberate operation performed by the experimenter, imposing a set of predetermined experimental conditions (the independent variable) on at least one group of subjects. The experimenter manipulates the levels of the independent variable by assigning subjects to varied conditions, usually administering the intervention to one group and withholding it from another. For example, we might be interested in the effect of medication to reduce hypertension. We can assign subjects to treatment and control groups and measure blood pressure changes that occur following a period of treatment or no treatment. It is possible to manipulate a single variable or a number of variables simultaneously.

Active and Attribute Variables

Independent variables can be distinguished as either active or attribute factors. An **active variable** is one that is manipulated by the experimenter so that subjects are assigned to levels of the independent variable. For instance, in a study where subjects can be assigned to receive medication or a placebo, treatment is an active variable. With an **attribute variable** the researcher is not able to assign subjects to groups, but must observe them within natural groupings according to inherent characteristics. Age group would be an attribute factor, as subjects automatically belong to one group or another, with no possibility for assignment. Pre-existing characteristics such as gender, occupation and diagnosis are other examples of attribute variables.

Attribute variables cannot be manipulated by the experimenter. Therefore, when the effect of one or more attribute variables is studied, the research cannot be considered a true experiment. For example, we could look at differences in strength and range of motion across various age groups or between males and females. Because age and gender are attributes in place before the study begins, we can consider relationships, but the design does not afford adequate opportunity for control, thereby limiting interpretation of cause and effect. This can be an important consideration for choosing statistical analyses.

It is possible to combine active variables and attribute variables in a single study. For instance, we could look at the effect of medication on hypertension combined with the influence of age. By dividing subjects into four age groups, the subjects within each age group could be assigned to one of the two treatment groups. Even though this study includes an attribute variable, it qualifies as an experiment because the researcher is able to manipulate the assignment of treatment levels for at least one independent variable.

Random Assignment

In Chapter 8 we discussed the importance of random selection for *choosing* subjects, to ensure that a sample was representative of the parent population and that it was not biased. Once a sample is selected, it is important to continue the process of randomization in *assigning* subjects to groups. **Random assignment** means that each subject has an equal chance of being assigned to any group, that is, assignments will be independent of personal judgment or bias. Random assignment is an essential feature of experimental research, providing the greatest confidence that no systematic bias exists with respect to a group's collective attributes that might differentially affect the dependent variable. If we can assume that groups are equivalent at the start of an experiment, then we can have confidence that differences observed at the end of the study are not due to intersubject variability that existed before the experiment began.

The concept of random assignment refers to groups being considered equivalent. Equivalence does not mean that every subject in one group is exactly equal to another subject in the other group. It does mean that any differences between the groups have been distributed as a function of chance alone. We can think of subjects as composites of personal characteristics such as motivation, intellectual ability, attitude, medical history, and strength. With random assignment, subjects with high or low values of these variables are just as likely to be assigned to one group or another. Random assignment is also expected to control for random events that might affect subjects during the course of the study; that is, subjects in both groups should be equally likely to experience illness, personal tragedy, happy occasions, or any other nonsystematic event that might affect the dependent variable. Thus, *overall,* intersubject differences should balance out.

Although random assignment is the preferred method for equalizing groups for scientific study, it does not guarantee equivalence. The concept of randomization is theoretical in that it applies to the probability of outcomes in the proverbial "long run." In other words, if we use random assignment to divide an infinitely large sample, the groups' average scores should not be different; however, because clinical samples tend to be limited in size, random assignment can result in groups that are quite disparate on certain important properties. Researchers often use statistical means of comparing groups on initial values that are considered relevant to the dependent variable, to determine if those extraneous factors did balance out. For example, it may be important to determine if relatively equal numbers of males and females were assigned to each group, or if groups are equivalent on age. When random assignment does not successfully balance the distribution of intersubject differences, there are several design variations that can be used. These will be discussed shortly.

Process of Assigning Subjects

The process of assigning subjects to groups can be carried out in several ways; however, the most effective method involves the use of a table of random numbers, like the one given in Table 8.1. The procedure for using a table of random numbers was introduced in Chapter 8 in relation to random selection. The reader is encouraged to review that process, as it is applicable for random assignment as well.

Suppose we are interested in comparing the effects of two exercises for strengthening knee extensors against a control group that receives no exercise. We assemble a list of 45 subjects, so that we can assign 15 subjects to each of the three groups. The names are numbered from 01 to 45. Because subjects are numbered with two-digit codes, we would use pairs of digits to identify them from the table. As subjects are chosen, they are assigned to Group 1, Group 2 or Group 3 on a rotating basis, until all subjects have been assigned.

In the assignment process, we designate groups as 1, 2, or 3, not by treatment. A good experimental strategy involves continuing the process of random assignment to assign levels of the independent variable to groups. If each treatment level is given a number, we can use the table of random numbers to carry out this assignment. By employing randomization techniques at each step, we have enhanced the validity of the study and fulfilled an essential requirement of experimental research.

Control Groups

The most effective design strategy for ruling out extraneous effects is the use of a **control group** against which the experimental group is compared. Subjects in a control group may receive a standard treatment that will act as a basis of comparison for a new intervention, a placebo or no intervention at all. To draw valid comparisons, we must be able to assume a reasonable degree of equivalence between the control and experimental groups at the start. Then, if we observe a change in the treatment group, but no change in the control group, we can reasonably attribute the change to treatment.

The operational definition of a control condition is important to the interpretation of outcomes. The difference between the two groups should be the essential element that is the independent variable. For example, Mulrow and associates[1] studied the effects of physical therapy intervention on mobility in frail elders in a nursing home. The control group did not receive therapy, but instead was assigned "friendly visitors" who visited with the same frequency as treatment was given. The visitors were intended to control for the effects of personal interaction and attention that were necessary parts of the physical therapy treatment, but not the essential component of the intervention.

The use of a control group may be unfeasible in some clinical situations, for practical or ethical reasons. Therefore, clinical researchers often evaluate a new experimental treatment against conventional methods of care. This does not diminish the validity or usefulness of the study, but it does change the question that can be asked of the data. Instead of assessing whether the new treatment *works*, this approach assesses whether the new treatment is more effective than standard methods. Unless the standard treatment has previously been tested against an untreated control, this type of question does not allow us to determine if the interventions are actually responsible for observed change. If such a study results in improvement in both groups, it would not be possible to determine if both treatments were equally effective or if both groups would have improved spontaneously without any intervention. It is justifiable to design studies with comparative treatments as controls when previous research has clearly established their effectiveness against a true control group, or when it is considered unreasonable to leave patients untreated.

THE RESEARCH PROTOCOL

To control for the effect of extraneous factors that occur within the experimental situation, the researcher must either eliminate them or provide assurance that they will affect all groups equally. In field settings, this type of control can be illusive. Clinical situations cannot always be altered to meet experimental requirements, and, indeed, it may be undesirable to do so. To consider a study a true experiment, however, the researcher must be able to exercise sufficient control over the experimental situation, so that the effect of confounding variables can be ruled out with confidence. Therefore, the clinical researcher must determine which factors are most likely to contaminate the independent variable and attempt to minimize their effects as much as possible. For instance, in studies of patients with rheumatoid arthritis, investigators have recommended that the time of day measurements are taken be kept constant because of circadian rhythms for pain and stiffness.[2]

Although it is impossible to make every subject's experience exactly alike, it is often possible to achieve a reasonable level of constancy for many relevant extraneous variables through delineation of a standardized research protocol. The protocol should specify the positioning of subjects, the timing of all treatments and measurements, the methods of calibrating equipment and any other specifications necessary to ensure the most consistent performance of experimental activities. Researchers often read instructions to subjects (or have subjects read them), so that each one receives exactly the same information. Criteria for assessing the dependent variable should be clear, and those performing data collection should be trained and tested for their reliability.

The realities of the clinical environment suggest, however, that we should weigh the merits of control over experimental conditions versus relevance to practice. If we design protocols that are more restrictive than typical practice, we may find that results are not readily applicable to real world situations. This is most pertinent in studies where the essential nature of treatment cannot reasonably be uniform for all patients. Sometimes we must be able to develop specific treatment plans and progress a patient according to individualized goals, or set the dosage of medication for individual needs. In this case, protocols should be made as consistent as possible, providing a standardized set of guidelines that would make it reproducible.[3] For instance, in the study by Mulrow and associates[1] examining the effect of physical therapy on mobility of nursing home residents, intervention plans were developed by setting specific treatment goals for each patient and organizing all treatments around range of motion, strength, balance and mobility techniques. This approach resulted in individualized treatment sessions, but used the same decision making model for all patients, which should be reproducible.

Handling Incomplete or Lost Data

In addition to controlling for confounding variables, it is important to maximize adherence to the research protocol to limit loss of data. Incomplete data compromise the effect of random assignment and decrease the power of a study (see Chapter 18 for a discussion of power). Loss of data can occur for several reasons.

- **Subjects may drop out of the study or terminate treatment before the study is complete.**   This is a problem because those who remain in a study often differ in an important way from those who drop out.[4] For instance, researchers studied the drug diacerein to relieve symptoms of osteoarthritis (OA), specifically to slow progressive decrease in joint space width in patients with hip OA.[5] In a randomized trial over 3 years, 47% of the patients discontinued the study. Members of the diacerein group dropped out because of adverse events and those in the placebo group left because their clinical status did not improve. In this situation, the attrition was related to group membership, and therefore, those who remained in the study presented a biased view of the outcome.

  In a different example, Winters and co-workers[6] studied the differential effects of active and passive stretching in patients with hip flexor muscle tightness. They recruited 45 subjects for their study, randomly assigning them to two groups. In the end, job conflicts, moving away, and unrelated injuries caused 8 drop-outs in the active stretching group and 4 in the passive stretching group. In this case, although attrition occurred in both groups, the reasons were not related to group assignment, thereby not biasing the outcome.

- **Subjects may cross over to another treatment during the course of the study.** In this situation, subjects do not get the treatment to which they were originally assigned. This may be due to patient preference or a patient's condition may change and the assigned treatment is no longer appropriate. For instance, a study was done to compare use of single-chamber ventricular pacemakers and dual-chamber pacemakers for patients who required cardiac pacing.[7] Patients were randomly assigned to receive one treatment or the other; however, 26% of those who were assigned ventricular pacing experienced symptoms that required changing to the dual-chamber pacemaker, and 2% of those initially assigned to dual-chamber pacing had their pacemakers reprogrammed to ventricular pacing.

- **Subjects may refuse the assigned treatment after allocation.**   A patient may initially consent to join a study, knowing that she may be assigned to either group, but after assignment is complete, the patient decides she wants the other treatment. For example, patients were entered into a randomized trial to compare the effects of epidural analgesia with intravenous analgesia on the outcome of labor.[8] The study included 1,330 women, but only 65% of each group accepted the randomly allocated treatment. Ethically, these patients must be allowed to receive the treatment they want.

- **Subjects may not be compliant with assigned treatments.**   Although they may remain in a study, subjects may not fulfill requirements of their group assignment, negating the treatment effect. For example, a study was done to improve walking and physical function in patients with multiple sclerosis through a progressive 6-month exercise program.[9] Patients were randomly assigned to an exercise or control group. The researchers found, however, that adherence to the strengthening regimen was only 59% in the exercise group.

- **Subjects may be excluded after randomization because they don't meet eligibility requirements.**   The issue of post-randomization exclusion is distinguished from patients dropping out because of noncompliance, withdrawal or loss to follow-up.[10] Some research protocols call for random assignment prior to the point where eligibility can be determined. If some subjects are later excluded from the study, the balance of random assignment will be distorted. For example, Gagnon and associates[11] compared the effects of an early postpartum discharge program versus standard postpartum care on maternal competence, infant weight gain and breastfeeding. Women were randomly assigned to two groups during their pregnancy. However, the researchers specified that complications in childbirth would be cause for exclusion for reasons of safety. Based on intrapartum or postpartum complications, they ended up excluding 46% of those randomized to the early postpartum group and 42% of those assigned to the usual care group. This would clearly unbalance the effect of randomization.

On-Protocol or Completer Analysis

Each of these situations causes a problem for analysis, as the composition of the groups is biased from the initial random assignment, especially if the number of subjects involved is large. There is no clean way to account for this difficulty. At first glance, it might seem prudent to just eliminate any subjects who did not get or complete their assigned treatment, and include only those subjects who sufficiently complied with the trial's protocol. This is called **on-protocol** or **on-treatment analysis**. Compliance refers to getting the assigned treatment, being evaluated according to the protocol, and adherence to protocol requirements.[12] Because this method includes only those who completed the study, it has also been called **completer analysis.**

Generally, the on-protocol approach will tend to bias results in favor of a treatment effect, as those who succeed at treatment are most likely to stick with it.[13,14] For example, in the exercise study with multiple sclerosis, it is possible that those who complied with the strengthening regimen were those who tended to see positive results and those who stopped exercising were not seeing any benefits. Therefore, when analyzing the data using only those subjects who complied, the exercise program would look successful compared to a control group.

It might also seem logical to analyze all subjects according to the treatment that they actually did receive, regardless of their original group assignment. This has been called **treatment-received analysis.**[12] This approach also results in bias, however, because the effect of the random assignment has been compromised. The two groups can no longer be seen as equivalent prior to receiving treatment.

Intention to Treat Analysis

A more conservative approach uses a principle called **intention to treat (ITT)**, which means that data are analyzed according to the original random assignments, regardless of the treatment subjects actually received; that is, we analyze data according to the way we *intended* to treat the subjects. This analysis ideally includes all subjects. The ITT approach serves several purposes. It guards against the potential for bias if dropouts are related to outcomes or group assignment, and preserves the original balance of random assignment. This approach is also considered reflective of routine clinical situations, in which some patients will be noncompliant.

Research has shown that many published randomized trials do not report an intention-to-treat analysis, or if they do, they don't explain how deviations from randomization or missing outcomes are actually handled.[13,15] Current guidelines for reporting randomized trials have been endorsed by an international community of medical journals, recommending use of intention to treat analysis whenever possible, with a flow diagram that documents how subjects were included or excluded through different phases of the study (see Figure 9.1).[16,17]

Fergusson et al[10] suggest that subjects who are excluded from a study after randomization may be omitted from an intention to treat analysis when ineligible patients are mistakenly randomized into a group, or when random assignment was premature. They stress that this strategy is appropriate only when the group assignment did not

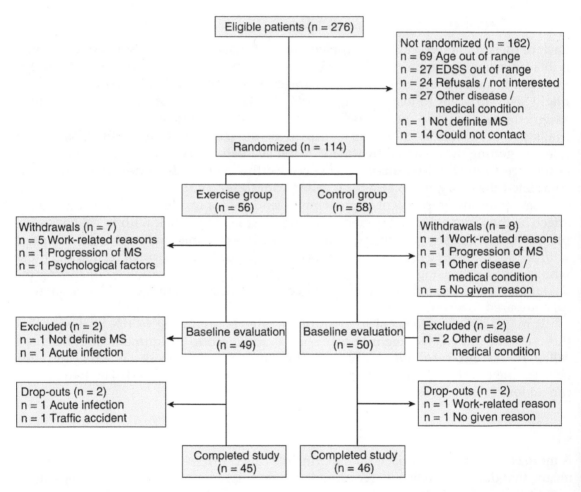

FIGURE 9.1 Sample flow chart showing subject progress through the phases of a randomized trial. Note that the final analysis includes those who completed the study as well as two subjects from each group that dropped out, using an intention to treat analysis. In this study, those who withdrew after allocation were not analyzed. The flow chart provides information on the reasons for dropouts. This is a standard format recommended for reporting randomized trials.[17] Adapted from Romberg A et al. Effects of a 6-month exercise program on patients with multiple sclerosis: A randomized study. *Neurology* 2004; 63:2034–2038. Figure, p. 2036. Used with permission.

influence the likelihood that a patient would or would not receive the intervention. In the previous example of early postpartum discharge, patients in both groups experienced complications in similar proportions, and the researchers did not include them in their intention to treat analysis.[11]

As might be expected, an intention-to-treat analysis may result in an underestimate of the treatment effect, making it harder to find significant differences. This is one of the primary objections to using this approach. However, to be safe, many researchers will analyze data using both intention to treat and on-protocol analyses. For example, in the study of active and passive stretching, described earlier, the authors got the same result with both types of analyses.[6] When outcomes are the same, the researcher will have strong confidence in the results.[18] In another study, Mazieres and colleagues[19] assessed the efficacy of chondroitin sulfate for treating knee osteoarthritis. They found no significant difference in improvement between treatment and placebo groups using the intention to treat approach, but did see a difference with a completer analysis. If the two methods yield different results, the researcher is obliged to consider what factors may be operating to bias the outcome.

Analysis Strategies for Handling Missing Data

Strategies for handling missing data should be specified as part of the research plan, and different approaches may be justified in different situations. Sometimes carrying out more than one strategy is helpful to see if conclusions will differ.

Completer Analysis.   Probably the most common approach is completer analysis. This analysis will represent efficacy of an intervention for those who persist with it, but may be open to serious bias. Using only complete cases can be justified if the number of incomplete cases is small, and if data are missing at random; that is, missing data are independent of group assignment or outcome. Therefore, researchers should report all reasons for missing data. Otherwise, this approach violates the principle of intention to treat and will tend to overestimate the treatment effect.[20]

Noncompleter Equals Failure.   For an intention to treat analysis, when the outcome is dichotomous (success/failure), those who drop out can be considered a "failure." Corcos et al.[21] used this approach in their randomized trial comparing surgery and collagen injections for treatment of female stress urinary incontinence. Success as the primary outcome after 12 months was defined as a dry 24-hour pad test. Patients who refused their assigned intervention, those who received an additional intervention, and those with missing final measures were scored as a failure in the ITT analysis. This is the most conservative approach, so if the treatment group is better we can be confident that the results are not biased by dropouts.[22] If the results show no difference, however, we would not know if the treatment was truly ineffective, or if the dropouts confounded the outcome because they were classified as failures.

Last Observation Carried Forward.   A preferred method for continuous data is called **last observation carried forward (LOCF)**, which means that the subject's last data point before dropping out is used as the outcome score. With multiple test points, the assumption is that patients improve gradually from the start of the study until the end, so that carrying forward an intermediate value is a conservative estimate of how well the person would have done had he or she remained in the study. If the subject drops out right after the pretest, however, this last score could be the baseline score. The LOCF approach allows the analysis to account for trends over time. It does not take into account that some dropouts may have shown no change up to their last assessment, but might have improved had they continued. Overall, however, the LOCF method is better than eliminating large numbers of subjects from the analysis.[22] Lachin[23] suggests that this type of analysis is especially powerful when an effective treatment arrests the progression of a disease, since even after a patient becomes noncompliant, the treatment may still have some long term effect.

Follow-up.   It may be possible to contact subjects who have withdrawn from treatment. Outcome measures can often be obtained from these subjects to make the analysis more complete.[22] Subjects are analyzed as part of the group to which they were originally assigned, even if they did not comply with the treatment. The rationale for this strategy is that it reflects patient behavior in real practice. For example, in the study of urinary incontinence just described, researchers collected additional information by telephone for women who did not have their final evaluation.[21] These women were then included in the intention to treat analysis.

Because missing data can be so disruptive to the interpretation of results of a clinical trial, researchers should take steps to limit this problem in the design and conduct of a study.[12] Efforts should be made to reduce noncompliance, dropouts, crossover of subjects, or loss to follow-up. Eligibility criteria should be as specific as possible to avoid exclusions. A thorough consent process, including adequate warning of potential side effects and expectations, may help to inform subjects sufficiently to avoid noncompliance. Ongoing support for subjects during a trial may also foster continuous participation. Although the true spirit of intention to treat analysis can only be achieved when complete outcome data are available for all subjects, current wisdom in the reporting of randomized trials supports the use of this approach as much as possible.[13]

BLINDING

The potential for observation bias is an important concern in experimental studies. The participants' knowledge of their treatment status or the investigator's expectations can, consciously or unconsciously, influence performance or the recording and reporting of outcomes. Protection against this form of bias is best achieved by using a **double-blind study**, where neither the subjects nor the investigators are aware of the identity of the treatment groups until after data are collected.

In its most complete form, a blind design can involve hiding the identity of group assignments from subjects, from those who provide treatment, from those who measure outcome variables, and from those who will reduce and analyze the data. It is useful to insulate each of these components by having different personnel involved at each level. It is also advisable to blind those responsible for treatment and assessment from the research hypothesis, so that they do not approach their tasks with any preconceived expectations and so that such knowledge cannot influence their interactions with the subjects.

The necessity for and feasibility of blinding depends on the nature of the experimental treatment and the response variables. To blind subjects, the experimental treatment must be able to be offered as a placebo. For many rehabilitation procedures this is not possible. In that case, a **single-blind study** can be carried out, where only the investigator or measurement team is blinded.

Some types of response variables are totally objective, so that blinding is not really necessary. For example, studies that examine survival rates look at death as an outcome variable, an assessment that is obviously not prone to bias; however, as assessments become more subjective, the need for blinding increases. To whatever extent is possible within an experiment, blinding will substantially strengthen the validity of conclusions.

The technique of blinding requires that treatments be coded in some way, so that when data collection is complete, the code can be broken and group assignments revealed. Because the potential for biases in data collection is so strong, blindness should be preserved carefully during the course of the study.

DESIGN STRATEGIES FOR CONTROLLING INTERSUBJECT DIFFERENCES

Clinical research is often concerned with measuring changes in behavioral responses that are potentially influenced by personal traits of those being studied. Several design strategies can be incorporated into a study that will control for these intrinsic variables. The most fundamental of these is random assignment, which eliminates bias by creating a balanced distribution of characteristics across groups. As we have suggested, however, random assignment is not a perfect system, and may result in groups that are not balanced on important variables. When one or two extraneous factors are of special concern, the researcher may not want to depend on randomization.

When a researcher suspects that specific subject traits may interfere with the dependent variable, the simplest way to control for them is to eliminate them by choosing subjects who are **homogeneous** on those characteristics. In that case, the extraneous variables are not allowed to vary, that is, they are eliminated as variables. For instance, if we think males and females will respond differently to the experimental treatment, we can choose only male subjects for our sample. If age is a potential confounder, male subjects can be restricted to a specific age range, such as between 20 and 30 years of age. Once a homogeneous group of subjects is selected, those subjects can be randomly assigned to treatment conditions. In that way, the effects of gender and age are controlled, with all other characteristics equally distributed. The major disadvantage of this approach is that the research findings can be generalized only to the type of subjects who participate in the study, in this case to men between 20 and 30 years of age. This often limits the application of results.

Another means of controlling for extraneous effects is to systematically manipulate attribute variables by building them into the experimental design as an independent variable. For instance, if we are concerned with the effect of age, we could divide subjects into three age groups: under 30, 30 to 40, and over 40. Then, in addition to treatment, we would have a second independent variable, age, with three levels. Each category of age is called a *block*, and the attribute variable, age, is called a **blocking**

variable. This procedure lets us control for age effects by allowing us to analyze the differential effect of age on treatment within the design.

A third strategy for dealing with extraneous variables involves **matching** subjects on the basis of specific characteristics. For example, if we were concerned with the effect of gender and age on our dependent variable, we could use a matching procedure to guarantee an equivalent group of males and females within different age ranges in the experimental and control groups. Studies that use identical twins to compare outcomes are using the ultimate matching process. Matching limits interpretation of research findings because the differential effect of the matching variables cannot be analyzed. For example, if we match subjects on age and gender, then we cannot determine if the effect of treatment is different across age ranges or across males and females. For most clinical studies, matching is not recommended when other methods of controlling extraneous variables are appropriate and practical.

Using Subjects as Their Own Control

Research designs can be structured to facilitate comparisons between independent groups of subjects, or they may involve comparisons of responses across treatment conditions within a subject. When the levels of the independent variable are assigned to different groups, with an active or attribute variable, the independent variable is considered an **independent factor**.* For example, if we compare the effect of two types of splints for reducing hand deformities in patients with rheumatoid arthritis, each type of splint would be worn by a different set of patients. Therefore, the variable of "splint" is an independent factor with two levels. If we compare the effect of splints between males and females, "gender" would also be an independent factor.

When all levels of the independent variable are experienced by all subjects, the independent variable is considered a **repeated factor** or a **repeated measure**. For instance, if we look at the effect of splinting over time, measuring each subject at 1-week intervals for 3 weeks, the variable of "time" becomes a repeated factor with three levels. If we were interested in functional abilities using each type of splint, we might allow each subject to use both splints and test specific hand tasks with each one to compare their responses. In this case, type of splint would be a repeated factor because both splints would be worn by all subjects. The use of a repeated measure is often described as *using subjects as their own control*.

A *repeated measures design* is one of the most efficient methods for controlling intersubject differences. It ensures the highest possible degree of equivalence across treatment conditions because subjects are matched with themselves. We can assume that stable individual characteristics such as gender, intelligence, physical characteristics, and age remain constant for each treatment, so that any differences observed among the treatment conditions can be attributed solely to treatment. Although this assumption is not completely valid for all variables (subjects do differ in mood, hunger, fatigue, and so on, from time to time), the variability of subjects from trial to trial will certainly be

---

*The term *independent factor* should not be confused with *independent variable*. An independent variable can be either an "independent factor," or a "repeated factor," depending on how its levels are defined.

minimal compared with differences between independent groups of subjects. Issues related to the design of repeated measures studies are explored further in Chapter 10.

Analysis of Covariance

The last method of controlling for confounding effects does not involve a design strategy, but instead uses a statistical technique to equate groups on extraneous variables. The **analysis of covariance (ANCOVA)** is based on concepts of analysis of variance and regression, which will be described in Chapters 20 and 24. Without going into details of statistical procedure at this time, we describe the conceptual premise for analysis of covariance for a hypothetical study involving a measure of step length in patients wearing two types of lower extremity orthoses.

Suppose we randomly assign 40 subjects to the two treatment groups, thereby assuming that extraneous factors are equally distributed between the groups. When we compare the subjects' step lengths, we find that the average step for those wearing Orthosis A is longer than the average step for those wearing Orthosis B. We would like to attribute this difference to the differential effects of the orthoses; however, step length is also related to characteristics such as height and leg length. Therefore, if the subjects in Group A happen to be taller than those in Group B, the observed difference in step length may be a function of height, not orthosis.

The purpose of the analysis of covariance is to statistically eliminate the influence of extraneous factors, so that the effect of the independent variable can be seen more clearly. These identified extraneous variables are called *covariates*. Conceptually, the ANCOVA removes the confounding effect of covariates by making them artificially equivalent across groups, and by estimating what the dependent variable *would have been* under these equivalent conditions. For instance, if the patients wearing orthosis A are taller than those in the other group, the analysis figures out what the step lengths would most likely have been had the heights been equally distributed. The analysis of differences between the two groups will then be based on these *adjusted scores*.

To be sure that certain variables are distributed equally across experimental conditions, control can be increased by selecting homogeneous subjects, matching subjects, using subjects as their own control, blocking, or by statistical manipulation using analysis of covariance (see Table 9.1). Each of these strategies requires that the investigator be able to predict which extraneous factors are relevant to the study in advance.

TABLE 9.1   DESIGN STRATEGIES FOR CONTROLLING INTERSUBJECT DIFFERENCES

---

1. *Selection of homogeneous subjects:* Choose only subjects who have the same characteristics of the extraneous variable.
2. *Blocking:* Build extraneous attribute variables into the design by using them as independent variables, creating *blocks* of subjects that are homogeneous for the different levels of the variable.
3. *Matching:* Match subjects on specific characteristics across groups.
4. *Using subjects as their own control:* Expose subjects to all levels of the independent variable, creating a *repeated measures* design.
5. *Analysis of covariance:* Select an extraneous variable as a *covariate*, adjusting scores statistically to control for differences on the extraneous variable.

Such predictions may be based on theory, past studies, or simply the researcher's intuition. The extent of control offered by these methods depends on which extraneous factors are measured and how strong the relationship is between those factors and the dependent variable.

THREATS TO VALIDITY

The goals of experimental research can be summarized by four major questions (see Figure 9.2): (1) Is there a relationship between the independent and dependent variables? (2) Given that a relationship does exist, is there evidence that one causes the other? (3) Given that a cause-and-effect relationship is probable, to what theoretical constructs can the results be generalized? (4) Can the results be generalized to persons, settings, and times that are different from those employed in the experimental situation? These four questions correspond to four types of design validity that form a framework for evaluating experiments: statistical conclusion validity, internal validity, construct validity, and external validity (see Table 9.2).[24]

Statistical Conclusion Validity

Is there a relationship between the independent and dependent variables?

Statistical conclusion validity concerns the potential inappropriate use of statistical procedures for analyzing data, leading to invalid conclusions about the relationship between independent and dependent variables. Some specific threats to statistical conclusion validity are listed here. Because these threats involve concepts of statistical inference that will be covered later in the text, we provide only brief definitions here.

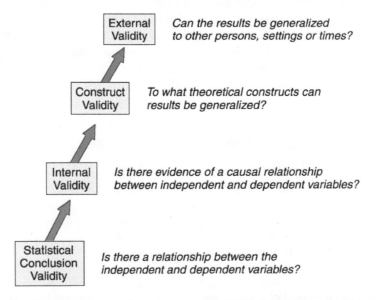

FIGURE 9.2   Four types of design validity. Each form of validity is cumulatively dependent on the components below it.

TABLE 9.2	THREATS TO DESIGN VALIDITY

1. ***Statistical conclusion validity:*** Refers to the appropriate use of statistical procedures for analyzing data.
   - Low statistical power
   - Violated assumptions of statistical tests
   - Error rate
   - Reliability
   - Variance

2. ***Internal validity:*** Refers to the potential for confounding factors to interfere with the relationship between the independent and dependent variables.

Single Group Threats	Multiple Group Threats (Selection Interactions)	Social Threats
• History	• Selection–history	• Diffusion or imitation of treatments
• Maturation	• Selection–maturation	• Compensatory equalization of treatment
• Attrition	• Selection–attrition	• Compensatory rivalry
• Testing	• Selection–testing	• Resentful demoralization
• Instrumentation	• Selection–instrumentation	
• Regression	• Selection–regression	

3. ***Construct validity of causes and effects:*** Refers to the theoretical conceptualization of the independent and dependent variables.
   - Operational definitions of independent and dependent variables
   - Time frame within operational definitions
   - Multiple-treatment interactions
   - Experimental bias
   - Hawthorne effect

4. ***External validity:*** Refers to the extent to which results of a study can be generalized outside the experimental situation.
   - Interaction of treatment and selection
   - Interaction of treatment and setting
   - Interaction of treatment and history

Low Statistical Power.   The power of a statistical test concerns its ability to reject the null hypothesis, that is, to document a real relationship between independent and dependent variables. Significant effects may be missed because of inadequate sample size or failure to control extraneous sources of variation.

Violated Assumptions of Statistical Tests.   Most statistical procedures are based on a variety of assumptions about the experimental data and the sample from which they are collected. If these assumptions are not met, statistical outcomes may lead to erroneous inferences.

Error Rate.   With certain tests, the probability of drawing incorrect conclusions increases as the number of repeated tests increases. Statistical procedures are generally available to control for this threat.

Reliability and Variance.   Statistical conclusions are threatened by any extraneous factors that increase variability within the data, such as unreliable measurement, failure to standardize the protocol, environmental interferences, or heterogeneity of subjects.

These threats contribute to statistical *error variance*, which is a function of all variance in the data that cannot be explained by treatment effects.

Failure to Use Intention to Treat Analysis.   Earlier in this chapter, we discussed the concept of intention to treat as a way to avoid bias in the analysis of data when original random assignment is not maintained, for any number of reasons. Researchers who only use an on-treatment analysis risk overestimating a treatment effect.

Internal Validity

Given a statistical relationship between the independent and dependent variables, is there evidence that one causes the other?

Internal validity focuses on cause and effect relationships. The assumption of causality requires three components.

Temporal Precedence.   First, we must be able to document that the cause precedes the effect; that is, any change in outcome must be observed only after a treatment is applied. This is the age-old metaphor of the chicken and the egg, and is often an issue with cyclical variables. For example, a classic question from economics asks: Does unemployment cause inflation, or does inflation cause unemployment? Temporal relationships can be controlled in prospective studies when the order of treatment and outcome are known.

Covariation of Cause and Effect.   Second, we must be able to document a relationship between independent and dependent variables, showing that the outcome only occurs in the presence of the intervention, or that the degree of outcome is related to the magnitude of the intervention. This type of relationship is clear with an observed change in a treatment group and no change in a control group.

No Plausible Alternative Explanations.   Finally, we must be able to demonstrate that alternative explanations for observed change are not plausible. Confounding variables present threats to internal validity because they offer competing explanations for the observed relationship between the independent and dependent variables; that is, they interfere with cause-and-effect inferences. Several types of alternative explanations must be considered. These can be grouped in three categories: single group threats, multiple group threats, and social threats.[25]

Single Group Threats

Single group threats are those that may affect the relationship between the independent and dependent variables when only one group of subjects is tested.

History.   **History** refers to the confounding effect of specific events, other than the experimental treatment, that occur after the introduction of the independent variable or between a pretest and posttest. For example, if we study the effect of exercise on knee extensor strength, history effects may include some subjects' participation in other athletic activities or other therapies that affect knee extensor strength. If the clinical staff involved in the study is replaced with new personnel during the course of the study, responses may be affected. History can also refer to more global events. For instance, suppose we were interested in studying the effect of an educational program for increasing the use of seat belts by teenagers. If our state passes a law mandating seat belt use during the course of the study, that represents a history effect.

History may not be as serious a concern in studies where data collection is completed within a short period, like a single session.[26] For example, if range of motion of shoulder flexion is measured, followed by 10 minutes of mobilization exercises, and then immediately remeasured, there is little opportunity for confounding events to influence the dependent variable. Even in this type of situation, however, the effects of conversation, the subject's moving around, or other disturbances in the environment may introduce history effects.

Maturation.
A second threat to internal validity concerns processes that occur simply as a function of the passage of time and that are independent of external events. **Maturation** may cause subjects to respond differently on a second measurement because they have grown older, stronger, healthier, more experienced, tired, or bored since the first measurement. For example, if we want to examine the effects of therapy on communication disorders following a stroke, we would have to take into account the fact that spontaneous changes often occur without any intervention.

Maturation is a relevant concern in many areas of clinical research, especially in studies where intervals between measurements are long. Those who study children often encounter physical and mental developmental changes, unrelated to therapeutic intervention, that may influence performance. Wound healing, remission of arthritic symptoms, regeneration in neurological injury, and postoperative recovery are all examples of potential maturation effects.

Attrition.
Clinical researchers are often faced with the fact that subjects drop out of a study before it is completed. **Attrition**, also called experimental mortality, is of concern when it results in a differential loss of subjects, dropouts that occur for specific reasons related to the experimental situation. For example, suppose we studied a program of breathing exercises for patients with emphysema. Subjects who find the exercises more difficult or those who are less motivated may drop out, leaving a group that is no longer representative of the original sample. Researchers may be able to compare pretest scores for those who remain and those who drop out to determine if there is a biasing effect.

Testing.
Testing effects concern the potential effect of pretesting or repeated testing on the dependent variable. In other words, the mere act of collecting data changes the response that is being measured. Testing effects can refer to improved performance or increased skill that occurs because of familiarity with measurements. For example, in educational tests, subjects may actually learn information by taking a pretest, thereby changing their responses on a posttest, independent of any instructional intervention. If a coordination test is given before and after therapy, patients may get higher scores on the posttest because they were able to practice the activity during the pretest. Testing effects also refer to situations where the measurement itself changes the dependent

variable. For instance, if we take repeated measurements of range of motion, the act of moving the joint through the range to evaluate it may actually stretch it enough to increase its range.

Tests that have the potential for changing the response they are measuring are called **reactive measurements**. Reactive effects occur whenever the testing process stimulates change, rather than acting as a passive record of behavior. For instance, placing a video camera in a room to record patient–therapist interactions may alter the observed responses because the subjects know they are being watched. This type of testing effect can be minimized by practice sessions and warm-up trials, to make subjects more comfortable in the testing environment. Unobtrusive or passive measures should be used whenever possible to avoid reactive effects.[27] Techniques such as watching subjects through a two-way mirror qualify as unobtrusive.

Instrumentation. **Instrumentation** effects are concerned with the reliability of measurement. Observers can become more experienced and skilled at measurement between a pretest and posttest. Changes that occur in calibration of hardware or shifts in criteria used by human observers can affect the magnitude of the dependent variable, independent of any treatment effect. Mechanical and bioelectronic instruments can threaten validity if linearity and sensitivity are not constant across the full range of responses and over time. For instance, a force gauge may be designed to register linear forces between 50 and 100 kg. Average scores for subjects who are very strong (near 100 kg) or very weak (near 50 kg) will not be measured as accurately as for those whose average falls between 50 and 100 kg. This threat to internal validity can be addressed by calibration and documenting test–retest and rater reliability.

Regression toward the Mean. **Regression** is also associated with reliability of a test. When measures are not reliable, there is a tendency for extreme scores on the pretest to regress toward the mean on the posttest. This effect occurs even in the absence of intervention. Extremely low scores tend to increase; extremely high scores tend to decrease; and scores that fall around the average tend to stay the same. Statistical regression is of greatest concern when individuals are selected on the basis of extreme scores. For instance, if we wanted to examine the effect of a specific exercise on weaker patients, we might choose a group of subjects with low strength scores on their pretest. The effect of regression will be to increase the group mean on the posttest due to chance variation. The amount of statistical regression is directly related to the degree of measurement error in the dependent variable. Therefore, this effect is minimized when reliability is strong. Examples of this concept were presented in Chapter 5.

Multiple Group Threats

The most effective strategy for ruling out single group threats to internal validity is through the research design, by including a control or comparison group. If the only difference between the intervention and control groups is the treatment, then observation of a difference between the groups following treatment may be attributed to the treatment. The essential point here is the need for groups to be equivalent on all other characteristics at the start of the study. If the groups are not equivalent, we would not be able to determine if the outcomes are due to treatment or to initial differences.

The threat of **selection interaction** refers to factors other than the experimental intervention that can influence posttest differences between groups. When groups are not comparable, the single group threats to internal validity may affect the groups differentially.

Selection–history effects result when experimental groups have different experiences between the pretest and posttest. This is especially important in multicenter studies or where groups are chosen to represent different geographical areas. **Selection–maturation effects** occur when the experimental groups experience maturational change at different speeds. For instance, if we compare changes in motor learning skills following a course of therapy in 3- and 10-year-olds, we can expect a different rate of developmental change that could confound treatment effects. **Selection–testing effects** occur when the pretest affects groups differently. **Selection–instrumentation interaction** occurs when the test is not consistent across groups, often due to variances in reliability. **Selection–regression** interaction is of concern if the groups are specifically divided based on higher and lower pretest scores.

The potential effect of differential selection is obviously controlled when random assignment is used; however, it becomes an issue when intact groups are used, or when the independent variable is an attribute variable. Designs that do not allow random assignment are considered quasi-experimental, in that differences between groups cannot be balanced out. There may be several reasons that subjects belong to one group over another, and these factors can contribute to differences in their performance. Researchers can exert some degree of control for this effect when specific extraneous variables can be identified that vary between the groups. The strategy of matched pairs or the analysis of covariance may be able to account for initial group differences.

Social Threats

Research results are often affected by the interaction of subjects and investigators. **Social threats** to internal validity refer to the pressures that can occur in research situations that may lead to differences between groups. Most of these threats occur because those involved are aware of the other groups' circumstances or are in contact with one another.

Diffusion or Imitation of Treatments. Sometimes the independent variable involves information or activities that are not intended to be equally available to all groups. Because the nature of many interventions makes blinding impractical, control subjects are often aware of the interventions intended for another group, and may attempt to change their behaviors accordingly.[28] For instance, we might want to compare the effect of an exercise program on patients' back pain. The experimental group would attend classes and read packets of information related to exercise, while a control group is given a neutral experience involving no exercise information. If the two groups have an opportunity to communicate, subjects in one group may learn the information intended for the others. Subjects in the control group may become aware of the need for exercise based on the experimental group's activities, and become motivated to begin their own exercise programs. This communication or knowledge will diffuse the treatment effect and make it impossible to distinguish the behaviors of the two groups (see Box 9.1).

BOX 9.1 **The Context of a Clinical Trial: The Lesson of "Mr. Fit"**

Understanding validity in experimental design requires that we consider results within the social context of the intervention. This context includes not only the environment, but the interaction of clinician and patient. One of the most classic examples of this phenomenon is the Multiple Risk Factor Intervention Trial, popularly known as MRFIT, which was conducted at 22 U.S. clinical centers from 1973 to 1982. The trial was designed to test whether lowering elevated serum cholesterol and diastolic blood pressure and ceasing cigarette smoking would reduce coronary heart disease mortality. Over 12,000 men were randomly assigned to either a special intervention (SI) program consisting of drug treatment for hypertension, counseling for cigarette smoking, and dietary advice for lowering blood cholesterol levels, or to their usual sources of health care in the community (UC). Over an average follow-up period of 7 years, the mortality from CHD for SI men was 17.9 deaths/ 1,000 men, and for UC men was 19.3 CHD deaths/1,000 men, a difference that was not significant ($p > .10$). The difference in mortality for all causes was only 2%, also not significant. Reductions in plasma cholesterol levels and smoking were also observed in both groups.

In retrospect, researchers have attributed this lack of difference between the two groups to the fact that men in both groups were originally selected in part because they were willing to participate in a risk factor modification program, knowing they could be assigned to either an intervention or control group. This, along with widespread public efforts in the 1970s to educate people about the benefits of risk factor modification, could have contributed to the observed changes in the UC group. At a cost of well over $100 million for the original trial, this was an expensive lesson.

Source: Multiple Risk Factor Intervention Trial. Risk factor changes and mortality results. *JAMA* 1982; 248:1465–1477.

Compensatory Equalization of Treatments.   When an experimental treatment is considered a desirable service or condition, those who work with and care for the subjects may try to even out experiences by providing compensatory services to the control group. For example, suppose we wanted to study the effect of continuous passive motion on knee range of motion following total knee replacement. Therapists who work with the control patients might work extra hard on range of motion exercises or joint mobilization to compensate for their patients' missing out on the "better" treatment. The effect of such compensatory attention will be to make the groups look more alike, and obscure the experimental effects of treatment.

Compensatory Rivalry and Resentful Demoralization of Respondents Receiving Less Desirable Treatments.   These two effects represent opposite reactions to the same situation. When one group's assigned treatment is perceived as more desirable than the other's, subjects receiving the less desirable treatment may try to compensate by working extra hard to achieve similar results. This is similar to compensatory equalization, described earlier, except that here the subject is responsible for equalizing effects.

In an alternative reaction to this type of situation, subjects receiving less desirable treatments may be demoralized or resentful. Their reaction may be to respond at lower levels of performance. The effect of such responses will be to artificially inflate group differences, which may then be incorrectly attributed to a significantly greater treatment effect.

One way to control this effect is to be sure that there is no interaction among subjects. Sometimes this is difficult, depending on the experimental environment. For instance, if a study were designed to compare the effect of early mother–newborn contact and usual care on mother–child bonding, it might be difficult to prevent interaction if those assigned to different groups were on the same hospital floor or in the same room. Their interaction would tend to contaminate the treatment effect.[29] When this effect is a potential threat, the researcher may choose to randomly assign treatments to different floors, rather than to individuals. The researcher would have to weigh the impact of this approach, as this *en bloc* randomization will control for the compensatory interactions, but may be less desirable in terms of truly balancing individual characteristics.[28]

Ruling Out Threats to Internal Validity

Threats to internal validity are likely to be present in every experiment to some degree. As this list suggests, the task of ruling out alternative explanations for observed changes and documenting the effect of the independent variable is not a small one. It can, however, be addressed as a logical process, one that requires insight, subject matter expertise, and the capacity for self-criticism.[29] Many threats, such as history, maturation, selection, statistical regression, testing, instrumentation, and selection interactions, can be ruled out by the use of random assignment and control groups. These issues are canceled out when both groups are equivalent at the start and are equally likely to be affected by events occurring during the course of the study. Random assignment cannot rule out the effects of attrition, imitating treatments, or compensatory reactions. Blinding subjects and investigators, however, will control many of these effects. The researcher must examine all possible threats and eliminate them or recognize their influence when they are inevitable. When they cannot be eliminated, it may not be possible to demonstrate causal relationships.

Construct Validity of Causes and Effects

Given that a cause and effect relationship is probable, to what theoretical constructs can the results be generalized?

Threats to validity can also be characterized in terms of the construct validity of the independent and dependent variables. As we have discussed before, constructs are abstract behaviors or events that cannot be directly observed, but that can be inferred from other relevant observable variables (see Chapters 2 and 6). **Construct validity of causes and effects** concerns the theoretical conceptualizations of the intervention and response variables and whether these have been developed sufficiently to allow reasonable interpretation and generalization of their relationship.[24]

Most of the treatments and responses that are used in clinical research are based on constructs that must be conceptualized by the researcher in terms of their operational definitions. The levels of the independent variable and measurement methods for the dependent variable will delimit their relationship. If we study "exercises to improve gait," we must conceptualize these variables in terms of specific activities and measurement tools. Outcomes will be interpreted differently, for example, if we study isometric knee exercises and measure gait speed, than if we study walking as an exercise and measure distance walked. Construct validity concerns the researcher's goals and how well experimental results can be generalized within the desired clinical context. Studies that are internally sound may have no practical application beyond the experimental situation if the researcher has not taken the time to explore conceptual questions and the theoretical basis for asking them.

Threats to construct validity are related to how variables are operationally defined within a study and to potential biases introduced into a study by subjects or experimenters.[†]

Operational Definitions

Cook and Campbell suggest that full explication of most constructs requires use of multiple treatment methods and multiple measurement methods.[24] When studies incorporate only one form of measurement or examine only one form of treatment, the results will apply only to a limited aspect of the construct. For example, the construct of pain is truly multidimensional. Therefore, if a study addresses only one form of treatment or one form of measurement, generalization of the results of that study is limited. This limitation is increased when some levels of the independent variable interact differently with various types of dependent variables. For instance, if we treat pain using relaxation exercises or transcutaneous electrical nerve stimulation (TENS), measures of success may vary depending on whether we assess pain by using a visual analog scale (VAS), by measuring range of motion of involved joints or by observing the efficiency of functional tasks. The VAS reflects the patient's subjective and relative feelings of pain intensity, the range of motion test reflects physiological concomitants of pain and functional evaluation is influenced by personality, attitude, motivation, and lifestyle. Therefore, each of these assessments measures a different aspect of pain that reflects components of the total construct.

Generalization is also limited by the time frame within operational definitions. For instance, if we study the effect of TENS over a 2-week period, we cannot generalize outcomes to events that might occur over a longer period of treatment. If treatment shows no effect within this time period, we would be inaccurate to conclude that TENS does not work. The duration of treatment cannot be ignored in defining the construct of intervention, and treatment may need to be carried out over various durations to determine the time necessary to achieve maximal effectiveness.

[†]These threats were originally defined by Campbell and Stanley under the category of *external validity*.[26] Cook and Campbell have subdivided that original categorization into construct validity and external validity.[24]

Construct validity is also affected when a study involves the administration of multiple treatments or multiple measurements. Generalization is limited by the possibility of **multiple-treatment interaction**, creating carryover or combined effects. **Order effects** can result when treatments or measurements are consistently given in the same order, creating possible influences on subsequent responses. The researcher cannot generalize these findings to the situation where only a single treatment or measurement is given; that is, the effect of one response cannot be interpreted out of the context of several responses.

Length of Follow-Up

When a study addresses the response of subjects over time, the length of follow-up will be important to the interpretation of results. Basing decisions on short-term data can be misleading if the observed effects are not durable or if they are slow to develop. For example, studies of continuous passive motion (CPM) following total knee replacement have shown a greater increase in knee range of motion within the first few days after surgery with CPM compared to standard therapy, although this differentiation was no longer evident after 1–3 months.[30,31] This is an important distinction is drawing conclusions about the effect of the intervention. This knowledge would not have been obtained if data collection was not continued beyond the first week. Conclusions should be based on the available data, and not interpreted beyond the scope of the study. For instance, if data are collected over one month, and the treatment does not show a significant effect, there is no way to determine if improvement might have been observed if data were collected over a longer period of time. Similarly, if improvement is seen within the first month, we cannot determine if the trend would be maintained over a longer time period. The construct validity of the independent variable must include reference to the timeframe used for data collection.

Experimental Bias

A third aspect of construct validity concerns biases that are introduced into a study by expectations of either the subjects or the experimenter. Subjects often try their best to fulfill the researcher's expectations or to present themselves in the best way possible, so that responses are no longer representative of natural behavior. This effect was documented in classical studies performed from 1924 to 1927 at the Hawthorne plant of the Western Electric Company in Chicago.[32,33] Researchers were interested in studying how various levels of illumination affected workers' output. What they found was that whether they lowered or raised lights, the workers increased production. Further studies involved introducing changes in work schedules, such as coffee breaks and a shorter work week, all resulting in better output, even when conditions were later returned to original schedules! No matter what the researchers did, productivity improved in regular and test groups. This phenomenon has become known as the **Hawthorne effect**, which is the tendency of persons who are singled out for special attention to perform better merely because they are being observed.

For example, this effect was documented in a study of post-operative pain following knee arthroscopy.[34] Patients who were told pre-operatively that they were part of a study scored significantly better on post-op measures of knee pain and psychological well-being compared to patients who were not given the same information. Researchers should acknowledge this effect when appropriate to the interpretation of results.

The Hawthorne experiments have been criticized for flaws in research design, lack of control groups, small samples, noncompliance and attrition of subjects, and misinterpretation of results.[35] Nonetheless, many researchers continue to explain their findings based on this effect.[34,36,37] Gale[38] provides a wonderful summary and description of the managerial lessons of the original Hawthorne studies, and their contributions to industrial psychology and organizational behavior theory.

Experimenters may also have certain expectancies that can influence how subjects respond. They may react more positively to subjects in the experimental group or give less attention to those in the control group, because of an emotional or intellectual investment in their hypothesis. Rosenthal described several types of **experimenter effects** in terms of the experimenter's *active behavior* and interaction with the subject, such as verbal cues and smiling, and *passive behaviors,* such as those related to appearance.[39] This threat to construct validity can be avoided by employing testers who are blinded to subject assignment and the research hypothesis.

External Validity

Can the results be generalized to persons, settings and times that are different from those employed in the experimental situation?

External validity refers to the extent to which the results of a study can be generalized beyond the internal specifications of the study sample. Whereas internal validity is concerned specifically with the relationship between the independent and dependent variables within a specific set of circumstances, external validity is concerned with the usefulness of that information outside the experimental situation. The generalizability of a study is primarily related to the specific patient context and conditions under investigation.[40]

Threats to external validity involve the interaction of treatment with the specific type of subjects tested, the specific setting in which the experiment is carried out, or the time in history when the study is done.

Interaction of Treatment and Selection

One of the major goals of clinical research is to apply results to a target population, that is, to individuals who are not experimental subjects but who are represented by them. If subjects are sampled according to specific characteristics, those characteristics define the target population. For instance, subjects may be restricted to a limited age range, one gender, a specific diagnosis, or a defined level of function. When samples are confined to certain types of subjects, it is not reasonable to generalize results to those who do not have these characteristics. Because patient characteristics and eligibility requirements can vary, generalizability will depend on how closely the study sample represents the clinical situation.

External validity is threatened when documented cause-and-effect relationships do not apply across subdivisions of the target population, that is, when specific interventions result in differential treatment effects, depending on the subject's characteristics. For instance, suppose we want to demonstrate the benefits of a particular exercise program for improving function following a stroke. The effect of the program may not be generalizable across groups that exhibit various levels of spasticity, those affected on the left or right, patients of different ages, or those with speech disorders. Studies are especially vulnerable to this threat when volunteers are used as subjects. Those who choose to volunteer may do so because of certain personal characteristics that ultimately bias the sample. When studies demonstrate conflicting results, it is often because of the differences within the accessible populations.

A related effect can occur if subjects do not comply with the experimental protocol. A study that is internally valid may still be compromised in relation to external validity under these circumstances. Researchers should examine adherence as they interpret findings, to determine if results are realistic and have clinical applicability.[41] From a sampling perspective, some investigators screen potential subjects prior to randomizing them into groups, to eliminate those who are not adherent. For example, the Physicians' Health Study, which investigated the effect of aspirin and beta carotene in the prevention of ischemic heart disease, used an 18-week "run-in period" and eliminated 33% of the subjects from the final study based on noncompliance.[42] This practice may help to build a compliant study sample, but it may also dilute external validity of the findings.[43] It is the researcher's responsibility to evaluate its potential effect in demonstrating the applicability of the findings.[44]

Interaction of Treatment and Setting

If we demonstrate a causal relationship between an exercise program and functional improvement using patients in a rehabilitation hospital, can we generalize these findings to a nursing home or to home care? This question can only be answered by replicating effects in different settings.

Interaction of Treatment and History

This threat to external validity concerns the ability to generalize results to different periods of time in the past or future. For instance, if we look at the results of nutritional studies for reducing cholesterol in the diet, results may be quite different today from results obtained 20 years ago, when knowledge about the effect of diet and exercise on cardiovascular fitness was less developed, and when society and the media were less involved in promoting fitness and health. This type of generalization is supported when results are replicated in subsequent studies and when previous research corroborates the established causal relationship.

THE CONSORT STATEMENT

Understanding randomized trials requires attention to how the elements of control and design are reported in published studies. Guidelines for reporting have been developed by an international community of researchers and statisticians. The Consolidated Standards for Reporting Trials, or the **CONSORT statement**, has been published on the web[45] and in several journals[46–48] to help authors and readers determine why a study was undertaken, and how it was conducted and analyzed.

The statement is composed of a checklist of 22 items pertaining to the content of the Title, Abstract, Introduction, Methods, Results and Discussion sections of an article (see Table 9.3). A flowchart is also included that details how participants are enrolled and carried through the trial (refer to Figure 9.1). The adoption of the CONSORT statement has improved the reporting of RCTs, enabling readers to better assess the validity of results.[49]

TABLE 9.3 **THE CONSORT STATEMENT**		
Checklist of items to include when reporting a randomized trial.		
PAPER SECTION and topic	**Item**	**Description**
TITLE & ABSTRACT	1	How participants were allocated to interventions (e.g., "random allocation," "randomized," or "randomly assigned").
INTRODUCTION Background	2	Scientific background and explanation of rationale.
METHODS Participants	3	Eligibility criteria for participants and the settings and locations where the data were collected.
Interventions	4	Precise details of the interventions intended for each group and how and when they were actually administered.
Objectives	5	Specific objectives and hypotheses.
Outcomes	6	Clearly defined primary and secondary outcome measures and, when applicable, any methods used to enhance the quality of measurements (e.g., multiple observations, training of assessors).
Sample size	7	How sample size was determined and, when applicable, explanation of any interim analyses and stopping rules.
Randomization— Sequence generation	8	Method used to generate the random allocation sequence, including details of any restriction (e.g., blocking, stratification).
Randomization— Allocation concealment	9	Method used to implement the random allocation sequence (e.g., numbered containers or central telephone), clarifying whether the sequence was concealed until interventions were assigned.
Randomization— Implementation	10	Who generated the allocation sequence, who enrolled participants, and who assigned participants to their groups.
Blinding (masking)	11	Whether or not participants, those administering the interventions, and those assessing the outcomes were blinded to group assignment. If done, how the success of blinding was evaluated.
Statistical methods	12	Statistical methods used to compare groups for primary outcome(s); methods for additional analyses, such as subgroup analyses and adjusted analyses.

TABLE 9.3	THE CONSORT STATEMENT	
PAPER SECTION and topic	**Item**	**Description**
RESULTS Participant flow	13	Flow of participants through each stage (a diagram is strongly recommended). Specifically, for each group report the numbers of participants randomly assigned, receiving intended treatment, completing the study protocol, and analyzed for the primary outcome. Describe protocol deviations from study as planned, together with reasons.
Recruitment	14	Dates defining the periods of recruitment and follow-up.
Baseline data	15	Baseline demographic and clinical characteristics of each group.
Numbers analyzed	16	Number of participants (denominator) in each group included in each analysis and whether the analysis was by "intention-to-treat." State the results in absolute numbers when feasible (e.g., 10/20, not 50%).
Outcomes and estimation	17	For each primary and secondary outcome, a summary of results for each group, and the estimated effect size and its precision (e.g., 95% confidence interval).
Ancillary analyses	18	Address multiplicity by reporting any other analyses performed, including subgroup analyses and adjusted analyses, indicating those prespecified and those exploratory.
Adverse events	19	All important adverse events or side effects in each intervention group.
DISCUSSION Interpretation	20	Interpretation of the results, taking into account study hypotheses, sources of potential bias or imprecision, and the dangers associated with multiplicity of analyses and outcomes.
Generalizability	21	Generalizability (external validity) of the trial findings.
Overall evidence	22	General interpretation of the results in the context of current evidence.

Available at <http://www.consort-statement.org/Statement/revisedstatement.htm#checklist> Accessed May 5, 2007.

COMMENTARY

The Relative Validity of Evidence

Design validity is an important consideration in all forms of research. Although the threats to validity described here have been presented in the context of experimental research, they are also relevant to exploratory and quasi-experimental designs, which are discussed in subsequent chapters. The only threat that is unique to experiments is internal validity, as it is specifically concerned with cause-and-effect relationships.

Because there are so many potential threats to validity, researchers must examine priorities among them. Not all threats to validity are of equal concern in every study. When steps are taken to increase one type of validity, it is likely that another type will be decreased. The specific research situation will dictate how specific extraneous factors impact on a given design. For instance, if we attempt to control for extraneous factors by using a homogeneous sample, we will improve internal validity, but at the expense of external validity. If we increase statistical conclusion validity by limiting variability in our data, the sample will be less representative of a general population. This will probably reduce external and construct validity. Similarly, if we work toward increasing construct validity by operationalizing variables in multiple dimensions, we run the risk of decreasing reliability with an increasing number of measurements. When theoretical issues are of special importance, construct validity should be of great concern. When cause-and-effect relationships are sought, internal validity is of primary importance.

The context of the research question will guide priorities in research design. Is the question related to public health concerns, with the primary intention of generalizing to a large population? Does the question target a new intervention and the need to document its effectiveness? Does the question focus on differential effects of a treatment in subgroups of a population? The progress of a line of research may dictate which elements of design validity are most important at a particular point. As studies are replicated and modified, all types of validity will eventually be addressed in a particular area of investigation.

After describing all the above threats to experimental validity, the clinical researcher might wonder how it is ever possible to design a completely valid study. In fact, there is no such thing in clinical research. Every study contains some shortcomings. Clinical researchers operate in an environment that demands consideration of ethical and practical issues, as well as the unpredictable and often immeasurable factors of human nature, error, emotion and thought. The clinical researcher can control neither the environment nor the consistency of a subject's interaction with that environment to the same extent that the laboratory researcher can control an animal's genetic makeup, diet, or physiological characteristics. It is virtually impossible to conduct a clinical experiment so that every facet of behavior, environment and personal interaction is exactly the same for every subject.

Does this mean that we cannot create experimental situations with sufficient control to be able to make valid judgments about human responses? Not at all. We can still conduct experiments and draw meaningful conclusions from them by adhering to the elements of experimental control with as much rigor as possible, accounting for variations in the experimental situation with every reasonable effort, and ultimately recognizing those factors over which we have no control.

Clinical studies cannot be expected to produce results that are perfectly controlled or directly relevant to all patients and settings.[50] Therefore, authors should provide sufficient details on the design of the study that will allow clinicians to judge how and to whom evidence can be reasonably applied. This is of special importance in external validity, to determine if interventions are safe. If study samples are too homogeneous (inclusion criteria are very narrow), findings will not be relevant to many patients who fit the overall diagnostic category. Limitations of a study should be discussed in a research report so that readers have a complete understanding of the circumstances in which results were obtained. To have confidence in results, however, the researcher must be able to justify the experimental conditions as a fair test of the experimental treatment within the context of the research question. When the researcher can anticipate that important extraneous factors cannot be controlled, to the point that they will have a serious impact on the interpretation and validity of outcomes, it is advisable to consider alternatives to experimental research, such as descriptive or correlational approaches.

REFERENCES

1. Mulrow CD, Gerety MB, Kanten D, Cornell JE, DeNino LA, Chiodo L, et al. A randomized trial of physical rehabilitation for very frail nursing home residents. *JAMA* 1994;271:519–524.
2. Bellamy N, Sothern RB, Campbell J, Buchanan WW. Circadian rhythm in pain, stiffness, and manual dexterity in rheumatoid arthritis: Relation between discomfort and disability. *Ann Rheum Dis* 1991;50:243–248.
3. Silverman WA. *Human Experimentation: A Guided Step into the Unknown*. New York: Oxford University Press, 1985.
4. Mahaniah KJ, Rao G. Intention-to-treat analysis: Protecting the integrity of randomization. *J Fam Pract* 2004;53:644.
5. Dougados M, Nguyen M, Berdah L, Mazieres B, Vignon E, Lequesne M. Evaluation of the structure-modifying effects of diacerein in hip osteoarthritis: ECHODIAH, a three-year, placebo-controlled trial. Evaluation of the chondromodulating effect of diacerein in OA of the hip. *Arthritis Rheum* 2001;44:2539–2547.
6. Winters MV, Blake CG, Trost JS, Marcello-Brinker TB, Lowe L, Garber MB, et al. Passive versus active stretching of hip flexor muscles in subjects with limited hip extension: A randomized clinical trial. *Phys Ther* 2004;84:800–807.
7. Lamas GA, Orav EJ, Stambler BS, Ellenbogen KA, Sgarbossa EB, Huang SKS, et al. Quality of life and clinical outcomes in elderly patients treated with ventricular pacing as compared with dual-chamber pacing. *New Engl J Med* 1998;338:1097–1104.
8. Ramin SM, Gambling DR, Lucas MJ, Sharma SK, Sidawi JE, Leveno KJ. Randomized trial of epidural versus intravenous analgesia during labor. *Obstet Gynecol* 1995;86: 783–789.
9. Romberg A, Virtanen A, Ruutiainen J, Aunola S, Karppi SL, Vaara M, et al. Effects of a 6-month exercise program on patients with multiple sclerosis: A randomized study. *Neurology* 2004;63:2034–2038.
10. Fergusson D, Aaron SD, Guyatt G, Hebert P. Post-randomisation exclusions: The intention to treat principle and excluding patients from analysis. *BMJ* 2002;325:652–654.
11. Gagnon AJ, Edgar L, Kramer MS, Papageorgiou A, Waghorn K, Klein MC. A randomized trial of a program of early postpartum discharge with nurse visitation. *Am J Obstet Gynecol* 1997;176:205–211.
12. Heritier SR, Gebski VJ, Keech AC. Inclusion of patients in clinical trial analysis: The intention-to-treat principle. *Med J Aust* 2003;179:438–440.
13. Hollis S, Campbell F. What is meant by intention to treat analysis? Survey of published randomised controlled trials. *BMJ* 1999;319:670–674.
14. Newell DJ. Intention-to-treat analysis: Implications for quantitative and qualitative research. *Int J Epidemiol* 1992;21:837–841.
15. Kruse RL, Alper BS, Reust C, Stevermer JJ, Shannon S, Williams RH. Intention-to-treat analysis: Who is in? Who is out? *J Fam Pract* 2002;51:969–971.

16. Moher D, Schulz KF, Altman DG. The CONSORT statement: Revised recommendations for improving the quality of reports of parallel-group randomised trials. *Clin Oral Investig* 2003;7:2–7.
17. CONSORT website. Available at <http://www.consort-statement.org/> Accessed August 19, 2005.
18. Motulsky H. *Intuitive Biostatistics*. New York: Oxford University Press, 1995.
19. Mazieres B, Combe B, Phan Van A, Tondut J, Grynfeltt M. Chondroitin sulfate in osteoarthritis of the knee: A prospective, double blind, placebo controlled multicenter clinical study. *J Rheumatol* 2001;28:173–181.
20. Choi SC, Lu IL. Effect of non-random missing data mechanisms in clinical trials. *Stat Med* 1995;14:2675–2684.
21. Corcos J, Collet JP, Shapiro S, Herschorn S, Radomski SB, Schick E, et al. Multicenter randomized clinical trial comparing surgery and collagen injections for treatment of female stress urinary incontinence. *Urology* 2005;65:898–904.
22. Streiner D, Geddes J. Intention to treat analysis in clinical trials when there are missing data. *Evid Based Ment Health* 2001;4:70–71.
23. Lachin JM. Statistical considerations in the intent-to-treat principle. *Control Clin Trials* 2000;21:167–189.
24. Cook TD, Campbell DT. *Quasi-experimentation: Design and Analysis Issues for Field Settings*. Boston: Houghton Mifflin, 1979.
25. Research methods knowledge base. Internal validity. Available at <http://www.socialresearchmethods.net/kb/intval.php> Accessed May 23, 2007.
26. Campbell DT, Stanley JC. *Experimental and Quasi-experimental Designs for Research*. Chicago: Rand McNally, 1963.
27. Webb EJ, Campbell DT, Schwartz RD, Sechrest L. *Unobtrusive measures*. Skokie, IL: Rand McNally, 1966.
28. Thomson ME, Kramer MS. Methodologic standards for controlled clinical trials of early contact and maternal-infant behavior. *Pediatrics* 1984;73:294–300.
29. Kirk RE. *Experimental Design: Procedures for the Behavioral Sciences* (2nd ed.). Belmont, CA: Brooks/Cole, 1982.
30. Bennett LA, Brearley SC, Hart JA, Bailey MJ. A comparison of 2 continuous passive motion protocols after total knee arthroplasty: A controlled and randomized study. *J Arthroplasty* 2005;20:225–233.
31. Lau SK, Chiu KY. Use of continuous passive motion after total knee arthroplasty. *J Arthroplasty* 2001;16:336–339.
32. Roethlisberger J, Dickson WJ. *Management and the Worker*. Cambridge, MA: Harvard University Press, 1966.
33. Gillespie R. *Manufacturing Knowledge: A History of the Hawthorne Experiments*. Cambridge ed. New York: Cambridge University Press, 1991.
34. De Amici D, Klersy C, Ramajoli F, Brustia L, Politi P. Impact of the Hawthorne effect in a longitudinal clinical study: The case of anesthesia. *Control Clin Trials* 2000;21:103–114.
35. Kolata G. Scientific myths that are too good to die. *The New York Times*, 1998 December 6, 1998; 18.
36. The Burton Report: Informatives on health care. The Hawthorne Effect. Available at: <http://www.burtonreport.com/InfHealthCare/Info&UseHawthorne.html> Accessed November 3, 2006.
37. Zinman R, Bethune P, Camfield C, Fitzpatrick E, Gordon K. An observational asthma study alters emergency department use: The Hawthorne effect. *Pediatr Emerg Care* 1996; 12:78–80.
38. Gale EA. The Hawthorne studies—A fable for our times? *QJM* 2004;97:439–449.

39. Rosenthal R. *Experimenter Effects in Behavioral Research.* New York: Appleton-Century-Crofts, 1966.
40. Gartlehner G, Hansen RA, Nissman D, Lohr KN, Carey TS. Criteria for distinguishing effectiveness from efficacy trials in systematic reviews. Technical Review 12 (Prepared by the RTI-International-University of North Carolina Evidence-Based Practice Center under Contract No. 290-02-0016.) AHRQ Publication No. 06-0046. Rockville, MD: Agency for Healthcare Research and Quality. April 2006. Available at: <http://www.ahrq.gov/downloads/pub/evidence/pdf/efftrials/efftrials.pdf> Accessed June 11, 2006.
41. Guyatt GH, Sackett DL, Cook DJ. Users' guides to the medical literature. II. How to use an article about therapy or prevention. B. What were the results and will they help me in caring for my patients? Evidence-Based Medicine Working Group. *JAMA* 1994;271:59–63.
42. Final report on the aspirin component of the ongoing Physicians' Health Study. Steering Committee of the Physicians' Health Study Research Group. *N Engl J Med* 1989;321:129–135.
43. Kramer MS, Shapiro SH. Scientific challenges in the application of randomized trials. *JAMA* 1984;252:2739–2745.
44. Pablos-Mendez A, Barr RG, Shea S. Run-in periods in randomized trials: Implications for the application of results in clinical practice. *JAMA* 1998;279:222–225.
45. CONSORT website. Available at: <http://www.consort-statement.org/> Accessed August 19, 2005.
46. Moher D, Schulz KF, Altman D. The CONSORT statement: Revised recommendations for improving the quality of reports of parallel-group randomized trials. *JAMA* 2001;285:1987–1991.
47. Moher D, Schulz KF, Altman DG. The CONSORT statement: Revised recommendations for improving the quality of reports of parallel-group randomised trials. *Lancet* 2001;357:1191–1194.
48. Altman DG, Schulz KF, Moher D, Egger M, Davidoff F, Elbourne D, et al. The revised CONSORT statement for reporting randomized trials: Explanation and elaboration. *Ann Intern Med* 2001;134:663–694.
49. Plint AC, Moher D, Morrison A, Schulz K, Altman DG, Hill C, et al. Does the CONSORT checklist improve the quality of reports of randomised controlled trials? A systematic review. *Med J Aust* 2006; 185:263–267.
50. Rothwell PM. External validity of randomised controlled trials: "To whom do the results of this trial apply?" *Lancet* 2005;365:82–93.

CHAPTER 10
Experimental Designs

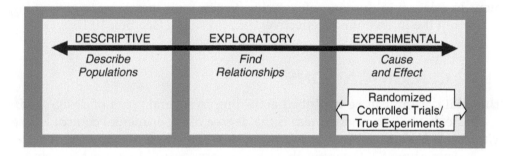

DESCRIPTIVE	EXPLORATORY	EXPERIMENTAL
Describe Populations	*Find Relationships*	*Cause and Effect*
		Randomized Controlled Trials/ True Experiments

The purpose of an experimental design is to provide a structure for evaluating the cause-and-effect relationship between a set of independent and dependent variables. Within the design, the researcher manipulates the levels of the independent variable and incorporates elements of control, so that the evidence supporting a causal relationship can be interpreted with confidence.

Although experimental designs can take on a wide variety of configurations, the important principles can be illustrated using a few basic structures. The purpose of this chapter is to present these basic designs and to illustrate the types of research situations for which they are most appropriate. For each design, we discuss strengths and weaknesses in terms of experimental control and internal and external validity. In addition, we include a short statement suggesting general statistical procedures for analysis. These suggestions do not represent all statistical options for a particular design, but they do represent the more commonly used techniques. This information demonstrates the intrinsic relationship between analysis and design.

CLINICAL TRIALS

The term **clinical trial** is often used to describe experimental studies that examine the effect of interventions on patient or community populations. Clinical trials are frequently designed on a large scale, involving subjects from a range of geographic areas or from several treatment centers. Clinical trials can be classified as either therapeutic or preventive. *Therapeutic trials* examine the effect of a treatment or intervention on a particular disease. For example, 25 years of clinical trials, begun in the 1970s, have shown that radical mastectomy is not necessary for reducing the risk of recurrence or spread of breast cancer, and that limited resection can be equally effective in terms of recurrence and mortality.[1] A *preventive trial* evaluates whether a procedure or agent reduces the risk of developing a disease. One of the most famous preventive trials was the field study of poliomyelitis vaccine in 1954, which covered 11 states.[2] The incidence of poliomyelitis in the vaccinated group was over 50 percent less than among those children who received the placebo, establishing strong evidence of the vaccine's effectiveness. In a more contemporary example, scientists continue to design trials in an effort to develop a vaccine to prevent HIV infection.[3]

In the investigation of new therapies, including drugs, surgical procedures and electromechanical devices, distinct sequences of clinical trials are typically carried out. The phases of trials are intended to provide different types of information about the treatment in relation to dosage, safety and efficacy, with increasingly greater rigor in demonstrating the intervention's effectiveness and safety (see Box 10.1).

DESIGN CLASSIFICATIONS

Experimental designs can be described according to several types of design characteristics. A basic distinction among them is the degree of experimental control.[4,5] In a **true experimental design**, subjects are randomly assigned to at least two comparison groups. An experiment is theoretically able to exert control over most threats to internal validity, providing the strongest evidence for causal relationships. The **randomized controlled trial (RCT)** is considered the gold standard of true experimental designs.

A **quasi-experimental design** does not meet the requirements of a true experiment, lacking random assignment or comparison groups, or both. Even though quasi-experimental designs cannot rule out threats to internal validity with the same confidence as experimental designs, many such designs are appropriate when stronger designs are not feasible. Quasi-experimental designs represent an important contribution to clinical research, because they accommodate for the limitations of natural settings, where scheduling treatment conditions and random assignment are often difficult, impractical or unethical. These designs will be covered in Chapter 11.

Experimental designs may be differentiated according to how subjects are assigned to groups. In **completely randomized designs**, also referred to as **between-subjects designs**, subjects are assigned to independent groups using a randomization procedure. In a **randomized block design** subjects are first classified according to an attribute variable (a blocking variable) and then randomized to treatment groups. A design in which subjects act as their own control is called a **within-subjects design** or a **repeated measures design**.

These designs can also be described according to the number of independent variables, or *factors*, within the design. *Single-factor designs* have one independent variable with any number of levels. *Multi-factor designs* contain two or more independent variables.

SELECTING A DESIGN

Once a research question is formulated, the researcher must decide on the most effective design for answering it. Although experimental designs represent the highest standard in scientific inquiry, they are not necessarily the best choice in every situation. When the independent variable cannot be manipulated by the experimenter, or when

BOX 10.1 Trial Phases in Investigational Studies

Preclinical Research

Before a new therapy is used on humans, it is tested under laboratory conditions, often using animal models. This may take many years, to screen different chemical compounds for drugs, or to refine interventions. When a new drug or device shows promise at this phase, researchers will then request permission to begin human trials from the Food and Drug Administration (FDA).

Phase I Trial

In a phase I trial, researchers work to show that a new therapy is safe. Data are collected on dosage, timing and side effects. Typically done on small samples of 20–80 subjects, phase I trials help us to understand the mechanisms of action of the therapy, and set the stage for controlled clinical trials.

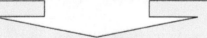

Phase II Trial

Once a therapy has been shown to be safe in humans, it is studied in a phase II trial to demonstrate that it is effective. Also done on relatively small samples, these trials may take up to 2 years. The response rate should be the same or better than standard treatment to warrant further testing.

Phase III Trial

A phase III clinical trial is a randomized, usually blinded, experiment that compares a new therapy with a standard treatment or placebo. These are large scale studies with hundreds or thousands of subjects. Successful outcomes will lead to seeking approval from the FDA.

Phase IV Trial

Once a drug or intervention has been approved, researchers may continue to investigate its effects in other populations, specifically to learn about risk factors, benefits and optimal use patterns.

important extraneous factors cannot be controlled, an observational or exploratory design may be more useful (see Chapter 13).

When an experimental design is deemed appropriate, the choice of a specific design will depend on the answers to six critical questions about how the study is conceptualized:

1. How many independent variables are being tested?
2. How many levels does each independent variable have, and are these levels experimental or control conditions?
3. How many groups of subjects are being tested?
4. How will subjects be assigned to groups?
5. How often will observations of responses be made?
6. What is the temporal sequence of interventions and measurements?

When each of these issues is considered, the range of potential designs will usually be narrowed to one or two appropriate choices. As specific designs are presented, these questions will be addressed within the context of research questions from the literature.

DESIGNS FOR INDEPENDENT GROUPS
Single-Factor Designs for Independent Groups

A single-factor design, also called a **one-way design**, is used to structure the investigation of one independent variable. The study may include one or more dependent variables.

Pretest-Posttest Control Group Design

The **pretest-posttest control group design** is the basic structure of a randomized controlled trial. It is used to compare two or more groups that are formed by random assignment. One group receives the experimental variable and the other acts as a control. These independent groups are also called **treatment arms** of the study. Both groups are tested prior to and following treatment. The groups differ solely on the basis of what occurs between measurements. Therefore, changes from pretest to posttest that appear in the experimental group but not the control group can be reasonably attributed to the intervention. This design is considered the scientific standard in clinical research for establishing a cause-and-effect relationship.

The pretest-posttest control group design can be configured in several ways. Figure 10.1 illustrates the simplest configuration, with one experimental group and one control group.

Example of a Pretest-Posttest Control Group Design
Researchers conducted a randomized controlled trial to study the effect of a supervised exercise program for improving venous hemodynamics in patients with chronic venous insufficiency.[6] They randomly assigned 31 patients to two groups. The experimental group received physical therapy with specific exercises for calf strengthening and joint mobility. The control group received no exercise intervention. Both groups received compression hosiery. Dynamic strength, calf pump function and quality of life were assessed at baseline and after 6 months of exercise.

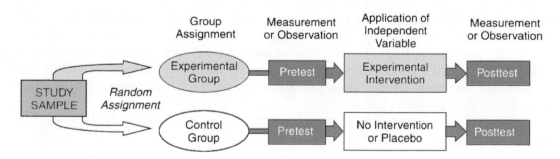

FIGURE 10.1   Pretest-posttest control group design; the basic structure of a randomized controlled trial (RCT).

Measurements for the control group are taken within intervals that match those of the experimental group. The independent variable has two levels, in this case exercise intervention and control. The absence of an experimental intervention in the control group is considered a level of the independent variable. As this example illustrates, a study may have several dependent variables that are measured at pretest and posttest.

The pretest-posttest design can also be used when the comparison group receives a second form of the intervention. The *two-group pretest-posttest design* (see Figure 10.2) incorporates two experimental groups formed by random assignment.

Example of a Two-Group Pretest-Posttest Design
Researchers conducted a randomized controlled trial to study the effect of semantic treatment on verbal communication in patients who experienced aphasia following a stroke.[7] They randomly assigned 58 patients to two groups. Speech therapists provided semantic treatment to the experimental group. The control group received speech therapy focused on word sounds. Verbal communication was assessed using the Amsterdam Nijmegen Everyday Language Test. Both groups were assessed at the start of the study and following 7 months of treatment.

Researchers use this approach when a control condition is not feasible or ethical, often comparing a "new" treatment with an "old" standard or alternative treatment. Even though there is no traditional control group, this design provides experimental control because we can establish initial equivalence between groups formed by random

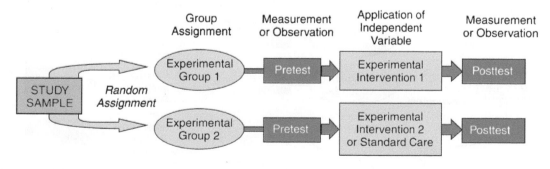

FIGURE 10.2   Two-group pretest-posttest design.

assignment. In this example, the word sound group acts as a control for the semantic treatment group and vice versa. If one group improves more than the other, we can attribute that difference to the fact that one treatment was more effective. This design is appropriate when the research question specifically addresses interest in a difference between two treatments, but it does not allow the researcher to show that treatment works better than no intervention.

The *multigroup pretest-posttest control group design* (see Figure 10.3) allows researchers to compare several treatment and control conditions.

> **Example of a Multigroup Pretest-Posttest Design**
> Researchers wanted to determine the effectiveness of aquatic and on-land exercise programs on functional fitness and activities of daily living (ADLs) in older adults with arthritis.[8] Participants were 30 volunteers, randomly assigned to aquatic exercise, on-land exercise or a control group. The control group was asked to refrain from any new physical activity for the duration of the study. Outcomes included fitness and strength measures, and functional assessments before and after an 8-week exercise program.

As these examples illustrate, the pretest-posttest control group design can be expanded to accommodate any number of levels of one independent variable, with or without a traditional control group. This design is strong in internal validity. Pretest scores provide a basis for establishing initial equivalence of groups, strengthening the evidence for causal factors. Selection bias is controlled because subjects are randomly assigned to groups. History, maturation, testing, and instrumentation effects should affect all groups equally in both the pretest and posttest. The only threat to internal validity that is not controlled by this design is attrition.

The primary threat to external validity in the pretest-posttest control group design is the potential interaction of treatment and testing. Because subjects are given a pretest, there may be reactive effects, which would not be present in situations where a pretest is not given.

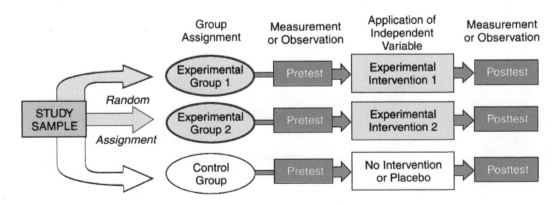

FIGURE 10.3   Multigroup pretest-posttest design.

Analysis of Pretest-Posttest Designs.   Pretest-posttest designs are often analyzed using change scores, which represent the difference between the posttest and pretest.* With interval-ratio data, difference scores are usually compared using an unpaired *t*-test (with two groups or a one-way analysis of variance (with three or more groups). With ordinal data, the Mann-Whitney *U*-test can be used to compare two groups, and the Kruskal-Wallis analysis of variance by ranks is used to compare three or more groups. The analysis of covariance can be used to compare posttest scores, using the pretest score as the covariate. The design can be analyzed as a two-factor design, using a two-way analysis of variance with one repeated factor, with treatment as one independent variable and time (pretest and posttest) as the second (repeated) factor. Discriminant analysis can also be used to distinguish between groups with multiple outcome measures.

Posttest-Only Control Group Design

The **posttest-only control group design** (see Figure 10.4) is identical to the pretest-posttest control group design, with the obvious exception that a pretest is not administered to either group.

> **Example of Posttest-Only Control Group Design**
> A study was designed to test the hypothesis that high-risk patients undergoing elective hip and knee arthroplasty would incur less total cost and shorter length of stay if inpatient rehabilitation began on postoperative day 3 rather than day 7.[9] Eighty-six patients who were older than 70 years were randomly assigned to begin rehabilitation on day 3 or day 7 The main outcome measures were total length of stay and cost from orthopedic and rehabilitation admissions.

In this study of hospital cost and length of stay, the dependent variables can only be assessed following the treatment condition. This design is a true experimental design which, like the pretest-posttest design, can be expanded to include multiple levels of the independent variable, with a control, placebo or alternative treatment group.

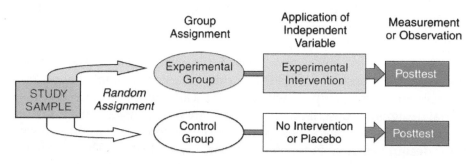

FIGURE 10.4   Posttest-only control group design.

---

*See discussion about the reliability of change scores in Chapter 6.

Because this design involves random assignment and comparison groups, its internal validity is strong, even without a pretest; that is, we can assume groups are equivalent prior to treatment. Because there is no pretest score to document the results of randomization, this design is most successful when the number of subjects is large, so that the probability of truly balancing interpersonal characteristics is increased.

The posttest-only design can also be used when a pretest is either impractical or potentially reactive. For instance, to study the attitudes of health care personnel toward patients with AIDS, we might use a survey instrument that asked questions about attitudes and experience with this population. By using this instrument as a pretest, subjects might be sensitized in a way that would influence their scores on a subsequent posttest. The posttest-only design avoids this form of bias, increasing the external validity of the study.

Analysis of Posttest-Only Designs.   With two groups, an unpaired *t*-test is used with interval-ratio data, and a Mann-Whitney *U*-test with ordinal data. With more than two groups, a one-way analysis of variance or the Kruskal-Wallis analysis of variance by ranks should be used to compare posttest scores. An analysis of covariance can be used when covariate data on relevant extraneous variables are available. Regression or discriminant analysis procedures can also be applied.

Multi-Factor Designs for Independent Groups

The designs presented thus far have involved the testing of one independent variable, with two or more levels. Although easy to develop, these single-factor designs tend to impose an artificial simplicity on most clinical and behavioral phenomena; that is, they do not account for simultaneous and often complex interactions of several variables within clinical situations. Interactions are generally important for developing a theoretical understanding of behavior and for establishing the construct validity of clinical variables. Interactions may reflect the combined influence of several treatments or the effect of several attribute variables on the success of a particular treatment.

Factorial Design

A *factorial design* incorporates two or more independent variables, with independent groups of subjects randomly assigned to various combinations of levels of the two variables. Although such designs can theoretically be expanded to include any number of variables, clinical studies usually involve two or three at most. As the number of independent variables increases, so does the number of experimental groups, creating the need for larger and larger samples, which are typically impractical in clinical situations.

Factorial designs are described according to their dimensions or number of factors, so that a *two-way* or two-factor design has two independent variables, a *three-way* or three-factor design has three independent variables, and so on. These designs can also be described by the number of levels within each factor, so that a 3×3 design includes two variables, each with three levels, and a $2 \times 3 \times 4$ design includes three variables, with two, three and four levels, respectively.

A factorial design is diagrammed using a matrix notation that indicates how groups are formed relative to levels of each independent variable. Uppercase letters, typically

A, B and *C*, are used to label the independent variables and their levels. For instance, with two independent variables, *A* and *B*, we can designate three levels for the first one (A_1, A_2 and A_3) and two levels for the second (B_1, B_2).

The number of groups is the product of the digits that define the design. For example, $3 \times 3 = 9$ groups; $2 \times 3 \times 4 = 24$ groups. Each cell of the matrix represents a unique combination of levels. In this type of diagram there is no indication if measurements within a cell include pretest-posttest scores or posttest scores only. This detail is generally described in words.

Two-Way Factorial Design. A *two-way factorial design* (see Figure 10.5) incorporates two independent variables, *A* and *B*.

Example of a Two-Way Factorial Design
Researchers were interested in studying the effect of intensity and location of exercise programs on the self-efficacy of sedentary women.[10] Using a 2×2 factorial design, subjects were randomly assigned to one of four groups, receiving a combination of moderate or vigorous exercise at home or a community center. The change in their exercise behavior and their self-efficacy in maintaining their exercise program was monitored over 18 months.

In this example, the two independent variables are intensity of exercise (*A*) and location of exercise (*B*), each with two levels (2×2). One group (A_1B_1) will engage in moderate exercise at home. A second group (A_2B_1) will engage in vigorous exercise at home. The third group (A_1B_2) will engage in moderate exercise at a community center. And the fourth group (A_2B_2) will engage in vigorous exercise at a community center. The two independent variables are *completely crossed* in this design, which means that

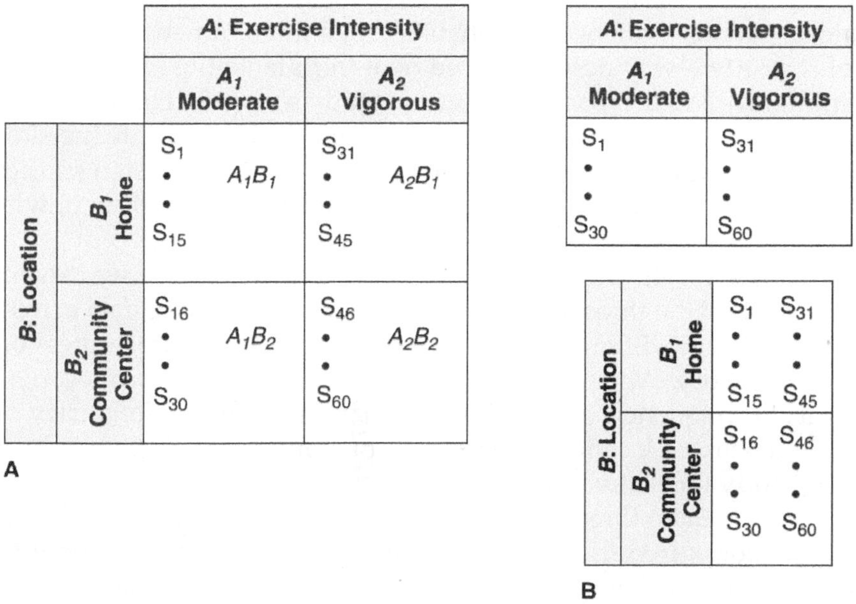

FIGURE 10.5   A. Two-way factorial design. **B.** Main effects for two-way factorial design.

every level of one factor is represented at every level of the other factor. Each of the four groups represents a unique combination of the levels of these variables, as shown in the individual cells of the diagram in Figure 10.5A. For example, using random assignment with a sample of 60 patients, we would assign 15 subjects to each group.

This design allows us to ask three questions of the data: (1) Is there a differential effect of moderate versus vigorous exercise? (2) Is there a differential effect of exercising at home or a community center? (3) What is the interaction between intensity and location of exercise? The answers to the first two questions are obtained by examining the **main effect** of each independent variable, with scores collapsed across the second independent variable, as shown in Figure 10.5B. This means that we can look at the overall effect of intensity of exercise without taking into account any differential effect of location. Therefore, we would have 30 subjects representing each intensity. The main effect of location is also analyzed without differentiating intensity. Each main effect is essentially a single-factor experiment.

The third question addresses the **interaction effect** between the two independent variables. This question represents the essential difference between single-factor and multifactor experiments. Interaction occurs when the effect of one variable varies at different levels of the second variable. For example, we might find that moderate exercise intensity is more effective in changing exercise behavior, but only when performed at a community center.

This example illustrates the major advantage of the factorial approach, which is that it gives the researcher important information that could not be obtained with any one single-factor experiment. The ability to examine interactions greatly enhances the generalizability of results.

Three-Way Factorial Design.   Factorial designs can be extended to include more than two independent variables. In a *three-way factorial design* (see Figure 10.6), the relationship among variables can be conceptualized in a three-dimensional format. We can also think of it as a two-way design crossed on a third factor.

For example, we could expand the exercise study shown in Figure 10.5 to include a third variable such as frequency of exercise. We would then evaluate the simultaneous effect of intensity, location and frequency of exercise. We could assign subjects to exercise 1 day or 3 days per week. Then we would have a $2 \times 2 \times 2$ design, with subjects assigned to one of 8 independent groups (see Figure 10.6).

A three-way design allows several types of comparisons. First, we can examine the main effect for each of the three independent variables, collapsing data across the other two. We can examine the difference between the two intensities, regardless of the effect of location or frequency. We can test the difference between the two locations, regardless of intensity or frequency. And we can evaluate the effect of frequency of exercise, regardless of intensity or location. Each of the three main effects essentially represents a single-factor study for that variable.

Then we can examine three *double interactions*: intensity × location, intensity × frequency, and location × frequency. For example, the interaction between intensity and location is obtained by collapsing data across the two levels of frequency of exercise. Each double interaction represents a two-way design. Finally, we can examine the *triple*

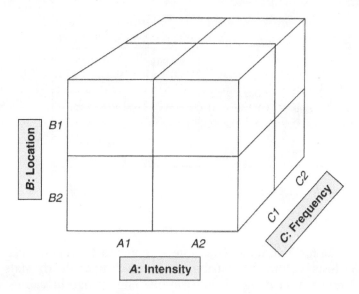

FIGURE 10.6   Three-way factorial design.

interaction of intensity, location and frequency. This interaction involves analyzing the differences among all 8 cells.

Many clinical questions have the potential for involving more than one independent variable, because response variables can be influenced by a multitude of factors. In this respect, the compelling advantage of multidimensional factorial designs is their closer approximation to the "real world." As more variables are added to the design, we can begin to understand responses, increasing construct validity of our arguments. The major disadvantages, however, are that the sample must be extremely large to create individual groups of sufficient size and that data analysis can become cumbersome.

Analysis of Factorial Designs.   A two-way or three-way analysis of variance is most commonly used to examine the main effects and interaction effects of a factorial design.

Randomized Block Design

When a researcher is concerned that an extraneous factor might influence differences between groups, one way to control for this effect is to build the variable into the design as an independent variable. The **randomized block design** (see Figure 10.7) is used when an attribute variable, or *blocking variable*, is crossed with an active independent variable; that is, homogeneous *blocks* of subjects are randomly assigned to levels of a manipulated treatment variable. In the following example, we have a 2×3 randomized block design, with a total of 6 groups.

> **Example of a Randomized Block Design**
> A study was performed to assess the action of an antiarrhythmic agent in healthy men and women after a single intravenous dose.[11] Researchers wanted to determine if effects were related to dose and gender. Twenty-four subjects were recruited, 12 men and 12 women. Each gender group was randomly assigned to receive 0.5, 1.5 or 3.0

		Gender Blocking Variable	
		Male	Female
Dose Randomized Variable	0.5 mg/kg		
	1.5 mg/kg		
	3.0 mg/kg		

FIGURE 10.7   Randomized block design.

mg/kg of the drug for 2 minutes. Therefore, 4 men and 4 women received each dose. Through blood tests, volume of distribution of the drug at steady state was assessed before and 72 hours after drug administration. The change in values was analyzed across the six study groups.

In studying the drug's effect, the researchers were concerned that men and women would respond differently. We can account for this potential effect by using gender as an independent variable. We can then assume that responses will not be confounded by gender.

We can think of this randomized block design as two single-factor randomized experiments, with each block representing a different subpopulation. Subjects are grouped by blocks (gender), and then random assignment is made within each block to the treatment conditions. When the design is analyzed, we will be able to examine possible interaction effects between the treatment conditions and blocks. When this interaction is significant, we will know that the effects of treatment do not generalize across the block classifications, in this case across genders. If the interaction is not significant, we have achieved a certain degree of generalizability of the results.

For the randomized block design to be used effectively, the blocking factor must be related to the dependent variable; that is, it must be a factor that affects how subjects will respond to treatment. If the blocking factor is not related to the response, then using it as an independent variable provides no additional control to the design, and actually provides less control than had random assignment been used. Randomized block designs can involve more than two independent variables, with one or more blocking variables.

Generalization of results from a randomized block design will be limited by the definition of blocks. For example, classification variables, such as gender or diagnosis, are often used as blocking variables. The number of levels of these variables will be inherent. When the blocking factor is a quantitative variable, however, such as age, two important decisions must be made. First, the researcher must determine the range of ages to be used. Second, the number and distribution of blocks must be determined. Generally, it is best to use equally spaced levels with a relatively equal number of subjects at each level. If the researcher is interested in trends within a quantitative variable, three or more levels should be used to describe a pattern of change. For instance, if four age groups are delineated, we would have a clearer picture of the trends that occur with age than if only two levels were used.

Analysis of Randomized Block Designs.   Data from a randomized block design can be analyzed using a two-way analysis of variance, multiple regression or discriminant analysis.

Nested Design

To this point, we have described multifactor designs in terms of two or three independent variables that are completely crossed; that is, all levels of variable A have occurred within all levels of variable B. This approach does not fit all multifactor analyses, however, when attribute variables are involved. Sometimes attribute variables cannot be crossed with all levels of other variables. Consider the following example.

> **Example of a Nested Design**
> An occupational therapist was interested in studying an intervention to facilitate motivational behaviors in individuals with psychiatric illness who had motivational deficits.[12] The intervention was based on strategies of autonomy support. Patients were randomly assigned to either an experimental or control group, and to one of two different groups of therapists who carried out the treatments.

To study the effectiveness of the intervention, scores would be compared across 10 "therapists," each providing either the experimental treatment or control condition. If we used a traditional two-way design (10×2), all 10 levels of therapists would be crossed with both levels of treatment. This would allow the researcher to look at the main effect of therapists, to determine if differences were due to their application of the treatment. If a significant interaction occurred between therapist and treatment, it would mean that the effectiveness of intervention was dependent on which therapist provided it.

If we wanted to follow up on this interaction, we might suspect that less experienced therapists provided a different quality of intervention than more experienced therapists. To test this, we could divide our sample of therapists into two groups based on their years of experience: "less experienced" and "more experienced." This introduces a third independent variable, experience, with two levels. But these two levels cannot be crossed with the 10 levels of therapists; that is, the same therapist cannot appear in both experience groups. Therefore, "therapists" are *nested* within "experience." All levels of therapist and experience can be crossed with the two methods in this **nested design** (see Figure 10.8). Although this resembles a three-way randomized block design, it must be analyzed differently because the interactions of therapist × experience and therapist × experience × method cannot be assessed.

Most variables in clinical studies can be completely crossed; however, with certain combinations of attribute variables, a nested arrangement is required. Nesting is commonly used in educational studies where classes are nested in schools or schools are nested in cities. For instance, Edmundson and associates studied an educational program to reduce risk factors for cardiovascular disease.[13] They evaluated the effect of the program on 6,000 students from 96 schools in four states. The schools were nested in

	Therapists									
	Group 1 Less Experienced					Group 2 More Experienced				
	1	2	3	4	5	6	7	8	9	10
Experimental Group										
Control Group										

FIGURE 10.8   Nested design.

states. Within each state the schools were randomly assigned to receive the program or a control condition.

Analysis of Nested Designs.   An analysis of variance is used to test for main effects and relevant interactions. The dimensions of that analysis depend on how many variables are involved in the study. Nested designs require a complicated approach to analysis of variance, which goes beyond the scope of this book. See Keppel for discussion of analysis of nested designs.[14 (pp. 550–565)]

REPEATED MEASURES DESIGNS

All of the experimental designs we have considered so far have involved at least two independent groups, created by random assignment or blocking. There are many research questions, however, for which control can be substantially increased by using a **repeated measures design**, where one group of subjects is tested under all conditions and each subject acts as his own control. Conceptually, a repeated measures design can be considered a series of trials, each with a single subject. Therefore, such a design is also called a **within-subjects design**, because treatment effects are associated with differences observed within a subject across treatment conditions, rather than between subjects across randomized groups.

The major advantage of the repeated measures design is the ability to control for the potential influence of individual differences. It is a fairly safe assumption that important subject characteristics, such as age, sex, motivation and intelligence, will remain constant throughout the course of an experiment. Therefore, differences observed among treatment conditions are more likely to reflect treatment effects, and not variability between subjects. Using subjects as their own control provides the most equivalent "comparison group" possible.

One disadvantage of the repeated measures approach is the potential for *practice effects*, or the learning effect that can take place when one individual repeats a task over and over. Another disadvantage is the potential for *carryover effects* when one subject is exposed to multiple-treatment conditions. Carryover can be reduced by allotting sufficient time between successive treatment conditions to allow for complete dissipation of previous effects. For instance, if we study the effect of different forms of heat on intramuscular temperature to relieve pain, we may need to repeat testing on different days to be sure that tissues have returned to resting temperatures. We would also have to be assured that the patient's pain level was constant across these days.

Therefore, repeated measures can only be used when the outcome measure will revert back to baseline between interventions, and the patient problem will remain relatively stable throughout the study period. There are many treatments for which carryover cannot be eliminated. For example, if we evaluate the effects of different exercise programs for increasing strength over a 4-week period, the effects of each exercise regimen will probably be long lasting, and rest periods will be ineffective for reversing the effect. With variables that produce permanent or long-term physiological or psychological effects, repeated measures designs are not appropriate.

Because repeated measures designs do not incorporate randomized comparison groups, they may not qualify as true experiments. However, they may be considered experiments when they incorporate randomization in the order of application of repeated conditions, and the comparison of one condition or intervention to another within one subject.

Single-Factor Designs for Repeated Measures

One-Way Repeated Measures Design

The simplest form of repeated measures design involves a single-factor experiment, where one group of subjects is exposed to all levels of one independent variable (see Figure 10.9).

Example of a One-Way Repeated Measures Design
Researchers were interested in the effect of using a cane on the intramuscular forces on prosthetic hip implants during walking.[15] They studied 24 subjects with unilateral prosthetic hips under three conditions: walking with a cane on the side contralateral to the prosthesis, on the same side as the prosthesis, and on the contralateral side with instructions to push with "near maximal effort." They monitored electromyographic (EMG) activity of hip abductor muscles and cane force under each condition. The order of testing under the three test conditions was randomly assigned.

For the study of cane use, the researchers wanted to examine EMG activity of the hip abductor muscles, with all subjects exposed to all three cane conditions. It would be possible to use a randomized design to investigate this question, by assigning different groups to each condition, but it doesn't make logical sense. By using a repeated measures format we can be assured that differences across conditions are a function of cane

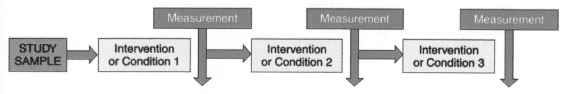

FIGURE 10.9 One-way repeated measures design.

use, and not individual physiological differences. In this example, the independent variable does not present a problem of carryover that would preclude one subject participating at all three levels. This design is commonly referred to as a *one-way repeated measures design*.

Order Effects.   Because subjects are exposed to multiple-treatment conditions in a repeated measures design, there must be some concern about the potentially biasing effect of test sequence; that is, the researcher must determine if responses might be dependent on which condition preceded which other condition. Effects such as fatigue, learning or carryover may influence responses if subjects are all tested in the same order.

One solution to the problem of **order effects** is to randomize the order of presentation for each subject, often by the flip of a coin, so that there is no bias involved in choosing the order of testing. In the study of cane use, the researchers were concerned that the subjects' responses could be affected if one condition was always tested first. This approach does theoretically control for order effects; however, there is still a chance that some sequences will be repeated more often than others, especially if the sample size is small. This design is sometimes considered a randomized block design, with the blocks being considered the specific sequences.

A second solution utilizes a **Latin Square**, which is a matrix composed of equal numbers of rows and columns, designating random permutations of sequence combinations.[†] For example, in the cane study, if we had 30 subjects, we could assign 10 subjects to each of three sequences, as shown in Figure 10.10. Using random assignment, we would determine which group would get each sequence, and then assign each testing condition to A, B or C.

Testing Conditions

	1	2	3
Block 1	A	B	C
Block 2	B	C	A
Block 3	C	A	B

FIGURE 10.10   A 3 × 3 Latin Square.

[†]For examples of Latin Squares of different sizes, see Fisher RA, Yates F. *Statistical Tables for Biological, Agricultural and Medical Research.* Longman Group UK, Ltd, 1974.

Analysis of One-Way Repeated Measures Designs. The one-way analysis of variance for repeated measures is used to test for differences across levels of one repeated factor.

Crossover Design

When only two levels of an independent variable are repeated, a preferred method to control for order effects is to *counterbalance* the treatment conditions so that their order is systematically varied. This creates a **crossover design** in which half the subjects receive Treatment A followed by B, and half receive B followed by A. Two subgroups are created, one for each sequence, and subjects are randomly assigned to one of the sequences.

> **Example of a Crossover Design**
> Researchers were interested in comparing the effects of prone and supine positions on stress responses in mechanically ventilated preterm infants.[16] They randomly assigned 28 infants to a supine/prone or prone/supine position sequence. Infants were placed in each position for 2 hours. Stress signs were measured following each 2 hour period, including startle, tremor, and twitch responses.

A crossover design should only be used in trials where the patient's condition or disease will not change appreciably over time. It is not a reasonable approach in situations where treatment effects are slow, as the treatment periods must be limited. It is similarly impractical where treatment effects are long term and a reversal is not likely. This design is especially useful, however, when treatment conditions are immediately reversible, as in the positioning of infants. When the treatment has some cumulative effect, however, a **washout period** is essential, allowing a common baseline for each treatment condition (see Figure 10.11). The washout period must be long enough to eliminate any prolonged effects of the treatment.

> **Example of a Crossover Design with Washout Period**
> Researchers were interested in the effectiveness of a cranberry supplement for preventing urinary tract infections in persons with neurogenic bladders secondary to spinal cord injury.[17] They treated 21 individuals, evaluating responses based on urinary bacterial counts and white blood cell counts. Subjects were randomly assigned to standardized 400-mg cranberry tablets or placebo 3 times a day for 4 weeks. After 4 weeks and an additional 1-week "washout period," participants were crossed over to the other group.

In this example, one week was considered sufficient for removal of effects from the patient's system.

Analysis of Crossover Designs. In the analysis of a crossover design, researchers will usually group scores by treatment condition, regardless of which order they were given. A paired *t*-test can then be used to compare change scores, or a two-way analysis of variance with two repeated measures can be used to compare pretest and posttest measures across both treatment conditions. The Wilcoxon signed-ranks test should be used to look at change scores when ordinal data are used. In some situations, the

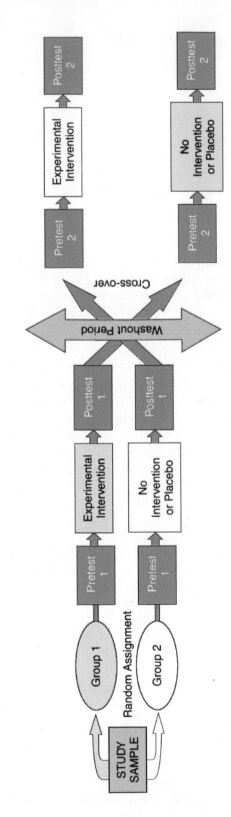

FIGURE 10.11 Crossover design with washout period.

researcher may want to see if order did have an effect on responses, and subjects can be separated into independent groups based on sequence of testing. This analysis may include a two-way analysis of variance with one repeated measure, with sequence as an independent factor and treatment condition as a repeated measure.

Multi-Factor Designs for Repeated Measures

Two-Way Design with Two Repeated Measures

Repeated measures can also be applied to studies involving more than one independent variable (see Figure 10.12).

Example of a Two-Way Repeated Measures Design
The use of back belts in industry is a subject of controversy. A study was designed to investigate the effect of back belts on oxygen consumption during lifting movements.[18] To study this question, researchers recruited 15 healthy subjects who were fitted with a semi-rigid lumbosacral orthosis. Oxygen consumption was measured while subjects participated in 6-minute submaximal lifting bouts of 10 kg. Each subject performed squat and stoop lifting, with and without the orthosis, for a total of four lifting bouts, in random order.

In the study of back belts, researchers created a 2×2 design with two repeated measures: type of lift (squat or stoop) and wearing of the orthosis (yes or no). Each subject was exposed to four test conditions. This design can be expanded to include three independent variables.

Analysis of Two-Way Repeated Measures Designs.   The two-way analysis of variance with two repeated measures is used to analyze differences across main effects and interaction effects.

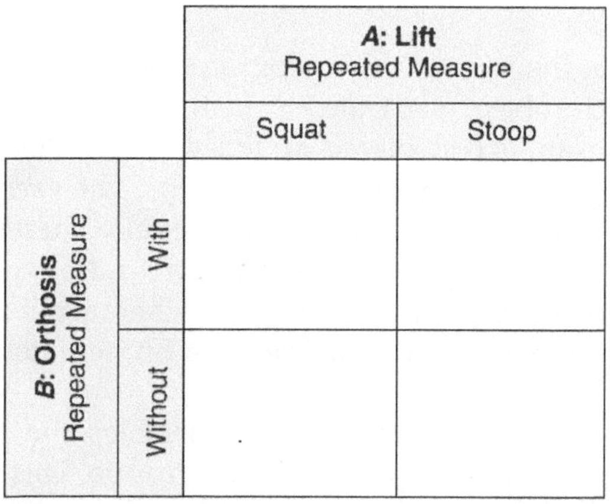

| | | A: Lift Repeated Measure | |
		Squat	Stoop
B: Orthosis Repeated Measure	With		
	Without		

FIGURE 10.12   Two-way design with two repeated measures.

	A: Time Repeated Measure		
	Pre	Post 1	Post 2
B: Intervention — Stabilizing Exercises			
B: Intervention — Standard Treatment			

FIGURE 10.13   Mixed design, with one repeated measure and one independent measure.

Mixed Design

A **mixed design** (see Figure 10.13) is created when a study incorporates two independent variables, one repeated across all subjects, and the other randomized to independent groups.

> **Example of a Mixed Design**
> A study was designed to evaluate the effectiveness of a treatment program of stabilizing exercises for patients with pelvic girdle pain after pregnancy.[19] The researchers based their design on the importance of activation of muscles for motor control and stability of the lumbopelvic region. Eighty women with pelvic girdle pain were assigned randomly to two treatment groups for 20 weeks. One group received physical therapy with a focus on specific stabilizing exercises. The other group received individualized physical therapy without specific stabilizing exercises. Assessments were administered by a blinded assessor at baseline, after intervention and at 1 year post partum. Main outcome measures were pain, functional status and quality of life.

In the comparison of the two exercise programs, subjects were randomly assigned to treatment groups. Each subject was tested three times (pretest and two posttests). The variable of exercise program is considered an *independent factor* because its levels have been randomly assigned, creating independent groups. The variable of time is a *repeated factor* because all subjects are exposed to its three levels. Therefore, this design is also called a *two-way design with one repeated measure*, or a 3 × 3 mixed design. This example illustrates a commonly used approach, where researchers want to establish if the effects of intervention are long lasting, and not just present immediately following completion of the program.

Mixed designs are often used with attribute variables. For instance, we could look at differences in pelvic girdle pain across three age groups. This would be a special case of a randomized block design, where subjects within a block act as their own controls. Mixed designs may incorporate more than two independent variables.

Analysis of Mixed Designs.   A two-way analysis of variance with one repeated measure is used to analyze main effects and interaction effects with a two-way design with one repeated factor.

SEQUENTIAL CLINICAL TRIALS

The **sequential clinical trial** is a special approach to the randomized clinical trial, which allows for continuous analysis of data as they become available, instead of waiting until the end of the experiment to compare groups. Results are accumulated as each subject is tested, so that the experiment can be stopped at any point as soon as the evidence is strong enough to determine a significant difference between treatments. Consequently, it is possible that a decision about treatment effectiveness can be made earlier than in a fixed sample study, leading to a substantial reduction in the total number of subjects needed to obtain valid statistical outcomes and avoiding unnecessary administration of inferior treatments. Sequential trials incorporate specially constructed charts that provide visual confirmation of statistical outcomes, without the use of formal statistical calculations.

The idea of sequential analysis was originally developed during World War II for military and industrial applications, and was for a time considered an official secret.[20] Soon after, it was recognized as a useful model for medical research, particularly in clinical trials of pharmacological agents. Even though there are a few examples of its application in rehabilitation literature,[21-23] sequential analysis remains a relatively unused technique in rehabilitation research. This is unfortunate because the sequential clinical trial is a convenient design that is applicable to many clinical research questions.

The specific purpose of a sequential trial is to compare two treatments, a "new" or experimental treatment (A) and an "old" or standard treatment (B). Treatment can also be compared with a control or placebo. The design is most often applied to independent samples, but may be used with repeated measures.

The process begins by admitting the first eligible patient into the study. This patient is assigned to either Treatment A or B, using the flip of a coin or some other randomization process. When the next eligible patient is admitted (and this may be days or months later), he or she is assigned to the alternate treatment. These two patients now form a *pair*, the results of which can be considered a "little experiment"; that is, we can determine for these two people whether Treatment A or B was better. The whole experiment is a *sequence* of these "little experiments," with each pair representing a comparison. The comparison between A and B is then assessed as **preference** for A or B. Preferences are based on subjective but clearly defined criteria for saying that one treatment is clinically more effective than the other.

Measuring Preferences

Preference is defined on the basis of clinically meaningful differences between two treatments. The specific criteria for expressing preference for one treatment over another can vary in objectivity. At one extreme, the patient can merely express subjective feelings that one treatment seems to work better or is more comfortable than the other. At the other extreme, outcomes can be totally objective, such as death–survival or

Outcome	Treatment A	Treatment B	Preference
1	Improvement	Improvement	None
2	No improvement	No improvement	None
3	Improvement	No Improvement	A
4	No improvement	Improvement	B

FIGURE 10.14   Four possible outcomes for evaluating preferences.

cured–not cured. In between are many subjective and objective types of measurements. A clinician might express preference based on a subjective evaluation of function or on the patient's general reaction to treatment. It is necessary, of course, to develop reliable criteria for making such dichotomous judgments.

It is also possible to reduce continuous data to a measure of preference. For instance, if we were measuring the effect of two treatments for increasing range of motion, we could specify that Treatment A would be preferred if it could produce at least 20 degrees *more* of an increase in range than Treatment B. In other words, any difference between treatments smaller than 20 degrees would not be clinically meaningful, and both treatments would be considered equally effective. This is a convenient approach, but the researcher must be aware that it results in a loss of information by reducing the data to a dichotomous outcome. Any difference greater than 20 degrees would indicate preference, whether that difference was 25 or 100 degrees. If analysis was based on the magnitude of differences, the amount of difference would be taken into account. The researcher must determine if the magnitude of difference is important or if the comparison between treatments is adequately assessed simply by expressing preference.

When two treatments are compared, there are four possible outcomes for classifying preference, as shown in Figure 10.14. In outcome 1, both treatments are equally successful, in which case we would not be able to specify a preference for A or B. In outcome 2, neither treatment is successful. In either of these two cases, we have no information as to which treatment is superior. These outcomes are considered *ties* and are dropped from the analysis. In outcomes 3 and 4, one treatment is preferred over the other, providing one piece of evidence in favor of either A or B.

The Sequential Chart

The result of each comparison within a pair of subjects is plotted on a *sequential chart*. Two types of charts have been used. The chart developed by Bross[24] has strong appeal because it has a fixed format (see Figure 10.15). The plot begins in the lower left corner square (a free square). As each comparison is made within a pair, an "x" is placed in the square either above the last occupied square (if A is superior) or to the right (if B is superior). If neither treatment is preferred within a pair, nothing is entered. The path continues until one of the boundaries is crossed. If the path goes upward, Treatment A is superior; if it goes to the right, Treatment B is superior. The middle boundary represents

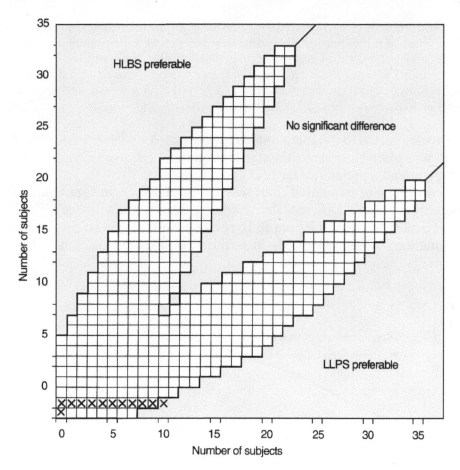

FIGURE 10.15 Sequential trial grid,[24] showing preference for low-load prolonged stretch (LLPS) over high-load brief stretch (HLBS) for treatment of knee flexion contractures. (From Light KE, Nuzik S, Personius W, et al. Low-load prolonged stretch vs. high-load brief stretch in treating knee contractures. *Phys Ther* 1984; 64:330–333, Figure 3, p. 332. Reprinted with the permission of the American Physical Therapy Association.)

the null hypothesis; that is, if the path moves diagonally, the conclusion is that no difference exists. The longest possible path in this plan is 58 squares (116 patients).[‡]

Example of a Sequential Clinical Trial
Researchers studied the differential effect of low-load prolonged stretch (LLPS) versus the more traditional high-load brief stretch (HLBS) for treating knee flexion contractures in elderly patients.[21] Subjects were admitted to the study based on the presence

---

[‡]This plan is based on *comparative success rates*, indicating whether Treatment A has an "advantage" over Treatment B. Bross includes a table that statistically defines "important advantage."[24] For instance, if Treatment B is known to "cure" 25% of the patients, Treatment A would demonstrate an important advantage over B if it could cure 44%. If B cures 50%, treatment A would be important if it could cure 70%; if Treatment B cures 75%, Treatment A should cure 88%. The power of this analysis is approximately 86% when Treatment A offers an important advantage over B; that is, 86% of the time the upper boundary will be correctly crossed.

of bilateral knee flexion contractures of at least 3 months' duration, and at least 30 degrees short of full extension. In addition, subjects had to be unable to walk or pivot transfer without maximal assistance. Subjects' limbs were randomly assigned to receive either LLPS or HLBS. Treatment was performed twice daily, 5 days a week, for 4 weeks. Range of motion was measured before and after 4 weeks, and preference was defined as a difference of at least 10 degrees between limbs.

In this example, the first patient tested demonstrated a preference for HLBS, and so the first "x" was placed just above the starting square. As shown in Figure 10.15, all further testing showed a preference for LLPS.

The second type of sequential chart was developed by Armitage,[25] and allows for more flexibility in design. Different size charts are drawn, allowing for different expectations of effects. The chart in Figure 10.16 shows results of one study to evaluate varied supplementary doses of opioids in terminally ill cancer patients.[26] The chart is

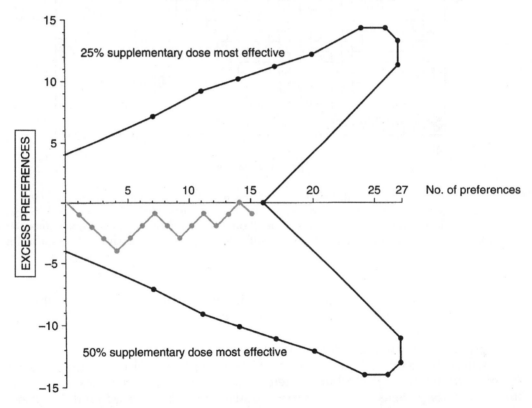

FIGURE 10.16 Sequential chart for analysis of treatment with an expected difference in 85% of the pairs, based on the procedures of Armitage.[25] Supplementary doses of opioids were given to terminally ill cancer patients at 25% and 50% of their 4-hour standard dose. The outcome measure was reduction in dyspnea. The study showed no final preference for either dose, leading the researchers to conclude that the lower 25% dose would be sufficient. (From Allard P, Lamontagne C, Bernard P, et al. How effective are supplementary doses of opioids for dyspnea in terminally ill cancer patients? A randomized continuous sequential clinical trial. *J Pain Symptom Manage* 1999;17:256–265. Used with permission).

drawn to detect a significant treatment difference if one drug regimen was better in at least 85% of the pairs.[§] In this format, the boundaries are drawn above and below a center baseline. Preferences for one treatment or the other are indicated by moving up or down from the last plotted point. The first four patients favored the 50% dose, the next three the 25% dose, the next two the 50% dose, and so on. This example shows an outcome that moves towards the middle boundary, indicating no significant difference.

Stopping Rules

After each successive "little experiment" is plotted, the researcher stops to consider the results of all the pairs completed thus far and makes one of three decisions: (1) Stop and make a *terminal decision* to recommend A or B; (2) stop the experiment and make a terminal decision that treatments A and B are not different; or (3) continue to collect data because the cumulated data are not yet sufficient to draw a conclusion. This process of considering cumulative results after each pair of subjects has been tested is called *sequential analysis.* The decision to stop or go on will depend on how strong the evidence is to that point in favor of one treatment. This is the primary benefit of a sequential analysis, in that a trial can be stopped as soon as it is evident that one treatment is superior to the other, or that no difference is going to be found.[27]

These boundaries represent three **stopping rules**: (1) If the upper boundary is crossed, we can make a terminal decision to recommend A; (2) if the lower boundary is crossed, we can make a terminal decision to recommend B; (3) if the middle boundary is crossed (either above or below the origin), there is no preference. In the stretching study (Fig. 10.15), 11 subjects were required to cross the lower boundary, indicating a significantly greater effect for LLPS. Had the first subject also "preferred" LLPS, only 8 subjects would have been needed to demonstrate significance. For the opioid study (Fig. 10.16), the first few subjects showed a preference for the 50% dose, but the final results showed a marked inconsistency, leading to the middle boundary. In this case, the line did not cross the boundary because of missing data in three of the pairs. The authors decided not to recruit additional subjects and concluded that the data did not support a difference between the two doses.

Considerations in Sequential Trials

A theoretical issue arises in the consideration of the effect of ties. When the difference between two treatments within a pair does not meet the criterion for demonstrating preference, that pair of subjects is discarded from the sequential analysis. If many ties occur, the final sample that is used for analysis is not a true random sample; that is, it is not a true representation of all tied and untied pairs that were originally chosen.[28] It

---

[§]See Armitage[25] for tables and figures for different effect sizes.

is useful to keep a record of ties, as they do provide information about the similarity of treatments. If the researcher finds that too many pairs result in ties, it might be reasonable to end the trial, as very little information will be gained by continuing to collect data. Such a decision is considered a *conditional decision* (as opposed to a terminal decision that occurs when a boundary is crossed). A conditional decision is rendered without crossing a boundary, but is based on practical considerations and observation of the plotted path.

Sequential trials are also somewhat limited by the time frame within which treatment effects can be expected to occur. The response should be observable relatively soon after treatment is begun. The outcome should at least be available within an observation period that is short relative to the total time of the study.[28] Otherwise, at any point in time, there will be a large number of subjects entered into the trial, but only a small proportion of results will be available. For instance, if a treatment effect is not expected for 1 year, within 6 months many subjects may have started treatment, but hardly any results would have been obtained. Consequently, the sequential rationale for economizing on time and subjects is subverted.

A major advantage of sequential analysis is that it more readily fits a clinical research model, allowing for subjects to enter the study as they are admitted for treatment and providing a structure for administering treatment within a clinical context; that is, the experimental treatments can be applied as they would be during normal practice, without having to create an artificial experimental environment. The sequential trial also provides a useful mechanism for studying qualitative outcomes, using the measure of preferences. In a practical sense, this approach can be quite effective as an adjunct to clinical decision making, because it allows the decision to be based on a variety of empirical criteria.

EFFICACY VS. EFFECTIVENESS

The randomized controlled trial is generally considered the gold standard for evaluating the effects of treatment. Researchers will often distinguish between efficacy and effectiveness in clinical studies. **Efficacy** is generally defined as the benefit of an intervention as compared to a control or standard program. It provides information about the behavior of clinical variables under controlled, randomized conditions. This lets us examine theory and draw generalizations to large populations. **Effectiveness** refers to the benefits and use of the procedure under "real world" conditions. It is the expectation that when we apply treatments, we do so without being able to control all the circumstances around us, and our results may not be the same as those obtained with a randomized experiment. This distinction is often seen as one reason for the perceived gap between research and practice, based on the mistaken assumption that effectiveness logically follows from a successful efficacy study.[29]

Studies may be closer to one end of this continuum or the other, depending on many factors in the design of the trial.[30] Gartlehner et al[31] have proposed seven criteria to help researchers and clinicians to distinguish between efficacy and effectiveness studies, as shown in Table 10.1. Which patients are eligible, degree of control over the

TABLE 10.1 CRITERIA TO DISTINGUISH EFFICACY AND EFFECTIVENESS STUDIES

Criterion	Efficacy Study	Effectiveness Study
Health care setting	Frequently conducted in large tertiary care referral settings.	Conducted in primary care settings available to a diverse population with the condition of interest.
Eligibility criteria	Highly selective, stringent eligibility criteria; sample may not be representative of the general population.	Source population reflects the heterogeneity of external populations. Comorbidities are not exclusion criteria.
Outcome measures	Common use of objective and subjective outcomes, such as symptom scores, lab values, disease recurrence.	Use of functional capacity, quality of life and other health outcome measures relevant to the condition of interest.
Study duration and clinically relevant treatment	Research protocol manipulated. Study duration often based on time needed to demonstrate safety and demonstrate an effect. Compliance must be assessed to determine if intervention works.	Research protocol based on clinical reality. Duration based on minimum length of treatment to allow assessment of health outcomes. Compliance may be unpredictable and should be defined as an outcome measure.
Assessment of adverse events	Not typically reported.	Objective scales used to define and measure adverse event rates.
Sample size	Large trials with few levels of analysis provide ideal design to detect small but clinically meaningful treatment effects.	Sample size sufficient to detect at least a minimally important difference on a health outcome scale.
Intention to treat (ITT) analysis	Research protocol will seek to limit factors that can alter treatment effects; may use completer analysis.	Factors such as compliance, adverse events, drug regimens, comorbidities, other treatments and costs are taken into account using ITT.

Source: Gartlehner et al.[31]

delivery of the intervention, what outcomes are assessed, which patients are included in the final analysis, how missing data are handled, and which statistical procedures are appropriate—all of these influence whether the results of a trial can be considered measures of efficacy or effectiveness. These two types of trials may yield very different results, but both are important to our understanding of patient responses to treatment.

These concepts help us understand the situation where the findings of a controlled trial demonstrate that a treatment works, but clinicians find that it does not have the same effect when used on their individual patients in actual treatment conditions. The efficacious treatment was tested on a defined sample, with inclusion and exclusion criteria, and was applied under controlled and defined conditions. It then becomes imperative to determine if the same result can be obtained when personnel, patients and the environment cannot be manipulated. Factors that potentially limit application across settings, populations, and intervention staff need to be addressed in both types of trials.

COMMENTARY

Matching the Research Question and Design

The importance of understanding concepts of experimental design cannot be overemphasized in the planning stages of an experimental research project. There is a logic in these designs that must be fitted to the research question and the scope of the project, so that meaningful conclusions can be drawn once data are analyzed. Alternative designs should be considered on the basis of their relative validity, and the strongest designs should be chosen whenever possible. The design itself is not a guarantee of the validity of research findings, however. Process must be controlled within the structure. Attention to measurement issues is especially important to ensure that outcomes will be valid. It is also important to note that the strongest design for a given question need not be the most complicated design. In many cases, using the simpler designs can facilitate answering the research question, where a more complex design creates uninterpretable interactions. The choice of a design should ultimately be based on the intent of the research question:

> . . . the question being asked determines the appropriate research architecture, strategy, and tactics to be used—not tradition, authority, experts, paradigms, or schools of thought.[32]

The underlying importance of choosing an appropriate research design relates to consequent analysis issues that arise once data are collected. Many beginning researchers have had the unhappy experience of presenting their data to a statistician, only to find out that they did not collect the data appropriately to answer their research question. Fisher[33] expressed this idea in his classical work, *The Design of Experiments*:

> Statistical procedure and experimental design are only two different aspects of the same whole, and that whole comprises all the logical requirements of the complete process of adding to natural knowledge by experimentation.

The relevant point is the need to use a variety of research approaches to answer questions of clinical importance. Although the clinical trial or experiment is considered a gold standard for establishing cause and effect, it is by no means the best or most appropriate approach for many of the questions that are most important for improving practice. The real world does not operate with controls and schedules the way an experiment can. Quasi-experimental and observational studies, using intact groups or nonrandom samples, play an important role in demonstrating effectiveness of interventions.[31] As we continue our emphasis on evidence-based practice, we must consider many alternatives to the traditional clinical trial in order to discover the most "effective" courses of treatment.[34]

REFERENCES

1. Fisher B, Jeong JH, Anderson S, Bryant J, Fisher ER, Wolmark N. Twenty-five-year follow-up of a randomized trial comparing radical mastectomy, total mastectomy, and total mastectomy followed by irradiation. *N Engl J Med* 2002;347:567–575.
2. Francis T, Korns FT, Voight RB, et al. An evaluation of the 1954 poliomyelitis vaccine trials: Summary report. *Am J Public Health* 1955;45:1–63.
3. Stratov I, DeRose R, Purcell DF, Kent SJ. Vaccines and vaccine strategies against HIV. *Curr Drug Targets* 2004;5:71–88.
4. Campbell DT, Stanley JC. *Experimental and Quasi-experimental Designs for Research.* Chicago: Rand McNally, 1963.
5. Cook TD, Campbell DT. *Quasi-experimentation: Design and Analysis Issues for Field Settings.* Boston: Houghton Mifflin, 1979.
6. Padberg FT, Jr., Johnston MV, Sisto SA. Structured exercise improves calf muscle pump function in chronic venous insufficiency: A randomized trial. *J Vasc Surg* 2004;39:79–87.
7. Doesborgh SJ, van de Sandt-Koenderman MW, Dippel DW, van Harskamp F, Koudstaal PJ, Visch-Brink EG. Effects of semantic treatment on verbal communication and linguistic processing in aphasia after stroke: A randomized controlled trial. *Stroke* 2004;35:141–146.
8. Suomi R, Collier D. Effects of arthritis exercise programs on functional fitness and perceived activities of daily living measures in older adults with arthritis. *Arch Phys Med Rehabil* 2003;84:1589–1594.
9. Munin MC, Rudy TE, Glynn NW, Crossett LS, Rubash HE. Early inpatient rehabilitation after elective hip and knee arthroplasty. *JAMA* 1998;279:847–852.
10. Cox KL, Gorely TJ, Puddey IB, Burke V, Beilin LJ. Exercise behaviour change in 40- to 65-year-old women: The SWEAT Study (Sedentary Women Exercise Adherence Trial). *Br J Health Psychol* 2003;8:477–495.
11. Salazar DE, Much DR, Nichola PS, Seibold JR, Shindler D, Slugg PH. A pharmacokinetic-pharmacodynamic model of d-sotalol Q-Tc prolongation during intravenous administration to healthy subjects. *J Clin Pharmacol* 1997;37:799–809.
12. Wu C. Facilitating intrinsic motivation in individuals with psychiatric illness: A study on the effectiveness of an occupational therapy intervention. *Occup Ther J Res* 2001;21:142–167.
13. Edmundson E, Parcel GS, Feldman HA, Elder J, Perry CL, Johnson CC, et al. The effects of the Child and Adolescent Trial for Cardiovascular Health upon psychosocial determinants of diet and physical activity behavior. *Prev Med* 1996;25:442–454.
14. Keppel G. *Design and Analysis: A Researcher's Handbook* (4th ed.). Englewood Cliffs, NJ: Prentice Hall, 2004.
15. Neuman DA. Hip abductor muscle activity as subjects with hip prostheses walk with different methods of using a cane. *Phys Ther* 1998;78:490–501.
16. Chang YJ, Anderson GC, Lin CH. Effects of prone and supine positions on sleep state and stress responses in mechanically ventilated preterm infants during the first postnatal week. *J Adv Nurs* 2002;40:161–169.
17. Linsenmeyer TA, Harrison B, Oakley A, Kirshblum S, Stock JA, Millis SR. Evaluation of cranberry supplement for reduction of urinary tract infections in individuals with neurogenic bladders secondary to spinal cord injury: A prospective, double-blinded, placebo-controlled, crossover study. *J Spinal Cord Med* 2004;27:29–34.
18. Duplessis DH, Greenway EH, Keene KL, Lee IE, Clayton RL, Metzler T, et al. Effect of semi-rigid lumbosacral orthosis use on oxygen consumption during repetitive stoop and squat lifting. *Ergonomics* 1998;41:790–797.

19. Stuge B, Laerum E, Kirkesola G, Vollestad N. The efficacy of a treatment program focusing on specific stabilizing exercises for pelvic girdle pain after pregnancy: A randomized controlled trial. *Spine* 2004;29:351–359.
20. Wald A. *Sequential Analysis*. New York: Wiley, 1947.
21. Light KE, Nuzik S, Personius W, Barstrom A. Low-load prolonged stretch vs. high-load brief stretch in treating knee contractures. *Phys Ther* 1984;64:330–333.
22. Bohannon RW. Knee extension torque during repeated knee extension-flexion reversals and separated knee extension-flexion dyads. *Phys Ther* 1985;65:1052–1054.
23. Gault SJ, Spyker MJ. Beneficial effect of immobilization of joints in rheumatoid and related arthritides: A splint study using sequential analysis. *Arthritis Rheum* 1969; 12:34–44.
24. Bross IDJ. Sequential clinical trials. *J Chron Dis* 1958;8:349–365.
25. Armitage P. *Sequential Medical Trials* (2nd ed.). New York: Wiley, 1975.
26. Allard P, Lamontagne C, Bernard P, Tremblay C. How effective are supplementary doses of opioids for dyspnea in terminally ill cancer patients? A randomized continuous sequential clinical trial. *J Pain Symptom Manage* 1999;17:256–1265.
27. Whitehead J. Monotherapy trials: Sequential design. *Epilepsy Res* 2001;45:81–87.
28. Mainland D. Statistical ward rounds 4. *Clin Pharmacol Ther* 1967;8:615–623.
29. Glasgow RE, Lichtenstein E, Marcus AC. Why don't we see more translation of health promotion research to practice? Rethinking the efficacy-to-effectiveness transition. *Am J Public Health* 2003;93:1261–1267.
30. Streiner DL. The 2 "Es" of research: Efficacy and effectiveness trials. *Can J Psychiatry* 2002;47:552–556.
31. Gartlehner G, Hansen RA, Nissman D, Lohr KN, Carey TS. Criteria for distinguishing effectiveness from efficacy trials in systematic reviews. Technical Review 12 (Prepared by the RTI-International–University of North Carolina Evidence-based Practice Center under Contract No. 290-02-0016.) AHRQ Publication No. 06-0046. Rockville, MD: Agency for Healthcare Research and Quality. April 2006. Available at: <http://www.ahrq.gov/downloads/pub/evidence/pdf/efftrials/efftrials.pdf> Accessed June 11, 2006.
32. Sackett DL, Wennberg JE. Choosing the best research design for each question. *BMJ* 1997;315:1636.
33. Fisher RA. *The Design of Experiments* (6th ed.). New York: Hafner, 1951.
34. Concato J, Shah N, Horwitz RI. Randomized, controlled trials, observational studies, and the hierarchy of research designs. *N Engl J Med* 2000;342:1887–1892.

CHAPTER 11
Quasi-Experimental Designs

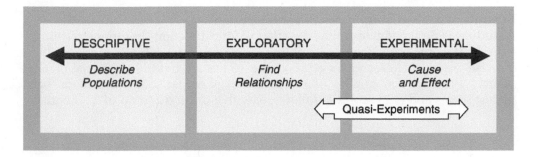

Although the randomized trial is considered the optimal design for testing cause-and-effect hypotheses, the necessary restrictions of a randomized trial are not always possible within the clinical environment.[1] Depending on the nature of the treatment under study and the population of interest, use of randomization and control groups may not be feasible. The specification of inclusion and exclusion criteria will often reduce generalizability and limit the range of patients that can be included.

Quasi-experimental designs utilize similar structures to experimental designs, but will lack either random assignment or comparison groups, or both. They often involve nonequivalent groups that may differ from each other in many ways in addition to differences between treatment conditions.[2] Therefore, the degree of control is reduced. Many studies incorporate quasi-experimental elements because of the limitations of clinical conditions. These designs present reasonable alternatives to the randomized trial, as long as the researcher carefully documents subject characteristics, controls the research protocol, and uses blinding as much as possible. The conclusions drawn from these studies must take into account the potential biases of the sample, but may provide important information, nonetheless.[3]

ONE-GROUP DESIGNS
One-Group Pretest-Posttest Design

The **one-group pretest-posttest design** is a quasi-experimental design that involves one set of repeated measurements taken before and after treatment on one group of subjects (see Figure 11.1). The effect of treatment is determined by measuring the difference between pretest and posttest scores. In this design, the independent variable is time, with two levels (pretest and posttest). Treatment is not an independent variable because all subjects receive the intervention.

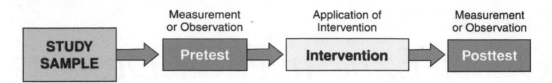

FIGURE 11.1   A one-group pretest-posttest design. Because only one group is tested and all subjects receive the intervention, time becomes the independent variable.

Example of a One-Group Pretest-Posttest Design

A study was designed to examine the effect of four-direction shoulder stretching exercises for patients with idiopathic adhesive capsulitis.[4] All subjects received the same exercise protocol. Researchers studied the effects of treatment on pain, range of motion, function and quality of life measures. Comparisons were made between pretest scores and final scores at follow-up, with a mean duration of 22 months.

In this study, the researchers saw significant improvements in outcome variables, and concluded that the treatment was successful. We must hold conclusions drawn from this design as suspect, however. The design is weak because it has no comparison group, making it especially vulnerable to threats to internal validity. Although the researcher can demonstrate change in the dependent variable by comparing pretest and posttest scores, there is always the possibility that some events other than the experimental treatment occurred within the time frame of the study that caused the observed change. Therefore, this design is particularly threatened by history and maturation effects. In addition, the influence of testing, instrumentation, statistical regression, and selection interaction effects cannot be ruled out. External validity is also limited by potential interactions with selection because there is no comparison group.

The one-group pretest-posttest design may be defended, however, in cases where previous research has documented the behavior of a control group in similar circumstances. For instance, other studies may have shown that shoulder pain does not improve in this population over a 4-week period without intervention. On that basis, we could justify using a single experimental group to investigate just how much change can be expected with treatment. This documentation might also allow us to defend the lack of a control group on ethical grounds. The design is also reasonable when the experimental situation is sufficiently isolated so that extraneous environmental variables are effectively controlled, or where the time interval between measurements is short so that temporal effects are minimized.[2] For instance, in studies where data collection is completed within a single testing session, temporal threats to internal validity will be minimal, although testing effects remain uncontrolled. Under all circumstances, however, this design is not considered a true experiment, and should be expanded whenever possible to compare two groups.

Analysis of One-Group Pretest-Posttest Designs.   A t-test for paired comparisons is usually used to compare pretest and posttest mean scores. With ordinal data or small samples, the sign test or the Wilcoxon signed-ranks test can be used.

One-Way Repeated Measures Design Over Time

Many research questions that deal with the effects of treatment on physiological or psychological variables are concerned with how those effects are manifested over time. As an extension of the pretest-posttest design, the repeated measures design is naturally suited to assessing such trends.[5] Multiple measurements of the dependent variable are taken within prescribed time intervals. The intervention may be applied once, or it may be repeated in between measurements (see Figure 11.2).

Example of a One-Way Repeated Measures Design Over Time
Researchers studied the effects of low-impact aerobic exercise on fatigue, aerobic fitness, and disease activity in adults with rheumatoid arthritis.[6] Measures were obtained preintervention, midtreatment (after 6 weeks of exercise), at the end of treatment (after 12 weeks of exercise), and at a 15-week follow-up.

Once again, in this example time is the independent variable. Every subject is evaluated at each time interval, making it a repeated measure. The design is quasi-experimental because there is no randomization of the order of treatment and no comparison group. Without a control group internal validity is threatened, as it is not possible to discern if changes would have occurred over time without the intervention.

This design may be appropriate, however, when the time course of a disease or condition is predictable. For example, several studies have shown that strength declines in a linear fashion in patients with amyotrophic lateral sclerosis (ALS).[7,8] Therefore, studies using this population for trials of drugs or other interventions may reasonably follow patients over time without needing a control or placebo group.[9]

Analysis of One-Way Repeated Measures Designs Over Time. When time is the independent variable, a one-way repeated measures analysis of variance can be performed. Analysis may also include polynomial contrasts to describe trends over time.

Time Series Design

Time-series designs are based on the application of multiple measurements, before and after treatment, to document patterns or trends of behavior (see Figure 11.3). These designs are often used to study community interventions[10] and policy changes.[11] They have also been adapted by behavioral analysts for the study of single subjects'

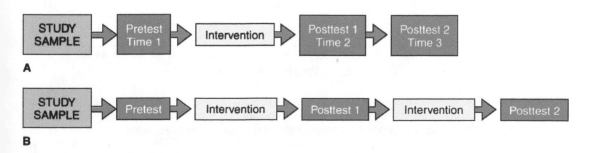

FIGURE 11.2 One-way repeated measures design with time as the repeated measure.

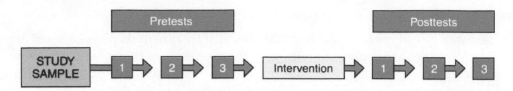

FIGURE 11.3   Interrupted time-series design.

responses over time (see Chapter 12). Basic time series designs have been defined by Cook and Campbell.[2]

> **Example of an Interrupted Time-Series Design**
> Researchers evaluated an intervention to reduce inappropriate use of key antibiotics by hospital staff.[11] They initiated a policy for appropriate use of specific drugs through concurrent feedback by clinical pharmacists for individual patients. Drug use and costs were assessed monthly for 2 years before and after the policy was implemented.

This is an example of an *interrupted time-series design* (see Figure 11.4), so named because it involves a series of measurements over time that are "interrupted" by one or more treatment occasions. It is considered a quasi-experimental design because only one

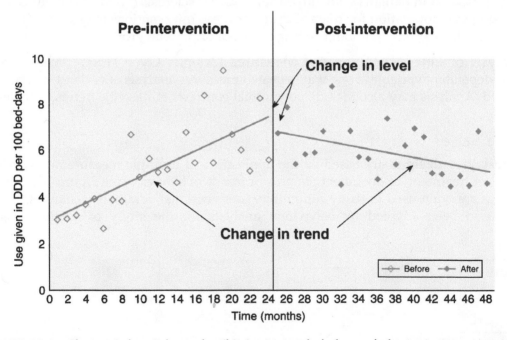

FIGURE 11.4   Changes in hospital use of antibiotics 24 months before and after instituting a prescription policy. The two regression lines, representing data before and after intervention, show changes in level (from end of pre-intervention to start of post-intervention) and trend (slope of line). (Adapted from Ansari F, Gray K, Nathwani D, et al. Outcomes of an intervention to improve hospital antibiotic prescribing: Interrupted time series with segmented regression analysis. *J Antimicrobial Chemotherapy* 2003; 52:842–848, Figure 2, p. 844. Reprinted with permission. Copyright 2003, British Society for Antimicrobial Chemotherapy.)

group is studied. The independent variable is time; that is, each measurement interval represents one level of time.* The research question concerns trends across these time intervals. The number of observations can vary, depending on the stability of the dependent variable. In some studies, researchers may extend pretest or posttest periods if the data are very variable, in an effort to stabilize responses before initiating treatment or ending the observations.

This design may be considered an extension of the one-group pretest-posttest design. It offers more control, however, because the multiple pretests and posttests act as a pseudocontrol condition, demonstrating maturational trends that naturally occur in the data or the confounding effects of extraneous variables. It is most effective when serial data can be collected at evenly distributed intervals, avoiding confounding by extraneous temporal factors.[12] To illustrate, consider several possible outcomes for an interrupted time-series design, shown in Figure 11.5. A series of observations are taken at times 1 through 8 (O_1–O_8), with the introduction of treatment at point X. In all three patterns, a similar increase in the dependent variable is seen from O_4 to O_5. In Pattern A we would be justified in assuming that treatment has an effect, as no change occurred prior to intervention. In Pattern B, however, it would be misleading to make this interpretation, as the responses are continually increasing within the baseline measures. Although Pattern C also shows an increase in the dependent variable from O_4 to O_5,

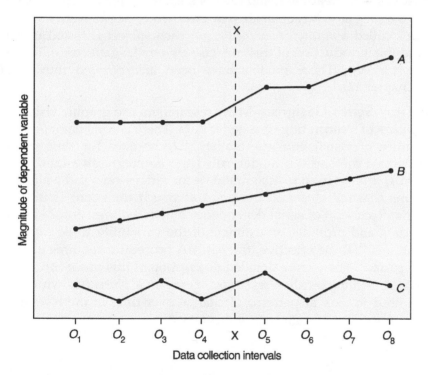

FIGURE 11.5   Illustration of three possible outcome patterns in the interrupted time-series design.

*Time series designs are distinguished from repeated measures designs by the large number of measurements that are taken continuously across baseline and intervention phases. See Chapter 12 for a description of time series experiments as they are constructed for single-subject research.

which would look like a treatment effect if these were the only two measurements taken, we can see from the erratic pattern changes before and after treatment that this conclusion is unwarranted.

The greatest threat to internal validity in the time series design is history. There is no control over the possible coincidental occurrence of some extraneous event at the same time that treatment is initiated. The level and trend of the pre-intervention data, however, do present a form of control for the post-intervention segment[11] (see Chapter 12 for further discussion of level and trend). This is illustrated in the data in Figure 11.4.

Most other threats to internal validity are fairly well controlled by the presence of multiple measurements; that is, their effects are not eliminated, but we can account for them. For instance, if instrumentation or testing effects are present, we should see changes across the pretest scores. External validity of a time-series design is limited to situations where repeated testing takes place.

Several variations can be applied to this design. Comparisons may include two or more groups. Treatment may be administered one time only with follow-up measurements, or intervention may be continued throughout the posttest period. In a third variation, treatment may be started after a series of pretest measurements, and then withdrawn after a specified time period, with measurements continuing into the withdrawal period. The *withdrawal design* does help to account for history effects. If the behavior improves with treatment, and reverts back to baseline levels when treatment is withdrawn, a strong case can be made that extraneous factors were not operating. In a fourth model, called a *multiple baseline design*, each subject is tested under baseline conditions, and the introduction of treatment is staggered, again controlling for history and maturation effects. These models have been incorporated into single-subject designs (see Chapter 12).

Analysis of Time Series Designs.   Many researchers use graphic visual analysis as the primary means of interpreting time-series data. There is considerable disagreement as to the validity of visual analysis. Statistical techniques for time-series analysis involve multivariate methods. A model called the autoregressive integrated moving average (ARIMA) is often used to accommodate for serial scores and weighs heavily on the observations that fall closer to the point at which treatment is introduced (see Chapter 12 for a discussion of serial dependency and autocorrelation).[13] It analyzes the trends in the data and provides an estimate of the variability to be expected among future observations.[14] To be effective, the ARIMA procedure requires at least 25 data points in each phase.[15] For a more detailed description of this procedure, consult Cook and Campbell.[2] A technique called *segmented regression analysis* (shown in Figure 11.4) has also been used to look at patterns of change over time in the level and slope of regression lines for different segments of the data.[16]

MULTIGROUP DESIGNS

Nonequivalent Pretest-Posttest Control Group Design

There are many research situations in the social, clinical, and behavioral sciences where groups are found intact or where subjects are self-selected. The former case is common in a clinic or school where patients or students belong to fixed groups or classes. The

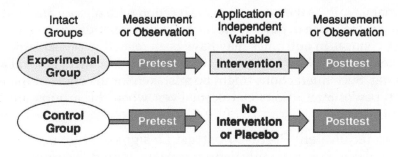

FIGURE 11.6   Nonequivalent pretest-posttest control group design.

latter case will apply when attribute variables are studied or when volunteers are recruited. The **nonequivalent pretest-posttest control group design** (see Figure 11.6) is similar to the pretest-posttest experimental design, except that subjects are not assigned to groups randomly. This design can be structured with one treatment group and one control group or with multiple treatment and control groups.

Example of a Nonequivalent Pretest-Posttest Control Group Design Based on Intact Groups

A study was done to determine the effectiveness of an individualized physical therapy intervention in treating neck pain.[17] One treatment group of 30 patients with neck pain completed physical therapy treatment. The control group of convenience was formed by a cohort group of 27 subjects who also had neck pain but did not receive treatment for various reasons. There were no significant differences between groups in demographic data or the initial test scores of the outcome measures. A physical therapist rendered an intervention to the treatment group based on a clinical decision making algorithm. Treatment effectiveness was examined by assessing changes in range of motion, pain, endurance and function. Both the treatment and control groups completed the initial and follow-up examinations, with an average duration of 4 weeks between tests.

Example of a Nonequivalent Pretest-Posttest Control Group Design Based on Subject Preferences

A study was designed to examine the influence of regular participation in chair exercises on postoperative deconditioning following hip fracture.[18] Subjects were distinguished by their willingness to participate, and were not randomly assigned to groups. A control group received usual care following discharge. Physiological, psychological, and anthropometric variables were measured before and after intervention.

In the study of therapy for neck pain, the patients are members of intact groups by virtue of their diagnosis. In the chair exercise study, subjects self-selected their group membership.

Although the nonequivalent pretest-posttest control group design is limited by the lack of randomization, it still has several strengths. Because it includes a pretest and a control group, there is some control over history, testing and instrumentation effects. The pretest scores can be used to test the assumption of initial equivalence on the dependent variable, based on average scores and measures of variability. The major threat to internal validity is the interaction of selection with history and maturation. For instance, if those who chose to participate in chair exercises were stronger or more motivated patients, changes in outcomes may have been related to physiological or psychological characteristics of subjects. These characteristics could affect general activity level or rate of healing. Such interactions might be mistaken for the effect of the exercise program. These types of interactions can occur even when the groups are identical on pretest scores.

Analysis of Nonequivalent Pretest-Posttest Designs.   Several statistical methods are suggested for use with nonequivalent groups, including the unpaired *t*-test (with two groups), analysis of variance, analysis of covariance, analysis of variance with matching, and analysis of variance with gain scores. Ordinal data can be analyzed using the Mann-Whitney *U* test. Nonparametric tests may be more appropriate with nonequivalent groups, as variances are likely to be unequal. Preference for one approach will depend in large part on how groups were formed and what steps the researcher can take to ensure or document initial equivalence. Tests such as the *t*-test, analysis of variance and chi square are often used to test for differences in baseline measures. Regression analysis or discriminant analysis may be the most applicable approach to determine how the dependent variable differentiates the treatment groups, while adjusting for other variables. Statistical strategies must include mechanisms for controlling for group differences on potentially confounding variables.

Historical Controls

Another strategy for comparing treatments involves the use of **historical controls** who received a different treatment during an earlier time period.

> **Example of a Nonequivalent Design Based on Historical Controls**
> Concern exists that prednisone-free maintenance immunosuppression in kidney transplant recipients will increase acute and/or chronic rejection. Over a 5-year period from 1999 to 2004, researchers worked with 477 kidney transplant recipients who discontinued prednisone on postoperative day 6, followed by a regimen of immunosuppressive therapy.[19] The outcomes were compared with that of 388 historical controls from the same institution (1996 to 2000) who did not discontinue prednisone. Outcomes included changes in serum creatinine levels, weight and cholesterol, as well as patient and graft survival rates.

As this example illustrates, a nonconcurrent control group may best serve the purpose of comparison when ethical concerns may preclude a true control group. When the researcher truly believes that the experimental intervention is more effective than standard care, the use of historical controls provides a reasonable alternative.[20] This approach has been used in cancer trials, for example, when protocols in one trial act as a control for subsequent studies.[21] The major advantage of this approach is its efficiency. Because all subjects are assigned to the experimental condition, the total sample will be smaller and the results can be obtained in a shorter period of time.

The disadvantages of using historical controls must be considered carefully, however. Studies that have compared outcomes based on historical controls versus randomly allocated controls have found positive treatment effects with historical controls that randomized trials have not been able to replicate.[22,23] The most obvious problem, therefore, is the potential for confounding because of imbalances in characteristics of the experimental and historical control groups. For this approach to work, then, the researcher must be diligent in establishing a logical basis for group comparisons. This means that the historical controls should not simply be any patients described in the literature, or those treated at another time or another clinic.[20,24] It is reasonable, however, as in the kidney transplant example, to consider using groups that were treated within the same environment, under similar conditions, where records of protocols were kept and demographics of subjects can be obtained. This approach may prove useful as large clinical data bases are accumulated within a given treatment setting.

Analysis of Designs with Historical Controls.   Researchers often use the independent samples *t*-test to compare current subjects with historical subjects, although there is an inherent flaw in this approach because there is no assumption of equivalence between the groups. The Mann-Whitney *U* test may be used with ordinal data. Chi square will allow the researcher to determine if there is an association among categorical variables. Multiple regression, logistic regression or discriminant analysis can be done, using group membership as a variable, to analyze differences between the groups while accounting for other variables.

Nonequivalent Posttest-Only Control Group Design

Nonequivalent designs are less interpretable when only posttest measures are available. The **nonequivalent posttest-only control group design** (see Figure 11.7), also called a **static group comparison**,[25] is a quasi-experimental design that can be expanded to include any number of treatment levels, with or without a control group. This design uses existing groups who have and have not received treatment.

> **Example of a Nonequivalent Posttest-Only Control Group Design**
> Researchers were interested in studying the effects of a cardiac rehabilitation program on self-esteem and mobility skill in 152 patients who received cardiac surgery.[26] They studied 37 subjects who participated in a 2-month exercise program, and another 115 subjects who chose not to attend the program, forming the control group. Measurements were taken at the end of the 2-month study period. Outcomes were based on the Adult Source of Self-esteem Inventory and the New York Heart Association Classification.

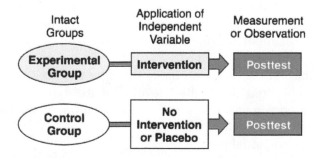

FIGURE 11.7   Nonequivalent posttest-only control group design.

To draw conclusions from this comparison, we would have to determine if variables other than the exercise program could be responsible for outcomes. Confounding factors should be identified and analyzed in relation to the dependent variable. For instance, in the cardiac rehabilitation example, researchers considered the subjects' age, years of education and occupational skill.[26] Although the static group comparison affords some measure of control in that there is a control group, internal validity is severely threatened by selection biases and attrition. This design is inherently weak because it provides no evidence of equivalence of groups before treatment. Therefore, it should be used only in an exploratory capacity, where it may serve to generate hypotheses for future testing. It is essentially useless in the search for causal relationships.

Analysis of Nonequivalent Posttest-Only Designs.   Because this design does not allow interpretation of cause and effect, the most appropriate analysis is a regression approach, such as discriminant analysis. Essentially, this design allows the researcher to determine if there is a relationship between the presence of the group attribute and the measured response. An analysis of covariance may be used to account for the effect of confounding variables.

COMMENTARY

Generalization to the Real World

In the pursuit of evidence-based practice, clinicians must be able to read research literature with a critical eye, assessing not only the validity of the study's design, but also the generalizability of its findings. Published research must be applicable to clinical situations and individual patients to be useful. The extent to which any study can be applied to a given patient is always a matter of judgment.

Purists will claim that generalization of intervention studies requires random selection and random assignment—in other words, a randomized controlled trial (RCT). In this view, quasi-experimental studies are less generalizable because they do not provide sufficient control of extraneous variables. In fact, such designs may be especially vulnerable to all the factors that affect internal validity.

One might reasonably argue, however, that the rigid structure and rules of the RCT do not represent real world situations, making it difficult for clinicians to apply or generalize research findings. The results of the RCT may not apply to a particular patient who does not meet inclusion or exclusion criteria, or who cannot be randomly assigned to a treatment protocol. Many of the quasi-experimental models will provide an opportunity to look at comparisons in a more natural context. In the hierarchy of evidence that is often used to qualify the rigor and weight of a study's findings, the RCT is considered the highest level. But the quasi-experimental study should not be dismissed as a valuable source of information. As with any study, however, it is the clinician's responsibility to make the judgments about the applicability of the findings to the individual patient.

REFERENCES

1. D'Agostino RB, Kwan H. Measuring effectiveness. What to expect without a randomized control group. *Med Care* 1995;33:AS95–105.
2. Cook TD, Campbell DT. *Quasi-experimentation: Design and Analysis Issues for Field Settings.* Boston: Houghton Mifflin, 1979.
3. Johnston MV, Ottenbacher KJ, Reichardt CS. Strong quasi-experimental designs for research on the effectiveness of rehabilitation. *Am J Phys Med Rehabil* 1995;74:383–392.
4. Griggs SM, Ahn A, Green A. Idiopathic adhesive capsulitis. A prospective functional outcome study of nonoperative treatment. *J Bone Joint Surg Am* 2000;82-A:1398–1407.
5. Green SB, Salkind NJ, Akey TM. *Using SPSS for Windows: Analyzing and Understanding Data.* Upper Saddle River, NJ: Prentice Hall, 1997.
6. Neuberger GB, Press AN, Lindsley HB, Hinton R, Cagle PE, Carlson K, et al. Effects of exercise on fatigue, aerobic fitness, and disease activity measures in persons with rheumatoid arthritis. *Res Nurs Health* 1997;20:195–204.
7. Brooks BR. Natural history of ALS: Symptoms, strength, pulmonary function, and disability. *Neurology* 1996;47:S71–81.
8. Caroscio JT, Mulvihill MN, Sterling R, Abrams B. Amyotrophic lateral sclerosis. Its natural history. *Neurol Clin* 1987;5:1–8.
9. Bryan WW, Hoagland RJ, Murphy J, Armon C, Barohn RJ, Goodpasture JC, et al. Can we eliminate placebo in ALS clinical trials? *Amyotroph Lateral Scler Other Motor Neuron Disord* 2003;4:11–15.
10. Biglan A, Ary D, Wagenaar AC. The value of interrupted time-series experiments for community intervention research. *Prev Sci* 2000;1:31–49.
11. Ansari F, Gray K, Nathwani D, Phillips G, Ogston S, Ramsay C, et al. Outcomes of an intervention to improve hospital antibiotic prescribing: Interrupted time series with segmented regression analysis. *J Antimicrob Chemother* 2003;52:842–848.
12. Matowe LK, Leister CA, Crivera C, Korth-Bradley JM. Interrupted time series analysis in clinical research. *Ann Pharmacother* 2003;37:1110–1116.
13. Nelson BK. Statistical methodology: V. Time series analysis using autoregressive integrated moving average (ARIMA) models. *Acad Emerg Med* 1998;5:739–744.
14. Allard R. Use of time-series analysis in infectious disease surveillance. *Bull World Health Organ* 1998;76:327–333.
15. Ottenbacher KJ. Analysis of data in idiographic research. *Am J Phys Med Rehabil* 1992;71:202–208.
16. Wagner AK, Soumerai SB, Zhang F, Ross-Degnan D. Segmented regression analysis of interrupted time series studies in medication use research. *J Clin Pharm Ther* 2002;27:299–309.
17. Wang WT, Olson SL, Campbell AH, Hanten WP, Gleeson PB. Effectiveness of physical therapy for patients with neck pain: An individualized approach using a clinical decision-making algorithm. *Am J Phys Med Rehabil* 2003;82:203–218; quiz 219–221.
18. Nicholson CM, Czernwicz S, Mandilas G, Rudolph I, Greyling MJ. The role of chair exercises for older adults following hip fracture. *S Afr Med J* 1997;87:1131–1138.
19. Matas AJ, Kandaswamy R, Humar A, Payne WD, Dunn DL, Najarian JS, et al. Long-term immunosuppression, without maintenance prednisone, after kidney transplantation. *Ann Surg* 2004;240:510–516.
20. Moser M. Randomized clinical trials: Alternatives to conventional randomization. *Am J Emerg Med* 1986;4:276–285.
21. Gehan EA, Freireich EJ. Non-randomized controls in cancer clinical trials. *N Engl J Med* 1974;290:198–203.

22. Sacks HS, Chalmers TC, Smith H, Jr. Sensitivity and specificity of clinical trials. Randomized v. historical controls. *Arch Intern Med* 1983;143:753–755.
23. Micciolo R, Valagussa P, Marubini E. The use of historical controls in breast cancer. An assessment in three consecutive trials. *Control Clin Trials* 1985;6:259–270.
24. Bridgman S, Engebretsen L, Dainty K, Kirkley A, Maffulli N. Practical aspects of randomization and blinding in randomized clinical trials. *Arthroscopy* 2003;19:1000–1006.
25. Campbell DT, Stanley JC. *Experimental and Quasi-experimental Designs for Research.* Chicago: Rand McNally, 1963.
26. Ng JY, Tam SF. Effect of exercise-based cardiac rehabilitation on mobility and self-esteem of persons after cardiac surgery. *Percept Mot Skills* 2000;91:107–114.

CHAPTER 12
Single-Subject Designs

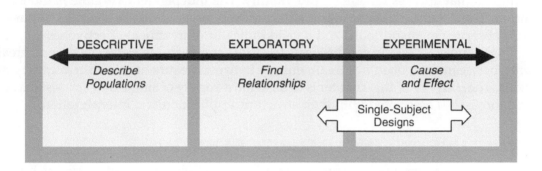

The demands of traditional experimental methods are often seen as barriers to clinical inquiry for several reasons. Because of their rigorous structure, experiments require control groups and large numbers of homogenous subjects, often unavailable in clinical settings. In addition, group studies typically take measurements at only two or three points in time, potentially missing variations in response that occur over time. Finally, the experimental model deals with group averages and generalizations across individuals, which may not allow the researcher to differentiate characteristics of those patients who responded favorably to treatment from those who did not improve. Therefore, although generalizations are important for explaining behavioral phenomena, clinicians understand that group performance is relevant only if it can be used to understand and predict individual performance.

To illustrate this dilemma, consider a study that was done to determine if the occurrence of stuttering would be different if adults read aloud at "usual" or "fast as possible" rates.[1] A group of 20 adults was tested, and no significant difference was seen between the two conditions based on a comparison of group means. However, a closer look at individual results showed that 8 subjects actually decreased their frequency of stuttering, one didn't change, and 11 demonstrated an increase during the faster speaking condition. The group analysis obscured these individual variations.[2] These results could mean that there is no consistent effect, but they may also point to specific subject characteristics that account for the differences.

Single-subject designs* provide an alternative approach that allows us to draw conclusions about the effects of treatment based on the responses of a single patient under controlled conditions. Through a variety of strategies and structures, these designs provide a clinically viable, controlled experimental approach to the study of a single case or several subjects, and the flexibility to observe change under ongoing treatment conditions. Given the focus of evidence-based practice on clinical decision making for individual patients, these designs are especially useful.

Single-subject designs require the same attention to logical design and control as other experimental designs, based on a research hypothesis that indicates the expected relationship between an independent and dependent variable and specific operational definitions that address reliability and validity. The independent variable is the intervention. The dependent variable is the patient response, defined as a **target behavior** that is observable, quantifiable, and a valid indicator of treatment effectiveness.

Single-subject designs can be used to study comparisons between several treatments, between components of treatments, or between treatment and no-treatment conditions. The purpose of this chapter is to describe a variety of single-subject designs and to explore issues associated with their structure, application and interpretation.

STRUCTURE OF SINGLE-SUBJECT DESIGNS

Single-subject designs are structured around two core elements that distinguish them from a case study or group studies: repeated measurement and design phases.

Repeated Measurement

Single-subject designs involve the systematic collection of *repeated measurements* of a behavioral response over time, usually at frequent and regular intervals, such as at each treatment session (which may be more than once a day), each day or once a week. These repeated assessments are required to observe trends and patterns in the data and to evaluate variability of the behavioral response over time. This type of variability is obscured in group studies when behavior is measured only before and after treatment. The advantage of repeated assessment is that the researcher can observe response patterns and modify the design as the study progresses to obtain the most meaningful outcome.

Design Phases

The second core element of a single-subject design is the delineation of at least two testing periods, or phases: a **baseline phase**, prior to treatment, and an **intervention phase**. The target behavior is measured repeatedly across both baseline and intervention phases. The baseline phase provides information about responses during a period

---

*These designs have also been called *single system strategies*,[3] N of 1 studies,[4] and *time series designs*.[5] Cook and Campbell[6] describe time series designs as quasi-experimental designs with multiple measurements over time. They present several variations of these designs, which are analogous to the withdrawal and multiple baseline designs presented in this chapter. The subject or system used most often is a single individual, but the sampling unit may be any unit of interest, such as a small group, a community, a department or an institution.

of "no treatment," or a control condition. This initial observation period reflects the natural state of the target behavior over time in the absence of the independent variable. The assumption is that baseline data reflect the ongoing effects of background variables, such as daily activities, other treatments and personal characteristics on the target behavior. When treatment is initiated, changes from baseline to the intervention phase should be attributable to intervention. Therefore, baseline data provide a standard of comparison for evaluating the potential cause-and-effect relationship between the intervention and target behavior.

Design phases are traditionally plotted on a line graph, as shown in Figure 12.1, with magnitude of the target behavior along the *Y*-axis and time (sessions, trials, days, weeks) along the *X*-axis. Using conventional notation, the baseline period is represented by the letter *A* and the intervention period by the letter *B*. To facilitate description, this design, with one baseline phase and one intervention phase, is called an **A–B design**.

The collection of baseline data is the single feature of a single-subject design that particularly distinguishes it from clinical practice, case studies and traditional experimental designs, where treatment is initiated immediately following assessment. From a research standpoint, the traditional approach makes it impossible to determine which components of treatment actually caused observed changes, or more important, if observed changes would have occurred without intervention. Just as we need a control group to validate group comparisons, we must have a control period to make these determinations for a single-subject experiment.

Ethical objections often arise when the baseline concept is introduced, just as they do when a control group is proposed for a group comparison study. Two points must be made in this regard. First, we can argue that it is not unethical to withhold treatment for a relatively short period when we are unsure about the effectiveness of the intervention in the first place. Indeed, it may actually be unethical to continue to provide an

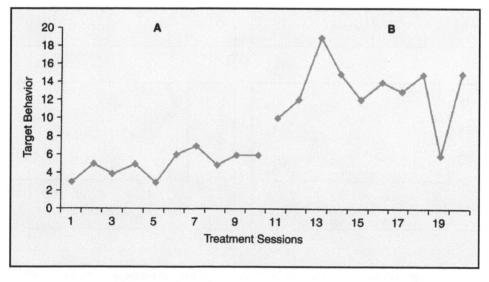

FIGURE 12.1   Example of a basic A–B design, showing baseline and intervention phases.

inferior or ineffective treatment without testing it experimentally. It is, however, important to realize that this approach is not appropriate for studying every type of intervention, such as treatments for critical or life-threatening situations, where treatment effects are not questioned and withholding treatment would be harmful. Second, collecting baseline data does not mean that the clinician is denying all treatment to the patient. It only means that one portion of the patient's total treatment is being isolated for study while all other treatments and activities are continued as background.

Baseline Characteristics

Two characteristics of baseline data are important for interpretation of clinical outcomes: **stability**, which reflects the consistency of response over time, and **trend**, or slope, which shows the rate of change in the behavior. The most desirable baseline pattern demonstrates a constant level of behavior with minimal variability, indicating that the target behavior is not changing (see Figure 12.2A). Therefore, changes that are observed after the intervention is introduced can be confidently attributed to a treatment effect. If treatment has no effect, we would expect to see this baseline pattern continue into the intervention phase.

A variable baseline (Figure 12.2B) can present a problem for interpretation. When this type of pattern emerges, it is generally advisable to continue to collect baseline data until some stability is achieved. With extreme variability, the researcher is obliged to

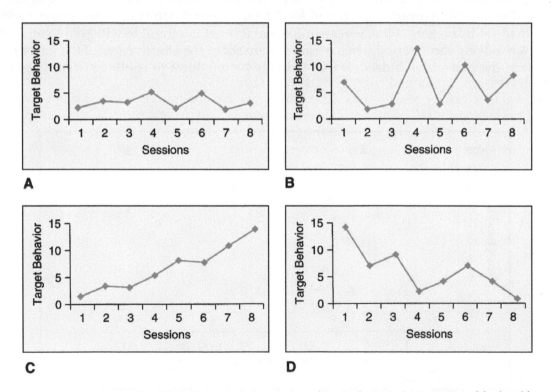

FIGURE 12.2   Types of baselines that may be encountered in single-case designs: (**A**) stable, level baseline, (**B**) variable baseline, (**C**) stable accelerating trend, (**D**) variable decelerating trend.

consider what factors might be influencing the target behavior to create such an erratic response. Sometimes cyclical patterns are evident, perhaps with variations corresponding to days of the week, time of day, or regular events occurring in the subject's life. If these factors continue to operate during intervention, they could easily obscure treatment effects.

An *accelerating* baseline (Figure 12.2C) or a *decelerating* baseline (Figure 12.2D) indicates that a change in the target behavior is occurring without intervention. Either type of trend may represent improvement or deterioration, depending on the target behavior. Trends can also be characterized as stable or unstable; that is, the rate of change may be constant (as in Figure 12.2C) or variable (as in Figure 12.2D). Trends in baseline data must be identified to determine if responses that are observed following treatment represent true change.

Length of Phases

One of the first questions clinicians ask when planning single-subject experiments concerns how long phases should be. Single-subject designs provide some flexibility in these choices, allowing for consideration of the type of patient, the type of treatment, and the expected rate of change in the target behavior. This flexibility differentiates the single-subject design from traditional designs where onset and duration of treatment are established and fixed prior to experimentation, regardless of how the patient responds. There are some guidelines that can be followed to assist in these decisions.

It is generally desirable to use relatively equal phase length. It is not uncommon, for example, to find that researchers preset intervals of 1 week for each phase in a design when daily measurements are taken. This practice helps to control for potential time-related factors such as maturation or the motivational influence of continued attention over prolonged treatment periods. Despite these plans, however, it is usually advisable to extend baseline or intervention phases until stability is achieved, or at least until one is sure that responses are representative of the true condition under study. Most important, it is essential that the length of time within each phase is sufficient to capture any changes that will occur over time.

Because trend is an important characteristic of repeated measurements, there must be a minimum of three to four data points in each phase. The application of some analysis procedures is enhanced by having 12 or more points within each phase to establish stability.[7] Clearly, the greater the number of data points, the more obvious trends will become. It is useful to remember that the intervals used for repeated measurements need not represent single days. When patient behaviors change rapidly in response to intervention, more than one session can be plotted within a day, so that a sufficient number of data points can be obtained in a short period.

THE TARGET BEHAVIOR

Target behaviors can reflect different response systems and may focus on impairments, activity limitations or measures of disability. Measurements may deal with overt motor behaviors, such as functional performance, range of motion (ROM), strength or gait characteristics. We can also assess physiological reactions, such as blood pressure or exercise responses, and verbal reactions, such as the number of correct responses to specific questions or subjective feelings of pain. Assessment techniques vary, depending on the types of variables designated as target behaviors. One benefit of the single-subject approach is the ability to develop individualized measurement systems that reflect a patient's performance in a clinically relevant way. For instance, specific functional tasks may be emphasized that indicate a patient's major limitations. The choice of a target behavior can be an important first step in making a single-subject study meaningful.

Measuring the Target Behavior

Although many clinical variables are typically assessed using qualitative values, they must be quantified in some way to be used as experimental data. One of the major advantages of the single-subject approach is that it provides a mechanism for quantifying even the most subjective clinical behaviors. The most common techniques for measuring behaviors within single-subject designs are frequency, duration and magnitude measures.

A **frequency count** indicates the number of occurrences of the behavior within a fixed time interval or number of trials. For example, we can count the number of times a particular gait deviation occurs, the number of times a patient can correctly name objects, or the number of times a patient loses her balance during a defined treatment session. Operational definitions for frequency counts must specify how the target behavior is distinguished from other responses and exactly what constitutes an occurrence and nonoccurrence of the behavior. For instance, if a patient attempts an exercise and achieves only partial range, is that counted as an occurrence? If a patient begins to fall over but catches herself by reaching for the wall, is that considered loss of balance?

Frequency can be expressed as a percentage, by dividing the number of occurrences of the target behavior by the total number of opportunities for the behavior to occur. This method is often used in studies where accuracy of performance (percentage correct) is of primary interest. Frequency counts can also be translated into *rates*. Rate refers to the number of times a behavior occurs within a specified time period. It is calculated by dividing the total number of occurrences of the behavior by the total time (seconds, minutes or hours) during which the behavior was observed. For example, we can measure ambulation in steps per minute or endurance in repetitions per minute.

A useful procedure for measuring repetitive behavior is called **interval recording**, which involves breaking down the full measurement period into preset time intervals, and determining if the behavior occurs or does not occur during each interval. For instance, Dave[8] studied the effects of vestibular stimulation on stereotypic body-rocking behaviors in three adults with profound mental retardation. He monitored the behavior for a total of 5 minutes, looking at the occurrence or nonoccurrence of rocking within consecutive 15-second intervals.

Target behaviors can also be evaluated according to how long they last. **Duration** can be measured either as the cumulative total duration of a behavior during a treatment session or as the duration of each individual occurrence of the behavior. Operational definitions for duration measures must specify criteria for determining when the behavior starts and when it ends. For example, we can measure how long a patient stays in a balanced standing posture within a single trial or over a treatment session, or we can time how long it takes for a patient to complete a specific functional task, such as buttoning a shirt.

Many clinical variables are measured using some form of instrumentation that provides a **quantitative score,** which may be a summary score, a subscale score or a single test value. For example, Shumway-Cook and co-workers[9] used a forceplate to assess the effect of balance training on movement of the center of pressure and time to stabilization in six children with cerebral palsy. Bastille and Gill-Body[10] used scores on the Berg Balance Scale and the Stroke Impact Scale as an indicators of the effectiveness of yoga-based exercise program for patients with chronic poststroke hemiparesis. These examples illustrate the potential for using single-subject designs to study changes in outcomes, including impairments, activity limitations and disability measures.

Choosing a Target Behavior

Because patients usually present several clinical problems, choosing one specific problem as the focus of an experiment can be difficult. To focus on one target behavior, it is often necessary to define complex behaviors and determine which component of the behavior is most problematic. It is useful to consider the relative stability with which a behavior is expected to respond. It is also important to establish that a specific intervention is readily available to address the target behavior, that the behavior is a valid indicator of that intervention's effectiveness, and that the treatment will cause an observable change in the behavior. Finally, choice of a target behavior may be influenced by available instrumentation and clinical goals. Researchers can also look at several target behaviors simultaneously, to examine their potential interaction or to document the relationship between impairments and functional measures.

In addition, a measurement method must be chosen that will reflect the element of performance that is of primary concern. Is it how often a patient can perform a particular task, or how long a behavior can be maintained? Is the number of correct responses or incorrect responses of interest? Or is it simply whether or not the behavior occurred? Each measurement method will provide a different perspective of the target behavior, which will obviously influence how the data will be interpreted.

RELIABILITY

Reliability is important in single-subject research as it is in any form of clinical inquiry. Because the single-subject experiment focuses on observation of behaviors in a clinical setting, reliability is usually assessed concurrently with data collection, rather than in a separate pilot study. Researchers usually report interrater reliability using a measure of percentage agreement between observers (see Chapter 26). Reliability checks are performed by having two testers simultaneously observe the target behavior at several sessions across each phase of the study. An agreement score is obtained for each session, and results are then reported as a range of agreement scores or as an average.[†]

[†]With magnitude data, reliability can also be established using correlational methods, such as the intraclass correlation coefficient (see Chapter 26).

EXPERIMENTAL CONTROL: LIMITATIONS OF THE A–B DESIGN

The element that most clearly characterizes an experimental research design is its ability to control for threats to internal validity (see Chapter 9). Unfortunately, the basic A–B single-subject design is limited in this respect. Consider the following example:

> Researchers explored the relationship between language development and sensory integration using a single case experimental study of four aphasic children ranging in age from 4 years, 0 months to 5 years, 3 months.[11] Other agencies had assessed all the children in the area of language development at least 6 months before the start of occupational therapy. Three of the four children had received either speech therapy, special education specific to aphasia, or both, before starting occupational therapy. Additional baseline data on language expression and comprehension, as well as on sensory integrative functioning, were gathered before beginning a year of occupational therapy that involved sensory integration procedures.

Figure 12.3 shows the development of language comprehension for one child in this study. Stable responses were observed over a 9-week baseline phase. Immediately following the onset of occupational therapy, scores rise markedly, suggesting at first glance that the therapy was instrumental in achieving this change. But is this conclusion definitive? Did other events or changes within the subject occur coincidentally at the same time treatment was initiated that could have accounted for the observed change? In other words, is this conclusion internally valid?

Note that several other events may be associated with this change. Speech therapy was begun 1 week later (D), an aphasia class started at 16 weeks (E), and a developmental therapy program began at 25 weeks (F). With this design, it is impossible to conclude that the occupational therapy treatment was the causative factor in improving language comprehension scores.

To strengthen the control in this design, we must include some other form of evidence that the treatment was indeed responsible for observed changes, evidence that will discredit alternative hypotheses for explaining treatment outcomes. Within a single-subject strategy, this additional control is provided by **replication of effects**, which can be accomplished in several ways. Phases can be repeated by withdrawing and reinstating baseline and treatment conditions or by alternating two or more interventions. We can also replicate effects across more than one subject or within one subject across multiple conditions or behaviors. The more often an effect can be replicated within a design, the stronger the design controls against potential threats to internal validity. These strategies form the basis for structuring single-subject designs.

WITHDRAWAL DESIGNS

Experimental control within a single-subject design can be achieved through withdrawal of intervention, to demonstrate that the target behavior occurs only in the presence of treatment. The **withdrawal design** includes a second baseline period, but may also include a second intervention period.

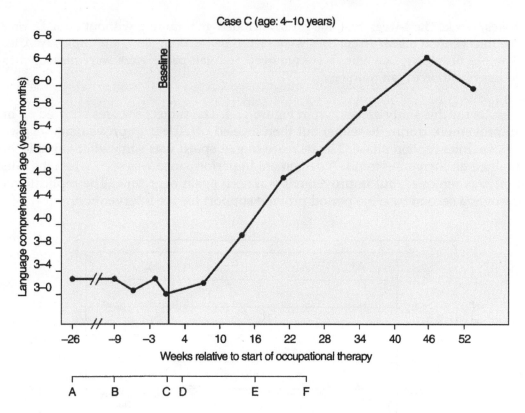

FIGURE 12.3   Example of an A–B design, illustrating potential threats to internal validity: scores on a language comprehension test in an aphasic child before and after the onset of occupational therapy. Relevant events: (A) initial testing, (B) first baseline data gathered, (C) started occupational therapy, (D) started individual speech therapy, (E) entered public school aphasia class, (F) started developmental therapy. (Adapted from Ayres AJ, Mailloux Z. Influence of sensory integration procedures on language development. *Am J Occup Ther* 1981; 35:383–90, Fig 3, p. 187. Copyright 1981 by the American Occupational Therapy Association. Reprinted with permission.)

A–B–A Design

The **A–B–A design** replicates one baseline phase following intervention. The premise of this design lies in its ability to show that behavioral changes are evident only in the presence of the intervention, during Phase B. If changes in the target behavior are not maintained during the second baseline period, one can logically conclude that the treatment was the factor causing the changes observed during the intervention phase. Internal validity is controlled because it is highly unlikely that confounding factors would coincidentally occur at both the onset and the cessation of treatment. If other variables were responsible for changes seen in the target behavior during the first two phases, the behavior would not be expected to revert to baseline levels during the withdrawal phase.

> Researchers studied the effect of using visual cues during gait training in an individual with Parkinson disease.[12] They assessed gait speed as the subject walked a distance of 10 meters as many times as she could in 30 minutes. The subject was seen three

times/week. The 4-week baseline phase included gait training without cues. During the intervention phase, visual cues were placed on the floor along the walkway. After 4 weeks of intervention, cues were removed and gait parameters were measured to assess retention of gait training.

The results for this study are shown in Figure 12.4. The subject's scores showed an initial improvement during baseline, but then leveled off. Clear improvement was seen during the intervention phase. The increase in gait speed was somewhat variable, but maintained an increasing trend. A decrement in performance was seen when the intervention was removed, but improvement was seen again over time. The replication of effects over a second baseline period provide support for the intervention.

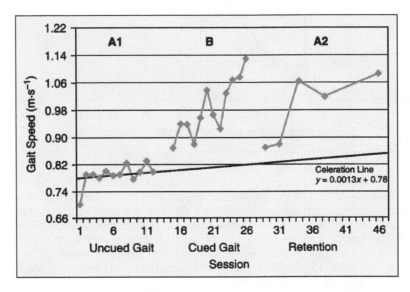

FIGURE 12.4 Example of an A–B–A design, showing gait speed during uncued and cued gait in a patient with Parkinson disease. The second baseline phase is considered a period of retention, to determine if the patient's performance would be maintained when cues were withdrawn. (From Sidaway B, Anderson J, Danielson G. Effects of long-term gait training using visual cues in an individual with Parkinson disease. *Phys Ther* 2006; 86:186–194, Figure 2, p. 190. Reprinted with permission of the American Physical Therapy Association.)

The obvious problem with the A–B–A design is that the behavior must be reversible. This is often not the case. Any response that is learned or that creates permanent change will not show a decrement when treatment is withdrawn. Consider the following example:

A study was done to determine if manual therapy, therapeutic exercise and patient education would be an effective strategy to reduce pain for a patient with disc displacement without reduction of both temporomandibular joints.[13] Pain was measured using a visual analog scale over 15 visits.

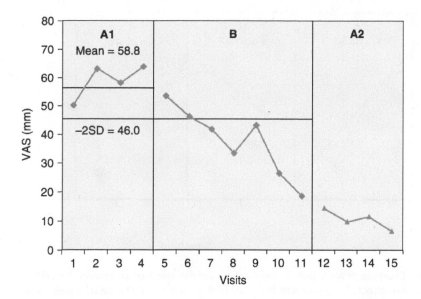

FIGURE 12.5 Pain data recorded in an A–B–A design using a 10-cm visual analog scale in a patient with temporomandibular joint pain. Intervention included manual therapy, exercise and patient education. Data show a maintenance of pain relief during the withdrawal phase. (From Cleland J, Palmer J. Effectiveness of manual physical therapy, therapeutic exercise, and patient education on bilateral disc displacement without reduction of the temporomandibular joint: A single-case design. *J Orthop Sports Phys Ther* 2004; 34: 535–548, Figure 3, p. 540. Reproduced with permission of the Orthopaedic and Sports Physical Therapy Sections of the American Physical Therapy Association.)

As shown in Figure 12.5, pain was relatively stable during the first baseline, showed a linear decline during intervention, and continued to decline during the second baseline phase. Pain level was clearly decreased starting at the point of intervention, but because of the effectiveness of the treatment, continued to decrease during the second baseline phase.

A–B–A–B Design

Experimental control and clinical relevance can be strengthened through the use of an **A–B–A–B design**, which provides initial baseline data and ends on an intervention phase. The major advantage of this design is that it provides two opportunities to evaluate the effects of the intervention. If effects can be replicated during two separate intervention phases, controlling for internal validity, the evidence is quite strong that behavioral change was directly related to the treatment.

Asymmetrical posture during static stance has been identified as a common problem in persons with hemiplegia. Researchers examined the effect of an activity-based therapy regimen on symmetric weight bearing in three adult subjects with hemiplegia.[14] An A–B–A–B design was used. The intervention program, including playing a bean bag game, was introduced for 30 minutes each day during each intervention phase. Quantitative measurements of weight distribution were taken with the Balance Master System.

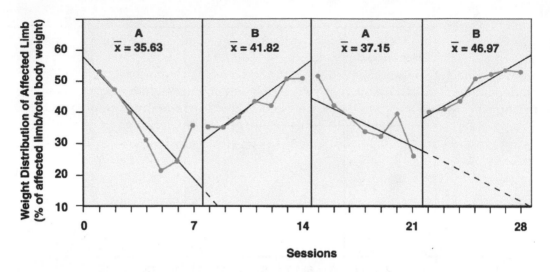

FIGURE 12.6 Example of an A-B-A-B design, showing the effect of an activity-based therapy on weight distribution over the affected leg (percent body weight) during static stance in a patient with hemiplegia. (From Wu S, Huang H, Lin C, and Chen M. Effects of a program on symmetrical posture in patients with hemiplegia: A single-subject design. *Am J Occup Ther* 1996; 50:17–23, Figure 1, p. 20. Reprinted with permission of the American Occupational Therapy Association.)

Figure 12.6 shows results for one subject for this study. Weight distribution was plotted as a ratio of the percent weight on the affected limb over total body weight; therefore, the goal was to achieve higher ratios. Although performance is variable, there is clearly a declining ratio during both baseline phases, and an increasing ratio during both intervention phases.

The A–B–A–B design faces the same limitations as the A–B–A design, in that behaviors must be reversible to see treatment effects. If, however, the target behavior does not revert to original baseline values, but stays level during the second baseline, the A–B–A–B strategy still makes it possible to demonstrate change if there is further improvement during the second intervention phase.

MULTIPLE BASELINE DESIGNS

The use of withdrawal is limited in situations where ethical considerations of withdrawal prevail and where behaviors are either nonreversible or prone to carryover effects. When practical replication cannot be achieved, a **multiple baseline design** can be used, where effects are replicated across subjects, across treatment conditions, or across multiple target behaviors. The multiple-baseline approach allows for use of the basic A–B format as well as withdrawal variations.

The multiple baseline design demonstrates experimental control by first requiring the concurrent collection of baseline data across a minimum of three data series. When all baselines exhibit sufficient stability, the intervention is applied only to the first series, while the other baselines are continued. When the first series achieves stability during treatment, intervention is introduced into the second series. Stability can be achieved either as a constant trend (acceleration or deceleration) or as a level response. This process is repeated on a staggered basis for all remaining baselines. By allowing each baseline to run for a different number of data points, systematic changes in the target behavior that are correlated with the onset of intervention can be reliably attributed to a treatment effect. Experimental control is strengthened by demonstrating that baselines are independent; that is, change is observed only when intervention is applied and does not occur during baseline periods. Some examples will help to illustrate this process.

Sometimes it is of interest to study the effect of one intervention on several related clinical behaviors. In the **multiple baseline design across behaviors,** the researcher monitors a minimum of three similar yet functionally independent behaviors in the same subject that can be addressed using the same intervention. Each target behavior is measured concurrently and continuously, until a stable baseline is achieved. The intervention is then introduced sequentially across the different behaviors.

Warren and coworkers[15] studied the effect of an interactive teaching approach on the acquisition of prelinguistic skills in a child with Down syndrome and language delay. They focused on three specific components of communication: prelinguistic requesting, vocal imitation and commenting. They tallied the number of appropriate responses observed during each session. After an initial baseline, training addressed requesting toys within the environment, while other behaviors were monitored. Training strategies were later introduced for imitation and commenting behaviors in a staggered fashion.

The results shown in Figure 12.7 demonstrate treatment effects most clearly for commenting behavior, with moderate gains in vocal imitation and dramatically variable changes in requests. Obviously, the multiple baseline design across behaviors requires that the targeted behaviors are similar enough that they will all respond to one treatment approach, and that they are functionally independent of one another so that baselines will remain stable until treatment is introduced. With many social and physical variables, this assumption can be problematic.

If we had used the A–B format for only one of these strategies, these results would not have been so definitive because of potential threats to internal validity; however, because the results have been replicated across three conditions at staggered times, it is highly unlikely that external factors could have coincidentally occurred at the time each treatment was initiated to cause the response change. One of the major advantages of the multiple-baseline approach is that replication and experimental control can be achieved without withdrawal of treatment.

In a **multiple baseline design across subjects,** one intervention is applied to the same target behavior across three or more individuals who share common relevant characteristics.

Researchers studied the effectiveness of an intermittent intensive physical therapy program for children with cerebral palsy.[16] They wanted to demonstrate that rest periods within the schedule of treatment could be well tolerated. Using an A–B multiple baseline design, baseline phases were staggered from 8 to 20 weeks, during which time the children received treatment 2 times/week. During the intervention phase, they received four treatments/week for 4 weeks, alternated with an 8-week rest

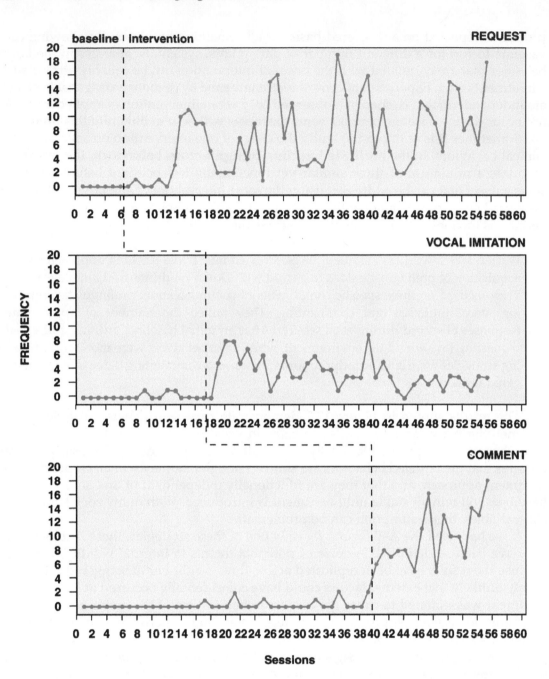

FIGURE 12.7 Example of a multiple baseline design across behaviors, showing the effect of effect of an interactive teaching approach on the frequency of requests, vocal imitations and comments by a child with Down Syndrome and language delay. (From Warren SF, Yoder PJ, Gazdag GE, Kim K, Jones HA. Facilitating prelinguistic communication skills in young children with developmental delay. *J Speech Hear Res* 1993; 36: 83–97, Fig. 1, p. 88. Reprinted with permisison of the American Speech-Language-Hearing Association.)

period. Children were seen over a total of 24 weeks. Changes in motor performance were assessed using the Gross Motor Function Measure (GMFM).

In this study, all subjects showed at least a consistent level of response, with no decrement in GMFM scores. The authors concluded that the intermittent intensive therapy schedule was well tolerated and effective compared to the standard schedule of 2 treatments/week.

In the **multiple baseline design across conditions,** one behavior is monitored on one individual, with the same treatment applied sequentially across two more environmental conditions. These may be different treatment settings, different instructional arrangements, or different clinicians. Experimental control in this design can be demonstrated only if the target behavior is independent of the environment. Therefore, behavioral change in one environment will not influence behavior in other settings.

> Researchers studied the effects of a computer-based intervention program on communication functions in children with autism.[17] Software was developed based on daily life activities in three settings. Five children between 8 and 12 years old were evaluated during play time, during food activities at breakfast or snack time, and during hygiene activities following snacks. Computer intervention was introduced on a staggered basis in each setting. Frequency of appropriate or inappropriate responses was measured within an A–B multiple baseline design.

In this study, the researchers saw that the frequency of relevant sentences clearly increased with the use of the software program during play. The level of response was minimal during hygiene activities, and the authors commented that this was not an activity the children enjoyed.

Nonconcurrent Multiple Baseline Design

A basic premise of the multiple baseline design across subjects is that baseline data are available for all subjects simultaneously so that temporal effects cannot contaminate results. A variation of this design, called a **nonconcurrent multiple baseline design,** can be used in the common clinical situation in which similar subjects are not available for concurrent monitoring.[18] This approach requires that the researcher arbitrarily determines the length of several baselines, such as 5, 10 and 15 days. When a subject who matches the study criteria becomes available, he is randomly assigned to one of the predetermined baseline lengths. Baseline data are collected, and treatment is introduced at the appropriate time, assuming baselines are sufficiently stable. If baseline data are too variable, the subject is dropped from the study. As other subjects become available, they are randomly assigned to the remaining baselines.

> Bailey and coworkers[19] studied the treatment of visual neglect in elderly patients with stroke. They used a nonconcurrent A–B–A multiple baseline design to examine the effect of a scanning and cueing strategy on unilateral visual neglect as measured by a written inventory, the Star Cancellation Test (SCT). Seven patients, aged 60 to 85 years, were recruited from a stroke rehabilitation unit. Baselines were staggered between 3 and 4 weeks. Intervention and second baseline (withdrawal) phases each lasted 3 weeks.

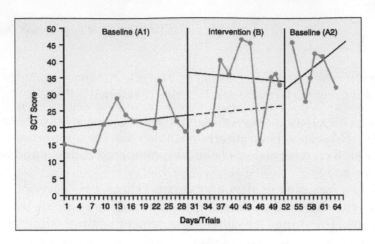

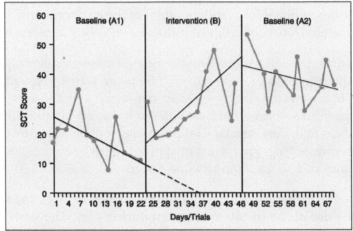

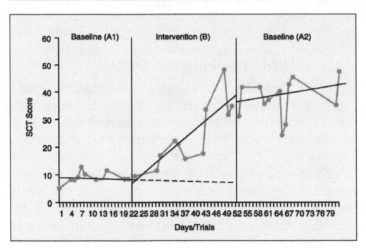

FIGURE 12.8 Example of a nonconcurrent multiple baseline design across three subjects, showing the effects of a scanning and cueing strategy on visual neglect in patients with stroke. The study uses an A-B-A design, demonstrating the effect of withdrawing the intervention. Data represent scores on the Star Cancellation Test (SCT), which measures accuracy of finding stars across a page. Baselines were staggered between 20 and 28 days. Data for all subjects are quite variable, although retention does appear evident for subjects 1 and 3. (From Bailey MJ, Riddoch MJ, Crome P. Treatment of visual neglect in elderly patients with stroke: A single-subject series using either a scanning and cueing strategy or a left-limb activation strategy. *Phys Ther* 2002;82:782–797, Figures 1, 2 and 4, p. 793. Reprinted with permission of the American Physical Therapy Association.)

The results for three patients are shown in Figure 12.8. We can see that the responses in these subjects are quite variable, making it more difficult to understand the effect of intervention. The trend lines in each intervention phase, however, do suggest that higher scores (decreased neglect) were evident for each subject. We will discuss interpretation of these trend lines shortly.

The benefit of the nonconcurrent baseline approach is obvious in terms of practical research requirements; however, it is a weaker design than the standard multiple baseline approach because external factors related to the passage of time may be different for each baseline. For instance, patients may be tested during different seasons of the year, or the clinical environment may change over time. Therefore, the nonconcurrent multiple baseline design should be used only when a sufficient number of subjects are not available for concurrent study. Because of this potential weakness as an experimental design, the number of subject replications should be increased as an additional element of control.

DESIGNS WITH MULTIPLE TREATMENTS

Withdrawal designs represent treatment-no treatment comparisons. Single-subject designs can also be used to compare the effects of two treatments.

Alternating Treatment Design

One strategy for studying multiple treatments involves the **alternating treatment design**. The essential feature of this design is the rapid alternation of two or more interventions or treatment conditions, each associated with a distinct stimulus. Treatment can be alternated within a treatment session, session by session, or day by day. This design can be used to compare treatment with a control or placebo or to compare two different interventions, to determine which one will be more effective. Data for each treatment condition are plotted on the same graph, allowing for comparison of data points and trends between conditions.

Scheduling of alternated treatments will depend on the time needed to complete the treatment condition at each session and the potential for carryover from trial to trial. Because treatment conditions are continuously alternated, sequence effects are of primary concern. This concern must be addressed either by random ordering of the treatment applications on each occasion or by systematic counterbalancing. In addition, other conditions that might affect the target behavior, such as the clinician, time of day, or setting should be counterbalanced.

> Yoo and Chung[20] investigated the effect of visual feedback and mental practice on symmetrical weight bearing in three individuals with hemiparetic stroke. They used a multiple baseline design across subjects to compare strategies of visual feedback alone or feedback with mental practice on the proportion of body weight borne by the affected limb. Interventions were applied using an alternating treatment approach, with treatments systematically alternated between morning and afternoon occupational therapy sessions.

Figure 12.9 illustrates the outcome for this study. With relatively stable baselines staggered from 4 to 10 sessions, we can see clear changes at the initiation of the interventions. The advantage of using the alternating treatment design over an A–B–A–B design for this type of question is that a prolonged withdrawal is unnecessary, and results can be obtained more quickly.

The alternating treatment design is also called a *between-series strategy,* indicating that analysis is not specifically concerned with trends over time, but that the primary focus is comparison of data points between treatment conditions at each session. For instance, in Figure 12.9 we see that the visual feedback condition was generally lower than the combined condition on each day. This design will work even under conditions where responses are very variable or where treatment conditions exhibit similar trends.

It is actually unnecessary to include a baseline phase in an alternating treatment design, just as a control group may not be included in group designs in which two treatments are compared. Baseline data can, however, be useful in situations where both treatments turn out to be equally effective, to show that they are better than no treatment at all.

Because target behaviors are measured in rapid succession, the alternating treatment design is appropriate where treatment effects are immediate and where behavior is a clear consequence of one specific treatment. The target behavior must be capable of changing quickly, and the interventions must be able to trigger those changes as they are applied and withdrawn. The alternating treatment design is not useful in situations where behavior takes time to change, where learning effects or physiological changes are cumulative and long term or where multiple-treatment interference is likely. In those situations, it would be difficult to separate out the effects of each intervention in alternated trials. The major advantage of the alternating treatment design is that it will usually provide answers to questions of treatment comparison in a shorter time frame than designs that require introduction and withdrawal of multiple treatment phases over time.

Multiple Treatment Designs

Using a variation of the withdrawal design, a **multiple treatment design** typically involves the application of one treatment (B) following baseline, the withdrawal of that treatment, and introduction of another treatment (C). These two interventions can represent two different treatments or one intervention and a placebo. In an A–B–C–A design, assuming the two treatments have independent and differential effects, we should be able to see differences in the target responses across the four phases of the study. By replicating the A phase, we provide the control needed to document differences between the two treatments.

> Clopton et al.[21] studied the effect of axial weight loading on gait parameters in individuals with cerebellar ataxia. Five subjects with ataxic gait ambulated along a fixed walkway for five trials in each of four conditions: unweighted (baseline), with 10% body weight at the shoulders, with 10% body weight at the waist and a final unweighted phase, creating an A–B–C–A design. Several gait parameters were measured, including velocity, cadence, step length and double support time.

Figure 12.10 shows the results for the first subject's double support time. Results show great variability, with some increase during the period of weight at the waist. This

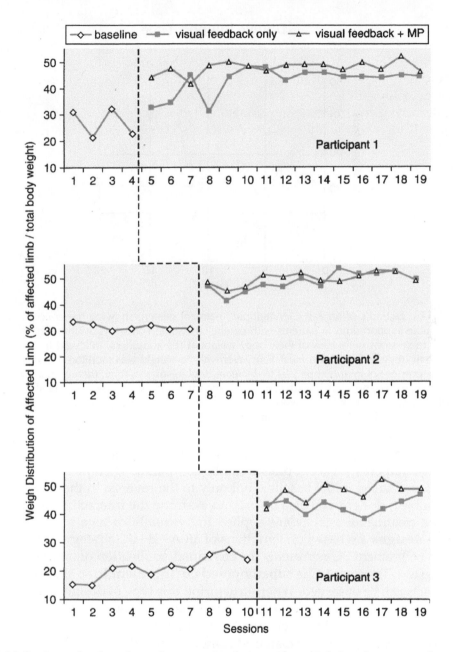

FIGURE 12.9   Example of an alternating treatment design with multiple baselines across three subjects. The intervention consisted of visual feedback or visual feedback with mental practice (MP). The proportion of the patient's weight bearing by the affected limb was measured. Data clearly show changes in weight distribution immediately following training. The visual feedback plus mental practice condition resulted in consistently higher scores for all three participants. (From Yoo E, Chung B. The effect of visual feedback plus mental practice on symmetrical weight-bearing training in people with hemiparesis. *Clin Rehabil* 2006;20:388–397, Figure 2, p. 394. Reprinted with permission.)

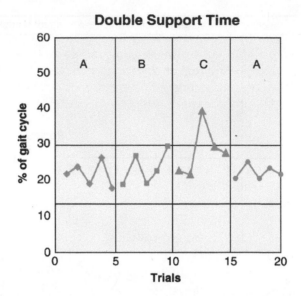

FIGURE 12.10 Example of an A-B-C-A multiple treatment design, showing the effect of axial weight loading on double support time in patients with cerebellar ataxia. Following an initial baseline, patients were exposed to sessions with 10% of their body weight at the shoulders, followed by several sessions with 10% of their body weight at the waist. Carryover with no weight was monitored in the second base-line phase. The purpose of intervention was to decrease double support time; therefore, a higher response is considered a poorer performance. (Adapted from Clopton N, Schultz D, Boren C. et al. Effects of axial weight loading on gait for subjects with cerebellar ataxia: Preliminary findings. *Neurology Report* 2003;27:15–21, Figure 1, p. 18. Reprinted with permission.)

was considered a deterioration in the response. It is important to note in multiple treat-ment designs, that only adjacent phases can be compared. Therefore, the C phase can-not be compared to the initial baseline, but only to the reversal in the final phase.

Single-subject designs can also be used to examine the interactive or joint effect of two or more treatments as they are applied individually or as a treatment package. **Interactive designs** are based on variations of an A−B−BC strategy (sometimes writ-ten A−B−B+C), where BC represents the combined application of interventions B and C. In this design, Treatment C is superimposed on Treatment B, so that combined and separate effects can be observed. When structuring this type of design, treatment effects should be replicated at least once to achieve internal validity. The study of interactions requires that only one variable be changed at a time from phase to phase, such as BC–B or B–BC, so that changes from isolated to combined conditions can be assessed across adjacent phases.

DATA ANALYSIS IN SINGLE-SUBJECT RESEARCH

Data analysis in single-subject research is based on evaluation of measurements within and across design phases, to determine if behaviors are changing and if observed changes during intervention are associated with the onset of treatment. Visual analysis of the graphic display of data is the most commonly used method. Many researchers prefer to use a form of statistical analysis to corroborate visual analysis of time-series data, to determine whether differences between phases are meaningful, or if they could have occurred by chance alone. Several authors have described methods for analyzing these designs.[3,22–24] Statistical analysis provides a more quantitative approach to determine whether observed changes are real or chance occurrences. In this section we examine both approaches and discuss some of the more commonly used methods for analyzing data from single-subject experiments.

Visual Analysis

Visual analysis is used most often to analyze single-subject data because it is intuitively meaningful. In contrast to statistical analysis in group designs, this approach focuses on the clinical significance of outcomes.[25] Data collected in a single-subject experiment can be analyzed in terms of within-phase and between-phase characteristics. Data within a phase are described according to **stability**, or variability, and **trend**, or direction of change. An analysis of changes between phases is used to evaluate the research hypothesis. *Phase comparisons can be made only across adjacent phases.* These comparisons are based on changes in three characteristics of the data: level, trend and slope. Figure 12.11 shows several common data patterns that reflect different combinations of these characteristics.

Level

Changes in **level** refer to the value of the dependent variable, or magnitude of performance, at the point of intervention. It is judged by comparing the value of the target behavior at the last data point of one phase with its value at the first data point of the next adjacent phase. For example, Figures 12.11A and B show a change in level from the baseline to the intervention phase.

Level can also be described in terms of the *mean* or average value of the target behavior within a phase. This value is computed by taking the sum of all data points within a phase and dividing by the number of points. Mean levels can be compared across phases, as a method of summarizing change. For instance, in Figure 12.11A, mean levels for each condition are shown by dotted lines. Means are useful for describing stable data that have no slope, as stable values will tend to cluster around the mean; however, when data are very variable or when they exhibit a sharp slope, means can be misleading. For example, in Figure 12.11C, the dotted lines represent the mean score within each phase. On the basis of these values, one might assume that performance did not change once intervention was introduced. Obviously, this is not the case. Mean values should always be shown on a graph of the raw data to reduce the chance of misinterpretation.

Trend

Trend refers to the direction of change within a phase. Trends can be described as accelerating or decelerating and may be characterized as stable (constant rate of change) or variable. Trends can be linear or curvilinear. Changes in linear trend across phases are displayed in Figures 12.11A and C. In Figure 12.11D, no trend is observed during baseline, and a curvilinear trend is seen in the intervention phase; that is, the data change direction within the intervention phase.

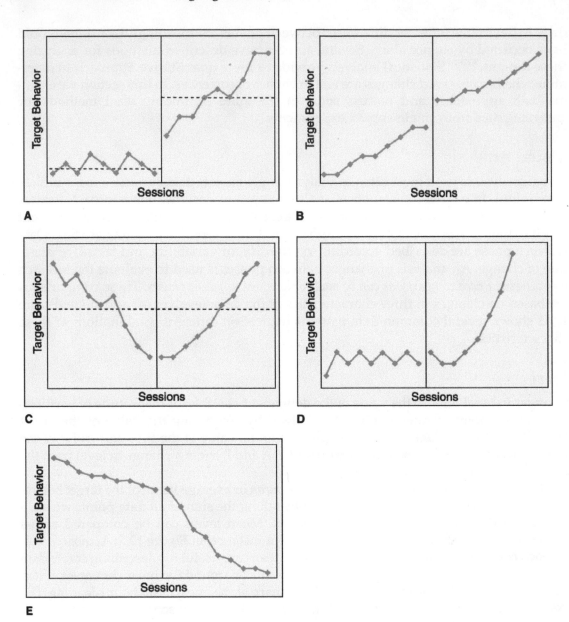

FIGURE 12.11   Examples of data patterns across baseline and intervention phases, showing changes in level and trend: (**A**) change in level and trend (dotted lines represent means for each phase); (**B**) change in level, no change in trend; (**C**) change in trend (dotted lines represent means for each phase); (**D**) change in trend, with a curvilinear pattern during phase *B*; (**E**) no change in level or trend, but a change in slope.

A trend in baseline data does not present a serious problem when it reflects changes in a direction opposite to that expected during intervention. One would then anticipate a distinct change in direction once treatment is initiated; however, it is a problem when the baseline trend follows the direction of change expected during treatment. If the improving trend is continued into the intervention phase, it would be difficult to assess treatment effects, as the target behavior is already improving without treatment. It is important to consider what other factors may be contributing to this improvement. Perhaps changes reflect maturation, a placebo effect or the effect of other treatments. Instituting treatment under these conditions would make it difficult to draw definitive conclusions. When trends occur in the baseline, it is usually advisable to extend the baseline phase, in hopes of achieving a plateau or reversal in the trend, and to try to identify causative factors. Those factors may be useful interventions in their own right and may provide the basis for further study.

The **slope** of a trend refers to its angle, or the rate of change within the data. Slope can only be determined for linear trends. In Figure 12.11B, trends in both phases have approximately the same slope (although their level has changed). In Figure 12.11E, both phases exhibit a decelerating trend; however, the slope within the intervention phase is much steeper than that in the baseline phase. This suggests that the rate of change in the target behavior increased once treatment was initiated.

Data analysis in single-subject research has traditionally focused on visual interpretation of these characteristics. Unfortunately, real data can be sufficiently variable that such subjective determinations are often tenuous and unreliable. For instance, look back at the data in Figure 12.8 for measures of unilateral neglect. Although it is relatively easy to determine that the level of response changed between the baseline and the treatment phase, it would not be so easy to determine the trend or slope in these data based solely on visual judgment.

Although interrater reliability of visual analysis is not necessarily strong,[22,26,27] the reliability of assessing trend is greatly enhanced by drawing a straight line that characterizes rate of change.[28–31] Several procedures can be used. Lines drawn freehand are generally considered unacceptable for research purposes. The most popular method involves drawing a line that represents the linear trend and slope for a data series. This procedure results in a **celeration line**, which describes trends as accelerating or decelerating. Linear regression procedures can be used to draw a *line of best fit*, although this technique is used less often (see Chapter 24).

Celeration Line

A celeration line is used to estimate the trend within a data series. We will demonstrate the steps in drawing a celeration line using the hypothetical data shown in Figure 12.12A. Although we will go through the process for the baseline phase only, in practice a separate celeration line can be computed for each phase in the design. Celeration lines are illustrated in Figures 12.4, 12.6 and 12.8.

The first step is to count the number of data points in the phase and then to divide those points into two equal halves along the X-axis. A vertical line is drawn to separate the two halves, as shown by the dotted line in Figure 12.12B. In this example, there are 10 data points in the baseline phase. Therefore, 5 points fall in each half of the phase. If an odd number of data points were plotted, the line would be drawn directly through the middle point. The second step is to divide these halves in half again, as shown by the broken vertical lines in Figure 12.12C. With 5 data points, the line is drawn through the third point in each half. If there were an even number of data points in each half, the line would be drawn directly between the two middle points.

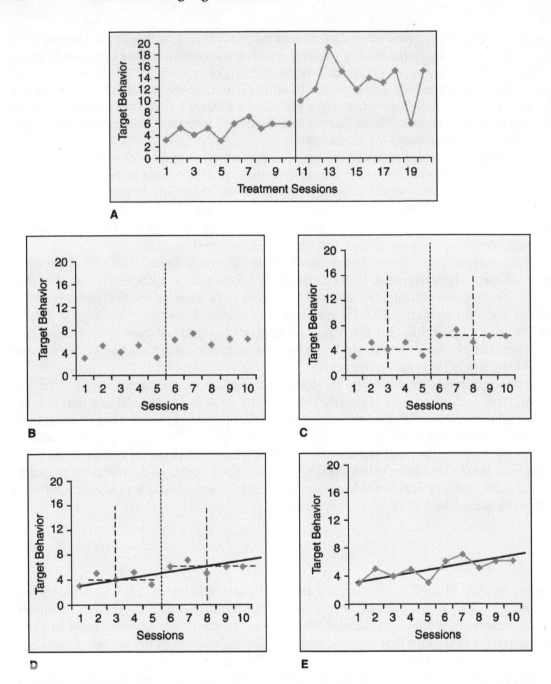

FIGURE 12.12 Computation of the "split-middle line," or celeration line, for baseline data only: (**A**) original data, showing baseline and intervention series; (**B**) baseline points are divided in half along the X-axis; (**C**) baseline points in each half-phase are divided in half again (broken lines); median values for each half-phase are marked with horizontal lines; (**D**) celeration line is drawn; (**E**) celeration line is shown with continuous baseline data.

The next step is to determine the *median score* for each half of the phase (using the halves created by the dotted vertical line). The median score divides the data in half along the Y-axis. This point is obtained by counting from the bottom up toward the top data point within each half phase. The point that divides the series in half vertically is the median score. For instance, in Figure 12.12B, there are 5 data points in the first half of the phase. Therefore, the third score will divide the series in half vertically. If there were an even number of points, the median would be midway between the two middle points. For our example, counting from the bottom up, these scores are 3, 3, 4, 5 and 5. The median score is 4. For the second half of the phase, scores are 5, 6, 6, 6, and 7, with a median of 6. A horizontal line is then drawn through each median point until it intersects the broken line, as shown in Figure 12.12C. Finally, a straight line is drawn connecting the two points of intersection. This is the celeration line, shown in Figure 12.12D.

Calculating Slope

The slope of the celeration line can be calculated to estimate the rate of change in the target behavior. Slope is computed by taking Y values on two points along the celeration line, usually spaced 1 week apart (although any useful time period can be used). The numerically larger value is divided by the smaller value to determine the slope. For example, in Figure 12.12E, the line is at 4 on Day 3 and at 6 on Day 9. Therefore, the slope of the line is 6/4 = 1.50. By looking at the direction of the trend line, we can determine that this target behavior is increasing at an average rate of 1.50 times per week. Slopes can be calculated for each phase in the design, and compared to determine if the rate of change in the target behavior is accelerating or decelerating. The difference between slopes of adjacent phases can be used to provide a numerical estimate of how intervention changes the rate of response.

Split Middle Line

The celeration line demonstrates trend in the data. The line can also be used to represent a measure of central tendency using the split-middle technique. The **split middle line** divides the data within a phase into two equal parts; therefore it represents a median point within the phase. To determine if the celeration line fits this model, the final step is to count the number of points on or above and on or below the line, and then to adjust the celeration line up or down if necessary so that the data are equally divided. The adjusted line must stay parallel to the original line; that is, the slope of the line does not change. In many cases, the line will not have to be adjusted. In Figure 12.12, for example, there are four points below the celeration line, four points above it and two points directly on the line. Therefore, we do not have to make any adjustments.

The split-middle line can be used to compare the trend of data across two adjacent phases.[‡] To illustrate this method, we have taken the split-middle line that was drawn for baseline data in Figure 12.12, and recreated it in Figure 12.13. The line has been

---

[‡]The celeration line can be limited as a means of analysis if the data within a phase are not linear. Ottenbacher recommends using an alternative approach to account for nonlinear trends in data called the *running medians procedure*.[32] This procedure breaks the data within a phase into three segments, so that nonlinear trends can be observed. Refer to Ottenbacher's informative paper for a clear description of this method.

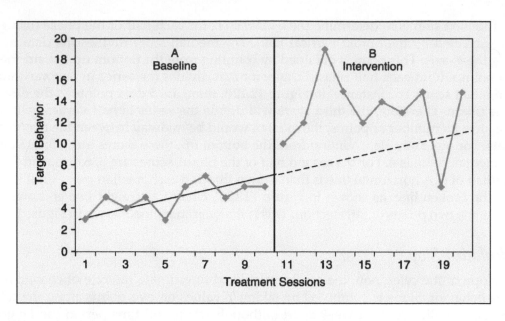

FIGURE 12.13   Celeration line for baseline and intervention phases. The split-middle line for the baseline data is extended into the intervention phase to test the null hypothesis. One point in the intervention phase falls below the line.

extended from the baseline phase into the intervention phase. If there is no difference between the phases, then the split-middle line for baseline data should also be the split-middle line for the intervention phase. Therefore, 50% of the data in the intervention phase should fall on or above that line, and 50% should fall on or below it. If there is a difference, and treatment has caused a real change in observed behavior, then the extended baseline trend should not fit this pattern.

Statistically, we propose a null hypothesis (H_0) which states that there is no difference across phases; that is, any changes observed from baseline to the intervention phase are due to chance, not treatment. We also propose an alternative to H_0, which can be phrased as a nondirectional or directional hypothesis; that is, we can state that we expect a difference between phases (nondirectional) or that responses will increase (or decrease) from baseline (directional). For the example shown in Figure 12.13, let's assume we propose that there will be an increase in response with intervention.

To test H_0, we apply a procedure called the **binomial test**, which is used when outcomes of a test are dichotomous; in this case data points are either above or below the split middle line. To do the test, we count the number of points in the intervention phase that fall above and below the extended line (ignoring points that fall directly on the line). In our example, one point falls below the line and nine points fall above the line. Clearly, this is not a 50–50 split. On the basis of these data, we would like to conclude that the treatment did effect a change in response; however, we must first pose a statistical question: Could this pattern, with one point below and nine points above the line, have occurred by chance? Or can we be confident that this pattern shows a true treatment effect?

We answer this question by referring to Appendix Table A.11, which lists probabilities associated with the binomial test. Two values are needed to use this table. First, we find the appropriate value of *n* (down the side), which is the total number of points in the intervention phase that fall above and below the line (not counting points on the line). In this case, there is a total of 10 points. We then determine if there are *fewer* points above or below the extended line. In our example, there are fewer points (one) below the line. The number of fewer points is given the value *x*; therefore, $x = 1$. The probability associated with $n = 10$ and $x = 1$ is .011, that is, $p = .011$.

The probabilities listed in Table A.11 are *one-tailed probabilities*, which means they are used to evaluate directional alternative hypotheses, as we have proposed in this example. If a nondirectional hypothesis is proposed, a *two-tailed test* is performed, which requires doubling the probabilities listed in the table.

The probability value obtained from the table is interpreted in terms of a conventional upper limit of $p = .05$. Probabilities that exceed this value are considered *not significant*; that is, the observed pattern could have occurred by chance. In this example, the probability associated with the test is less than .05 and, therefore, is considered significant. The pattern of response in the intervention phase is significantly different from baseline. The concept of probability testing and statistical significance is covered in detail in Chapter 18.

Two Standard Deviation Band Method

Another useful method of analysis is the **two standard deviation band method**. This process involves assessing variability within the baseline phase by calculating the mean and standard deviation of data points within that phase (see Chapter 17 for calculation methods for these statistics). Use of the two standard deviation band method is shown in Figures 12.5 and 12.10.

To illustrate this procedure, we have again used the hypothetical data reproduced in Figure 12.14. The solid line represents the mean level of performance for the baseline phase, and the shaded areas above and below this line represent two standard deviations above and below the mean. As shown in the figure, these lines are extended into the intervention phase. If at least two consecutive data points in the intervention phase fall outside the two standard deviation band, changes from baseline to intervention are considered significant. In this example, the mean response for baseline is 5.0, with a standard deviation of 1.33. The shaded areas show two standard deviations above and below the baseline mean (±2.66). Eight consecutive points in the intervention phase fall above this band. Therefore, we would conclude that there was a significant change from the baseline to the intervention phase.

Serial Dependency

It is also possible to use conventional statistical tests, such as the *t*-test and analysis of variance (see Chapters 19 and 20), with time-series data; however, these applications are limited when large numbers of measurements are taken over time. Under these conditions, data points are often interdependent, as is often the case in single-subject research.[32,33] This interdependence is called **serial dependency**, which means that successive observations in a series of data points are related or correlated; that is, knowing the level of performance at one point in time allows the researcher to predict the

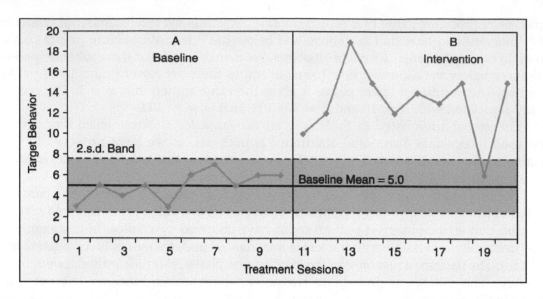

FIGURE 12.14 Two–standard deviation band method, showing mean performance level for baseline (dashed line) and shaded area two standard deviations above and below the mean. Because 8 consecutive points in the intervention phase fall out of this band, the difference between phases is considered significant.

value of subsequent points in the series. Serial dependency can interfere with several statistical procedures, and may also be a problem for making inferences based on visual analysis.[34,35]

The degree of serial dependency is reflected by the **autocorrelation** in the data, or the correlation between data points separated by different intervals, or lags. For example, a lag 1 autocorrelation is computed by pairing the first data point with the second, the second with the third, and so on for the entire series. Using lag 2, the first data point is paired with the third, the second with the fourth, and so on. The higher the value of autocorrelation, the greater the serial dependency in the data. Ottenbacher[3] presents a method for computing autocorrelation by hand, but the process is easily performed by computer, especially with large numbers of data points. For further discussion of this analysis, see the section on time series designs in Chapter 10.

C Statistic

The **C statistic** is a method of estimating trends in time-series data.[36] This statistic can be computed with as few as eight observations in a phase, and is not affected by autocorrelation in the data series.[3]

Calculations begin with baseline data only, to determine if there is a significant trend in Phase A. If there is no significant trend, the baseline and intervention data are combined, and the C statistic is computed again to determine if there is a significant change in trend across both phases. If the baseline data do show a significant trend, the C statistic is less useful.[3]

The process for calculating the *C* statistic is illustrated in Tables 12.1A and 12.1B. In this case, the baseline data do not show a significant trend. The combined data, however, do show a significant trend. Therefore, we conclude that there is a difference in performance from baseline to intervention.

Statistical Process Control

Pfadt and colleagues[37] introduced a unique application of a statistical model to evaluate variability in single-subject data. This model, called **statistical process control (SPC)**, was actually developed in the 1920s at Bell Laboratories as a means of quality control in the manufacturing process.[38] The basis of this process lies in the desire to reduce variation in outcome; that is, in manufacturing, consistency in production is desirable. One can always expect, however, some variation in quality. Cars come off the assembly line with some defects; clothing will have irregularities. A certain amount of variation is random, expected and tolerable. This variation is considered background "noise," or what has been termed **common cause variation**.[23] Statistically, such variation is considered to be "in control"; that is, the variation is predictable.

There will be a point, however, at which the variation will exceed acceptable limits, and the product will no longer be considered satisfactory for sale; that is, such variation identifies problems in production. Such deviation is considered "out of control," and is called **special cause variation**. This is variation that is unexpected, intermittent and not part of the normal process. Consider, for instance, the variation in your own signature. If you sign your name 10 times there will be a certain degree of expected or common cause variation, due to random effects of fatigue, distraction or shift in position. If, however, someone comes by and hits your elbow while you are writing, your signature will look markedly different—a special cause variation. We can think of this variation in the context of reliability. How much variation is random error, and how much is meaningful, due to true changes in response?

Applying SPC to Single-Subject Data

We can apply this model to single-subject designs in two ways. First, by looking at baseline data, we can determine if responses are within the limits of common cause variation (expected variability).[37] This would allow us to assess the degree to which the data represent a reasonable baseline. Sometimes extreme variability within a baseline can obscure treatment effects.[39] We may also find that one point exceeds the limits of common cause, and can be accounted for by special circumstances, thereby discounting the variation as important. For instance, we may find that a patient's responses over the baseline period are consistent except for one day when he did not feel well, or a different clinician took measurements. By analyzing the circumstances of special cause, we can often determine if the response is significant. Consider, for example, the data in Figure 12.5. A steadily decreasing trend is noted during the intervention phase, except for one point on day 9. The concept of special cause obliges the researcher to reflect on possible reasons for this variation.

We can also look at the degree to which intervention responses vary from baseline, with the intent of assigning special cause to the intervention. In other words, we want

TABLE 12.1A   STEPS IN CALCULATION OF THE *C* STATISTIC-BASELINE DATA (DATA FROM FIGURE 12.14)

	Baseline Scores X	Difference Scores[a] ❶ D	Squared Difference Scores D^2	PURPOSE: Test the hypothesis that there is no significant trend across phases. Start by determining if there is a significant trend in baseline data only.
1	3	—	—	
2	5	2	4	❶ Calculate the difference (D) for each adjacent pair of baseline scores ($n_2 - n_1$ and $n_3 - n_2$ and so on). Signs are ignored.
3	4	1	1	
4	5	1	1	
5	3	2	4	
6	6	3	9	
7	7	1	1	❷ Square each of the range scores and calculate the sum of the squared values (ΣD^2).
8	5	2	4	
9	6	1	1	
10	6	0	0	
		❷ $\Sigma D^2 = 25$		

	Baseline Scores X	Baseline Mean $\overline{X}$	Mean Difference Score $(X - \overline{X})$	Squared Mean Difference $(X - \overline{X})^2$	❸ Calculate the mean baseline score
1	3	❸ 5	❹ −2	❺ 4	$\overline{X} = \dfrac{\Sigma X}{n} = \dfrac{50}{10} = 5.0$
2	5	5	0	0	
3	4	5	−1	1	❹ Calculate the difference between each score and the baseline mean $(X - \overline{X})$
4	5	5	0	0	
5	3	5	−2	4	
6	6	5	1	1	❺ Square these values $(X - \overline{X})^2$
7	7	5	2	4	
8	5	5	0	0	❻ Calculate the sum of the squared difference scores, $\Sigma(X - \overline{X})^2$
9	6	5	1	1	
10	6	5	1	1	
	$\Sigma X = 50$		❻ $\Sigma(X - \overline{X})^2 = 16$		

❼ Calculate the C statistic

$$C = 1 - \frac{\Sigma D^2}{2(\Sigma(X - \overline{X})^2)} \qquad C = 1 - \frac{25}{2(16)} = 1 - \frac{25}{32} = 1 - .78 = .22$$

❽ Calculate the standard error (SE) of the baseline scores, based on the number of baseline values

$$SE = \sqrt{\frac{n - 2}{(n - 1)(n + 1)}} = \sqrt{\frac{8}{(9)(11)}} = .284$$

❾ Calculate a z score to determine if the C statistic is significant

$$z = \frac{C}{SE} = \frac{.22}{.284} = 0.77 \qquad \text{If } z \geq 1.645, \text{ there is a significant trend in baseline (one-tailed).}$$

CONCLUSION: Because $z < 1.645$, there is no significant trend in baseline scores.

[a]There will be one fewer difference scores than baseline scores.

TABLE 12.1B   CALCULATION OF THE *C* STATISTIC-BASELINE AND INTERVENTION DATA COMBINED (DATA FROM FIGURE 12.14)

	Baseline and Intervention Scores X	Difference Scores D	Squared Difference Scores D^2	Mean $\bar{X}$	Mean Difference Score $(X - \bar{X})$	Squared Mean Difference $(X - \bar{X})^2$
1	3	—	—	9.2	6.2	38.44
2	5	2	4	9.2	4.2	17.64
3	4	1	1	9.2	5.2	27.04
4	5	1	1	9.2	4.2	17.64
5	3	2	4	9.2	6.2	38.44
6	6	3	9	9.2	3.2	10.24
7	7	1	1	9.2	2.2	4.84
8	5	2	4	9.2	4.2	17.64
9	6	1	1	9.2	3.2	10.24
10	6	0	0	9.2	3.2	10.24
11	10	4	16	9.2	-0.8	0.64
12	12	2	4	9.2	-2.8	7.84
13	19	7	49	9.2	-9.8	96.04
14	15	4	16	9.2	-5.8	33.64
15	12	3	9	9.2	-2.8	7.84
16	14	2	4	9.2	-4.8	23.04
17	13	1	1	9.2	-3.8	14.44
18	15	2	4	9.2	-5.8	33.64
19	9	6	36	9.2	0.2	0.04
20	15	6	36	9.2	-5.8	33.64
	$\Sigma X = 184$		$\Sigma D^2 = 200$			$\Sigma(X - \bar{X})^2 = 443.20$

Calculate the *C* statistic

$$C = 1 - \frac{\Sigma D^2}{2(\Sigma(X - \bar{X})^2)}$$

$$C = 1 - \frac{200}{2(443.20)} = 1 - \frac{200}{886.40} = 1 - .23 = .77$$

Calculate the standard error (SE) based on the total number of scores

$$SE = \sqrt{\frac{n-2}{(n-1)(n+1)}} = \sqrt{\frac{18}{(19)(21)}} = .212$$

Calculate a *z* score to determine if the *C* statistic is significant

$$z = \frac{C}{SE} = \frac{.77}{.212} = 3.63 \quad \text{If } z \geq 1.645, \text{ there is a significant trend (one-tailed).}$$

CONCLUSION: There is a significant trend from baseline to intervention.

the treatment to cause a meaningful change in the subject's response. Statistical process control offers a mechanism to determine if variations in response are of sufficient magnitude to warrant interpretation as special cause.[23]

Upper and Lower Control Limits

Statistical process control is based on analysis of graphs called control charts. These are the same as the graphs we have been using to show the results of single-subject data, although some differences exist depending on the type of data being measured. The "X-moving range chart" (X-mR)[§] is used with continuous variables, and will be used most often with single-subject data. Other charts should be used when data are binary outcomes or counts.[24] Statistical process control charts can be drawn using SPSS® software under the Graph function.

In SPC, the interpretation of data is based on variability around a mean value. A central line is plotted, representing the mean response for the phase. An **upper control limit (UCL)** and **lower control limit (LCL)** are then plotted at 3 standard deviations above and below the mean.[**] Regardless of the underlying distribution, almost all data will fall within ±3 sd from the mean if the data are stable; that is, if the process is in statistical control.[40] Therefore, these boundaries define the threshold for special cause.[††]

Although there is some variability in defining the criteria for special cause, the most common set of rules is:[23,39,40]

1. Any one point that falls outside the upper or lower control limits (see Figure 12.15A).
2. Seven or more consecutive points all above or all below the center mean line, called a "run" (see Figure 12.15B).
3. Six or more consecutive points moving up or down across the center mean line, called a "trend" (see Figure 12.15C).

Consider once again the hypothetical data in Figure 12.16. Calculation of the UCL and LCL values are shown in Table 12.2. The baseline data all fall within the upper and lower control limits, demonstrating common cause or chance variation. This is what we would hope to see in a stable baseline. We then extend the control limits into the intervention phase to determine if special cause is present once we have initiated treatment. We can see that 9 points fall outside the UCL, indicating that there is a significant difference in the response during the intervention phase.

[§]The moving range is analogous to the difference score used to calculate the C statistic. The difference between each pair of adjacent scores is calculated. The mean of the moving range scores is used to determine the standard deviation to determine the upper and lower control limits (see Table 12.2).

[**]A 3–standard deviation band around the mean theoretically represents 99.74% of all the data around that mean. Note that the standard deviation used for this model is not the same as the standard deviation typically calculated for a distribution of scores (as illustrated in Chapter 17). See Table 12.2 for calculations.

[††]The upper and lower control limits set boundaries that are analogous to the level of significance in standard statistical testing. Using a band of 2 standard deviations, the limit of Type I error is held to less than 5%, which fits conventional significance tests. With a time series design, however, each plotted point is a basis of comparison, and therefore each one contributes to the overall probability of Type I error.[40] To control for this potential inflation the 3–standard deviation band is used, keeping the potential for Type I error at 0.26%. For additional discussion of Type I error, see Chapters 18 and 21.

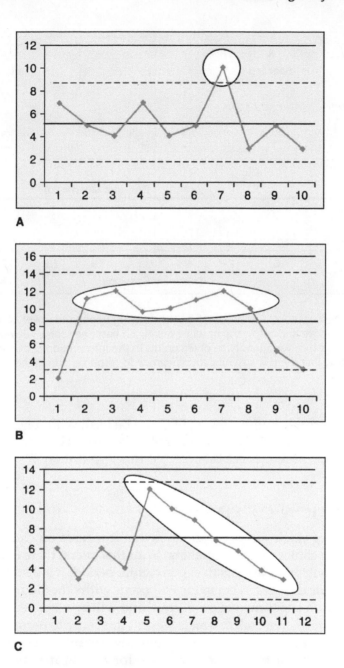

FIGURE 12.15 Illustration of criteria for special cause in a statistical process control chart: **(A)** Any one point that falls outside the upper or lower control limits; **(B)** Seven or more consecutive points all above or below the center mean line; **(C)** Six or more consecutive points moving up or down across the center mean line. Broken lines represent upper and lower control limits.

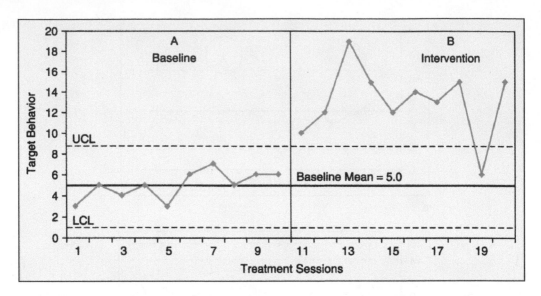

FIGURE 12.16   Statistical control chart (X-mR chart) showing upper and lower control limits based on 3 standard deviations above and below the baseline mean. All baseline scores fall within the control limits, indicating common cause variation. Nine of ten points in the intervention phase fall outside the upper control limit, indicating that there is a significant difference in response during the intervention phase.

As a process for total quality control, SPC can be used within healthcare settings to monitor variation in service delivery and health outcomes. The reader is encouraged to consult several excellent references that discuss this application.[40–44]

GENERALIZATION OF FINDINGS

The special appeal of single-subject research is that it focuses on clinical outcomes and can provide data for clinical decision making. With this intent, then, it is not sufficient to demonstrate these outcomes during an experimental period. It is also necessary to show that improvements or changes in behavior will occur with other individuals under conditions that differ from experimental conditions, and will be sustained after the intervention has ended. The term **generalization** is used in this sense to represent a limited form of external validity for the single case. Although significant effects on a single patient provide no "proof" that a treatment will work for others, it is not unreasonable to assume that the treatment will work for other patients with similar characteristics.

The important contribution of single-subject research is that the specific characteristics of the treatment and the circumstances in which the treatment is successful can be delineated, so that this assumption can be tested. Clinicians can begin to ask questions about which specific patient traits are relevant. In addition, visual inspection of individual performance allows the researcher to observe clinically strong effects that would not necessarily have been statistically significant (and would therefore have been ignored). Therefore, results from single case designs may actually provide more "real world" insight and understanding of individual responses than data from group studies.

TABLE 12.2   CALCULATION OF CONTROL LIMITS FOR THE X-MOVING RANGE CHART (X-Mr) FOR DATA IN FIGURE 12.14.

	Baseline Score X	❷ Moving Range Score R
1	3	—
2	5	2
3	4	1
4	5	1
5	3	2
6	6	3
7	7	1
8	5	2
9	6	1
10	6	0

❶ $\Sigma X = 50$ ❸ $\Sigma R^2 = 13$

❶ Compute the mean baseline score, $\overline{X}$

$$\overline{X} = \frac{\Sigma X}{n} = \frac{50}{10} = 5.0$$

❷ Compute the moving range (R) of each two adjacent data points.[a] Signs are ignored.

❸ Compute the mean moving range, $\overline{R}$

$$\overline{R} = \frac{\Sigma R^2}{n-1} = \frac{13}{9} = 1.44$$

❹ Compute the standard deviation of the moving range, s[b]

$$s = \frac{\overline{R}}{1.128} = \frac{1.44}{1.128} = 1.28$$

❺ Calculate the upper and lower control limits for baseline scores

$$\textbf{UCL} = \overline{X} + 3s = 5.0 + 3(1.28) = 8.84$$

$$\textbf{LCL} = \overline{X} - 3s = 5.0 - 3(1.28) = 1.16$$

[a]There will be one fewer R values than data points. This is the same process as described for the difference scores (D) in Table 12.1A.

[b]The denominator for calculation of the standard deviation based on the moving range is a constant, 1.128.[24]

Direct Replication

To demonstrate external validity, it is necessary to replicate the results of single-subject experiments across several subjects or by repeating the study on the same subject. This is called **direct replication.** The setting, treatment conditions, and patient characteristics should be kept as constant as possible. External validity becomes stronger as results accumulate across subjects, establishing what types of patients respond favorably to the treatment. One successful single-subject experiment and three successful replications are considered sufficient to demonstrate that findings are not a result of chance.[45,46] Multiple baseline designs provide direct replication.

Systematic Replication

Systematic replication is used to demonstrate that findings can be observed under conditions different from those encountered in the initial experiment. Systematic replication should occur after generalization across subjects has been established through direct replication. The purpose of systematic replication is to define the conditions under which the intervention will be successful or fail. It is, in essence, a search for exceptions.[45] It involves the variation of one or two variables from the original study in an attempt to generalize to other similar, but not identical, situations. For instance, the target behavior can be monitored in different settings than the original study; different clinicians, support personnel, or family members can perform the intervention; the treatment may be given at different times of day; or different types of equipment may be used. The continued success of intervention under these changed conditions provides strong evidence supporting application of the treatment under clinical conditions that typically cannot incorporate experimental controls.

For example, in a study of children who suffered from asthma, the children were tested for their ability to use inhalation equipment.[47] They were given specific rewards for proper use of the equipment within special training sessions, and demonstrated successful learning. It was then of interest to establish that the children could maintain their performance when they were actually exhibiting asthmatic symptoms. To evaluate this generalization, the investigators told the children that the "intervention," the reward strategies, would continue if they used the equipment properly whenever it was really needed. Follow-up data, provided by the nursing staff, supported the generalization of the target behavior to actual treatment situations.

We can also incorporate a *follow-up* or *maintenance* phase in a single-subject design, which involves monitoring the target behavior after the intervention is stopped, often weeks or months later. For example, in a study of naming deficits in patients with aphasia, accuracy was assessed at baseline, during intervention, and again at 6 and 10 weeks following completion of the study.[48] These single measures can be shown on the graphs, indicating the level of retention. Follow-up is important when the intent of treatment is to effect a permanent change in behavior.

Clinical Replication

Although we have attempted to define the process of single-subject research using a clinical model, in reality the fit is less than perfect. Treatment plans are not developed around isolated patient problems, nor are they based on partitioned treatment components. In the long run, then, the true applicability of research data will depend on our ability to demonstrate that treatment packages can be successfully applied to patients with multiple behaviors that tend to cluster together. Barlow and Hersen[45] have called this process **clinical replication**. Such a procedure may be considered field testing; that is, clinical replication becomes one with actual practice.

Clinical replication is an advanced replication procedure, which can occur only after direct replication and systematic replication have supplied the researcher with well defined relationships between treatment components and patient characteristics. After testing these relationships one at a time, the researcher can begin to build clinical strategies by combining and recombining successful treatments for coexisting problems. For example, consider the multitude of problems inherent in disorders such as stroke, cerebral palsy, autism, and low back dysfunction. Many of the "treatments" that are used to address these problems incorporate a variety of techniques, with expected overlapping and combined effects. In fact, these treatment programs are not always successful. A comprehensive process of clinical replication is really the only way to establish the conditions under which we can expect positive results.

Social Validation

Beyond the question of external validity, which concerns generalization of findings to different subjects and settings, behavioral analysts are also interested in the importance of treatment effects within a social context. **Social validity** is based on the significance of the goals of interventions, the acceptability of procedures by target groups, and the importance of the treatment's effect.[49] These determinations may be made by patients, families or caregivers, or they may be applied within a broader framework by epidemiologists and clinicians.[50] Social validity is considered important especially with regard to behavior change strategies, to assure that interventions will be appreciated and adopted.

This is a practical issue, based on whether interventions are satisfactory and perceived as useful. Procedures that are intrusive or impractical are less likely to be used, and therefore, less important to study. For example, researchers used a single-subject withdrawal design to study the effect of using therapy balls as seating for young children with autism spectrum disorder on their classroom behavior.[51] The study showed improved behavior, and at the completion of the study, surveys of teachers, staff and parents working with participants showed that they were satisfied with the results and wanted to use the balls for classroom and home seating.

Although social validation is not required for establishing treatment effectiveness, it has always been recognized as an important element of treatment planning and decision making. It serves a valuable function in the interpretation of clinical research findings as evidence for practice. Measures of social validation should be encouraged as a critical link between single-subject research and the treatment planning process.

COMMENTARY

Documenting Wisely

The maturation of single-subject research methodology has been an important step in the development of clinical research. It provides an opportunity for the practitioner to evaluate treatment procedures within the context of clinical care, and to share insights about patient behavior and response that are typically ignored or indiscernible using traditional research approaches. The single-subject design offers a logical method for judging clinical significance of data.[52] The process of single-subject research should eventually diminish the role of trial and error in clinical practice and provide useful guidelines for making clinical choices. The underlying message in all of this is that the clinician, working in the practice setting, is uniquely qualified to perform these studies. This is especially true in terms of the importance of clinical replication.

Statistical procedures can be a useful adjunct to visual analysis for interpreting the results of single-subject experiments, although there is no agreement on one appropriate method for all studies. This is especially true in situations where data variability makes subjective assessments of change difficult and inconsistent.

Because many analysis procedures are available, clinical researchers must be able to decide what type of documentation is appropriate for a particular study. This decision must be based on the nature of the target behavior, the expected direction of change, variability in the data, the extent of treatment effects, and the way clinical outcomes will be interpreted. Using more than one method within a study is often advisable to determine the degree of consistency in findings.

Of course, single-subject designs are not a panacea for all clinical research woes. Many research questions cannot be answered adequately using these designs. Single-subject designs can be limited in that they require time to document outcomes. They are not readily applicable to acute situations where baseline periods are less reasonable and treatment does not continue for long periods. In addition, researchers often find that patient responses are too unstable, making attempts at analysis very frustrating. Nonetheless, single-subject designs serve a distinct purpose in the ongoing search for scientific documentation of therapeutic effectiveness. They offer a practical methodology for exploring cause-and-effect relationships in clinical phenomena and for sorting out the effects of individual patient characteristics on treatment outcomes.

These designs are flexible enough to provide opportunities for examining the relationships among impairments, activity limitations and disability measures. As the emphasis on evidence-based practice continues in rehabilitation research, the single-subject strategy provides a unique opportunity to explore these relationships and to ask questions about those factors that may impact individual patients. Group designs will often hide these factors or cancel their effect, giving us no information with which to critically examine the differences among our patients. Because of the emphasis on visual presentation and continuous description of responses over time, single-subject experiments can be the source of empirical hypotheses that lead to new avenues of study and to the discovery of clinical implications that would not otherwise be seen or shared. This process will force us to challenge clinical theories and to document the benefits of our interventions in a convincing scientific way, for ourselves and for others. Pooled results from several individual single subject trials could extend the conclusions beyond the individual patient, and help to characterize a subset of responders to a specific treatment or clarify the heterogeneity of the disease.[53]

REFERENCES

1. Kalinowski J, Armson J, Stuart A. Effect of normal and fast articulatory rates on stuttering frequency. *Fluency Disorders* 1995;20:293–302.
2. Ingham RJ. Valid distinctions between findings obtained from single-subject and group studies of stuttering: some reflections on Kalinowski et al. (1995). *Fluency Disorders* 1997;22:51–56.
3. Ottenbacher KJ. *Evaluating Clinical Change: Strategies for Occupational and Physical Therapists*. Baltimore: Williams & Wilkins, 1986.
4. Hasson S. Guest editorial: Making a case for single case research. *J Orthop Sports Phys Ther* 1996;24:1–3.

5. Hayes SC. Single case experimental design and empirical clinical practice. *J Consult Clin Psychol* 1981;49:193–211.
6. Cook TD, Campbell DT. *Quasi-experimentation: Design and Analysis Issues for Field Settings.* Boston: Houghton Mifflin, 1979.
7. Wheeler DJ. *Understanding Variation: The Key to Managing Chaos* (2nd ed.). Knoxville, TN: SPC Press, 2000.
8. Dave CA. Effects of linear vestibular stimulation on body-rocking behavior in adults with profound mental retardation. *Am J Occup Ther* 1992;46:910–915.
9. Shumway-Cook A, Hutchinson S, Kartin D, Price R, Woollacott M. Effect of balance training on recovery of stability in children with cerebral palsy. *Dev Med Child Neurol* 2003;45:591–602.
10. Bastille JV, Gill-Body KM. A yoga-based exercise program for people with chronic post-stroke hemiparesis. *Phys Ther* 2004;84:33–48.
11. Ayres AJ, Mailloux Z. Influence of sensory integration procedures on language development. *Am J Occup Ther* 1981;35:383–390.
12. Sidaway B, Anderson J, Danielson G, Martin L, Smith G. Effects of long-term gait training using visual cues in an individual with Parkinson disease. *Phys Ther* 2006;86: 186–194.
13. Cleland J, Palmer J. Effectiveness of manual physical therapy, therapeutic exercise, and patient education on bilateral disc displacement without reduction of the temporo-mandibular joint: a single-case design. *J Orthop Sports Phys Ther* 2004;34:535–548.
14. Wu S, Huang H, Lin C, Chen M. Effects of a program on symmetrical posture in patients with hemiplegia: A single-subject design. *Am J Occup Ther* 1996;50:17–23.
15. Warren SF, Yoder PJ, Gazdag GE, et al. Facilitating prelinguistic communication skills in young children with developmental delay. *J Speech Hearing Res* 1993; 36:83–97.
16. Trahan J, Malouin F. Intermittent intensive physiotherapy in children with cerebral palsy: A pilot study. *Dev Med Child Neurol* 2002;44:233–239.
17. Hetzroni OE, Tannous J. Effects of a computer-based intervention program on the communicative functions of children with autism. *J Autism Dev Disord* 2004;34:95–113.
18. Watson PJ, Workman EA. The non-concurrent multiple, baseline across-individuals design: An extension of the traditional multiple baseline design. *J Behav Ther Exper Psychiat* 1981;12:257–259.
19. Bailey MJ, Riddoch MJ, Crome P. Treatment of visual neglect in elderly patients with stroke: A single-subject series using either a scanning and cueing strategy or a left-limb activation strategy. *Phys Ther* 2002;82:782–797.
20. Yoo E, Chung B. The effect of visual feedback plus mental practice on symmetrical weight-bearing training in people with hemiparesis. *Clin Rehabil* 2006;20:388–397.
21. Clopton N, Schultz D, Boren C, Porter J, Brillhart T. Effects of axial weight loading on gait for subjects with cerebellar ataxia: Preliminary findings. *Neurology Report* 2003;27: 15–21.
22. Nourbakhsh MR, Ottenbacher KJ. The statistical analysis of single-subject data: A comparative examination. *Phys Ther* 1994;74:768–776.
23. Callahan CD, Barisa MT. Statistical process control and rehabilitation outcome: The single-subject design reconsidered. *Rehabil Psychol* 2005;50:24–33.
24. Orme JG, Cox ME. Analyzing single-subject design data using statistical process control charts. *Soc Work Res* 2001;25:115–127.
25. Kearns KP. Back to the future with single-subject experimental designs in aphasia treatment research. *Neurophysiology and Neurogenic Speech and Language Disorders. ASHA Special Interest Division 2* 2005;15:14–22.

26. Ottenbacher KJ. Reliability and accuracy of visually analyzing graphed data from single-subject designs. *Am J Occup Ther* 1986;40:464–469.
27. Harbst KB, Ottenbacher KJ, Harris SR. Interrater reliability of therapists' judgements of graphed data. *Phys Ther* 1991;71:107–115.
28. Bobrovitz CD, Ottenbacher KJ. Comparison of visual inspection and statistical analysis of single-subject data in rehabilitation research. *Am J Phys Med Rehabil* 1998;77:94–102.
29. Hojem MA, Ottenbacher KJ. Empirical investigation of visual-inspection versus trend-line analysis of single-subject data. *Phys Ther* 1988;68:983–988.
30. Johnson MB, Ottenbacher KJ. Trend line influence on visual analysis of single-subject data in rehabilitation research. *Int Disabil Stud* 1991;13:55–59.
31. Ottenbacher K. Interrater agreement of visual analysis in single-subject decisions: Quantitative review and analysis. *Am J Ment Retard* 1993;98:135–142.
32. Ottenbacher KJ. Analysis of data in idiographic research. *Am J Phys Med Rehabil* 1992;71:202–208.
33. Jones RR, Baught RS, Weinrott MR. Time-series analysis in operant research. *J Appl Behav Anal* 1977;10:151.
34. Jones RR, Weinrott MR, Vaught RS. Effects of serial dependency on the agreement between visual and statistical inference. *J Appl Behav Anal* 1978;11:277–283.
35. Bengali MK, Ottenbacher KJ. The effect of autocorrelation on the results of visually analyzing data from single-subject designs. *Am J Occup Ther* 1998;52:650–655.
36. Tryon WW. A simplified time-series analysis for evaluating treatment interventions. *J Appl Behav Anal* 1982;15:423–429.
37. Pfadt A, Cohen IL, Sudhalter V, Romanczyk RG, Wheeler DJ. Applying statistical process control to clinical data: An illustration. *J Appl Behav Anal* 1992;25:551–560.
38. Berwick DM. Controlling variation in health care: A consultation from Walter Shewhart. *Med Care* 1991;29:1212–1225.
39. Pfadt A, Wheeler DJ. Using statistical process control to make data-based clinical decisions. *J Appl Behav Anal* 1995;28:349–370.
40. Benneyan JC, Lloyd RC, Plsek PE. Statistical process control as a tool for research and healthcare improvement. *Qual Saf Health Care* 2003;12:458–464.
41. Hantula DA. Disciplined decision making in an interdisciplinary environment: Some implications for clinical applications of statistical process control. *J Appl Behav Anal* 1995;28:371–377.
42. Solodky C, Chen H, Jones PK, Katcher W, Neuhauser D. Patients as partners in clinical research: A proposal for applying quality improvement methods to patient care. *Med Care* 1998;36:AS13–20.
43. Diaz M, Neuhauser D. Pasteur and parachutes: When statistical process control is better than a randomized controlled trial. *Qual Saf Health Care* 2005;14:140–143.
44. Mohammed MA. Using statistical process control to improve the quality of health care. *Qual Saf Health Care* 2004;13:243–245.
45. Barlow DH, Hersen M. *Single Case Experimental Designs: Strategies for Studying Behavior Change* (2nd ed.). New York: Pergamon Press, 1984.
46. Chambless DL, Hollon SD. Defining empirically supported therapies. *J Consult Clin Psychol* 1998;66:7–18.
47. Renne CM, Creer TL. Training children with asthma to use inhalation therapy equipment. *J Appl Behav Anal* 1976;9:1–11.
48. Kiran S, Thompson CK. The role of semantic complexity in treatment of naming deficits: Training semantic categories in fluent aphasia by controlling exemplar typicality. *J Speech Lang Hear Res* 2003;46:773–787.

49. Wolf MM. Social validity: The case for subjective measurement or how applied behavior analysis is finding its heart. *J Appl Behav Anal* 1978;11:203–214.
50. Winett RA, Moore JF, Anderson ES. Extending the concept of social validity: Behavior analysis for disease prevention and health promotion. *J Appl Behav Anal* 1991;24: 215–230.
51. Schilling DL, Schwartz IS. Alternative seating for young children with Autism Spectrum Disorder: Effects on classroom behavior. *J Autism Dev Disord* 2004;34:423–432.
52. da Prato R. Large-group fantasies versus single-subject science. *Topics in Early Childhood Special Education* 1992;12:54–62.
53. Madsen LG, Bytzer P. Review article: Single subject trials as a research instrument in gastrointestinal pharmacology. *Aliment Pharmacol Ther* 2002;16:189–196.

CHAPTER 13
Exploratory Research: Observational Designs

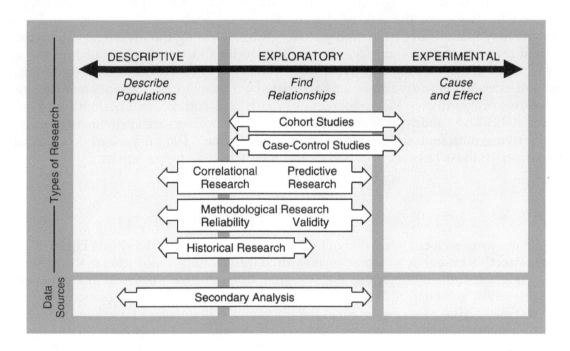

The complexity of human behavior and clinical phenomena present a considerable challenge to the clinician and researcher. In many situations, the impetus for a research study is the need to understand how human attributes and environmental characteristics interact to control behavioral responses. As clinical scientists continue to question how we can achieve optimal outcomes under defined clinical conditions, we must examine the multiple factors that influence our patients' and clients' lives. Studies that help us gather this information are considered **observational** because data are collected as they naturally exist, rather than through manipulation of variables as in experiments. Observational studies may be considered descriptive or exploratory. Descriptive studies will be described in the next chapter.

Exploratory research is the systematic investigation of relationships among two or more variables. Researchers use this approach to predict the effect of one variable on another, or to test relationships that are supported by clinical theory. Diagnostic and prognostic factors are identified through exploration of their relationships with the results of specific tests and patient outcomes. This type of research is usually guided by a set of hypotheses that help to structure measurements and interpretation of findings. For example, researchers have used this approach to study the relationship between long-term medical conditions and depression,[1] and to demonstrate the association of decreased muscle mass and strength with loss of mobility and function in older men and women.[2] Miles and colleagues[3] used a predictive model to identify outcomes and risks associated with different subgroups of autism, to assist with prognostication and counseling.

Observational studies may involve prospective data collection or retrospective analysis of existing data, and may be designed using longitudinal or cross-sectional methods. Correlational methods are generally used to develop predictive models, which may be used for diagnostic or prognostic purposes. Observational studies may be used to determine the risk of disease associated with specific exposures. Such designs may include an explicit comparison group, allowing the investigator to determine if the rate of disease or disability is different for those exposed or unexposed to the factor of interest. Case-control and cohort studies are observational analytic designs that are intended to study risk factors associated with disease or disability and specific exposures or conditions. Methodological research uses correlational methods to focus on reliability and validity of measurement tools. Historical research provides an opportunity to use data from the past to analyze current issues. The purpose of this chapter is to describe these research approaches and their various configurations.

RETROSPECTIVE AND PROSPECTIVE RESEARCH

Exploratory research can be carried out retrospectively or prospectively (see Figure 13.1). In **prospective research** variables are measured through direct recording in the present. The researcher follows subjects as they progress through their treatment or evaluation. The researcher is thereby able to identify the factors that precede given outcomes.

Retrospective research involves the examination of data that have been collected in the past, often obtained from medical records, databases or surveys. With retrospective studies the researcher does not have direct control of the variables under study because they have occurred in the past or they represent attribute variables that cannot be manipulated. The researcher cannot control operational definitions of variables or the reliability or completeness with which data were collected. Therefore, the accuracy and credibility of the data source are important considerations. Retrospective data, however, represent an important source of information because many research questions can only be answered using data that have already been collected.

As an example, Sellers and co-workers[4] were interested in developing criteria to predict prolonged ventilator dependence in patients who have experienced severe burns. They reviewed medical records of patients who had been admitted over a 4-year period who required ventilator support, and successfully documented a series of objective factors that were effective predictors.

Prospective studies are more reliable than retrospective studies because of the potential for greater control of data collection methods and the ability to document a temporal sequence of events.

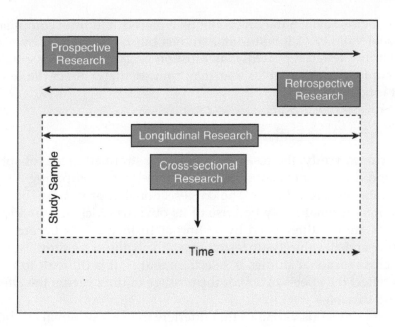

FIGURE 13.1 Graphic representation of the direction of inquiry for prospective and retrospective designs, and the relationship between longitudinal and cross-sectional research.

LONGITUDINAL AND CROSS-SECTIONAL RESEARCH

Longitudinal Research

In a **longitudinal study** the researcher follows a cohort of subjects over time, performing repeated measurements at prescribed intervals (see Figure 13.1). The advantage of the longitudinal method is its ability to accumulate data through intensive documentation of growth and change on the same individuals. Longitudinal data are collected in a time sequence that allows for documentation of the direction as well as the magnitude of change over time. This lets the researcher describe patterns of change and suggest causal relationships between variables.[5] Some researchers argue that longitudinal designs must be prospective,[6] although others assert a broader view that both prospective and retrospective methodologies can be incorporated into longitudinal research.[5]

Many longitudinal studies involve large databases that follow a cohort of subjects over an extended period. These include ongoing surveys such as those under the aegis of the National Center for Health Statistics,[7] including the National Health Interview Survey,[8] the National Survey of Early Childhood Health,[9] and the National Health and Nutrition Examination Survey.[10] Other examples of longitudinal databases include the Nurses Health Study,[11] the National Spinal Cord Injury Database,[12,13] and the Medicare Current Beneficiary Survey.[14,15] One of the most famous longitudinal studies is the continuing Framingham Heart Study, begun in 1948, now crossing two generations.[16] These surveys represent decades of data that have been used in the study of disease, physical function and health care.

Researchers using a longitudinal approach face many practical difficulties, most notably the extended obligation to a single project, requiring long-term commitment of funds and resources. Once a longitudinal study is begun, changes can jeopardize the validity of all previous data. Subjects cannot be replaced, and their compliance must be ensured. Internal validity of longitudinal studies can be threatened by testing effects because subjects are tested repeatedly, by attrition because of the long data collection time, and by confounding variables that may coincidentally affect the developmental sequence that is being evaluated.

Cross-Sectional Research

In a **cross-sectional study**, the researcher studies a stratified group of subjects at one point in time and draws conclusions about a population by comparing the characteristics of those strata (see Figure 13.1). The cross-sectional approach has been used more often than the longitudinal study because of its obvious efficiency. In addition, cross-sectional studies are not threatened by testing or history effects because subjects are tested only once, and all subjects are tested at relatively the same time. The major threat to validity in cross-sectional studies is selection; that is, it is difficult to know to what extent results reflect the effects of age or the passage of time versus the effects of extraneous sampling variables.

Many of the extraneous variables that interfere in cross-sectional studies pertain to **cohort effects**, that is, effects that are not age specific but are due to a subject's generation or time of birth. Subjects can differ in quality, style or duration of education, exposure to information about health, or historical events that influenced life choices and practices. For example, suppose we were interested in studying the development of cardiovascular risk factors using a cross-sectional approach. We include present-day elders who were born at the beginning of the 20th century, adults who were born after World War II, and younger subjects born after 1960. We might observe significant variation in health variables across these three age groups; however, based on this evidence alone we cannot conclude that these factors normally change with age. The differences may have some age-related basis, but it is also likely that life experiences play an important role. For instance, the elders did not have the benefits of growing up in a world of improved medical technology and media campaigns about physical fitness and diet. Therefore, conclusions about age effects may be threatened by the extraneous effects of cohort differences

CORRELATION AND PREDICTION

The foundation of exploratory study is the process of **correlation**, a measure of the degree of association among variables. Correlation is a function of *covariation* in data, that is, the extent to which one variable varies directly or indirectly with another variable. We measure the strength of this relationship using a correlation statistic. The reader is referred to Chapters 23, 24 and 29 for descriptions of specific correlation methods.

In exploratory studies, researchers do not attempt to control or manipulate the variables under study, only to measure how they vary with respect to each other. Therefore, exploratory studies are not used to test differences between groups or to establish the presence of cause-and-effect relationships between independent and dependent variables. This is an important distinction when interpreting correlational outcomes. There may appear to be a strong correlation between two variables, X and Y, because there is actually some third variable, Z, that causes both X and Y. For instance, we might find that the inability to climb stairs is correlated with poor knee strength in patients with osteoarthritis; however, the cause of the functional limitation may actually be knee pain, which is also related to measurable weakness in knee muscles. Exploratory research will often provide evidence of a relationship that can then be tested using experimental techniques to determine if one variable can be considered the cause of the other.

Correlational and Predictive Studies

The purpose of a **correlational study** is to describe the nature of existing relationships among variables. Data from this type of study often provide the rationale for clinical decisions or the generation of hypotheses. Researchers will often look at several variables at once to determine which ones are related. For instance, in a prospective study, Higgins[17] examined the perception of fatigue in chronically ill patients who were undergoing long-term mechanical ventilation. She examined the effect of nutritional status, depression and sleep on fatigue, and found a strong relationship only between fatigue and depression. This relationship can be used to foster appropriate interventions for this population.

A **predictive correlational study** is designed to predict a behavior or response based on the observed relationship between that behavior and other variables. Predictive designs can be used to develop models that can serve as a basis for clinical decision making, to understand factors that impact the success of interventions. This approach is especially useful for validation of diagnostic and prognostic information. A statistical technique called **regression** is used to establish the accuracy of prediction (see Chapters 24 and 29).

Predictive studies are also often used in the process of diagnosis for validation of a measurement tool. For instance, Rutledge et al[18] identified problems in using the Glasgow Coma Scale (GCS) in intubated patients, because the scale requires verbal responses that are blocked by intubation. The purpose of their study, therefore, was to develop a basis for predicting the verbal score using only the motor and eye responses of the scale. The authors designed a prospective study to assess patients in an intensive care unit who could provide verbal responses. They used a multiple regression procedure to determine if the motor and eye variables were strong predictors of the verbal score, resulting in the following regression equation:

$$\text{Verbal score} = 2.3976 + (0.9253 \times \text{GCS motor}) + (-0.9214 \times \text{GCS eye})$$

$$+ (0.2208 \times \text{GSCmotor}^2) + (0.2318 \times \text{GSC eye}^2)$$

To evaluate this equation, we could take a single patient's eye and motor responses and, by substituting them in the equation, predict the expected verbal score. The predicted value will not be totally accurate; that is, there is likely to be some degree of error in the equation. We can look at the actual verbal score for that patient and determine the difference between the observed and expected values. A strong model will demonstrate little discrepancy between these values. In this study, the accuracy of the model was extremely high, predicting 83% of the variance in the verbal score. The ultimate purpose of developing the model is to extend its use to a different set of subjects. Therefore, the model must be cross-validated by testing it on different groups. For example,

Meredith et al[19] tested this equation using a retrospective sample of over 14,000 patients taken from a trauma registry by comparing their predicted and actual GCS scores. Their findings supported the predictive validity of the model, confirming the ability to determine an accurate GCS score in the absence of a verbal component. Based on these findings, the equation could be used with some confidence with patients who are intubated to predict their verbal score.

Prediction has become an important research goal in outcomes research as well, with a focus on determining those factors that contribute to or detract from successful clinical outcomes. As an example, Saposnik et al[20] studied factors that were related to the degree of improvement within 24 hours following acute stroke in patients who received thrombolytic therapy. They found that elevated glucose level, time to thrombolytic therapy, and cortical involvement were predictors of lack of improvement at 24 hours, and that this lack of improvement was also associated with poor outcome and death at 3 months. As clinicians continue to explore models of health and function, these types of studies will prove essential for testing assumptions about the relationships among impairments, activity limitations and disability.

Theory Testing

Another purpose for correlational study is the testing of theory. With this approach, the researcher chooses specific variables for study, based on expected relationships derived from deductive hypotheses. This approach is illustrated in a study by Rauch et al,[21] who used regression statistics to test the theory that developmental changes in bone strength are secondary to the increasing loads imposed by larger muscle forces. They hypothesized, therefore, that increases in muscle strength should precede increases in bone strength. They investigated the relationship between lean body mass (as a surrogate measure of muscle strength) and bone mineral content (as a measure of bone strength) in 138 boys and girls who were longitudinally examined during pubertal development. They were able to demonstrate a consistent temporal pattern of peak body mass preceding peak bone mineral content. Their analysis was able to establish an association between body mass and bone strength, independent of gender and height. These authors also understood the limitation of correlational analysis for deriving cause and effect conclusions, and speculated that their findings do not exclude the hypothesis that the two processes are independently determined by genetic mechanisms.

CASE-CONTROL STUDIES

A **case-control study** is a method of epidemiologic investigation in which groups of individuals are selected on the basis of whether or not they have the disorder under study. *Cases* are those classified as having the disorder, and *controls* are chosen as a comparison group without the disorder. The investigator then looks backward in time, via direct interview, mail questionnaire or chart review of previously collected data, to determine if the groups differ with respect to their exposure histories or the presence of specific characteristics that may put a person at risk for developing the condition of interest (see Figure 13.2). The assumption is that differences in exposure histories should explain why more cases than controls developed the outcome.

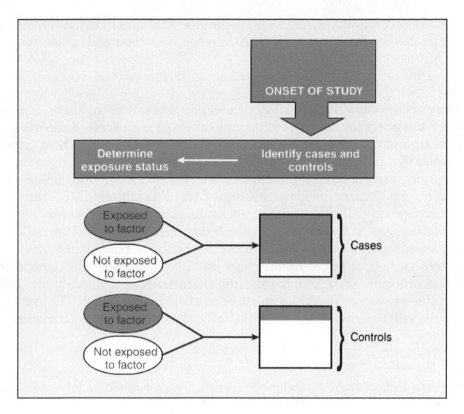

FIGURE 13.2   Illustration of a case-control design. Note the direction of inquiry is retrospective. Subjects are chosen based on their status as a case or control, and then exposure status is determined.

For example, a retrospective case-control design was used to investigate the hypothesis that the occurrence of knee osteoarthritis (OA) may be related to the duration of participation in some forms of sport and active recreation.[22] The only strong association found was a greatly increased risk of knee OA with a previously sustained knee injury. The researchers found that subjects who had had a knee injury were 8 times more likely to have knee OA than those who did not have an injury. The exercise/sports variables did not demonstrate such a significant relationship. Therefore, the authors concluded that there was little evidence to suggest that increased levels of regular physical activity throughout life lead to an increased risk of knee OA later in life. Procedures for calculating risk estimates for case control studies are described in Chapter 28.

The advantage of the case-control design is that samples are relatively easy to gather. Therefore, case-control studies are useful for studying disorders that are relatively rare, because they start by finding cases in a systematic manner. Case-control methods are especially applicable for analyzing disorders with long latency periods, where longitudinal studies would require years to identify those who developed the disease. A disadvantage of case-control studies is the potential for uncertainty in the temporal relationship between exposure and disease. In addition, the proportion of cases and controls in the study is not related to the proportion of cases in the population. Therefore, findings must be subjected to scrutiny in terms of the potential for bias.

Results of case-control studies, however, do provide estimates that may support a causal relationship between risk factors and disease when combined with other evidence.

Selection of Cases and Controls

The validity of case-control studies is dependent on several design issues. Perhaps most obvious are the effects of case definition and case selection. **Case definition** refers to the diagnostic and clinical criteria that identify someone as a case. These criteria must be comprehensive and specific, so that cases are clearly distinguished from controls and so that the study sample is homogeneous. Case definitions for many diseases have been developed by the Centers for Disease Control and Prevention (CDC) and the World Health Organization (WHO). At times, these definitions are revised to reflect recent medical findings, as in the increasingly comprehensive definition of AIDS. Clinical diagnoses are sometimes more difficult to define or control. For instance, disorders such as birth defects, hemiplegia, cerebral palsy and low back pain can be manifested in many different forms. Therefore, the specific characteristics that qualify an individual as having the disease or disability must be spelled out in detail. The population to which results will be generalized is defined according to these characteristics.

Selection of Cases

Once the case definition is established, criteria for *case selection* must be developed. Cases may be identified from all those who have been treated for the disorder at a specific hospital or treatment center, or they may be chosen from the larger general population of those with the disorder. A **population-based study** involves obtaining a sample of cases from the general population of those with the disorder. In a **hospital-based study**, cases are obtained from patients in a medical institution. The latter approach is more common because samples are relatively easy to recruit and subjects are easy to contact. The population-based study affords greater generalizability, but is often too expensive and logistically unfeasible.

The researcher must also determine whether the study should include new or existing cases. The difference, of course, is that with existing cases duration of illness is not accounted for. If the duration of a condition is not related to exposure, then a case-control study using existing cases is justifiable. If exposure affects duration of the condition, however, results from a case-control study is more difficult to interpret. In general, it is preferable to use new cases or to restrict cases to those who were diagnosed within a specific period.

Selection of Controls

The most serious challenge to the researcher in designing a case-control study is the choice of a control group. The purpose of a case-control study is to determine if the frequency of an exposure or certain personal characteristics is different for those who did and did not develop the disease. Therefore, for the comparison to be fair, the controls should be drawn from the population of individuals who would have been chosen as cases had the disease been present. Any restrictions or criteria used to select cases must also be used to select controls. Often, researchers match cases and controls on a variety of relevant factors, such as age, race, gender or occupation.

Controls can be obtained from several sources. They are often recruited from the same hospital or institution as the cases, from those who have been admitted for conditions other than the disease of interest. For example, Altieri and associates[23] explored the relationship between leisure physical activity and the experience of a first myocardial infarction (MI). They studied individuals who were hospitalized for an MI during a specified period, and recruited controls from patients who had been admitted for other acute conditions. They found that individuals who engaged in leisure exercise were half as likely to experience an MI as those who did not exercise. The advantage of using hospital-based controls is that hospitalized patients are readily available and similarly motivated. The disadvantage, of course, is that they are ill and, therefore, potentially different from healthy subjects who might be exposed to the same risk factors. In addition, studies have shown that hospitalized patients are more likely to smoke cigarettes, use oral contraceptives and drink more alcohol than nonhospitalized individuals.[24,25] Therefore, if these risk factors are being studied or if they are related to the disease being studied, they could bias the results. It is also important to determine what disorders other than the case disorder are represented among controls. If the risk factors being studied are associated with these other disorders, the estimate of their effects on cases will be minimized. Despite the disadvantages, however, hospital controls are often used because of the convenience they offer.

Controls can be obtained from the general population by a variety of sampling methods, such as random-digit dialing, or by using available lists such as voter registration and membership directories. Population-based controls may also be sampled from special lists. For instance, in a case-control study to establish the risk associated with limited physical activity and ovarian cancer, community controls were selected randomly from lists of licensed drivers and Medicare reicipients.[26] Sometimes special groups can be contacted to provide controls, such as family members and friends of those with the disease. These controls provide some comparability in ethnic and lifestyle characteristics.

Analysis Issues

The analysis of results of case-control studies requires attention to bias in the selection and classification of subjects and in the assessment of exposure status. Because subjects are purposefully selected for case-control studies on the basis of their having or not having a disease, **selection bias** is of special concern. Cases and controls must be chosen regardless of their exposure histories. If cases and controls are differentially selected on some variable that is related to the exposure of interest, it will not be possible to determine if the exposure is truly related to the disease. When samples are composed of subjects who have consented to participate, self-selection biases can also occur.

An additional source of bias is introduced if subjects are misclassified, that is, if those who have the disease are mistakenly put in the control group or those who do not really have the disease are considered cases. If this **misclassification** is random, and equally present in both groups, it is considered *nondifferential misclassification*, which will tend to minimize the relationship between the exposure and disease.* With *differential misclassification*, however, when groups are not affected equally, the results may overestimate or underestimate that relationship.[27] For example, in a study evaluating risk factors associated with falling in hospitalized elderly, cases were identified from incident reports of a geriatric rehabilitation hospital for a 1-year period, and controls were selected at random from patients who were "nonfallers," that is, for whom incident reports had not been filed.[28] There may, however, have been cases of falling that were not reported, or nurses may have filed incident reports even when the patient was carefully lowered to the ground by a staff member, if they felt weak while ambulating. In either case, patients would have been misclassified, and in the former situation, some cases may have been chosen as controls.

Observation bias occurs when there is a systematic difference in the way information about disease or exposure is obtained from the study groups. **Interviewer bias** is introduced when the individual collecting data elicits, records, or interprets information differentially from controls and cases. **Recall bias** occurs when subjects who have experienced a particular disorder remember their exposure history differently from those who are not affected. This bias may result in an underestimate or an overestimate of the risk of association with a particular exposure. It is not unusual for individuals who have a disease to analyze their habits or past experiences with greater depth or accuracy than those who are healthy.

COHORT STUDIES

In clinical research, a cohort is defined as a group of individuals who are followed together over time. The most common types of cohorts are geographic cohorts, such as residents of a particular community, or birth cohorts, such as baby boomers. A historical cohort includes individuals who experience specific common events, such as veterans of a given war. Victims who are survivors of natural disasters would be considered members of environmental cohorts. Developmental cohorts are based on life changes, such as getting married or moving into a nursing home.

In a **cohort study** (also called a follow-up study), the researcher selects a group of subjects who do not yet have the outcome of interest and follows them to see if they develop the disorder (see Figure 13.3). Subjects are interviewed or observed to determine the presence or absence of certain exposures, risks or characteristics. Cohort studies may be purely descriptive, with the intent of describing the natural history of a disease. More often, however, they are analytic, identifying the risk associated with these exposures by comparing the incidence of specific outcomes in those who were and were not exposed.

One advantage of a cohort study over a case-control study is the ability to determine the onset of the condition. A temporal sequence can be established for the relationship between exposure to risk factors and development of a particular outcome. This sequence is necessary for drawing inferences about causative factors. The disadvantage of cohort studies is that they are not useful for studying disorders that are uncommon

---

*This is also referred to as biasing toward the null.

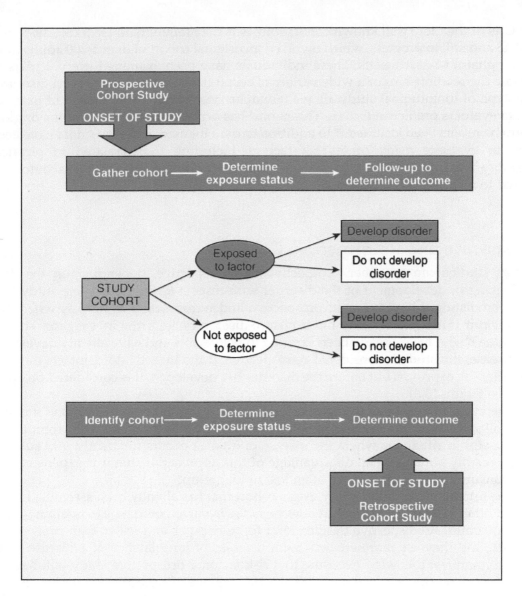

FIGURE 13.3   Illustration of a cohort design. Subjects are chosen based on their membership in a defined cohort. In a prospective cohort study, the investigator enters the study at the time of exposure, and follows subjects to determine who develops the disorder of interest. In a retrospective cohort study, the investigator enters the study after the outcomes have been determined, and tracks data from the past to determine exposure status.

in the population. If the disorder is rare, a large number of subjects would have to be followed for a long time to document a sufficient number of cases for analysis. In this situation, case-control studies would be more appropriate; however, cohort studies are useful when exposures are rare because the cohort can be assembled and classified according to their exposure status (where case-control subjects were classified according to disease status). Cohort studies are also very effective for studying multiple disorders.

One of the more well known cohort studies is the Framingham Heart Study, begun in 1948 and still in progress, which involved an original cohort of over 5,200 adults from Framingham, Massachusetts. These individuals have been examined every 2 years to explore the relationships of a wide variety of risk factors with coronary heart disease.[29] This type of longitudinal study allows researchers to examine consistency of patterns and to evaluate predictive factors. This cohort has expanded as children of the original group have also been included.[30] In addition to risks for cardiac disease, data have been used to evaluate many other risk factors, including those related to physical disability,[31,32] stroke,[33,34] low back pain,[35] and bone mineral density,[36] as outcomes related to a variety of exposures.

Prospective and Retrospective Cohorts

Cohort studies can be either prospective or retrospective, depending on the time sequencing of development of the disorder with respect to the start of the study. The basis for distinguishing between prospective and retrospective designs is where the investigator initiates entry into the exposure-disease cycle. If the investigator studies individuals who have already been exposed to risk factors and have already developed the disease, the study is considered retrospective. If the investigator contacts the subjects after the exposure, but before the disorder has developed, it is considered prospective (see Figure 13.3).

The main advantage of the prospective design is the ability to control and monitor data collection and to measure variables completely and accurately. This approach is most useful in situations where the disease of interest occurs frequently, and subjects can be readily obtained. The disadvantage of this approach is that it is expensive and time consuming, and subjects are often lost to follow-up.

The retrospective cohort study uses a cohort that has already been assembled (usually for other reasons), and looks at how variables occurred over time in relation to specific outcomes. Retrospective designs tend to be cheaper and faster than prospective designs, and they are more efficient with diseases of long latency. If a disease takes years to manifest following exposure to a risk factor, a prospective study will have to go on for a long time to document it. The disadvantage of retrospective designs is that they may have to deal with incomplete or inadequate data from medical records, the subject's memory, or the memories and perspectives of family members or caregivers.

Selection of Subjects

The selection of subjects for a cohort study must be appropriate for the research question. For purely descriptive studies, the sample must be representative of the target population to which results will be generalized. Probability samples would be ideal, but are rarely used because of expense and limited accessibility. For analytic studies, two groups must be identified, those who have been exposed and those who have not been exposed to the risk factors. The most important consideration is that the exposed group be of sufficient numbers to obtain meaningful outcome measures; that is, there must be enough subjects who eventually develop the disease.[†]

The group that has been exposed to the risk factors may come from several sources. For relatively common exposures, a large number of individuals may be available from the general population. Often, accessible groups, such as nurses in the previously mentioned Nurses' Health Study, residents of defined geographical areas, or employees of a specific company, are targeted as a cohort, not necessarily because of their exposure histories, but because they can be followed easily. The subjects in the Framingham Heart Study represent a classical example of this type of cohort, chosen because of the accessibility of a stable population. When exposures are rare in the population, special cohorts may be chosen because of their unique exposure histories. For example, in order to study the relationship of extremely vigorous physical activity and exercise to development of musculoskeletal injuries, a cohort was comprised of young men in Army infantry basic training.[37]

The comparison cohort must be as similar as possible to the exposed cohort in all factors related to the disease except for the specific exposures under study. It is important that all subjects who are chosen have a chance of developing the disorder. For instance, if one were studying risks associated with abnormal menstruation, women who have had hysterectomies or who have passed menopause would not be eligible.

Analysis Issues

The results of a cohort study will clearly be influenced by the misclassification of either exposure or disease, as described earlier. Bias is less of a concern in prospective cohort studies than in case-control or retrospective studies, because classification of exposure is made independently of knowledge about the subject's disease status.

Because of the longitudinal nature of prospective cohort studies, they are especially prone to attrition. The researcher must determine the validity of the study based on whether the loss of subjects is related to either the exposure, the disease or both. Researchers generally take great pains to ensure good rapport with participants, and must be aggressive in maintaining contact with them.

EVALUATING CAUSALITY IN OBSERVATIONAL STUDIES

The epidemiologist is ultimately concerned with identifying those factors or exposures that cause disease or disability. Because case-control and cohort studies do not involve direct experimentation or manipulation of variables, the validity of statistical association between exposure and disease with these observational designs must be made under conditions that are not strictly controlled. Therefore, the epidemiologist must

---

[†]Researchers can perform a power analysis when planning a study, to determine how many subjects should be included. The sample size determinations are based on the expected outcome, that is, the degree of association expected between the exposure and the disease. This expected relationship is called the *effect size*. The larger the effect size (a stronger relationship), the fewer subjects would be needed. For a fuller discussion of the concept of effect size see Appendix C.

first rule out influences of bias, confounding and chance variation, and then must assess the strength of cause and effect criteria.

Perhaps most important is the establishment of a *time sequence* that documents the exposure preceding the disease. In addition, the researcher can look at the *strength of the association* using a measure of relative risk. The stronger the association, the more likely a causative relationship exists. The relationship should also have *biologic credibility*. The researcher should be able to postulate some mechanism by which the exposure might reasonably alter the risk of developing the disease. This may not be possible, depending on the state of knowledge, but it will make the conclusion more plausible if a realistic explanation can be offered. It is also helpful to show *consistency* with other studies. The more times a relationship can be documented by different researchers using different samples and conditions, the more likely it is true. Lastly, the presence of a **dose–response relationship** provides evidence for causality. This means that the severity of the disease can be associated with varying levels of the exposures. If the risk of developing the disease does not vary with increases or decreases in exposure, it is unlikely that the exposure is the true risk factor. These five criteria, taken together, can be used to provide evidence for a cause-and-effect relationship.

METHODOLOGICAL RESEARCH: RELIABILITY AND VALIDITY

Methodological research involves the development and testing of measuring instruments for use in research or clinical practice. This approach is used extensively in health care research, as clinicians work toward establishing the reliability and validity of clinical measurement tools. In a research context, this approach does not involve the evaluation of treatment effectiveness, but rather, makes contributions to establishing the methods used to carry out research or support clinical assessment.

The outcomes movement has provided the impetus for comprehensive methodological study of health status and functional assessment tools. These studies emphasize the use of outcome instruments as a way of indicating quality of care and quality of life. Establishing reliability and validity of instruments requires multiple approaches and trials. The implications of the results of these studies are far reaching, as we decide which tools will serve us best to demonstrate the effectiveness of our services. It is essential, therefore, that we understand the designs and analyses of methodological study, so we can make the most appropriate choices and be able to defend them.

Reliability Questions

Issues of reliability are basic to the continued use of measurements for research or clinical practice. Reliability questions generally focus on two aspects of measurement: the rater and the tool itself. See Chapter 5 for a thorough discussion of types of reliability and Chapter 26 for coverage of statistical approaches.

Testing the Rater

Rater reliability is of primary importance when repeated measurements are taken by one or more individuals. Intrarater and interrater reliability should be established to support the accuracy of measurements taken in a clinical study. Theoretically, the demonstration of rater reliability is intended to generalize beyond the individuals in a methodological study; that is, the raters being tested are assumed to be representative of others who would perform the test.

Miano and associates[38] provide a useful example of this concern in their study of interrater reliability of a functional rating scale for amyotrophic lateral sclerosis (ALS). The scale is often applied by caregivers or patients when travel to a study site is not possible and final assessments may be performed by telephone. Therefore, it was important to determine if different raters would obtain substantially different scores. They found that clinician ratings were often lower than those of patients or caregivers; however, the degree of error was less than one point in statistical analyses if 25% of the final visit assessments were performed by the patient in place of the provider. They concluded that the ALS functional scale can be successfully used even if evaluators change.

Validity Questions

Perhaps the most comprehensive approach to methodological study is in the development of a new tool. Although many clinicians have been motivated to find effective ways of measuring things within their practice environment, creating a new tool is truly an extensive process. It starts with a clear description of a problem for which a good measurement is not available. If the measurement is a physical property, it may be necessary to build a prototype to test the feasibility of building an instrument that will serve the desired purpose. This can be both time consuming and expensive. If the variable is a construct, such as pain or function, the researcher must be able to delineate the theoretical foundation for the phenomenon to be measured.

For example, in the study of chronic obstructive pulmonary disease (COPD), Eisner and co-workers[39] described the need for a disease-specific measure of severity that could be used to identify risk factors for adverse health outcomes. They found that existing pulmonary function measures and quality of life instruments were not able to adequately assess the severity of disease. Therefore, they designed a new measurement, a comprehensive disease-specific COPD severity score, which was based on disease status, medication use, receipt of clinical treatments and recent hospitalization for COPD. They demonstrated the reliability, internal consistency, construct and concurrent validity of the instrument.

Methodological studies make major contributions to research efforts, as it is virtually impossible to conduct meaningful research without adequate measurement tools. These types of studies are of special importance to scientific disciplines that are engaged in human behavior research, for which objective and direct measuring tools are often unavailable. Reliability and validity studies are reported with increasing frequency in medical and rehabilitation journals, as clinicians continue to realize their importance for establishing measurement standards. We must stress, however, that methodological research is not intended as an end in and of itself; that is, the purpose of methodological study is to develop instruments that can be used in further testing, not to establish reliability or validity for its own sake. Therefore, it is important to examine reliability and validity within a context that will serve as a guide for interpretation of outcomes. Reliability or validity is a property that is achieved to some degree within each context. Instruments are never absolutely reliable or valid, but must be tested under a given set of conditions on a specific population. The concept of reliability is discussed in detail in Chapters 5 and 26. Validity testing is covered in Chapters 6 and 27.

HISTORICAL RESEARCH

Historical research involves the critical review of events, documents, literature and other sources of data to reconstruct the past in an effort to understand how and why past events occurred. This approach has its foundations in the discipline of history, where past world events are examined and analyzed to determine how present conditions evolved and, ultimately, to anticipate future events. In similar fashion, historical research can build a foundation for interpreting current clinical theory and practice, providing a context within which we can evaluate professional trends. Historical research has received little attention in rehabilitation literature, which is unfortunate, considering its potential for contributing to perspectives on professional issues, directions of professional growth and change, and effects of professional and societal trends on modes of practice. Historical research efforts in nursing are extensive. Lusk[40] has presented a primer on historical research methodology that, although written in the context of nursing, provides comprehensive guidelines for all health professionals.

The process of historical research starts with the determination of a research question that addresses a topic of interest within a particular time period.[41] For example, Krisman-Scott[42] was interested in reasons for the long-standing tradition in medicine of nondisclosure of terminal status to patients. She examined this concept within social, political and cultural contexts from 1930 to 1990, and discussed how societal changes have influenced individuals' perceptions of death and the right to make end-of-life decisions. In another example, Markel[43] has discussed an historical account of the AIDS epidemic from 1980 to 2001, analyzing why it has been of intense interest to medical, social and political communities, and how AIDS is an example of both a global pandemic and a chronic disease. Galas and McCormack[44] have questioned the impact of genomic technologies such as cloning and DNA sequencing on changes in the scientific community's view of biology through the latter quarter of the 20th century. These types of questions can only be answered retrospectively within the historical perspective of events that precipitated change.

Once a problem area is identified, an organizing framework is formed to guide the search for data. It is this element that distinguishes historical research from a critical review of literature or a chronological presentation of a series of events (although these will be major components of the historical research process). Historical research is not a collection of facts or dates, but is meant to incorporate judgments, analyses, and inferences in the search for relationships, by organizing and synthesizing data from the past, not just summarizing them.[40] For instance, Paris[45] described the development of joint manipulation as an accepted therapeutic technique in physical therapy in contrast to chiropractic philosophy and practice. In another example, Gutman[46] studied the development of occupational therapy and the influence of the relationship between orthopedists and reconstruction aides during the first World War, which marked an early willingness by occupational therapists to accept the medical model as one guide for clinical practice.

Sources of Historical Data

Historians use a variety of sources to accumulate data. The researcher must be critical in the acceptance of all that is read, recognizing that those who wrote in the past may have been selective in their presentation of facts or creative in their representation of the truth. For this reason especially, the historical researcher should distinguish between firsthand and secondhand sources of information. For the historian, *primary sources* include original documents, such as letters, videotapes, photographs, or minutes of a meeting, eyewitness accounts, and direct recordings of events. This does not guarantee the truth or accuracy of the report, only that no intervening account has colored the information. *Secondary sources* may include biographies, textbooks, encyclopedias, literature reviews, newspaper accounts and any summary of primary materials. As with all research, the historian should use primary sources whenever possible. The transmission of information from original to secondary accounts will invariably present some distortion or slant that could affect the validity of subsequent interpretations.[47]

Reliability and Validity

Historical data must also be evaluated for reliability and validity. Because historical information is subject to contamination, researchers will find that not all sources are of equal value.[48] The historian must be able to establish the authenticity of data, by subjecting the material to **external criticism**. This may involve determination that papers were indeed written by the ascribed author (not ghost written) or that documents have not been altered.

The data must also be subjected to **internal criticism,** which questions the truth or worth of the material's content within the context of the research question. Although it is not a scientifically rigorous procedure, to some extent internal validity of information can be examined on the basis of corroboration from other sources or by finding no substantial contrary evidence.[48] It is also important to understand the relevant definitions and concepts used during the historical period and to recognize that standards and terminology change over time.

Synthesis of Historical Data

The historical researcher must determine how much information is needed to draw valid conclusions, being careful not to make assumptions about the past merely because no information can be found. Some elements of data will be given more weight than others in their interpretation and application to the hypothesis. The historian attempts to incorporate a scientific logic into this process, so that interpretations are made as objectively as possible. Historians must also be alert to their own biases, so that unintended meanings are not ascribed to information.

Because sources, measurements, and organization of data are not controlled, cause-and-effect statements cannot be made in historical research. One can only synthesize what is already known into systematized accounts of the past, and discuss potential relationships between variables based on sequencing of events and associated underlying characteristics of variables.

A wonderful example of historical research and its potential for influence on practice was presented by Brush and Capezuti,[49] who analyzed the use of bed siderails in American hospitals through the 20th century. They examined social, economic and legal influences, and argued that the use of siderails was based on a gradual consensus between law and medicine, rather than empirical evidence in practice. Their study identified a continued use of siderails that contrasted sharply with documented patient accidents and contemporary ideas about the importance of mobility and functional independence, particularly in the elderly. They concluded that changes in this practice will have to be driven by data, and that alternative strategies will only become accepted once administrators, regulators, attorneys, patients and clinicians understand why siderails became common practice in the first place. This study illustrates the importance of understanding the past as professionals face current and future challenges.

SECONDARY ANALYSIS

Much of the research in health and social science involves the collection of large amounts of data, often more than the researcher actually analyzes. In **secondary analysis** a researcher uses an existing database to re-examine variables and answer questions other than those for which the data were collected. Investigators may analyze subsets of variables or subjects different from those analyzed in the initial study, or they may be interested in exploring new relationships among the variables. Sometimes the unit of analysis can be changed, so that one study might look at overall hospital characteristics, whereas another might look at individual responses of health care personnel. Researchers can also explore outcomes using different statistical techniques, either because initial findings were based on inappropriate statistical procedures or to test different hypotheses. When two or more comparable data sets can be combined for secondary analysis, researchers can expand the generalizability of outcomes. In this way secondary analysis can be especially useful for supporting theoretical hypotheses.

The major advantages of secondary analysis are the minimal expense involved, the ability to study large samples and the elimination of the most time-consuming part of the research process, data collection. Researchers can formulate hypotheses and proceed to test them immediately. For new researchers, secondary analysis may provide a useful way to start the research process, especially when funds are limited. For experienced researchers, existing data sets may provide unexpected but important findings at little or no cost.

The disadvantage of this approach relates to the researcher's lack of control over the data collection process. There is no way to ensure the quality of the data, how questions were asked, or which variables were tested. Data may be missing or incorrectly entered. The researcher interested in secondary analysis must consider possible sources of error and judge their effect according to the documentation available on the data and the necessary rigor of the research hypothesis.

Finding a Question to Fit the Data—or Finding Data to Fit the Question

Secondary data analysis can proceed in two directions. Perhaps the more direct approach is to look carefully at existing data, to determine what types of questions would fit. This requires familiarity with the data and the variables that were measured. The researcher can then start to consider the possible relationships that might be of interest. Often the effect of demographic factors, such as age, gender, race, income level and so on can generate questions about their influence on physiological or performance variables. As a question begins to evolve, the researcher must proceed to the literature, so that a theoretical framework can be developed and hypotheses can be proposed.

The alternative process involves searching for a database that will provide the needed information to answer a given research question. The researcher must first develop a list of variables that are germane to the question, so that the viability of a particular database can be determined. For this process to work, the researcher must have some familiarity with databases that are available. It may be necessary to contact other individuals who have access to data, such as people in industry or hospital administration, who would know what kinds of information was accessible. Computerized databases from medical records may provide a rich source of information for clinical research. The researcher may also explore collaborative relationships with other investigators.

Sources of Secondary Data

Secondary analysis has become increasingly common in recent years because of the availability of large computer data sets. Information about these data sets may be obtained through journal articles or conference presentations. A variety of large databases are supported by data libraries such as the International Data Library and Reference Service at the University of California at Berkeley, the Council of Social Science Data Archives in New York City, the Roper Public Opinion Research Center at Williams College and the Archive of the Inter-University Consortium for Political and Social Research at the University of Michigan. The U.S. government sponsors continued collection of health-related data through the National Center for Health Statistics (NCHS) and the U.S. Bureau of the Census, among others. Access to these databases can usually be obtained at minimal or no cost, often with direct online connections.

Databases such as the National Health Interview Survey, the National Hospital Discharge Survey, and the National Nursing Home Survey, all through NCHS, are continually used by researchers in public health, allied health, medicine and social science to document health care utilization, health status of various age groups and related personal and lifestyle characteristics. Data collected since 1950 as part of the Framingham Heart Study were originally intended to study risk factors for coronary heart disease, and have been used to study longitudinal changes in other factors, such as physical function,[31,50] stroke,[51] and cognition.[52] Started in 1973, the Multiple Risk Factor Intervention Trial (MRFIT) was a randomized primary prevention trial to test the effect of a multifactor intervention program on mortality from coronary heart disease (CHD) in 12,866 high-risk men.[53] This data set has been used extensively, however, to answer other questions, such as risk factors affecting of the wives of participants,[54,55] mortality from pulmonary disease,[56] risk associated with ethnicity,[57,58] risk factors for stroke,[59] and alcohol use.[60] As these examples illustrate, with the availability of data through computer access, secondary analysis is an important research option, providing a rich source of information for clinicians to investigate important clinical questions.

COMMENTARY

Advantages and Disadvantages of Exploratory Research

Even though exploratory studies are not able to establish cause-and-effect relationships, they play an important role in clinical research, especially considering the lack of documented evidence that exists concerning most clinical phenomena. Before one can begin to investigate causal factors for behaviors and responses using experimental methods, one must first discover which variables are related and how they occur in nature. For many phenomena, we will probably never be able to establish causality and can move ahead in our critical inquiry only if we can understand how those phenomena manifest themselves with regard to concurrent variables.

Many correlational studies are based on variables that have been measured in the past or that represent attributes of individuals that are beyond the control of the investigator. Under these conditions, exploratory research is limited in its interpretation because of the potential bias that exists in the data. Many secondary analyses are performed on databases that offer a great deal of information, but without the benefit of controlling measurement and operational definitions. The researcher is obliged to consider the implications of these potential biases when interpreting the outcomes of correlational analyses.

Finally, the complex nature of clinical phenomena and the intricate interrelationships that exist among attitudes, behaviors, physical and psychological characteristics and the environment present special interpretive problems for correlational analysis. It is often difficult to establish that two variables are associated without considering the multitude of other variables that would have to enter into any predictive or theoretical relationship. Correlational studies compel us to contemplate the theories that help explain observed relationships, and to approach analyses from a *multivariate* perspective. This means that analyses can become quite complex, but at the same time, this also presents exciting opportunities for exploring alternative explanations for our clinical observations.

REFERENCES

1. Patten SB, Beck CA, Kassam A, Williams JV, Barbui C, Metz LM. Long-term medical conditions and major depression: Strength of association for specific conditions in the general population. *Can J Psychiatry* 2005;50:195–202.
2. Visser M, Goodpaster BH, Kritchevsky SB, Newman AB, Nevitt M, Rubin SM, et al. Muscle mass, muscle strength, and muscle fat infiltration as predictors of incident

mobility limitations in well-functioning older persons. *J Gerontol A Biol Sci Med Sci* 2005; 60:324–333.

3. Miles JH, Takahashi TN, Bagby S, Sahota PK, Vaslow DF, Wang CH, et al. Essential versus complex autism: Definition of fundamental prognostic subtypes. *Am J Med Genet A* 2005;135:171–180.

4. Sellers BJ, Davis BL, Larkin PW, Morris SE, Saffle JR. Early prediction of prolonged ventilator dependence in thermally injured patients. *J Trauma* 1997;43:899–903.

5. Menard S. *Longitudinal research*. Newbury Park, CA: SAGE Publications, 1991.

6. Baltes PB, Reese HW, Nesselroade JR. *Introduction to Research Methods, Life-Span Developmental Psychology*. Hillsdale, NJ: Lawrence Erlbaum Associates, 1988.

7. Centers for Disease Control and Prevention. National Center for Health Statistics. <http://www.cdc.gov/nchs> Accessed January 1, 2005.

8. Gregg EW, Gerzoff RB, Caspersen CJ, Williamson DF, Narayan KM. Relationship of walking to mortality among U.S. adults with diabetes. *Arch Intern Med* 2003;163:1440–1447.

9. Bethell C, Reuland CH, Halfon N, Schor EL. Measuring the quality of preventive and developmental services for young children: National estimates and patterns of clinicians' performance. *Pediatrics* 2004;113:1973–1983.

10. Christmas C, Crespo CJ, Franckowiak SC, Bathon JM, Bartlett SJ, Andersen RE. How common is hip pain among older adults? Results from the Third National Health and Nutrition Examination Survey. *J Fam Pract* 2002;51:345–348.

11. The Nurses Health Study. <http://www.channing.harvard.edu/nhs/index.html> Accessed January 1, 2005.

12. University of Alabama at Birmingham, Department of Physical Medicine and Rehabilitation. National Spinal Cord Injury Statistical Center. <http://main.uab.edu/show.asp?durki=10766> Accessed January 1, 2005.

13. Charlifue S, Lammertse DP, Adkins RH. Aging with spinal cord injury: Changes in selected health indices and life satisfaction. *Arch Phys Med Rehabil* 2004;85:1848–1853.

14. Centers for Medicare and Medicaid Services. Medicare Current Beneficiary Survey. <http://www.cms.hhs.gov/MCBS/default.asp> Accessed January 1, 2005.

15. Freburger JK, Holmes GM. Physical therapy use by community-based older people. *Phys Ther* 2005;85:19–33.

16. National Heart, Lung and Blood Institute. Framingham Heart Study. <http://www.framingham.com/heart/> Accessed January 1, 2005.

17. Higgins PA. Patient perception of fatigue while undergoing long-term mechanical ventilation: Incidence and associated factors. *Heart Lung* 1998;27:177–183.

18. Rutledge R, Lentz CW, Fakhry S, Hunt J. Appropriate use of the Glasgow Coma Scale in intubated patients: A linear regression prediction of the Glasgow verbal score from the Glasgow eye and motor scores. *J Trauma* 1996;41:514–522.

19. Meredith W, Rutledge R, Fakhry SM, Emery S, Kromhout-Schiro S. The conundrum of the Glasgow Coma Scale in intubated patients: A linear regression prediction of the Glasgow verbal score from the Glasgow eye and motor scores. *J Trauma* 1998;44:839–844; discussion 844–845.

20. Saposnik G, Young B, Silver B, Di Legge S, Webster F, Beletsky V, et al. Lack of improvement in patients with acute stroke after treatment with thrombolytic therapy: Predictors and association with outcome. *JAMA* 2004;292:1839–1844.

21. Rauch F, Bailey DA, Baxter-Jones A, Mirwald R, Faulkner R. The "muscle-bone unit" during the pubertal growth spurt. *Bone* 2004;34:771–775.

22. Sutton AJ, Muir KR, Mockett S, Fentem P. A case-control study to investigate the relation between low and moderate levels of physical activity and osteoarthritis of the knee

using data collected as part of the Allied Dunbar National Fitness Survey. *Ann Rheum Dis* 2001;60:756–764.

23. Altieri A, Tavani A, Gallus S, La Vecchia C. Occupational and leisure time physical activity and the risk of nonfatal acute myocardial infarction in Italy. *Ann Epidemiol* 2004;14:461–466.

24. West DW, Schuman KL, Lyon JL, Robison LM, Allred R. Differences in risk estimations from a hospital and a population-based case-control study. *Int J Epidemiol* 1984;13:235–239.

25. Morabia A, Stellman SD, Wynder EL. Smoking prevalence in neighborhood and hospital controls: Implications for hospital-based case-control studies. *J Clin Epidemiol* 1996;49:885–889.

26. Bertone ER, Newcomb PA, Willett WC, Stampfer MJ, Egan KM. Recreational physical activity and ovarian cancer in a population-based case-control study. *Int J Cancer* 2002;99:431–436.

27. Hennekens CH, Buring JE. *Epidemiology in Medicine.* Boston: Little Brown, 1987.

28. Sorock GS. A case control study of falling incidents among the hospitalized elderly. *J Safety Res* 1983;14:47–52.

29. Karp I, Abrahamowicz M, Bartlett G, Pilote L. Updated risk factor values and the ability of the multivariable risk score to predict coronary heart disease. *Am J Epidemiol* 2004;160:707–716.

30. Murabito JM, Nam BH, D'Agostino RB, Sr., Lloyd-Jones DM, O'Donnell CJ, Wilson PW. Accuracy of offspring reports of parental cardiovascular disease history: The Framingham Offspring Study. *Ann Intern Med* 2004;140:434–440.

31. Visser M, Harris TB, Langlois J, Hannan MT, Roubenoff R, Felson DT, et al. Body fat and skeletal muscle mass in relation to physical disability in very old men and women of the Framingham Heart Study. *J Gerontol* 1998;53A:M214–221.

32. Allaire SH, LaValley MP, Evans SR, O'Connor GT, Kelly-Hayes M, Meenan RF, et al. Evidence for decline in disability and improved health among persons aged 55 to 70 years: the Framingham Heart Study. *Am J Public Health* 1999;89:1678–1683.

33. Janardhan V, Wolf PA, Kase CS, Massaro JM, D'Agostino RB, Franzblau C, et al. Anticardiolipin antibodies and risk of ischemic stroke and transient ischemic attack: The Framingham cohort and offspring study. *Stroke* 2004;35:736–741.

34. Wolf PA. Fifty years at Framingham: Contributions to stroke epidemiology. *Adv Neurol* 2003;92:165–172.

35. Edmond SL, Felson DT. Function and back symptoms in older adults. *J Am Geriatr Soc* 2003;51:1702–1709.

36. Booth SL, Broe KE, Peterson JW, Cheng DM, Dawson-Hughes B, Gundberg CM, et al. Associations between vitamin K biochemical measures and bone mineral density in men and women. *J Clin Endocrinol Metab* 2004;89:4904–4909.

37. Jones BH, Cowan DN, Tomlinson JP, Robinson JR, Polly DW, Frykman PN. Epidemiology of injuries associated with physical training among young men in the army. *Med Sci Sports Exerc* 1993;25:197–203.

38. Miano B, Stoddard GJ, Davis S, Bromberg MB. Inter-evaluator reliability of the ALS functional rating scale. *Amyotroph Lateral Scler Other Motor Neuron Disord* 2004;5:235–239.

39. Eisner MD, Trupin L, Katz PP, Yelin EH, Earnest G, Balmes J, et al. Development and validation of a survey-based COPD severity score. *Chest* 2005;127:1890–1897.

40. Lusk B. Historical methodology for nursing research. *Image J Nurs Sch* 1997;29:355–359.

41. Rees C, Howells G. Historical research: Process, problems and pitfalls. *Nurs Stand* 1999;13(27):33–35.

42. Krisman-Scott MA. An historical analysis of disclosure of terminal status. *J Nurs Scholarsh* 2000;32:47–52.

43. Markel H. Journals of the plague years: Documenting the history of the AIDS epidemic in the United States. *Am J Public Health* 2001;91:1025–1028.

44. Galas DJ, McCormack SJ. An historical perspective on genomic technologies. *Curr Issues Mol Biol* 2003;5:123–127.

45. Paris SV. A history of manipulative therapy through the ages and up to the current controversy in the United States. *J Manual Manipulative Ther* 2000;8:66–77.

46. Gutman SA. Influence of the U.S. military and occupational therapy reconstruction aides in World War I on the development of occupational therapy. *Am J Occup Ther* 1995;49:256–262.

47. Kerlinger FN. *Foundations of Behavioral Research* (3rd ed.). New York: Holt, Rinehart & Winston, 1985.

48. Christy TE. The methodology of historical research: A brief introduction. *Nurs Res* 1975;24:189–192.

49. Brush BL, Capezuti E. Historical analysis of siderail use in American hospitals. *J Nurs Scholarsh* 2001;33:381–385.

50. Guccione AA, Felson DT, Anderson JJ, Anthony JM, Zhang Y, Wilson PW, et al. The effects of specific medical conditions on the functional limitations of elders in the Framingham Study. *Am J Public Health* 1994;84:351–358.

51. Benjamin EJ, RB DA, Belanger AJ, Wolf PA, Levy D. Left atrial size and the risk of stroke and death. The Framingham Heart Study. *Circulation* 1995;92:835–841.

52. Elias MF, Elias PK, D'Agostino, RB, Silbershatz H, Wolf PA. Role of age, education, and gender on cognitive performance in the Framingham Heart Study: Community-based norms. *Exp Aging Res* 1997;23:201–235.

53. Multiple Risk Factor Intervention Trial Research Group. Multiple risk factor intervention trial. Risk factor changes and mortality results. *JAMA* 1982;248:1465–1477.

54. Sexton M, Bross D, Hebel JR, Schumann BC, Gerace TA, Lasser N, et al. Risk-factor changes in wives with husbands at high risk of coronary heart disease (CHD): The spin-off effect. *J Behav Med* 1987;10:251–261.

55. Svendsen KH, Kuller LH, Martin MJ, Ockene JK. Effects of passive smoking in the Multiple Risk Factor Intervention Trial. *Am J Epidemiol* 1987;126:783–795.

56. Kuller LH, Ockene JK, Townsend M, Browner W, Meilahn E, Wentworth DN. The epidemiology of pulmonary function and COPD mortality in the multiple risk factor intervention trial. *Am Rev Respir Dis* 1989;140:S76–S81.

57. Flack JM, Neaton JD, Daniels B, Esunge P. Ethnicity and renal disease: Lessons from the Multiple Risk Factor Intervention Trial and the Treatment of Mild Hypertension Study. *Am J Kidney Dis* 1993;21:31–40.

58. Connett JE, Stamler J. Responses of black and white males to the special intervention program of the Multiple Risk Factor Intervention Trial. *Am Heart J* 1984;108:839–848.

59. Neaton JD, Wentworth DN, Cutler J, Stamler J, Kuller L. Risk factors for death from different types of stroke. Multiple Risk Factor Intervention Trial Research Group. *Ann Epidemiol* 1993;3:493–499.

60. Folsom AR, Hughes JR, Buehler JF, Mittelmark MB, Jacobs DR, Jr., Grimm RH, Jr. Do type A men drink more frequently than type B men? Findings in the Multiple Risk Factor Intervention Trial (MRFIT). *J Behav Med* 1985;8:227–235.

CHAPTER 14
Descriptive Research

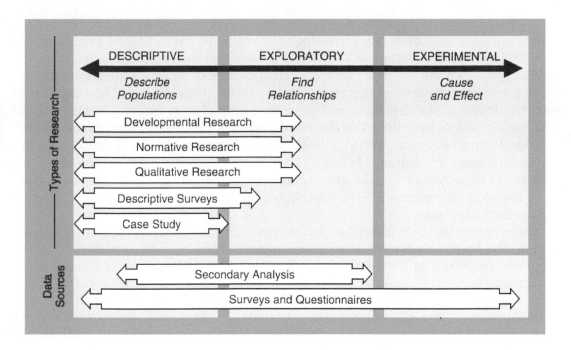

Descriptive research is designed to document the factors that describe characteristics, behaviors and conditions of individuals and groups. For example, researchers have used this approach to describe a sample of individuals with spinal cord injuries with respect to gender, age, and cause and severity of injury to see whether these properties were similar to those described in the past.[1] Descriptive studies have documented the biomechanical parameters of wheelchair propulsion,[2] and the clinical characteristics of stroke.[3] As our diagram of the continuum of research shows, descriptive and exploratory elements are commonly combined, depending on how the investigator conceptualizes the research question.

Descriptive studies document the nature of existing phenomena and describe how variables change over time. They will generally be structured around a set of guiding questions or research objectives to generate data or characterize a situation of interest. Often this information can be used as a basis for formulation of research hypotheses that can be tested using exploratory or experimental techniques. The descriptive data supply the foundation for classifying individuals, for identifying relevant variables, and for asking new research questions.

Descriptive studies may involve prospective or retrospective data collection, and may be designed using longitudinal or cross-sectional methods (see Chapter 13). Surveys and secondary analysis of clinical databases are often used as sources of data for descriptive analysis. Several types of research can be categorized as descriptive, including developmental research, normative research, qualitative research and case studies. The purpose of this chapter is to describe these approaches.

DEVELOPMENTAL RESEARCH

Concepts of human development, whether they are related to cognition, perceptual-motor control, communication, physiological change, or psychological processes, are important elements of a clinical knowledge base. Valid interpretation of clinical outcomes depends on our ability to develop a clear picture of those we treat, their characteristics and performance expectations under different conditions. **Developmental research** involves the description of developmental change and the sequencing of behaviors in people over time. Developmental studies have contributed to the theoretical foundations of clinical practice in many ways. For example, the classic descriptive studies of Gesell and Amatruda[4] and McGraw[5] provide the basis for much of the research on sequencing of motor development in infants and children. Erikson's studies of life span development have contributed to an understanding of psychological growth through old age.[6]

Developmental studies can be characterized by the method used to document change. The longitudinal method involves collecting data over an extended period, to document behaviors as they vary over time. Because the same individuals are tested throughout the study, personal characteristics remain relatively constant, and differences observed over time can be interpreted as developmental change. With the cross-sectional method, the researcher studies various developmental levels (usually age levels) within a particular cohort of subjects and describes differences among those levels as they exist at a single point in time.

One of the earliest developmental studies was actually a longitudinal case report of data collected between 1759 and 1777, chronicling the physical growth of a child at 6-month intervals, from birth to 18 years. These data still represent one of the most famous records of human growth.[7] Intellectual growth has been the subject of many longitudinal studies, in children[8] and adults.[9] Changes that occur in psychological and physiological processes with aging are also best described using longitudinal methods. For example, research has documented the development of personality through late adulthood[10] and cognitive effects of aging.[11] At the other end of the spectrum, researchers have described longitudinal patterns of development in infant heart transplant recipients, demonstrating mild motor delays and age-dependent variability in cognitive skills.[12]

Marsala and VanSant[13] used the cross-sectional approach to study toddlers as they rose to a standing position from the floor in a sample of 60 children aged 15 to 47 months. They classified movement patterns of the upper and lower extremities and trunk across different age groups. In this study, the investigators chose to examine the characteristics of a broad sample at one time, rather than follow a group over several years.

Developmental research provides an invaluable source of information for the production of correlational and experimental hypotheses. A foundation of descriptive data is needed for the generation of developmental theories and determination of which variables are most important for studying treatment effects. Cross-sectional data are most effective when the primary interest in a developmental study is the description of typical individuals at various stages of life or the description of existing groups in contemporary society. The cross-sectional method will provide a greater possibility of sampling large representative groups for such assessments. If, however, the primary interest is the study of patterns of change, the longitudinal method is preferred, as only this method can establish the validity of temporal sequencing of behaviors and characteristics.

Natural History

Longitudinal studies may focus on the **natural history** of disease states. This type of information is important in the future design of clinical trials and the generation of hypotheses about the etiology and progression of disease. For example, Godbolt and associates[14] documented the 10-year progression of symptoms of Alzheimer's disease in a familial cohort of 23 individuals, demonstrating the challenge of recording subtle early deficits and the later deterioration of spelling and naming. Howieson and co-workers[11] prospectively examined the occurrence and outcome of cognitive decline in healthy, community-dwelling elders. Ninety-five elders (mean age 84 years) who at entry had no cognitive impairments were followed for up to 13 years. Outcomes of aging were characterized as intact cognition, persistent cognitive decline without progression to dementia, and dementia.

In another example, Munsat and colleagues[15] followed 50 patients with amyotrophic lateral sclerosis (ALS) over 6 years, to document the rate and pattern of motor deterioration. They described a linear and symmetric rate of motor neuron loss (see Figure 14.1). Understanding the developmental nature of disease states is an important

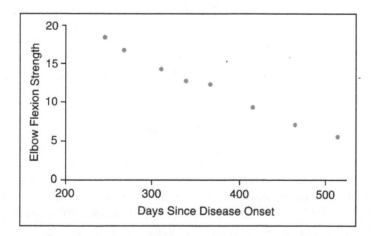

FIGURE 14.1 Composite measure of deterioration in upper extremity muscle strength for a patient with ALS, illustrating the natural history of the disease. (Adapted from Munsat TL, Andres PL, Finison L, et al. The natural history of motorneuron loss in amlyotrophic lateral sclerosis. *Neurol* 1988; 38:409–413, Figure 4, p. 412. Used with permission of the American Academy of Neurology.)

part of moving toward study of their management. For instance, the natural history data on ALS was used to generate hypotheses about specific drug interventions to slow the progression of the disease.[16-18] Without the natural history data, it would not have been possible to determine whether or not the drugs were effective.

NORMATIVE STUDIES

The utility of evaluative findings in the assessment of a patient's condition is based on the comparison of those findings with known standards of performance. For example, joint motion is compared with ranges "within normal limits,"[19] and nerve conduction velocities are interpreted with reference to "normal values."[20] Clinicians need these standards as a basis for documenting the existence and severity of weakness, limitations and patient problems as a guide for setting goals.

The purpose of **normative research** is to describe typical or standard values for characteristics of a given population. Normative studies are often directed toward a specific age group, gender, occupation, culture or disability. For example, researchers have established normative values for speech perception capacity in children aged 5 to 10 years;[21] the diagnosis of osteoporosis is based on "young normal" and "age-matched" norms;[22] age and sex-matched Constant scores have been developed as norms for shoulder function.[23,24]

Norms are usually expressed as an average, or mean, within a range of acceptable values. Therefore, the normal nerve conduction velocity of the ulnar nerve is expressed as 57.5 meters/sec, with a normal range of 49.5 to 63.6 m/s,[25] with corrections needed for limb temperature,[26] age and height.[27] The normal cadence of women walking in high heels is given as 117 steps/minute, with a range from 100 to 133 steps/minute.[28] Average values are often given with a standard deviation (see Chapter 17). Therefore, we can describe normal knee ranges for healthy adults during free speed walking as 60 ± 7 degrees.[29] Norms can also represent standardized scores that allow interpretation of responses with reference to an arbitrary "normal" value. For example, the Wechsler Intelligence Scales scores are "normed" against a mean of 100 and a standard deviation of 15.[30]

The importance of establishing the validity of normative values is obvious. The estimation of "normal" behavior or performance is often used as a basis for prescribing corrective intervention or for predicting future performance. If the interpretation of assessments and the consequent treatment plan are based on the extent of deviation from normal, the standard values must be valid reflections of this norm. Because no characteristics of a population can be adequately described by a single value, normal values are often established with reference to concomitant factors. For instance, several studies have established normative values for grip strength in children based on age and hand dominance.[31-33] Häger-Ross and Rösblad[34] studied 530 boys and girls aged 4 through 16, and found that there was no difference in grip strength between the genders until age 10, after which the boys were significantly stronger than the girls (see Figure 14.2). Another study established norms for 5–15 year olds based on age, gender and body composition.[35] Normative data for grip strength in adults[36] and older

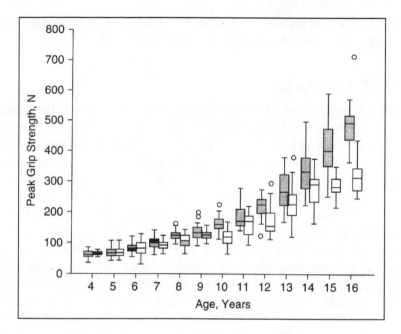

FIGURE 14.2   Box plots illustrating peak grip strength for boys (shaded boxes) and girls (white boxes) from 4 to 16 years of age. Each box represents the 25th–75th percentile, and the horizontal line across the box is the median (50th percentile). Whisker lines extending above and below each box indicate the total range. Small circles outside the whiskers indicate outliers (one 16-year-old male had practiced heavy weight lifting). (From Häger-Ross C, Rösblad B. Norms for grip strength in children aged 4–16 years. *Acta Paediatr* 2002; 91:617–625, Figure 2, p. 619. Used with permission of the Foundation Acta Paediatrica and Blackwell Publishing).

persons[37] is also distinguished by gender and level of fitness activity. These data provide a reference for making clinical decisions about the management of hand problems and for setting goals after hand injury or surgery.

There is still a substantial need for normative research in health-related sciences. As new measurement tools are developed, research is needed to establish standards for interpretation of their output. This is especially true in areas where a variety of instruments is used to measure the same clinical variables, such as balance, function and health status assessments. For example, norms have been published for health status instruments such as the SF-36 that help health care providers and clients assess health in several domains[38] and in different geographic populations.[39–41] It is also essential that these norms be established for a variety of diagnostic and age groups, so that appropriate standards can be applied in different clinical situations. For example, the functional reach test has been used extensively as a measure of stability in the elderly.[42] It has also been tested as a balance assessment for patients with spinal cord injury[43] and age-related normative values have been determined for children and adults without disabilities.[44,45]

Researchers should be aware of the great potential for sampling bias when striving to establish standard values. Samples for normative studies must be large, random and representative of the population's heterogeneity. The specific population of interest should be delineated as accurately as possible. Replication is essential to this form of research, to demonstrate consistency and, thereby, validate findings.

QUALITATIVE RESEARCH

Qualitative research paradigms offer a perspective to explore and understand human behavior that arises from a different philosophy than quantitative research designs. Quantitative methodology is linked to the philosophy of **logical positivism,** in which human experience is assumed to be limited to logical and controlled relationships between specific measurable variables. The rationale for studying these relationships can be defined in advance, based on hypotheses that guide the methods of inquiry. Accordingly, variables can be operationalized and assigned numerical values, independent of historical, cultural or social contexts within which performance is observed.[46] For example, many quality of life assessments, by virtue of their list of questions, are based on assumptions about measurable behaviors that reflect health status. By using a single rating scale for all subjects, investigators demonstrate the reductionist premise of quantitative research: that experience and clinical phenomena can be reduced to a set of specific questions and variables predetermined by the researcher.

The essence of the qualitative method, on the other hand, obliges the researcher to understand the person's perspective first. **Qualitative research** seeks to describe the complex nature of humans and how individuals perceive their own experiences within a specific social context. Qualitative methodology uses the subject's own words and narrative summaries of observable behavior to express data, rather than numerical data derived from predetermined rating systems. The qualitative approach emphasizes an understanding of human experience, exploring the nature of people's transactions with themselves, others and their surroundings. Qualitative designs and methods also allow the study of many simultaneous variables contained in a phenomenon. Questions that lend themselves to qualitative inquiry are generally broad, seeking to understand why something occurs, what certain experiences mean to a patient or client, or how the dynamics of an experience influence subsequent behaviors or decisions.[47]

For example, Carpenter[48] explored the experience of a spinal cord injury (SCI) with individuals who had sustained such an injury. This work demonstrated that the education about living with SCI provided by health care professionals did not match the lived experience of those with the injury, suggesting the need to transform educational approaches. The qualitative investigation into this phenomenon helped to uncover the meaning of SCI to those who experience it, and how it affects their behavior, emotions, body image, self-esteem and interactions. The purpose of qualitative inquiry is to examine such experiences using a holistic approach that is concerned with the true nature of "reality" as the participants understand it. Qualitative methodology has been a cornerstone of research in sociology and anthropology and has more recently received attention by clinical researchers.[49,50]

The need to understand the patient's view of the world is particularly important with the widespread adoption of principles of evidence-based practice, which compel the practitioner to consider the patient's values and circumstances in combination with clinical judgment and evidence from the literature. Qualitative designs are well suited to explore patients' preferences, giving practitioners the opportunity to understand the concepts of health, illness and disability from the direct perspective of the person who lives it.[51-53]

Combining Qualitative and Quantitative Approaches

Qualitative research is not just a description of a particular situation. To qualify as a research method, such inquiry must be tied to understanding, explaining, or developing theory about an observed phenomenon. From such insightful description, relevant variables can be uncovered, and questions can then be posed to study quantitative aspects of those variables in controlled settings. Qualitative and quantitative aspects can also be combined within one study to measure certain components of behavior and to see how such measurements relate to the nature of the actual experience.[54] Use of both qualitative and quantitative methods in the same study can increase the validity of the findings.[55]

For example, Tallon and colleagues[56] used a focus group of patients with osteoarthritis of the knee to design a questionnaire that exposed a mismatch between treatment priorities of patients and those of health care practitioners. Hayes et al[57] used both a descriptive questionnaire and qualitative interviews to better understand clinical instructors' perspectives of problematic student behaviors. Paterson et al[58] used both semi-structured interviews and standardized outcome tools to measure the outcomes of a program of massage in patients with Parkinson disease. The two approaches were used together to identify difficulties with the standardized tools and specific perceptions of the participants not available in those tools. Because of the richness of the combined data, the authors were able to recommend several very specific features for future research.

Perspectives in Qualitative Research

There are a number of different approaches one may take when using a qualitative research design. These include phenomenology, ethnography and grounded theory.[59] These methods are considered **naturalistic inquiry** because they require substantial observation and interaction with subjects in their own natural environment.

Phenomenology

The tradition known as **phenomenology** seeks to draw meaning from complex realities through careful analysis of first-person narrative materials.[60] The researcher begins this type of inquiry by identifying the clinical phenomenon to be studied. Illness, physical disability and childbirth are examples of phenomena that have been explored by health professionals. Within the phenomenological perspective, experience is constructed within the individual's social context and is, therefore, intersubjective.[61] As an example of this approach, DeGrace[62] studied the meaning of a family's experience of daily life with a child with severe autism. Her results showed that the family had difficulty engaging in daily activities that held positive meaning for them, and that they relied on stringent routines that revolved around the child to meet daily life demands.

In a phenomenological study in the workplace, Blau and colleagues[63] describe the responses of physical therapists to major changes in the healthcare system in which they practiced. They identified four common themes related to stress and discontentment, but also identified that participants were able to find positive affirmation in their work. In a similar study, Dale et al[64] investigated the influences of cost containment constraints on occupational therapists in a hand therapy clinic. They found that the therapists modified their skills, their professional settings, and implemented innovative interventions to function effectively.

Ethnography

A second common perspective, called **ethnography,** is the study of attitudes, beliefs and behaviors of a specific group of people within their own cultural milieu.[65] In ethnographic studies, the researcher becomes immersed in the subjects' way of life to understand the cultural forces that shape behavior and feelings. Questions often emerge as data are collected. The ethnographer begins this type of inquiry by identifying the setting or culture to be studied and may specify the types of phenomena that will be observed. Classic examples of ethnographic research are found in the well known anthropological works of Margaret Mead.[66,67]

This approach has been used to study the traditional beliefs and practices related to pregnancy and childbirth among Native American women.[68] Swigart and Kolb[69] interviewed sheltered and street-dwelling homeless persons to describe factors that influence their decisions to utilize or reject a public health disease-detection program. Wingate et al[70] studied the perceptions of activity and vocational status in women with cardiac illness. As these examples illustrate, the concept of culture in ethnographic research is taken broadly.

Qualitative research has also expanded to include the concept of research synthesis through the use of meta-ethnography. This approach uses analysis of multiple sources to develop new insights into the phenomenon being studied. For example, Smith et al[71] studied factors that delay a person's willingness to seek help for a potential cancer. Their synthesis of 32 papers was able to identify several factors that delay seeking help, including lack of recognition of the meaning of symptoms, fear, and gender of the patient.

Grounded Theory

One of the unique features of qualitative methodology is that it allows the researcher to develop theory to explain what is observed. This approach is called **grounded theory research,** in which the researcher collects, codes, and analyzes data simultaneously. This facilitates identification of relevant variables, and using an inductive process, identification of theoretical concepts that are "grounded" in the observations.[72] These concepts are not based on preconceived hypotheses, but instead grow out of an ongoing **constant comparative analysis** of each set of data collected. As data are gathered and coded, each idea or theme is compared to others to determine where they agree or conflict. At any point in the study, if data do not support the theory, the data are not discarded, but the theory is refined so that it fits the existing data; that is, the theory must come from the data.

As this process continues, interrelationships emerge that lead to the development of a theoretical framework. Data collection and analysis continues until data being collected become repetitious, affirming what has already been identified and no new concepts or relationships emerge. This method requires a sophisticated approach to coding and categorizing data.

A wonderful example of grounded theory research is found in the work of Jensen and colleagues,[73,74] who collected and analyzed data over a 10-year period to develop a theory of what constitutes expert practice in physical therapy. Working with recognized "experts" in a variety of specialty areas, they formulated a theoretical model with four dimensions, as shown in Figure 14.3. The theory suggests that these dimensions may exist in the novice practitioner, but not in an integrated manner. They propose that these elements become increasingly integrated as a therapist's competence and expertise grow, moving toward a well-developed philosophy of practice.

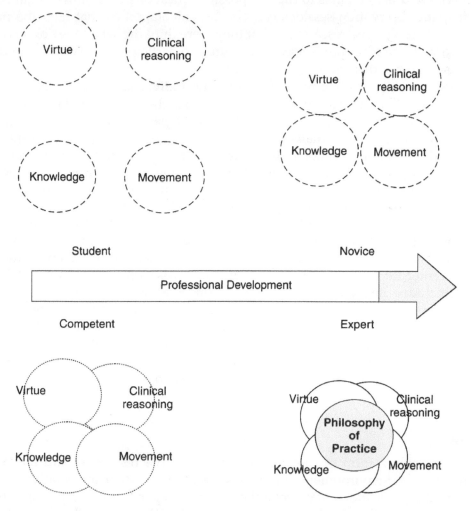

FIGURE 14.3   Model of core dimensions of expert practice in physical therapy. (From Jensen GM, Hack LM, Shepard KF. *Expertise in Physical Therapy Practice (2nd ed)*. Saunders, St. Louis, 2007, Figure 8-4, p. 168. Reprinted with permission of Saunders Elsevier.)

Methods of Qualitative Data Collection

Because qualitative data can come from a wide variety of sources and can take many different forms, the methods of data collection are also quite varied. The most common forms of data collection are observation and interviews.

Observation

Field observation of the phenomenon being studied is often conducted prior to interviews. The purpose of this observation is to identify people, interactions, the influence of sociocultural context and even artifacts that might be studied in depth to acquire relevant data to answer the research question. As a "nonparticipant" in the activities being monitored, the researcher quietly and as inconspicuously as possible simply observes. Immediately following the observation, the researcher records field notes about what was observed and uses memos to capture possible questions for follow-up interviews. Nonparticipant observation sessions can also be videotaped so that later the participants can discuss with the researcher what they were thinking while they observe their own behavior. This technique is used to capture the participant's reality while diminishing the sometimes distorting effects of recall.

The essence of qualitative research is that the individual's experience should be described as it is lived by that individual. Therefore, the researcher can also become embedded within the group, using the technique of **participant observation.** With this method, the researcher actually becomes a participant in the activities of the group being studied, so that observation of behaviors can be appreciated from the standpoint of those who are being observed. While this technique, as with other research techniques, is inherently biased by the researcher's own preconceptions, it does provide a mechanism to describe the interactions of individuals within a social context and to analyze behaviors as a function of the subjects' personal realities. The researcher is in a position to recognize feelings and thoughts that emerge from the subjects' frame of reference. For example, Hasselkus[75] studied the meaning of daily routines and activities at a day-care center for persons with Alzheimer disease, as experienced by the staff. Data collection included interviews and participant-observation, by working directly with the staff. Through this experience, the researcher determined that the foremost guiding principle for all activities during the day was prevention, that is, to prevent participant behavior that would be harmful to self or others. She was also able to identify characteristics of the staff's perception of a "good day" versus a "rough day." Participant-observer is a complex role, but one that is believed to enhance the validity of qualitative observations.[76]

Interviews

Interviews involve a form of direct contact between the researcher and the subjects within their natural environment. Interviews are used to gather information, with the researcher asking questions that probe the subject's experiences and perceptions. For example, Monninkhof and colleagues[77] interviewed patients with chronic obstructive pulmonary disease (COPD) in their homes. The data obtained was used to explain how and why standardized health related quality of life scales failed to capture accurately the patient's experience. Potter et al[78] used structured interviews and a nominal group technique to identify the kinds of patients perceived as difficult by physical therapists, as well as strategies for dealing with them. They identified behavioral problems and patient expectations as leading to the greatest difficulties, with improved communication as the primary strategy. Fogarty[79] used focus group interviews to identify the benefits of exercise for patients with schizophrenia who resided in a community care facility. In addition to reported gains in physical status, both staff and participants reported improvement in cohesion among residents and between residents and staff.

Interviews should be approached with a broadly structured script that will guide the discussion and provide a basis for comparing responses; however, they must also be flexible enough to allow the interviewer to probe and ask follow-up questions that are relevant to the specific individual's circumstances. For example, an interviewer might simply ask, "Tell me what it has been like for you to have a spinal cord injury? Such a question is usually followed by additional probes, such as "Can you tell me more about that?" and "Can you give me an example of _____?" to elicit the full richness and truth value of the data. This process requires that the interviewer have expertise in the subject matter that will be discussed. This should include prior observations of the participant in his or her natural setting so that the appropriate and relevant follow-up questions will be asked.

The quality of the data collected will depend on the knowledge and skill of the interviewer. Therefore, interviewers should be trained in both interviewing and observation skills, and must be sensitive to the issues that will be raised by respondents.[80] While interviews for qualitative research may seem similar to the clinical interview, it is important to remember a fundamental difference. Clinical interviews have as their primary focus to arrive at a diagnostic decision; qualitative interviews are designed to bring about a better understanding of the phenomenon from the participant's perspective.[81]

Data Analysis and Interpretation

Qualitative data analysis is primarily an inductive process, with a constant interplay between data that represent the reality of the study participants and theoretical conceptualization of that reality. Therefore, the process of analysis is ongoing as data are collected. Because observational and interview responses are recorded as narratives, qualitative data are typically voluminous. Data will usually be recorded through written memos or transcribed from audio or videotapes. The specific techniques of data analysis can vary from purely narrative descriptions of observations to creating a coding system from which categories can be developed, and in a systematic way, patterns or themes develop from the mass of information.[82]

Analysis of qualitative data by hand involves many hours of sifting through narratives, coding and organizing. There are computer programs that help the qualitative researcher manage the large amounts of data that are typically gathered. The available programs are user friendly and highly interactive and are designed to assist the researcher to record, store, index, cross-index, code, sort and interconnect text-based material.[83] There are also numerous programs available which are referred to as computer-assisted software. These are categorized into five main software families which reflect their primary function: text base managers, code programs, retrieval programs, code-based theory builders, and conceptual network builders.[84]

There is considerable debate in the field of qualitative research about the use of computer programs for data analysis. The debate focuses on the loss of intimacy with the data as well as issues of confidentiality and security of the participants. The key to researchers using these programs is to keep in mind that they are designed only to assist the researcher in managing the data, but not to analyze data, develop theory or draw conclusions about findings. It is of utmost importance that researchers not allow the computer program to direct the interpretive activity.[84]

Reliability and Validity

Reliability and validity are issues of concern in qualitative research just as they are in all types of research. For qualitative study, the concept of "measurement error" must be examined in terms of judgments rather than numerical equivalency.[85] Because the data sources are words rather than numbers, different terms and techniques are used to describe and determine the trustworthiness of the data. Lincoln and Guba[86] have suggested the terms "credibility" and "truth" to refer to internal validity, "transferability" to refer to external validity, and "consistency" and "dependability" to refer to reliability. They describe a number of techniques that can be used to increase credibility and consistency of qualitative data. Similar to techniques used in quantitative research, these approaches reflect a need to consider the rigor of data analysis and the potential for investigator bias.

Techniques for Ensuring Trustworthiness of Qualitative Data

Triangulation refers to a process whereby concepts are confirmed using more than one source of data, more than one data collection method, or more than one set of researchers. The concept actually originated as a technical term in surveying, to demonstrate how two visible points could be used to locate a third point. In social sciences, the concept has been adopted to reflect multiple methods or data sources to substantiate an outcome. For instance, a researcher may identify a specific concept through an interview, by direct observation of group performance, and by analysis of written materials. If comparable conclusions are drawn from each method, the internal validity or credibility of the interpretation is considerably strengthened. For example, Galantino and colleagues[87] demonstrated that use of exercise groups resulted in positive physical changes, enhanced coping and improved social interactions for a group of people living with HIV/AIDS. They supported the validity of their findings by showing common themes using focus groups, nonparticipant observation and journals.

The validity of findings can also be supported by a clear description and documentation of the thought processes used to interpret data. This process is referred to as an **audit trail,** allowing those who read the research to follow the investigator's logic. This provides an opportunity for others to agree or disagree with conclusions, and to reconstruct categorizations. In their study of therapists' reactions to changes in the health care system, Blau and colleagues[63] transcribed initial and follow-up interviews, used process notes, and other documentation of data reconstruction to carefully document their process of analysis.

Other strategies for improving accuracy include the involvement of more than one investigator to confirm ideas, confirmation of conclusions with the subject of the study through member checks, and analysis until data saturation (no new themes identified) is reached. For example, Jensen et al[73] used three non-physical therapist consultants to support their theoretical formulations. Blau et al[63] summarized the themes they extracted from their data and mailed them to participants several months later, interviewing them to validate their interpretations. These strategies are important to control for the potential bias in qualitative analysis.

Sampling

In qualitative research, subject selection proceeds in a purposeful way, as the investigator must locate subjects who will be effective informants, and who will provide a rich source of information.[88] Depending on the research question, the researcher may select one of many types of sampling strategies including typical, maximum variation or extreme. Another type of sampling, termed **theoretical sampling,** is based on the need to collect data to examine emerging categories and their relationships, and not on identifying specific age, gender or other characteristics of subjects.[89] In this type of sampling, a few subjects are initially chosen because they belong to a certain group, but further subjects are recruited based on their fit with theory that emerges from the initial data.[90]

A common misconception about sampling in qualitative research is that all samples are small. Sample size remains an important consideration. Samples that are too small will not support claims of having reached a point of saturation in the data. Samples that are too large will not permit the in-depth analysis that is the essence of qualitative inquiry. Sandelowski[91] suggests that determining adequate sample size in qualitative research is a matter of judgment and experience in evaluating the quality of the information collected and the purpose of the research.

We recognize that this brief introduction to qualitative analysis is by no means sufficient to demonstrate the scope of data collection and analysis methods that have been developed. This approach has great promise for generating understanding of health and how it is evaluated. Those interested in pursuing qualitative research are urged to read the references cited in this chapter. We also suggest reading professional literature, such as the journal *Qualitative Health Research*, to gain an appreciation for the breadth of qualitative research and to develop familiarity with the techniques and terminology of qualitative methodology.

DESCRIPTIVE SURVEYS

Surveys are often used as a source of data to collect information about a specific group, to describe their characteristics or risk factors for disease or dysfunction. These types of studies are generally focused on a particular issue or aspect of the group's behaviors or attitudes. The purpose of this approach is to provide an overall picture of the group's characteristics, but may involve some correlational interpretations regarding association among certain variables. As an example, Jensen and co-workers[92] used a survey to examine the nature and scope of pain in persons with neuromuscular disorders. They demonstrated that, while pain is a common problem in this population, there are some important differences between diagnostic groups in the nature and scope of pain and its impact. In another example, Miller et al[93] described the most prevalent disorders of older adults that were seen by physical therapists, and compared these across several regions of the United States. Giesbrecht[94] surveyed occupational therapists in 75 facilities across Canada to describe risk assessment tools, referral patterns and interventions related to management of pressure ulcers. We will discuss the design of surveys in Chapter 15.

CASE STUDIES

Clinicians and researchers have long recognized the importance of the **case study** or **case report** for developing a clinical knowledge base. A description of interesting, new and unique cases is necessary to build a foundation for clinical science and as a means of sharing special information among professional colleagues. Typically, case studies involve the in-depth description of an individual's condition or response to treatment; however, case studies can also focus on a group, institution, or other social unit, such as a particular school, healthcare setting, community or family. A **case series** is an expansion of a case study involving observations in several similar cases.

Purposes of Case Studies

Perhaps the greatest advantage of the case study as a form of clinical investigation is that it provides an opportunity for understanding the totality of an individual's condition outcomes of care. Rather than simply recording behavior, the depth of the case study allows the researcher to explore the subject's condition, emotions, thoughts, and past and present activities as they relate to the focus of the study. The researcher tries to determine which variables might be important to the subject's development or behavior, in an effort to understand why the subject responds or changes in a particular way, or why certain outcomes were achieved and others were not. The case study becomes a valuable source of information for evidence-based practice because it shares important aspects of clinicians' experiences with different patients. Case studies can serve several purposes.

Understanding Unusual Patient Conditions

Clinical case studies often emphasize unusual patient problems or diagnoses that present interesting clinical challenges. For instance, Gann and Nalty[95] highlighted the unusual diagnosis of a patient with a vertical patellar dislocation. The case was remarkable because the injury occurred without trauma. The authors documented their findings as a contribution to understanding mechanisms of patellar injury. As another example, Herrera and Stubblefield[96] reported on a case series of eight patients with rotator cuff tendonitis as an unusual complication of lymphedema, and discussed the possible etiology and treatment options.

Sometimes unique situations offer perspectives to support the implementation of guidelines for patient care. Laursen et al[97] report on a case of a 27-year-old male who suffered from acute delusional psychotic disorder and severe physical agitation. Following a period of physical restraint, the patient was diagnosed with bilateral deep venous thrombosis (DVT). The case report suggests an association between the occurrence of DVT and the immobilization by physical restraint in the absence of pre-existing risk factors. The authors used this case report as a forum to recommend that medical guidelines for prevention of DVT be considered when physical restraint is necessary in this patient population.

Providing Examples of Innovative or Creative Therapies

Case studies may focus on innovative approaches to treatment. For example, Sullivan and Hedman[98] reported on the use of a home program with electrical stimulation as an effective therapy for upper extremity tasks in the case of a patient 5 years after stroke. MacLachan et al[99] described the first case of the successful use of "mirror treatment" in a person with a lower limb amputation to treat phantom limb pain. They demonstrated that this approach, which had been successful with upper extremity amputation, was equally effective for improving lower extremity phantom pain.

Changes in technology provide an excellent opportunity to demonstrate resourceful approaches to patient care. For instance, Gillen[100] described a combination of occupational therapy interventions to improve mobility of a man with multiple sclerosis whose impairments included ataxia, and decreased strength and endurance. Through the use of assistive technology, positioning, orthotic prescription and adaptation of movement patterns, she observed improved postural stability and independent control of a power wheelchair. Case studies like this one allow clinicians to disseminate creative ideas that can contribute to successful patient outcomes.

Schuman and Abrahm[101] illustrate the use of the case study approach in describing implementation of educational and consensus-building strategies to engage hospital staff in providing palliative sedation for patients in intractable pain at the end of life. In this case, the unit of concern was not an individual patient, but a team of clinicians responsible for making decisions and administering pain management, including nurses, physicians and pharmacists, as well as family members. The focus of the case study was on the course of institutional change, using several patient histories to demonstrate the process. Descriptive case studies can be extremely useful for understanding institutional culture and change.

Generating and Testing Theory

Treatment and diagnostic decisions frequently require reference to theory in the absence of more direct evidence. Case studies are especially helpful for demonstrating how clinical theories can be applied. For example, Rosenbaum and co-workers[102] describe the case of a man who experienced widespread brain damage in a motor cycle accident 20 years earlier, and who has been followed because of his unusual memory impairment. The researchers have documented how this patient's experiences contribute to several aspects of memory theory, including understanding episodic and semantic memory, and the distinction between implicit and explicit memory.

Case studies can also offer insight into existing theories, providing opportunities to confirm or challenge specific hypotheses. For instance, Lott et al[103] used the physical stress theory (described in Chapter 2) to explain the effect of weight-bearing activities on healing of foot ulcers in a 66-year-old man with a history of diabetes. They accounted for the recurrence of ulcers based on cumulative plantar stresses that occurred with a rapid change in the patient's walking patterns after initial healing.

Providing Future Research Directives

Although case studies focus on the details of individual patients, the results can often highlight issues that require further inquiry, providing a rich source of research questions. One major contribution of the case study to research is its ability to provide information that can be used to generate inductive hypotheses. Because the case study allows for a thorough analysis of a single situation, it often leads to the discovery of relationships that were not obvious before. As more and more cases are reported, a form of "case law" gradually develops, whereby empirical findings are considered reasonable within the realm of accepted knowledge and professional experience.[104] Eventually, with successive documented cases, a conceptual framework forms, providing a basis for categorizing patients and for generating hypotheses that can be tested using exploratory or experimental methods.

As an example, Reinthal et al[105] examined the effectiveness of a postural control program in an adolescent who had problems walking and talking simultaneously following traumatic brain injury. They hypothesized that her difficulty was due to excessive co-activation of trunk, extremity and oral musculature. Following 2 years of speech and physical therapy, the patient was able to significantly improve her ability to communicate intelligibly while walking. The results of treatment suggested that improved postural control allowed less rigid compensation of oral musculature, allowing her to speak. This hypothesis can now be tested in other patients or under different conditions.

Format of a Case Study

A clinical case study is an intensive investigation designed to analyze and understand those factors important to the etiology, care and outcome of the subject's problems. It is a comprehensive description of the subject's background, present status, and responses to intervention.

A case study may begin with an introduction that describes background literature on the patient problem. Theoretical or epidemiologic information is often helpful to understand the scope and context of the disorder. A full history of the patient is then provided, delineating problems, symptoms, and prior treatments, as well as demographic and social factors that are pertinent to the subject's care and prognosis. Authors sometimes include photographs (with the patient's permission) to illustrate a patient's condition.

A section on methods presents elements of the treatment plan. Expectations should be presented as justification for the treatment approach chosen.[104] Where relevant, literature should be cited to support the rationale for treatment and interpretation of outcomes. If special assessments are used, they should be described in functional detail. Some case studies are actually geared to describing the applicability of new or unusual assessment instruments for diagnosing certain problems.

A results section will include the subject's responses and any follow-up data. When appropriate, tables or graphic presentation of data may be useful to explain the patient's progress. The discussion section of the report provides interpretation of outcomes and conclusions, including reference to research and other clinical information that may support or challenge the current findings. This section should include discussion of unique or special considerations in the patient's condition or responses that may explain unexpected outcomes, or that may distinguish the patient from others with the same condition. Finally, the author of a case study should present questions for further study, suggesting where the case study's findings may lead.

Generalizability of Case Studies

The case study is probably the most practical approach to research because of its direct applicability to patient care, but it is also the least rigorous approach because of its inherent lack of control and limited generalizability. The interaction of environmental and personal characteristics and the effect of multiple interventions make the case study weak in internal validity. Generalization from one case to a larger population is also limited because the responses of one individual or social unit may bear little resemblance to those of others in similar circumstances. In addition, case studies are often concerned with exceptional situations or rare disorders, and subjects are generally not representative of the "typical" patient seen in the clinic. Therefore, external validity is also limited.

The validity of inferences from a case study can be enhanced, however, by taking steps to objectify treatment effects and to demonstrate them under different conditions.[106,107] For instance, interpretations can be made stronger by direct quantified observation and by taking repeated measurements over the course of treatment. Treatment effects can be further supported by using multiple dependent variables and by choosing outcome measures that show large and immediate changes. Generalization can be enhanced by documenting the subject's behavior in more than one setting and by including information from the follow-up visit to establish the long-range success of treatment. Literature should be used to demonstrate how results support a particular theoretical approach to treatment. When validity is an important issue to demonstrate the effect of intervention, a single-subject design should be considered.

Case Reports in Epidemiology

An **epidemiologic case report** is a description of one or more individuals, documenting a unique or unusual occurrence or medical condition. The purpose of the case report is to present as complete a picture as possible about the characteristics of, and exposures faced by, that individual, often resulting in the presentation of a hypothesis about the causal factors that might account for the observed outcome. Many notable examples of this approach exist, such as the original report of a patient with unique dementia characteristics by Alzheimer in 1905;[108] the single case report in 1961 of a 40-year-old pre-menopausal woman who developed a pulmonary embolism 5 weeks after starting to use oral contraceptives;[109] and a series of reports documenting the first cases of AIDS in five young previously healthy homosexual males in Los Angeles.[110] These cases led to the formulation of important analytic hypotheses that have since been tested and supported.

In a more recent example, Jeong and coworkers[111] documented the first report of a "floating total knee," which resulted from fractures of the distal femur and proximal tibia after a total knee arthroplasty. The patient was an 80-year-old man with rheumatoid arthritis who fell in his home 3 years after the original procedure. The report described surgical revision of the joint replacement and postoperative follow-up. Given that periprosthetic fractures are rare following knee replacement, the authors used this case to discuss risk factors related to the patient and surgical technique. They described their choice of treatment options and successful short-term outcomes. This type of case report provides important information that can be used to minimize future risks and to prompt further study.

As is true with clinical case reports, case studies in epidemiology do not provide sufficient control to allow for generalizations or conclusions about causality. They can only act as a catalyst for further study; however, as the preceding examples illustrate, case reports can be vitally important for identifying new health hazards and facilitating further analytic research.

COMMENTARY

First Things First

The purpose of descriptive research is to characterize phenomena so that we know what *exists*. Without this fundamental knowledge, it would be impossible to ask questions about behaviors or treatment effects or to propose theories to explain them. This approach is clearly contrasted with traditional experimental research, which seeks to determine what *will* happen in a given set of controlled circumstances.

Although descriptive studies do not strive for the degree of control found in experimental studies, descriptive research serves an important role within the spectrum of research designs. The state of knowledge in the rehabilitation professions in relatively immature, and we still face the need to define clinical behaviors so that we can begin to explore them. Just like a child must learn to crawl before it can walk, clinical scientists must first discover how the world around them naturally behaves before they can manipulate and control those behaviors to test methods of changing them.

Despite the fact that descriptive studies do not involve manipulation of variables or randomization, descriptive research still requires rigor in defining and measuring variables of interest, whether they emerge as narrative descriptions or quantitative summaries. Unfortunately, there is a tendency to view conclusions from descriptive studies as weaker than conclusions from experimental studies, but this is only true in the context of establishing cause-and-effect relationships. Descriptive findings can be strong and meaningful as a basis for explanation and characterization of variables when they are the result of a well designed study and when they are interpreted within the context of an appropriate research question. The results of descriptive studies may provide essential evidence for understanding the benefits of clinical trials, and for describing or explaining why some subjects respond differently than others.

Experimental designs will not necessarily be "better" if the research question focuses on the development of understanding of clinical phenomena or if the study variables represent constructs that are poorly developed. With so many behavioral and clinical concepts not yet fully understood, descriptive research presents an extraordinary and vital challenge to the clinical researcher.

REFERENCES

1. Calancie B, Molano MR, Broton JG. Epidemiology and demography of acute spinal cord injury in a large urban setting. *J Spinal Cord Med* 2005;28:92–96.
2. Shimada SD, Robertson RN, Bonninger ML, Cooper RA. Kinematic characterization of wheelchair propulsion. *J Rehabil Res Dev* 1998;35:210–218.
3. Rathore SS, Hinn AR, Cooper LS, Tyroler HA, Rosamond WD. Characterization of incident stroke signs and symptoms: Findings from the atherosclerosis risk in communities study. *Stroke* 2002;33:2718–2721.
4. Gesell A, Amatruda CS. *The Embryology of Behavior*. New York: Harper & Brothers, 1945.
5. McGraw MB. *The Neuromuscular Maturation of the Human Infant*. New York: Hafner, 1963.
6. Erikson EH. *Childhood and Society* (2nd ed.). New York: Norton, 1963.
7. Tanner JM. Physical growth. In PH Mussen (ed.), *Carmichael's Manual of Child Psychology* (3rd ed). New York: Wiley, 1970.
8. Honzik MP, MacFarland JW, Allen L. The stability of mental test performance between two and eighteen years. *J Exp Educ* 1949;17:309.
9. Horn JL, Donaldson G. Cognitive development: II. Adulthood development of human abilities. In OG Brim, J Kagan (Eds.), *Constancy and change in Human Development*. Cambridge, MA: Harvard University Press, 1980.
10. Hogan R, Roberts BW. A socioanalytic model of maturity. *Career Assess* 2004;12:207–217.
11. Howieson DB, Camicioli R, Quinn J, Silbert LC, Care B, Moore MM, et al. Natural history of cognitive decline in the old old. *Neurology* 2003;60:1489–1494.
12. Freier MC, Babikian T, Pivonka J, Burley Aaen T, Gardner JM, Baum M, et al. A longitudinal perspective on neurodevelopmental outcome after infant cardiac transplantation. *J Heart Lung Transplant* 2004;23:857–864.
13. Marsala G, VanSant AF. Age-related differences in movement patterns used by toddlers to rise from a supine position to erect stance. *Phys Ther* 1998;78:149–159.
14. Godbolt AK, Cipolotti L, Watt H, Fox NC, Janssen JC, Rossor MN. The natural history of Alzheimer disease: A longitudinal presymptomatic and symptomatic study of a familial cohort. *Arch Neurol* 2004;61:1743–1748.
15. Munsat TL, Andres PL, Finison L, Conlon T, Thibodeau L. The natural history of motoneuron loss in amyotrophic lateral sclerosis. *Neurology* 1988;38:409–413.
16. Munsat TL, Taft J, Jackson IM, Andres PL, Hollander D, Skerry L, et al. Intrathecal thyrotropin-releasing hormone does not alter the progressive course of ALS: Experience with an intrathecal drug delivery system. *Neurology* 1992;42:1049–1053.
17. Miller RG, Bouchard JP, Duquette P, Eisen A, Gelinas D, Harati Y, et al. Clinical trials of riluzole in patients with ALS. ALS/Riluzole Study Group-II. *Neurology* 1996;47:S86–90; discussion S90–92.

18. Riviere M, Meininger V, Zeisser P, Munsat T. An analysis of extended survival in patients with amyotrophic lateral sclerosis treated with riluzole. *Arch Neurol* 1998;55: 526–528.

19. Norkin CC, White DJ. *Measurement of Joint Motion: A Guide to Goniometry* (3rd ed.). Philadelphia: FA Davis, 2003.

20. Delisa JA, Lee HJ, Baran EM, Lai K. *Manual of Nerve Conduction Velocity and Clinical Neurophysiology* (3rd ed.). New York: Raven Press, 1994.

21. Hnath-Chisolm TE, Laipply E, Boothroyd A. Age-related changes on a children's test of sensory-level speech perception capacity. *J Speech Lang Hear Res* 1998;41:94–106.

22. Lewiecki EM, Watts NB, McClung MR, Petak SM, Bachrach LK, Shepherd JA, et al. Official positions of the international society for clinical densitometry. *J Clin Endocrinol Metab* 2004;89:3651–3655.

23. Constant CR, Murley AH. A clinical method of functional assessment of the shoulder. *Clin Orthop Relat Res* 1987:160–164.

24. Yian EH, Ramappa AJ, Arneberg O, Gerber C. The Constant score in normal shoulders. *J Shoulder Elbow Surg* 2005;14:128–133.

25. McQuillen MP, Gorin FJ. Serial ulnar nerve conduction velocity measurements in normal subjects. *J Neurol Neurosurg Psychiatry* 1969;32:144–148.

26. Nelson R, Agro J, Lugo J, Gasiewska E, Kaur H, Muniz E, et al. The relationship between temperature and neuronal characteristics. *Electromyogr Clin Neurophysiol* 2004;44:209–216.

27. Rivner MH, Swift TR, Malik K. Influence of age and height on nerve conduction. *Muscle Nerve* 2001;24:1134–1141.

28. Murray MP, Kory RC, Sepic SB. Walking pattern of normal women. *Arch Phys Med Rehabil* 1970;51:637.

29. Brinkmann JR, Perry J. Rate and range of knee motion during ambulation in healthy and arthritic subjects. *Phys Ther* 1985;65:1055–1060.

30. Maddox T. *Tests: A Comprehensive Reference for Assessment in Psychology, Education and Business* (5th ed.). Austin, TX: Pro-Ed, 2001.

31. Lee-Valkov PM, Aaron DH, Eladoumikdachi F, Thornby J, Netscher DT. Measuring normal hand dexterity values in normal 3-, 4-, and 5-year-old children and their relationship with grip and pinch strength. *J Hand Ther* 2003;16:22–28.

32. Beasley BW, Woolley DC. Evidence-based medicine knowledge, attitudes, and skills of community faculty. *J Gen Intern Med* 2002;17:632–639.

33. Surrey LR, Hodson J, Robinson E, Schmidt S, Schulhof J, Stoll L, et al. Pinch strength norms for 5- to 12-year-olds. *Phys Occup Ther Pediatr* 2001;21:37–49.

34. Hager-Ross C, Rosblad B. Norms for grip strength in children aged 4–16 years. *Acta Paediatr* 2002;91:617–625.

35. Sartorio A, Lafortuna CL, Pogliaghi S, Trecate L. The impact of gender, body dimension and body composition on hand-grip strength in healthy children. *J Endocrinol Invest* 2002;25:431–435.

36. Hanten WP, Chen WY, Austin AA, Brooks RE, Carter HC, Law CA, et al. Maximum grip strength in normal subjects from 20 to 64 years of age. *J Hand Ther* 1999;12:193–200.

37. Horowitz BP, Tollin R, Cassidy G. Grip strength: Collection of normative data with community dwelling elders. *Phys Occup Ther Geriatr* 1997;15:53–64.

38. Ware JEJ, Snow KK, Kosinski M, et al. *SF-36 Survey: Manual and Interpretation Guide*. Boston: The Health Institute, New England Medical Center, 1993.

39. Hopman WM, Towheed T, Anastassiades T, Tenenhouse A, Poliquin S, Berger C, et al. Canadian normative data for the SF-36 health survey. Canadian Multicentre Osteoporosis Study Research Group. *CMAJ* 2000;163:265–271.

40. Loge JH, Kaasa S. Short form 36 (SF-36) health survey: Normative data from the general Norwegian population. *Scand J Soc Med* 1998;26:250–258.
41. Blake C, Codd MB, O'Meara YM. The Short Form 36 (SF-36) Health Survey: Normative data for the Irish population. *Ir J Med Sci* 2000;169:195–200.
42. Duncan PW, Weiner DK, Chandler J, Studenski S. Functional reach: A new clinical measure of balance. *J Gerontol* 1990;45:M192–197.
43. Lynch SM, Leahy P, Barker SP. Reliability of measurements obtained with a modified functional reach test in subjects with spinal cord injury. *Phys Ther* 1998;78:128–133.
44. Isles RC, Choy NL, Steer M, Nitz JC. Normal values of balance tests in women aged 20–80. *J Am Geriatr Soc* 2004;52:1367–1372.
45. Donahoe B, Turner D, Worrell T. The use of functional reach as a measurement of balance in boys and girls without disabilities ages 5 to 15 years. *Ped Phys Ther* 1994;6: 189–193.
46. Leininger MM. *Qualitative Research Methods in Nursing.* Orlando, FL: Grune & Stratton, 1985.
47. Sofaer S. Qualitative methods: What are they and why use them? *Health Serv Res* 1999;34:1101–1118.
48. Carpenter C. The experience of spinal cord injury: The individual's perspective— Implications for rehabilitation practice. *Phys Ther* 1994;74:614–628.
49. Hammell KW, Carpenter C. *Qualitative Research in Evidence-Based Rehabilitation.* Philadelphia: Churchill Livingston, 2004.
50. Morse JM, Swanson MN, Kuzel A. *The Nature of Qualitative Evidence.* Thousand Oaks, CA: Sage, 2001.
51. Downing AM, Hunter DG. Validating clinical reasoning: A question of perspective, but whose perspective? *Man Ther* 2003;8:117–119.
52. Johnson R, Waterfield J. Making words count: The value of qualitative research. *Physiother Res Int* 2004;9:121–131.
53. Swinkels A, Albarran JW, Means RI, Mitchell T, Stewart MC. Evidence-based practice in health and social care: Where are we now? *J Interprof Care* 2002;16:335–347.
54. Goering PN, Streiner DL. Reconcilable differences: The marriage of qualitative and quantitative methods. *Can J Psychiatry* 1996;41:491–497.
55. Morgan DL. Practical strategies for combining qualitative and quantitative methods: Applications to health research. *Qual Health Res* 1998;8:362–376.
56. Tallon D, Chard J, Dieppe P. Exploring the priorities of patients with osteoarthritis of the knee. *Arthritis Care Res* 2000;13:312–319.
57. Hayes KW, Huber G, Rogers J, Sanders B. Behaviors that cause clinical instructors to question the clinical competence of physical therapist students. *Phys Ther* 1999;79: 653–667.
58. Paterson C, Allen JA, Browning M, Barlow G, Ewings P. A pilot study of therapeutic massage for people with Parkinson's disease: The added value of user involvement. *Complement Ther Clin Pract* 2005;11:161–171.
59. Creswell JW. *Qualitative Inquiry and Research Design: Choosing Among Five Traditions.* Thousand Oaks, CA: Sage, 1998.
60. Moustakas C. *Phenomenological Research Methods.* Thousand Oaks, CA: Sage, 1994.
61. Gubrium JF, Holstein JA. Analyzing interpretive practice. In N Denzin, Y Lincoln (Eds.), *Handbook of Qualitative Research* (2nd ed.). Thousand Oaks, CA: Sage, 2000.
62. DeGrace BW. The everyday occupation of families with children with autism. *Am J Occup Ther* 2004;58:543–550.
63. Blau R, Bolus S, Carolan T, Kramer D, Mahoney E, Jette DU, et al. The experience of providing physical therapy in a changing health care environment. *Phys Ther* 2002;82: 648–657.

64. Dale LM, Fabrizio AJ, Adhlakha P, Mahon MK, McGraw EE, Neyenhaus RD, et al. Occupational therapists working in hand therapy: The practice of holism in a cost containment environment. *Work* 2002;19:35–45.

65. Fetterman DM. *Ethnography: Step by Step*. Newbury Park, CA: Sage, 1989.

66. Mead M. *Coming of Age in Samoa*. New York: Morrow, 1928.

67. Mead M. Ethnological aspects of aging. *Psychosomatics* 1967;8:Suppl:33–37.

68. Long CR, Curry MA. Living in two worlds: Native American women and prenatal care. *Health Care Women Int* 1998;19:205–215.

69. Swigart V, Kolb R. Homeless persons' decisions to accept or reject public health disease-detection services. *Public Health Nurs* 2004;21:162–170.

70. Wingate S, Loscalzo F, Hozdic T. Perceptions of activity and vocational status in women with cardiac illness. *Prog Cardiovasc Nurs* 2003;18:127–133,146.

71. Smith LK, Pope C, Botha JL. Patients' help-seeking experiences and delay in cancer presentation: A qualitative synthesis. *Lancet* 2005;366:825–831.

72. Strauss A, Corbin J. *Basics of Qualitative Research: Grounded Theory Procedures and Techniques*. Thousand Oaks, CA: Sage, 1990.

73. Jensen GM, Gwyer J, Shepard KF. Expert practice in physical therapy. *Phys Ther* 2000;80:28-43; discussion 44–52.

74. Jensen GM, Gwyer JA, Hack LM, Shepard KF. *Expertise in Physical Therapy Practice* (2nd ed.). St. Louis: Saunders Elsevier, 2007.

75. Hasselkus BR. The meaning of activity: Day care for persons with Alzheimer disease. *Am J Occup Ther* 1992;46:199–206.

76. Kielhofner G. Qualitative research: Part two. Methodological approaches and relevance to occupational therapy. *Occup Ther J Res* 1982;2:150–164.

77. Monninkhof E, van der Aa M, van der Valk P, van der Palen J, Zielhuis G, Koning K, et al. A qualitative evaluation of a comprehensive self-management programme for COPD patients: Effectiveness from the patients' perspective. *Patient Educ Couns* 2004; 55:177–184.

78. Potter M, Gordon S, Hamer P. The difficult patient in private practice physiotherapy: A qualitative study. *Aust J Physiother* 2003;49:53–61.

79. Fogarty M, Happell B. Exploring the benefits of an exercise program for people with schizophrenia: A qualitative study. *Issues Ment Health Nurs* 2005;26:341–351.

80. Patton MQ. *Qualitative Research and Evaluation Methods* (3rd ed.). Thousand Oaks, CA: Sage, 2002.

81. Britten N. Qualitative interviews in medical research. *Bmj* 1995;311:251–253.

82. Santasier AM. Factors That Influenced Individuals from Ethnically Diverse Groups to Become Physical Therapists. Dissertation. Temple University, 2004.

83. Denzin N, Lincoln Y. *Handbook of Qualitative Research* (2nd ed.). Thousand Oaks, CA: Sage, 2000.

84. Weitzman EA, Miles MB. *Computer Programs for Qualitative Data Analysis*. Thousand Oaks, CA: Sage, 1995.

85. Brink PJ. Issues in reliability and validity. In JM Morse (Ed.), *Qualitative Nursing Research: A Contemporary Dialogue*. Rockville, MD: Aspen, 1989:151–168.

86. Lincoln YS, Guba EG. *Naturalistic Inquiry*. Newbury Park, CA: Sage, 1985.

87. Galantino ML, Shepard K, Krafft L, Laperriere A, Ducette J, Sorbello A, et al. The effect of group aerobic exercise and t'ai chi on functional outcomes and quality of life for persons living with acquired immunodeficiency syndrome. *J Altern Complement Med* 2005;11:1085–1092.

88. Patton MQ. *Qualitative Evaluation and Research Methods* (2nd ed.). Newbury Park, CA: Sage, 1990.

89. Chenitz WC, Swanson JM. *From Practice to Grounded Theory: Qualitative Research in Nursing.* Menlo Park, CA: Addison-Wesley, 1986.

90. Coyne IT. Sampling in qualitative research. Purposeful and theoretical sampling; Merging or clear boundaries? *J Adv Nurs* 1997;26:623–630.

91. Sandelowski M. Sample size in qualitative research. *Res Nurs Health* 1995;18:179–183.

92. Jensen MP, Abresch RT, Carter GT, McDonald CM. Chronic pain in persons with neuromuscular disease. *Arch Phys Med Rehabil* 2005;86:1155–1163.

93. Miller EW, Ross K, Grant S, Musenbrock D. Geriatric referral patterns for physical therapy: A descriptive analysis. *J Geriatr Phys Ther* 2005;28:20–27.

94. Giesbrecht E. Pressure ulcers and occupational therapy practice: A Canadian perspective. *Can J Occup Ther* 2006;73:56–63.

95. Gann N, Nalty T. Vertical patellar dislocation: A case report. *J Orthop Sports Phys Ther* 1998;27:368–370.

96. Herrera JE, Stubblefield MD. Rotator cuff tendonitis in lymphedema: A retrospective case series. *Arch Phys Med Rehabil* 2004;85:1939–1942.

97. Laursen SB, Jensen TN, Bolwig T, Olsen NV. Deep venous thrombosis and pulmonary embolism following physical restraint. *Acta Psychiatr Scand* 2005;111:324–327.

98. Sullivan JE, Hedman LD. A home program of sensory and neuromuscular electrical stimulation with upper-limb task practice in a patient 5 years after a stroke. *Phys Ther* 2004;84:1045–1054.

99. MacLachlan M, McDonald D, Waloch J. Mirror treatment of lower limb phantom pain: A case study. *Disabil Rehabil* 2004;26:901–904.

100. Gillen G. Improving mobility and community access in an adult with ataxia. *Am J Occup Ther* 2002;56:462–466.

101. Schuman ZD, Abrahm JL. Implementing institutional change: An institutional case study of palliative sedation. *J Palliat Med* 2005;8:666–676.

102. Rosenbaum RS, Kohler S, Schacter DL, Moscovitch M, Westmacott R, Black SE, et al. The case of KC: Contributions of a memory-impaired person to memory theory. *Neuropsychologia* 2005;43:989–1021.

103. Lott DJ, Maluf KS, Sinacore DR, Mueller MJ. Relationship between changes in activity and plantar ulcer recurrence in a patient with diabetes mellitus. *Phys Ther* 2005;85:579–588.

104. Bromley DB. *A Case-Study Method in Psychology and Related Disciplines.* New York: John Wiley, 1986.

105. Reinthal AK, Mansour LM, Greenwald G. Improved ambulation and speech production in an adolescent post-traumatic brain injury through a therapeutic intervention to increase postural control. *Pediatr Rehabil* 2004;7:37–49.

106. Kazdin AE. Drawing valid inferences from case studies. *J Consult Clin Psychol* 1981;49:183–192.

107. Kratochwill RT, Mott SE, Dodson CL. Case study and single-case research in clinical and applied psychology. In AS Bellack, M Hersen (Eds.). *Research Methodology in Clinical Psychology.* New York: Pergamon Press, 1984.

108. Alzheimer A, Stelzmann RA, Schnitzlein HN, Murtagh FR. An English translation of Alzheimer's 1907 paper, "Uber eine eigenartige Erkankung der Hirnrinde." *Clin Anat* 1995;8:429–431.

109. Jordan WM. Pulmonary embolism. *Lancet* 1961;2:1146–1147.

110. Centers for Disease Control. Pneumocystis pneumonia—Los Angeles. *MMWR* 1981;30:250.

111. Jeong GK, Pettrone SK, Liporace FA, Meere PA. "Floating total knee": Ipsilateral periprosthetic fractures of the distal femur and proximal tibia after total knee arthroplasty. *J Arthroplasty* 2006;21:138–140.

CHAPTER 15
Surveys and Questionnaires

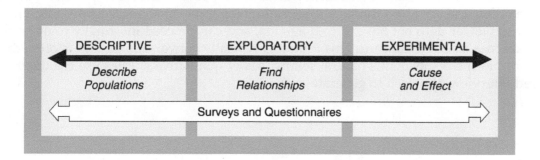

DESCRIPTIVE	EXPLORATORY	EXPERIMENTAL
Describe Populations	Find Relationships	Cause and Effect

Surveys and Questionnaires

One of the most popular methods for collecting descriptive or subjective data is the survey approach. A survey is composed of a series of questions that are posed to a group of subjects, and may be conducted as an oral interview or as a written or electronic questionnaire. Sometimes the data are intended for generalization to a larger population; other times they may be intended as a description of a particular group. Surveys in clinical research are often concerned with describing current practices, attitudes and values, or characteristics of specific groups. For example, survey questionnaires have been used to compare the effectiveness of medication, acupuncture and spinal manipulation for chronic low back pain,[1] to study physicians' attitudes and practices toward disclosure of prognosis for terminally ill patients,[2] and to describe the demographics and injury characteristics of patients with spinal cord injury.[3] Standardized questionnaires are also used extensively as instruments for assessing outcomes related to function, health status and quality of life. As these examples illustrate, survey data can be used in experimental, exploratory or descriptive studies.

The purpose of this chapter is to present an overview of the structure of survey instruments. We discuss essential elements of survey design, question writing, and some special assessment techniques associated with questionnaires, including several measurement scales.

INTERVIEWS AND QUESTIONNAIRES

Interviews

In an **interview** the researcher asks respondents specific questions and records their answers for later analysis. Interviews can take a few minutes or several hours, depending on the nature of the questions and the respondent's willingness to share information. Interviews can be conducted face to face or over the telephone, although face-to-face interviews tend to be more effective for establishing rapport between the interviewer and the respondent. This interaction can be important for eliciting forthright responses to questions that are of a personal nature. The advantage of the interview approach is the opportunity for in-depth analysis of respondents' behaviors and opinions because the researcher can probe responses and directly observe respondents' reactions. The major disadvantages of interviews include cost and time, the need for personnel to carry out the interviews, scheduling and the lack of anonymity of the respondents.

Most interviews are *structured* in that they consist of a standardized set of questions that will be asked. In this way, all respondents are exposed to the same questions, in the same order, and are given the same choices for responses. In an *unstructured* interview, the interviewer does not have a fixed agenda, and can proceed informally to question and discuss issues of concern. This format is typically conversational and is often carried out in the respondent's natural setting. Many qualitative studies use the unstructured interview approach to generate data.

Questionnaires

Questionnaires are structured surveys that are self-administered using pen and paper or electronic formats. The advantages of using questionnaires are many. They are generally more efficient than interviews because respondents complete them on their own time. Data can be gathered from a large sample in a wide geographical distribution in a relatively short period of time. Written forms are standardized, so that everyone is exposed to the same questions in the same way, reducing potential bias from interactions with an interviewer. Respondents to questionnaires can take time to think about their answers and to consult records for specific information. Questionnaires also provide anonymity, encouraging honest and candid responses. Questionnaires are particularly useful as a research method for examining phenomena that can be assessed through self-observation, such as attitudes and values. They are not as useful for studying behaviors that require objective observation. The primary disadvantages of the written questionnaire are the potential for misunderstanding or misinterpreting questions or response choices, and unknown accuracy or motivation of the respondent. In interviews, the researcher can clarify such misinterpretations.

The most common method of distributing questionnaires has traditionally been through the mail, although many research situations allow for in-person distribution. Electronic distribution of surveys is quickly becoming common practice. Survey software is available through many vendors, allowing for anonymity and automatic tallying of responses. Such questionnaires are economical and can reach a large population in a relatively short period.

A major disadvantage of mail or email questionnaires is that the return rate is often quite low. Responses from 60% to 80% of a sample are usually considered excellent. Realistically, researchers can expect return rates between 30% and 60% for most studies. Actual response rates are lowered further by having to discard returns that are incomplete or incorrectly filled out. Low returns can severely limit the external validity of survey results. Therefore, survey samples are usually quite large so that a sufficient percentage of usable responses will be obtained.

Self-Report

Survey data that are collected using either an oral interview or a written questionnaire are based on a form of **self-report**; that is, the researcher does not directly observe the respondent's behavior or attitudes, but only records the respondent's report of them. There is always some potential for bias or inaccuracy in self-reports, particularly if the questions concern personal or controversial issues. The phenomenon of **recall bias** can be a problem when respondents are asked to remember past events, especially if these events were of a sensitive nature. Research has shown, however, that self-report measures are generally valid. For instance, variables such as injury,[4] mobility function,[5] hypertension,[6] and smoking habits[7,8] have been reported accurately, although a few studies have shown a poor correlation between performance and self-report measures.[9,10] These differences point out the need to understand the target population and the respondents' abilities to answer the questions posed. For many variables, however, such as perceptions, fears, motivations and attitudes, self-report is the only direct way to obtain information.

DESIGN OF SURVEYS

The process of developing a survey instrument is perhaps more time consuming than most people realize. It involves several stages, within which the instrument is written and revised, until it is finally ready for use as a research tool.

The Research Question

The first consideration in every research effort is delineation of the overall research question (see Chapter 7). The research problem must be identified with reference to a target population. These decisions will form the structure for deciding the appropriate research design. A survey is appropriate when the question requires obtaining information from subjects, rather than measuring performance.

Guiding Questions

As with any other research approach, validity is a major concern in the design of a survey instrument; that is, the questionnaire or interview must measure what it was intended to measure. Questions are not asked out of casual interest or curiosity, but because they reflect specific pieces of information that taken as a whole will address the proposed research question. Therefore, the first step in developing the survey is to define its purpose through a series of **guiding questions**, or objectives that delineate what the researcher is trying to find out. The guiding questions may reflect purely descriptive interest, or they may address expected relationships among variables. For example, Couch and colleagues[11] examined the role that play occupies within occupational therapy practice with preschoolers. They proposed three guiding questions for their study:

1. *How do occupational therapists incorporate play into their practice?*
2. *Do occupational therapists assess play behaviors and what methods do they use?*
3. *Are there differences between school-based and non–school-based settings that influence the role of play within pediatric occupational therapy?*

These types of questions focus the content of a questionnaire.

Hypotheses

Survey instruments can also be designed to examine relationships. Some researchers will, therefore, specify hypotheses in addition to guiding questions. Hypotheses are important to direct statistical analyses and conclusions. To illustrate, Rozier and coworkers[12] looked at the relationship between gender and career success factors in physical therapists. One of the several guiding questions they posed was, "Are perceptions of career success different for male versus female physical therapists?" They proposed a series of hypotheses to answer this question, such as:

> Men and women will differ with respect to perceptions of career success.
> a. Men will rate themselves higher in career success compared with women.
> b. Men will report greater importance of salary and position compared with women.

By delineating the specific variables and expected outcomes, the authors were able to clearly structure the analysis and discussion of their findings.

Questionnaire Outline

Once the guiding questions or hypotheses are formulated, the researcher must develop a detailed outline, listing each item of information that will be needed to answer the guiding questions. Each item should relate back to at least one of the study's objectives. Often, more than one item will be needed to address a single question or hypothesis.

Stating useful guiding questions that support an overall research question requires that the researcher have a clear conceptualization of the phenomenon or characteristics being studied. In the study by Couch,[11] it would not be possible to ask questions that allow the researchers to determine if play was truly part of a therapist's practice without a good concept of "play." In Rozier's study,[12] the elements of career success must be understood to compare opinions of male and female respondents. Each individual question in a survey should add to a larger informational context that will answer the guiding questions.

Typically, researchers also include questions about important demographic information in a survey. Couch et al[11] asked occupational therapists about their academic degrees, years of experience and practice setting. Rozier et al[12] asked their sample for information about age, employment setting, length of employment and family responsibilities. Studies will also often include items related to income, race, marital status, living situation and so on. This type of information is needed to describe the characteristics of the respondents, to compare the characteristics of the sample with those of the population to which the results will be generalized, and to interpret how personal characteristics are related to the subject's responses. Guiding questions should be included to reflect how this information will be related to the overall research question.

Review of Existing Instruments

The next step in questionnaire development should be to review existing instruments, to determine if they are applicable or adaptable for the study. Many investigators have developed and validated instruments for a variety of purposes. For example, instruments have been developed for exploring attitudes,[13] health behaviors,[14] and functional status.[15,16] Often, these instruments can be borrowed directly or in part, or they can be modified to fit new research situations, saving a great deal of time. It is not wise to adopt previously used surveys blindly, without considering differences in populations being studied and the specific objectives of the instrument. It is, however, always possible to benefit from the review of literature and insights into development or validation issues that the creator of such an instrument can provide.

Designing the Instrument

The researcher begins to design a survey by writing a series of questions that address each behavior, knowledge, skill or attitude reflected in the guiding questions. Questions should be grouped and organized to reflect each category or topic. The first draft of a questionnaire should include several questions for each topic, so that these can eventually be compared and weeded out. Content should flow so that the respondent's thought processes will follow a logical sequence. Questions should proceed from the general to the specific. The format of questions will vary, depending on how the survey will be administered, that is, by phone or personal interview, or questionnaire. The initial questions should pique the respondent's interest, or at least be "neutral." Sensitive questions should come later. Some researchers put demographic questions at the beginning, but many prefer to keep these less interesting questions for the end.

The organization of the survey is extremely important to the success of its application. Respondents can easily be turned off by a format that is complicated or confusing. The document should be presented in as "friendly" a format as possible. The page should be uncluttered, printed in laser-quality print, and aligned so that it is easy to find the next question. The font size should be at least 11 or 12 point. The font should be simple to read, not fancy or unusual. Some researchers like to use colored paper, rather than white, for written questionnaires to make the survey stand out. Colors used in email surveys should be subtle.

Preliminary Drafts

The preliminary draft of the survey should now be distributed to a panel of colleagues who can review the document, identify problems with questions, including wording and organization. Ask for criticism and suggestions for constructive change. No matter how carefully the survey has been designed, the researcher is usually too close to it to see its flaws. Provide the panel with the study's guiding questions. Based on the panel's comments, the survey should be revised, and then presented to the panel again for further comment. The reviewers should try to answer the survey questions, and discuss how they interpreted each one. The revision process should continue, with additional feedback from evaluators, until the researcher is satisfied that the instrument is concise, clear and serves its intended purpose. This process is indeed time consuming, but necessary, and helps to establish the content validity of the instrument.

Pilot Testing and Revisions

The revised questionnaire should then be pilot tested on a small representative sample, perhaps 5 to 10 individuals from the target population. The researcher should interview these respondents to determine where questions were unclear or misleading. If the researcher is unsure about the appropriateness of specific wording, several versions of a question can be asked to elicit the same information in different ways, and responses can be compared for their reliability. Look for missing answers and inconsistencies. It is also useful to monitor the time it takes for respondents to complete the questionnaire. It may be helpful to administer the survey to this group on two occasions, perhaps separated by several days, to see if the responses are consistent, as a way of estimating test-retest reliability. Based on the results of pilot testing, the questionnaire may again be revised and retested until the final instrument attains an acceptable level of validity.

A major concern during this process will be the length of the survey. More often than not, the initial versions will be too long. Long questionnaires are less likely to maintain the respondent's attention and motivation, resulting in potentially invalid or unreliable responses or, in the case of mail surveys, nonresponses. The importance of each item for the interpretation of the study should be examined, and only those questions that make direct and meaningful contributions should be retained. Researchers have shown that shorter questionnaires are often more valid than longer ones, as items generally have some redundancy built into them.[17]

If the study involves the use of interviewers, a formal training process should be incorporated once the questions have been finalized. Interviewers must be consistent in how they present the survey, how questions are asked, and how probing follow-up questions are used (if they are to be allowed). They should be briefed on the purpose of the study, and their presentation should convey the proper attitude. The interviewers must understand the process of recording responses, an important skill when open-ended questions are used.

Selecting a Sample

Before the survey can be administered, the researcher must choose a sample. An accessible population must be identified. As much as possible, a probability sample should be selected. Stratified sampling is often used to control for variations within the sample, such as geographical area when national samples are used. Cluster sampling may be used to increase accessibility of respondents.

For interview surveys, the respondents will typically be within a local geographic area, and may be recruited from agencies or clinics. Before an interview is administered, the potential respondents should be contacted to elicit their cooperation. For telephone interviews, it is appropriate to send advance notice in the mail that the phone call will be coming as a means of introduction and as a way of establishing the legitimacy of the phone call. For mail surveys, the accessible population may be quite dispersed, and may be limited only by the availability of mailing addresses. Mailings lists can be purchased from professional associations or organizations. Published lists of schools or hospitals can usually be obtained from libraries or professional organizations.

Contacting Respondents

Survey respondents should be given an introduction to the survey so that they understand its purpose and how the data will be used. They should be given an idea of how long it will take to complete the survey. In a written questionnaire, this information will be included in the cover letter. In a mail survey, a self-addressed stamped envelope must be included. It is also appropriate to ask respondents if they would like a copy of the study results when it is completed. Because the survey will typically be anonymous, a separate form can be included for them to send back with their name and address for this purpose.

Because of low response rates in surveys, the researcher should plan to follow up on those who do not respond. To maintain anonymity, in mail surveys, researchers will often code the back of the return envelope, so they can keep a record of who has returned the questionnaire. It is appropriate to send out reminders—postcards, emails, or phone calls—about 2 weeks after the initial mailing to encourage a reply. Because online survey responses are anonymous, email reminders can be sent to the entire sample, (with apologies to those who did respond). Although the majority of responses will be obtained within the first 2 weeks, a reasonable improvement can usually be obtained through follow-up.

Cover Letter

Questionnaires must include a cover letter that orients the respondents to the survey and politely requests their participation. Because a questionnaire can easily be ignored, the cover letter becomes vitally important to encourage a return. An example of a cover letter is shown in Figure 15.1. The letter should include the following elements:

1. Start with the purpose of the study, including its importance. If the research is sponsored by an agency, this information should be included. If the project is a thesis or student project, the respondents should know this.
2. Indicate why the respondent has been chosen for the survey.
3. Assure the respondents that the survey will be anonymous. Encourage them to be honest in their answers, and assure them that they can refuse to answer any questions that make them uncomfortable.
4. Suggest how long it will take to complete the questionnaire.
5. Ask them to respond by sending back the survey in the enclosed self-address stamped envelope or by electronic submission. Provide a deadline date. It is reasonable to give 2 to 3 weeks for a response. A shorter time is an imposition, and longer may result in the questionnaire being put aside and forgotten.
6. Thank respondents for their cooperation. Stress the importance of their response for your work. Provide an opportunity for them to receive a summary of the report.
7. Sign the letter (or use an electronic signature), including your name, degrees and affiliation. If there are several investigators, it is appropriate to include all signatures.

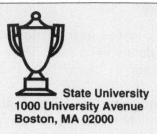

State University
1000 University Avenue
Boston, MA 02000

April 2, 2007

Dear Dr. Jones:

We are conducting a study to examine models of clinical education in occupational therapy programs in the United States. The purpose of the study is to document the various models that are used, to describe how they are implemented and to explore preferences of academic faculty, clinical instructors and clinical managers. The results of this study will help occupational therapy educators understand the issues that impact on the provision of clinical education within today's health care delivery system, and provide a basis for considering mechanisms for making clinical education more effective and efficient.

Your name was selected at random from a list of clinical faculty for accredited occupational therapy programs. We would appreciate your completing the enclosed questionnaire. The questionnaire is anonymous and will not identify respondents in any way. We are interested in your honest opinions. If you prefer not to answer a question, please leave it blank.

The questionnaire should take approximately 15 minutes to complete. A stamped envelope is included for your convenience in returning the questionnaire. We would appreciate your returning the completed questionnaire by April 24.

Thank you in advance for your cooperation with this important effort. Your answers will make a significant contribution to our understanding of contemporary issues that are affecting all of us involved in clinical education programs. If you would like a summary of our findings, please fill in your name and address on the enclosed request form, and we will be happy to forward our findings to you when the study is completed.

Sincerely,

Ann P. Smith, PhD, OTR
Assistant Professor

FIGURE 15.1   Sample cover letter for a mailed questionnaire.

CONSTRUCTING SURVEY QUESTIONS

Two types of questions can be asked in a survey: open-ended and closed-ended questions. **Open-ended questions** ask respondents to answer in their own words. **Closed-ended questions** provide multiple response choices.

Open-Ended Questions

Open-ended questions are useful for probing respondents' feelings and opinions, without biases or limits imposed by the researcher. For example, "What aspects of your job are most satisfying to you?" would require the respondent to provide specific examples of job characteristics. This format is useful when the researcher is not sure of all possible responses to a question. Therefore, respondents are given the opportunity to provide answers in their own words and from their own perspective. Sometimes researchers will use open-ended questions in a pilot study to determine a range of responses which can then be converted to a multiple choice item.

Open-ended questions are, however, difficult to code and analyze because so many different responses can be obtained. If open-ended questions are misunderstood, they may elicit answers that are essentially irrelevant to the researcher's goal. Respondents may not want to take the time to write a full answer, or they may answer in a way that is clear to them but uninterpretable, vague, or incomplete to the researcher. For instance, a question like, "What types of exercise do you do regularly?" could elicit a long list of specific movements or a general description of an exercise routine. If the purpose of the question is to find out if the respondent engages in particular exercise activities, it would be better to list certain exercises and ask if they are done. Open-ended questions can be effective in interviews because the interviewer can clarify the respondent's answers by follow-up questions. Open-ended questions are generally avoided in questionnaires, except where responses are fairly objective, such as asking for a person's yearly income, or where the researcher's purpose is to explore respondents' motivations or behaviors without presenting a predefined list of choices.

Closed-Ended Questions

Closed-ended questions ask respondents to select an answer from among several choices that are provided by the researcher.

> Which of the following aspects of your job do you find most satisfying?
>
> [ ] Patient contact
> [ ] Intellectual challenge
> [ ] Interaction with other medical personnel
> [ ] Opportunities for educational growth

This type of question is easily coded and provides greater uniformity across responses. Its disadvantage is that it does not allow respondents to express their own personal viewpoints and, therefore, may provide a biased response set. The list of choices may overlook some important responses, or they may bias answers by presenting a particular attitude.

There are two basic considerations in constructing closed-ended questions. First, the responses should be *exhaustive;* that is, they should include all possible responses that can be expected. As a protection, it is often advisable to include a category for "not applicable" (NA), "don't know," or "other (please specify ____)." In the preceding example, for instance, it is likely that respondents will have other reasons for job satisfaction that have not been listed. Second, the response categories should be *mutually exclusive;* that is, each choice should clearly represent a unique answer. The preceding example is inadequate on this criterion. For example, a respondent may see "intellectual challenge" and "opportunities for educational growth" as elements of the same concept. Where only one response is desired, it may be useful to add an instruction asking respondents to select the *one best answer* or the answer that is most important; however, this technique does not substitute for carefully worded questions and choices.

There should also be a rationale for ordering response choices. Sometimes, there is an inherent hierarchy in the responses, so that choices can be given in order of increasing or decreasing intensity or agreement. When there is no purposeful order, the researcher must be careful to avoid "leading" the respondent to a particular choice by the order or phrasing.

Sometimes the researcher is interested in more than one answer to a question. For instance, we might want to know all the reasons for a person's job satisfaction. Instructing the respondent to mark "all that apply" creates an interpretation problem in that the respondent may not choose a particular item because it does not apply, because it was not clear, or because it was missed. In addition, it is difficult to code multiple responses. When multiple choices are of interest, it is better to ask respondents to mark each choice separately, as in the following example:

Which of the following aspects of your job do you find satisfying?

	Yes	No	Unsure
Patient contact	[ ]	[ ]	[ ]
Intellectual challenge	[ ]	[ ]	[ ]
Interaction with other medical personnel	[ ]	[ ]	[ ]
Opportunities for educational growth	[ ]	[ ]	[ ]

Format of Closed-Ended Questions

Two common formats are used to list choices to closed-ended questions: (1) using brackets, as just presented, where respondents are asked to check the appropriate response, or (2) asking respondents to circle the number or letter that appears before the answer, as shown next.

The simplest form of closed-ended question is one that presents two choices, or *dichotomous* responses:

Are you presently enrolled in a degree program?

a. Yes
b. No

When questions address a characteristic that is on a continuum, such as attitudes or quality of performance, it is more useful to provide a range of responses, so that the respondent can find a choice that represents the appropriate intensity of response. Usually, three to five multiple-choice options are provided. An option for "Don't know" or "Unsure" should always be included.

How important do you think it is to include a research course in your professional program?

a. Very important
b. Important
c. Somewhat important
d. Not important
e. Unsure

When a series of questions use the same format, a *grid* or checklist can provide a more efficient presentation. With this approach, instructions for using the response choices need only be given once, and the respondent can quickly go through many questions without reading a new set of choices. For example, Figure 15.2 shows a checklist for a question concerning patients' level of knee pain during different activities.

For each of the following activities, please indicate the level of knee pain you have experienced during the past week:

	No pain	Minimal	Moderate	Severe
Walking a short distance				
Walking a long distance				
Ascending stairs				
Descending stairs				

FIGURE 15.2   Example of a grid for using one set of response choices for a series of questions.

An alternative question format is the *rank-order* question, where the respondent is presented with a series of responses and is asked to rank the responses on an ordinal scale.

The following are some of the reasons applicants choose to attend a particular school. Please order them in terms of importance, from 1 (most important) to 5 (least important).

_____ Location
_____ Faculty reputation
_____ Length of program
_____ Affiliation with a medical center
_____ Research opportunities

Some question sequences try to follow up on specific answers with more detailed questions, using a technique called *branching*. Depending on the response to an initial question, the respondent will be directed to answer additional questions or to skip ahead to a later question.

> 1. Do you perform any clinical consulting activities?
>
>   a. No ⟹ Skip to Question 3
>   b. Yes
>
> 2. Approximately how many hours per week do you work as a consultant? _____

This process saves time by avoiding questions that are irrelevant to a specific respondent.

Wording Questions

Simplicity is a key to good questionnaires. Sentences should be succinct and grammatically correct. Respondents will not be inclined to ponder the meaning of a long, involved question. The author of the questionnaire should assume that respondents will read and answer questions quickly and should provide choices that will be understood at a glance. Questions should be written in common language for the lowest educational level that might be encountered.

Language may be an issue if respondents do not speak English, or English is a second language. The researcher must know the sample well enough to accommodate language in the wording of questions. Idioms or subtle cultural expressions should be carefully avoided. The researcher may have the questionnaire translated into another language for specific sample groups. The translation must account for cultural biases.

It goes without saying that survey questions must be clear and unambiguous. Questions that require subtle distinctions to interpret responses are more likely to be misunderstood. For example, consider the question: "How many different sports do you participate in?" There are two ambiguous terms here. First, there may be different ways to define sports. Some may include any form of physical activity, including riding a stationary bicycle; others may include only legitimate field sports. Second, what constitutes participation? Does it have to be an organized schedule of play, or can it mean throwing a basketball in your yard on weekends or playing golf once a year? This type of ambiguity can be corrected by providing the respondent with appropriate definitions, as in the following example:

> Do you participate in any of the following team sports on a regular basis as part of amateur league play?
>
> | | Yes | No |
> |------------|------|------|
> | Softball | [ ] | [ ] |
> | Basketball | [ ] | [ ] |
> | Football | [ ] | [ ] |
> | Soccer | [ ] | [ ] |
> | Hockey | [ ] | [ ] |

Double-Barreled Questions

Each question should be confined to a single idea. Surveys should avoid the use of **double-barreled questions**, using "or" or "and" to assess two things within a single question. For instance, "How many times a week do you jog or ride a stationary bicycle?" It is obviously possible to perform both of these activities at different rates, making it impossible to answer the question. It is better to ask two questions to assess each activity separately.

Frequency and Time Measures

Researchers are often interested in quantifying behavior in terms of frequency and time. For example, it might be of interest to ask, "How many alcoholic drinks do you consume each day?" or "How many patients do you treat per day?" These types of questions may be very difficult to answer because the frequency of the behavior may vary greatly from day to day, month to month, or even season to season. The researcher should determine exactly what aspect of the behavior is most relevant to the study and provide an appropriate time frame for interpreting the question. For instance, the question could ask about a particular period, such as the maximum number of patients seen within the last week, or the respondent can be asked to calculate an average daily value. This assumes, of course, that this time period is adequately representative for purposes of the study. Alternatively, the question could ask for an estimate of "typical" or "usual" behaviors. This approach makes an assumption about the respondent's ability to form such an estimate. Some behaviors are much more erratic than others. For example, it may be relatively easy to estimate the number of patients treated in a day, but it may be more difficult to estimate typical behavior in consuming alcoholic beverages. Estimates of "typical" will also tend to ignore extremes, which may or may not be important to the purpose of the study.

   Questions related to time should also be specific. A question such as, "Has your back pain limited your ability to work?" may be difficult to answer if it is not a consistent problem. It is better to provide a time frame for reference. For example, "Has your back pain limited your ability to work within the past month?" Many function, pain and health status questionnaires specify time periods within the last month, last week, or last 24 hours.

Dealing with Sensitive Questions

Questionnaires often deal with sensitive or personal issues that can cause some discomfort on the part of the respondent. Although some people are only too willing to express personal views, others are hesitant, even when they know their responses are anonymous. Some questions may address social behaviors that have negative associations, such as smoking, sexual practices and drinking alcohol; others may inquire about behaviors that respondents are not anxious to admit to, such as ignorance of facts they feel they should know and compliance with medications or exercise programs. Sensitive questions may also be subject to recall bias. For example, respondents may be selective in their memory of risk factors for disease or disability. Respondents should be reminded in the introduction to the survey that they may refuse to answer any questions.

Sensitive questions should be phrased to put the respondent at ease. It may be useful to preface such questions with a statement as in these examples: "Many people forget to take their medications from time to time." "It is often very difficult for people to fit exercise sessions into their daily routines." "Clinicians are faced with a tremendous task in keeping up with the variety of treatment approaches that are being developed for low back pain. Depending on experience and practice, some clinicians have had an opportunity to learn these techniques more than others." These statements tell the respondent that it is okay if they fit into that category.

Phillips[18] suggests that questions that ask respondents to admit to socially unacceptable behaviors should be phrased in a manner that assumes the respondent engages in the behavior. For instance, rather than asking,

---

Do you ever forget to take your medication?

[ ] Yes [ ] No

If yes, how often?

[ ] Every day
[ ] Once a week
[ ] Once a month

---

we could ask one question:

How often do you forget to take your medication?

[ ] Every day
[ ] Once a week
[ ] Once a month
[ ] Never

SCALES

A **scale** is an ordered system based on a series of questions or items that provide an overall rating that represents the degree to which a respondent possesses a particular attitude, value or characteristic. The purpose of a scale is to distinguish among people who demonstrate different intensities of the characteristic that is being measured. Scales have been developed to measure attitudes, function, health and quality of life, pain, exertion and other physical, physiological and psychological variables.

Categorical scales are based on nominal measurement. A question asks the respondent to assign himself according to one of several classifications. This type of scale is used with variables such as gender, diagnosis, religion or race. These data are expressed as frequency counts or percentages.

Most scales represent a characteristic that exists on a continuum. **Continuous scales** may be measured using interval or ratio values, such as age, blood pressure or years of experience. An ordinal scale requires that a continuous variable be collapsed into ranks. For instance, pain can be measured as "minimal, moderate, severe," or function as "independent, minimal assist, moderate assist, maximal assist, dependent." Scale items should represent the full range of values that represent the characteristic being measured.

Scales are created so that a *summary score* can be obtained from a series of items, indicating the extent to which an individual possesses the characteristic of interest. Because item scores are combined to make this total, it is important that the scale is structured around only one dimension; that is, all items should reflect different elements of a single characteristic. A **summative scale** is one that presents a total score with all items contributing equal weight to the total. A **cumulative scale** demonstrates an accumulated characteristic, with each item representing an increasing amount of the attribute being measured.

We will describe several scaling models used to summarize respondent characteristics: Likert scales, the semantic differential, visual analogue scales, cumulative scales and Rasch models.

Likert Scales

A **Likert scale** is a summative scale, most often used to assess attitudes or values. A series of statements is presented expressing a viewpoint, and respondents are asked to select an appropriately ranked response that reflects their agreement or disagreement with each one. For example, Figure 15.3 shows a set of statements that evaluate students' opinions about including a research course in an entry-level professional curriculum. Likert's original scale included five categories: strongly agree (SA), agree (A), neutral (N), disagree (D), and strongly disagree (SD).[19] Many modifications to this model have been used, sometimes extending it to seven categories (including "somewhat disagree" and "somewhat agree") or four categories (eliminating "neutral").

For each statement given below, please indicate whether you strongly agree (SA), agree (A), are neutral (N), disagree (D), or strongly disagree (SD):

	SA	A	N	D	SD
a. Knowledge of research principles is important for the practicing clinician.	☐	☐	☐	☐	☐
b. Research and statistics should be taught in entry-level professional programs.	☐	☐	☐	☐	☐
c. Participation in a research project should be a requirement.	☐	☐	☐	☐	☐

FIGURE 15.3 A 5-point Likert Scale.

There is no consensus regarding the number of response categories that should be used. Some researchers believe the "neutral" option should be omitted so that the respondents are forced to make a choice, rather than allowing them an "out" so that they do not have to take sides on an issue. Others feel that respondents who do not have strong feelings should be given a viable option to express that attitude. When the forced choice method is used, responses that are left blank are generally interpreted as "neutral."

Each choice along the scale is assigned a point value, based on the degree to which the item represents a favorable or unfavorable characteristic. For example, we could rate SA = 5, A = 4, N = 3, D = 2, SD = 1, or we could use codes such as SA = 2, A = 1, N = 0, D = −1, SD = −2. The actual values are unimportant, as long as the items are consistently scored; that is, agreement with favorable items should always be scored higher than agreement with unfavorable items. Therefore, if positively phrased items are coded 5 through 1, then negatively phrased items must be coded 1 through 5.

An overall score is computed for each respondent by adding points for each item. Creating such a total assumes that the items are measuring the same things and that each item reflects equal elements of the characteristic being studied; that is, one item should not carry any more weight than the others.

Constructing a Likert scale requires more than just listing a group of statements. A large pool of items should be developed, usually 10 to 20, that reflect an equal number of both favorable and unfavorable attitudes. It is generally not necessary to include items that are intended to elicit neutral responses, because these will not help to distinguish respondents. The scale should be validated by performing item analyses that will indicate which items are truly discriminating between those with positive and those with negative attitudes. These items are then retained as the final version of the scale, and others are eliminated. If respondents are equally likely to agree with both favorable and unfavorable statements, then the scale is not providing a valid assessment of their feelings about a particular issue. The basis of the item analysis is that there should be correlation between an individual's total score and each item response. Those who score highest should also agree with positively worded statements, and those who obtain the lowest total scores should disagree. Those items that generate agreement from both those with high and low scores are probably irrelevant to the characteristic being studied, and should be omitted.

Semantic Differential

Attitudes have also been evaluated using a technique called the **semantic differential**.[20] This method tries to measure the individual's feelings about a particular object or concept based on a continuum that extends between two extreme opposites. For example, we could ask respondents to rate their feelings about natural childbirth by checking the space that reflects their attitude on the following scale:

Good |____|____|____|____|____|____|____| Bad

The semantic differential is composed of a set of these scales, using pairs of words that reflect opposite feelings. Typically a 7-point scale is used, as just shown, with the middle representing a neutral position. This scale is different from the Likert scale in

Myself			
Useful	___|___|___|___|___|___|___	Useless	(P)
Active	___|___|___|___|___|___|___	Passive	(A)
Ugly	___|___|___|___|___|___|___	Beautiful	(E)
Slow	___|___|___|___|___|___|___	Fast	(A)
Important	___|___|___|___|___|___|___	Unimportant	(E)
Delicate	___|___|___|___|___|___|___	Rugged	(P)
Warm	___|___|___|___|___|___|___	Cold	(E)
Sharp	___|___|___|___|___|___|___	Dull	(A)
Weak	___|___|___|___|___|___|___	Strong	(P)
Good	___|___|___|___|___|___|___	Bad	(E)

FIGURE 15.4 Example of a semantic differential for testing self-image. Dimensions of evaluation (E), potency (P), and activity (A) are indicated, although these designations would not appear in an actual test.

two ways. First, only the two extremes are labeled. Second, the continuum is not based on agree/disagree, but on opposite adjectives that should express the respondent's feelings about the concept. Figure 15.4 illustrates a semantic differential to explore self-image in a group of elderly women who reside in a nursing home.

Research has demonstrated that the adjective pairs used in this scale tend to fall along three underlying dimensions, which have been labeled evaluation, potency and activity.[20,21] **Evaluation** is associated with adjectives such as nice–awful, good–bad, clean–dirty, valuable–worthless and helpful–unhelpful. Some concepts that lie on the positive side of this dimension are doctor, family, peace, success and truth. Negative evaluation concepts include abortion, disease, war and failure. **Potency** ideas are big–little, powerful–powerless, strong–weak, large–small and deep–shallow. Strong potency concepts include bravery, duty, law, power and science. Negative concepts include baby, love and art. The **activity** dimension is characterized by fast–slow, alive–dead, noisy–quiet, young–old, active–passive and sharp–dull. Strong activity concepts are danger, anger, fire and child. Concepts that lie toward the negative activity side are calm, death, rest and sleep. The ratings shown in Figure 15.4 are labeled according to their respective dimensions. It is a good idea to mix up the order of presentation of the dimensions in listing the scales.

The semantic differential is scored by assigning values from 1 to 7 to each of the spaces within each adjective pair, with 1 representing the most negative response and 7 indicating the positive extreme. To avoid biases or a tendency to just check the same column in each scale, the order of negative and positive responses should be randomly varied. For instance, in Figure 15.4, ratings of weak–strong, slow–fast and ugly–beautiful place the negative value on the left; all other scales have the positive value on the left. A total score can be obtained by summing the scores for each rating. Lower total scores will reflect generally negative feelings toward the concept being assessed, and higher scores represent generally positive feelings. Statistical procedures, such as factor analysis, can be applied to the scale ratings to determine if the evaluation, potency, and activity ratings tend to go together (see Chapter 29 for a description of factor analysis). In this way, the instrument can be used to explore theoretical constructs.

Visual Analogue Scales

A **visual analogue scale (VAS)** is one of the simplest methods to assess the intensity of a subjective experience. A line is drawn, usually fixed at 100 mm in length, with word anchors on either end that represent extremes of the characteristic. The intermediate levels along the line are not defined. Respondents are asked to place a mark along the line corresponding to their perceived level for that characteristic. The VAS is scored by measuring the distance of the mark from the left-hand anchor in millimeters. This method has also been used to measure a variety of characteristics,[22] most extensively for pain,[23,24] as shown in Figure 15.5. The VAS can be used to evaluate a variable at a given point in time or its degree of change over time.

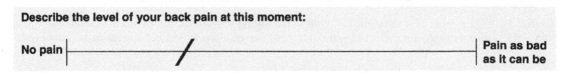

Describe the level of your back pain at this moment:

No pain |————————————/————————————————————————| Pain as bad as it can be

FIGURE 15.5   A 100 mm visual analogue scale for pain, showing a mark at 27 mm.

The scores obtained with a VAS have generally been treated as ratio level data, measured in millimeters.[25–27] This assumption permits VAS scores to be added to obtain a mean and subjected to parametric statistical procedures. Some have argued that the scores are only psuedo ratio, and should be treated as ordinal, handled with nonparametric statistics.[28] They suggest that the individual marking the line is not truly able to appreciate the full continuum, evidenced by ceiling effects[29] and a tendency to cluster marks at certain points.[30] Therefore, even though the actual readings from the scale are obviously at the ratio level, the true measurement properties may be less precise. This dilemma will continue to emerge in studies using the VAS.[31]

The simple format of the VAS continues to make it a popular method for assessing unidimensional characteristics. This points out one disadvantage of the technique, however, in that each VAS is only capable of evaluating one dimension of a trait. Researchers often incorporate several VAS lines, each with different anchors, to assess related aspects of the characteristic being measured.[32,33]

Cumulative Scales

In a summative scale, several item scores are added to create a total score. One of the limitations of this type of measure is that the total score can be interpreted in more than one way. Suppose we have a scale, scored from 0 to 100, that measures physical function, including elements related to locomotion, personal hygiene, dressing and feeding. Two individuals who achieve a score of 50 may have obtained this score for very different reasons. One may be able to walk, but is unable to perform the necessary upper extremity movements for self-care. Another may be in a wheelchair, but is able to take care of his personal needs. Therefore, a summed score can be ambiguous. This potential outcome reflects the fact that the items within the scale actually reflect different components or dimensions of the trait being measured, in this case physical function, which are not all equal.

Cumulative scales (also called Guttman scales) provide an alternative approach, wherein a set of statements is presented that reflects increasing intensities of the characteristic being measured. This technique is designed to ensure that there is only one dimension within a set of responses; that is, there is only one unique combination of responses that can achieve a particular score. For instance, in a cumulative scale a respondent who agrees with item 2 will also have had to agree with item 1; one who agrees with item 3 will have had to agree with items 1 and 2; and so on. Therefore, although there may be several combinations of responses that will result in a total score of 10 for a summative scale, there is only one way to achieve that score on a cumulative scale. Consider the following statements which were included in a self-assessment interview of elderly people concerning their functional health status.[34]

1. I can go to the movies, church or visiting without help.
2. I can walk up and down to the second floor without help.
3. I can walk half a mile without help.
4. I am not limited in any activities.
5. I have no physical conditions or illnesses now.
6. I am still healthy enough to do heavy work around the house without help.

If these items represent a cumulative scale, then all those who can walk half a mile can also climb stairs to the second floor and go out visiting. Those who cannot walk half a mile should not be able to do heavy housework and probably have some limiting illness or physical condition. The development of this scale is, therefore, based on a theoretical premise that there is a hierarchy to this dimension of health.

Each item in the cumulative scale is scored as 1 = agree or 0 = disagree. A total cumulative score is then computed for all items. The maximum score will be equal to the number of items in the scale. A respondent who achieves a score of 2 would have had to agree only with items 1 and 2. If he agreed with items 1 and 3 only, the scale would be faulty because the set of statements would not constitute a hierarchy in terms of the characteristic being assessed. In reality, such scales are not free of error, and some of the subjects can be expected to present inconsistent patterns of response. In the analysis of the response categories for functional health, researchers found that most of their subjects could participate in social activities (86%) and that the fewest could do heavy work around the house, like shoveling snow and washing walls (21%).[34] The frequencies for other responses ranged between these two extremes, supporting the cumulative scale.

Rasch Analysis

The issues of hierarchical assessment extend to many of the questionnaire instruments that have been developed to assess functional and health outcomes. In most such scales, items are marked using ordinal values, and a total score is generated. For example, we could ask elderly patients if their health limits their function based on several ADL items, as follows:

	(1) Limited a Lot	(2) Limited a Little	(3) Not Limited
Eating	☐	☐	☐
Walking indoors	☐	☐	☐
Climbing stairs	☐	☐	☐

Although this is an obviously abbreviated scale for the sake of example, a person who is independent in all three items would obtain a total score of 9. A person who is severely limited in all three tasks would receive a total score of 3. For this total score to be meaningful, however, three criteria must be met. First, the scale items must reflect a unidimensional construct. For instance, the ability to eat is not necessarily related to the ability to walk indoors or climb stairs; that is, these items may be part of different dimensions of function.[35] If so, the sum of scores on these items would not reflect a unified construct—sort of adding apples and oranges. Therefore, two patients who obtain a score of 5 may not demonstrate the same functional profile.

Second, the items must progress according to a hierarchical model from easy to difficult, so we can determine if someone has more or less of the trait. This would also mean that the order of difficulty for the items is consistent for all patients, and that the range of the scale incorporates the extremes.[36] Therefore, if our sample functional scale was properly arranged, eating would be easier than walking indoors, and walking indoors would be easier than climbing stairs for everyone.

Third, we need a scale that will allow us to measure change within or across patients. As we have noted before, ordinal values may present problems in this regard because they have limited sensitivity and precision. A patient might improve in his ability to climb stairs, but not enough to be scored at a higher level of independence. Therefore, for a score to be meaningful, units of measurement must have equal intervals along the scale, to account for magnitude of change. These objectives can be achieved using a technique called **Rasch analysis**, which statistically manipulates ordinal data to create a linear measure on an interval scale.[37-41]

We can describe this process using items from the Functional Independence Measure (FIM), a popular instrument for assessing function in rehabilitation settings. The FIM is an 18-item scale designed to evaluate the amount of assistance a patient needs to accomplish activities of daily living (ADLs).[42] The items measure both motor and cognitive functions. Each item is scored on an ordinal scale from 1 (total assist) to 7 (total independence). The larger the total score, the less assistance the patient requires. Theoretically, then, if the scale represents a singular construct of function, the total score should reflect an "amount" of independence; that is, we can think of individuals as being "more" or "less" independent.

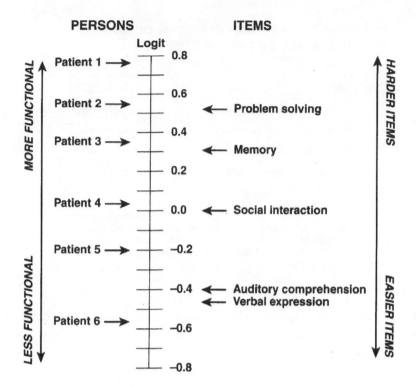

FIGURE 15.6 Example of a two-facet linear functional scale for mobility, showing the placement of scale items and patients according to a Rasch analysis. The increments represent item difficulty on the logit scale, with higher values representing greater difficulty.

The Rasch Model

Now let us conceive of function as a line, representing the continuum of function, as shown in Figure 15.6. For this example we will use the five items in the cognitive sub-scale, listed in Table 15.1.* We construct the line using items in the scale, with easier items at the base, and harder items at the top. Using data from a patient sample and specialized computer programs,[43] the Rasch analysis determines the order of difficulty of the items, and locates them along this continuum, to show how they fit a unidimensional model of function. The analysis will also position patients along this line according to "how much" or "how little" cognitive function they have. The arrangement of items in Figure 15.6 illustrates these concepts based on a study by Heinemann et al[44] who performed a Rasch analysis on the motor and cognitive portions of the FIM. The figure illustrates two facets of this scale: On the right, the items are ranked in relation to their difficulty; and on the left, the patients are positioned relative to their abilities.[45] The more difficult items have a higher score, and patients who have these abilities

---

*Some researchers have distinguished the motor and cognitive portions of the FIM as separate scales based on Rasch analysis.[44,46] For purposes of illustration, then, it is reasonable to consider the items on cognitive function as a separate scale.

TABLE 15.1   ITEMS FROM THE COGNITIVE SUBSCALE OF THE FUNCTIONAL INDEPENDENCE MEASURE

Item	Logit
1. Problem solving	0.53
2. Memory	0.30
3. Social interaction	0.00
4. Auditory comprehension	−0.40
5. Verbal expression	−0.45

Source: Heinemann AW, Linacre JM, Wright BD, Hamilton BB, Granger C. Relationships between impairment and physical disability as measured by the Functional Independence Measure. Arch Phys Med Rehabil 1993;74:566–573.

(they are more independent) will also be placed near the top of the scale. Patients who are less functional are placed toward the bottom of the scale, as they are only able to complete the easier items. In Figure 15.6, patient 5 was only able to achieve the auditory comprehension and verbal expression items, while patients 1 and 2 were able to achieve all five items.

If the scale truly represents one functional construct, it should meet three measurement principles.[14,45] First, the total score on the scale should reflect level of function implied by the items; second, the items will range in difficulty; and third, the rank order of difficulty will not change from person to person. The results of the computerized Rasch analysis will show where each individual respondent fits along the continuum; the level of difficulty achieved by each item on an interval scale; and goodness-of-fit of the model, showing how well each item matches the cumulative scale.[14]

Measurement Criteria

Several criteria are used to judge the adequacy of a scale as part of a Rasch analysis:

1. *Item difficulty* refers to the position of items within the hierarchical scale. It is expressed as a *logit*[†], or log-odds unit, with a central zero point, allowing items to be scaled as positive or negative. The items are ordered so that the degree of function becomes systematically greater as the items become harder; that is, patients who have greater functional ability will "pass" the more difficult items. Therefore, it becomes possible to determine how close or far apart items are in difficulty, not just their rank order

---

[†]To determine the position of an item along an interval scale, each item is examined for the probability that a person with a given level of ability will pass or fail, creating an odds ratio. These odds are then transformed to a logarithmic scale, creating a value called a *logit* that will range from minus to plus infinity. The logit is defined as the mean of the natural logarithm of the odds that the average ability patient will transition from one category to the next higher one (e.g., from a rating of 1 to 2, 2 to 3, etc.). It is considered an equal-interval measure, thereby creating an interval scale that has additive properties.

of difficulty. Ideally items are positioned equally across the scale, not leaving large gaps. As shown in Table 15.1 and Figure 15.6, the five items on the FIM range in difficulty from −0.45 to 0.53, with a reasonable spread of scores. The most difficult item is problem solving, and the easiest item is verbal expression. If gaps are identified, they suggest where items need to be added better to reflect the continuum.

2. *Item fit* is the extent to which the individual items conform to the unidimensional model. *Person fit* represents the extent to which individuals fit the model. The Rasch analysis develops a probability model that predicts what scores should be for each item and person. If we look at the continuum for the construct of cognitive function, for example, a good fit means that each item represents a level on the scale that will discriminate between those who require less assistance and those who require more assistance. Patients who are less functional will be placed toward the bottom, and those who are more functional will be placed toward the top; that is, the more functional individual will pass more of the items (and more of the difficult items), and the less functional individual will fail more of the items.

When expected relationships are not found, the responses are considered a *misfit*.[‡] For example, a Rasch analysis for the entire FIM scale has shown that combining all 18 items resulted in a large proportion of misfitting items;[44] that is, some of the more difficult items and more functional patients were not placed at the top (supporting the separation of motor and cognitive subscales).

Fit statistics are calculated for each item to reflect how well the items conform to the hierarchical model. These statistics are expressed as a *mean square residual (MNSQ)*, which is the difference between the observed scores and the scores expected by the model. If the observed and expected values are the same, the MNSQ will equal 1.0.[§] Higher MNSQ values indicate greater discrepancy from the model; that is, the item is not consistent in its level of difficulty across patients.[**] It would then be reasonable to consider revising the scale, either by eliminating the item or rewording it to remove ambiguity. If patients are misfit, the researcher must examine their characteristics, potentially identifying subgroups in the population. In the FIM study by Heinemann and colleagues,[44] several patient groups were evaluated, demonstrating that differently ordered cognitive scales were needed to represent groups with and without brain dysfunction. For instance, patients with right- and left-sided strokes did not demonstrate similar difficulty with verbal expression.

3. *Item separation* reflects the spread of items, and *person separation* represents the spread of individuals. Ideally, the analysis will show that items can be separated into at least three *strata* that represent low, medium and high difficulty,[48] although a good scale may actually delineate many strata to clarify the construct. Statistically, this spread is

---

[‡]Each item in the scale should reflect a given level of function. For a good fitting item, 50% of the sample at that functional level should "pass" that item.[39]

[§]The significance of item fit can be derived using the *t*-statistic, testing the difference of the mean square residual from 1.0.[47]

[**]Two indicators of fit may be reported.[36] *Infit* is sensitive to erratic response patterns for items that are close to a patient's functional level. Therefore, a large infit would indicate a problem with the item's fit with the unidimensional model. *Outfit* reflects the occurrence of extremely unexpected or rare responses. A large outfit value would indicate that some patients have unique patterns of impairment and probably reflect a different population.

related to measurement error or reliability; that is, the more reliable a scale, the more likely the item or person score represents the true score. Measurement error should be small so that segments of the scale are separated by distances greater than their measurement error alone. Separation statistics may be expressed as a reliability coefficient, or the ratio of the sample standard deviation to the standard error of the test.[39] Conceptually, this is a ratio of the true spread of scores divided by the measurement error.

An understanding of measurement principles applied to questionnaires is essential if we want to use scores as part of our patient evaluations or to look at group performance over time. We must consider the potential for misinference when ordinal scales are used. Rasch Item Response Theory provides an important technique for testing our assumptions in clinical measurement. Several useful examples of Rasch analysis can be found in the literature.[49-53]

Q-SORT

The **Q-sort** is an analytic technique used to characterize attitudes, opinions or judgments of individuals through a process of comparative rank ordering.[54] The technique involves presenting an individual with a set of cards containing a series of written items such as statements, ideas, phrases or pictures. The individual is asked to sort the cards into piles according to some scaled criterion. For example, cards may list areas of clinical research in rehabilitation, and the subject may be asked to sort the cards according to high versus low priority. The criterion is defined on a discrete continuum, such as an 11-point scale, with 0 representing no interest at all and 10 representing the highest priority. Scales of different widths may be appropriate for different variables; however, a wide enough continuum is necessary to see a clear distribution.

The subject must sort through the cards and place them in piles representing each rank along the continuum; however, the researcher specifies how many cards are to go into each pile, so that the subject is faced with forced choices. For example, we could present a deck of 60 cards, each with a topic of clinical research, and ask a subject to form piles according to the distribution shown in Table 15.2. The subject would be instructed to read through the entire set of cards, and to place in Pile 0 the one card containing the single least important topic and in Pile 10 the single topic of highest priority. Then, from the remaining 58 cards, the subject would place the two least important items in Pile 1 and the two most important in Pile 9. This process continues for Piles 2 and 8, 3 and 7, and 4 and 6. The remaining 12 cards are placed in Pile 5, essentially a neutral pile. The subjects are free to replace or move any card to another pile at any time during the sorting procedure until they are satisfied with results. Although Q-distributions are essentially arbitrary, for statistical convenience the distribution is

TABLE 15.2 DISTRIBUTION OF 60 CARDS FOR A Q SORT

	Low Priority									High Priority	
	0	1	2	3	4	5	6	7	8	9	10
Number of cards	1	2	4	7	10	12	10	7	4	2	1

usually arranged to resemble a normal distribution, with fewer and fewer items toward the extremes. Although the number of cards used will vary according to the research question, Q-sorts generally range from a low of 60 to a high of 100 to 120 items. Too large a deck is difficult to sort through, and too small a deck will not provide sufficient stability for statistical reliability.

Q-methodology provides an empirical basis for exploring abstract ideas and theories, generally with good reliability. It can be applied to a variety of research questions and is quite flexible. It is possible to use the technique to answer questions that require the use of two or more related sets of items, or a single set of items can be sorted on more than one scale. For instance, Biddle et al[55] used a Q-sort to establish key characteristics of effective primary care training experiences for third-year medical students. The students completed a Q-sort using three sets of items: preceptor characteristics, site characteristics and a combination of the two.

The approach to analysis of Q-sort data will depend on the research question. For some purposes, descriptive statistics, such as averages, percentages, and simple tallies of rank orderings, will be sufficient. For example, Q-sort has been used to rank applicants to a physical therapy program.[56] More complex statistical procedures can also be applied to the Q-methodology. Correlations are often used to determine if the sorts of several subjects are related, usually using a nonparametric procedure for correlating ranks. For instance, Kovach and associates[57] studied employees in long-term care facilities to describe factors that facilitate positive change in the care of patients with dementia. The employees were asked to rank personal factors and facility factors. Using Spearman correlation coefficients, the researchers found little congruence between real and ideal facility characteristics, but a strong relationship between real and ideal personal characteristics. Factor analysis and content analysis are also used to uncover underlying themes in the Q-sort. For example, in the study of medical students' perceptions of clinical experiences, Biddle et al[55] use content analysis to group responses into six categories, including patients, staff characteristics, preceptor's personal characteristics, programmatic issues, educational opportunities, and the strongest theme around preceptor teaching characteristics.

The Q-sort is limited in its generalizability because subjects are not randomly chosen. Samples tend to be small because of the logistic difficulties administering the technique. Replication of Q-sorts over many samples is necessary to demonstrate validity of findings. Use of already established Q-sorts (sets of items) is helpful to validate findings by replication. When Q-sorts do not exist, the researcher must establish the content validity of items used.

DELPHI SURVEY

Many questions of interest in medical and social sciences are related to practice, values or standards, and are best answered by developing consensus around a specific issue. In a **Delphi survey**, a panel of experts is asked to complete a series of questionnaires to identify their opinions.[58,59] The Delphi technique differs from typical questionnaires in several ways. The most distinguishing difference is the use of several rounds of questionnaires, typically two or three. In each round, the researcher reviews and collates the results, and then distributes these findings to the panel for their response. This process generally continues until the responses are consistent with the previous round, demonstrating consensus.

This technique was used, for example, in a study of opinions of physical therapist managers on the importance of specific knowledge and skills in leadership, administration, management and professionalism (LAMP).[60] In a first round, the panel was asked to respond to a list of LAMP components, modifying or adding items. Data from round one were compiled by a research team, resulting in 178 items. In the second round, panel members were asked to rank the importance of each item on a Likert scale. The purpose of the third and final round was to reach consensus on the level of knowledge and skills needed by a new graduate. The panel agreed that 44% of the items were important at a high to moderate level of skill, and that no skill was needed in 29% of the items. These findings present useful information for the design of professional curricula.

The Delphi survey has great potential for planning and problem solving for a variety of practice issues. Investigators have used this technique to establish consensus on indicators for assessing the severity of rheumatoid arthritis through medical records,[61] quality indicators for care of general medical conditions in nursing home residents,[62] clinically important differences in the evaluation of change in health-related quality of life for patients with asthma[63] and effective smoking prevention strategies for female adolescents.[64] It is an efficient method because the members of the panel do not need to come together, making large response groups feasible, including individuals at a distance. Consensus is developed without interaction among respondents, avoiding the potential for group biases, such as one dominant individual swaying others in the group. Responses are shared without any one individual being challenged by the group. The anonymity offered by this method will also encourage honest responses from the panel. The disadvantages include the cost of printing and mailing, and the need to maintain a commitment by the panel members over several rounds. Researchers will generally use follow-up reminders to encourage full participation.

ANALYSIS OF SURVEY DATA

The first step in the analysis of data is to collate responses and enter them into a computer. Each item on the survey is a data point, and must be given a variable name, often the item number. The researcher must sort through each questionnaire as it is returned, or through all responses from an interview, to determine if responses are valid. In many instances, the respondent will have incorrectly filled out the survey, and that respondent may have to be eliminated from the analysis. Some questions may have to be eliminated from individual questionnaires because they were answered incorrectly, such as putting two answers in for a question that asked for a single response. The researcher must keep track of all unusable questionnaires to report this percentage in the final report.

Responses to closed-ended questions are *coded;* that is, responses are given numeric codes that provide labels for data entry and analysis. For instance, sex can be coded 0 = male, 1 = female. We could code hospital size as 1 = less than 50 beds, 2 = 50 to 100 beds, and 3 = over 100 beds. These codes are entered into the computer to identify responses. Using codes, the researcher can easily obtain frequency counts and percentages for each question, to determine how many subjects checked each response.

The analysis of survey data may take many forms. Most often, descriptive statistics are used to summarize responses. When quantitative data such as age are collected, the researcher will usually present averages. With categorical data, the researcher reports the frequency of responses to specific questions. These frequencies are typically converted to a percentage of the total sample. For example, a researcher might report that 30% of the sample was male and 70% was female, or in a question about opinions, that 31% strongly agree, 20% agree, 5% disagree, and so on. Percentages should always be accompanied by reference to the total sample size, so that the reader can determine the actual number of responses in each category. Percentages are usually more meaningful than actual frequencies because sample sizes may differ greatly among studies.

Another common approach to data analysis involves the description of relationships between two or more sets of responses. For instance, a survey might contain a question asking a person's gender, and other questions might ask about attitudes toward abortion. The researcher can then examine the frequency of responses to the attitude questions in relation to each respondent's sex. **Cross-tabulations** are usually presented, showing the number of males and females who answered positively or negatively to each attitude question. The chi-square test (χ^2) can be used to examine this relationship statistically, to determine if there is a significant relationship between the two variables (see Chapter 25).

When questionnaires include a scale, researchers may want to look at sums as a reflection of the respondents' answers. These sums may be presented for the entire scale, or subscales may be analyzed. Measurement properties of such scales must be considered, such as the potential need for weighting items differently within a scale, or the decision on which items belong to a subscale.

Depending on the length and complexity of the questionnaire, researchers may present response percentages for all questions on the survey, or they may simply summarize the more important relationships that were studied. Some reports present purely narrative descriptions of the results; others include tables showing the responses to each question. The author must determine which type of presentation will be most effective for the data.

If a questionnaire is developed for the purpose of assessing a particular characteristic, such as function or pain, the researcher should evaluate the reliability and validity of the instrument. Different types of reliability and validity should be tested, depending on the type of questions and purpose of the assessment (see Chapters 5 and 6). The examination of an instrument's measurement properties is essential if the instrument will be used by others.

INFORMED CONSENT

Even though interviews or questionnaires do not require physical interaction with subjects, these studies must go through a formal process of review and approval by an Institutional Review Board (see Chapter 3). Researchers must be able to demonstrate the protection of subjects from psychological risk and the guarantee of confidentiality. The IRB will want assurances that all relevant individuals have been notified and are in support of the project. Surveys will often receive expedited reviews by a review board.

Individuals who participate in face-to-face interviews can be given an informed consent form to sign in the presence of the interviewer and a witness. Consent to participate in telephone interviews is implied by the individual's participation. The researcher is obliged to give telephone respondents full information at the beginning of the call, so that they can decide whether they want to continue with the interview. Similarly, consent for mail questionnaires is implied by the return of the questionnaire. The cover letter provides the information needed.

COMMENTARY

They Have a Thousand and One Uses

Survey research represents a technique of data collection that can actually be applied across a wide range of research designs and approaches. Surveys may be purely descriptive, or they may be focused on variables that are expected to demonstrate specific relationships. Surveys and interviews can be the main form of data collection in quantitative or qualitative studies. They may be included as part of the data collection in an experimental study, to gather demographic information as part of the study, or they can be used as an outcome instrument. Surveys can be used for retrospective or prospective studies as well. Most often, surveys are based on a cross-sectional sample, meaning that a large group of respondents are tested at relatively the same point in time. Surveys can, however, be used in longitudinal studies by giving follow-up interviews or questionnaires to document changes in attitudes or behaviors.

Although surveys seem relatively easy to use as a research tool, this approach carries with it methodologic challenges. For descriptive studies, the researcher must construct a new measuring tool. This is no small accomplishment, and requires attention to principles of reliability and validity. Item reliability of questions, rater reliability for interviewers, and content and construct validity are all concerns for survey researchers. Generalizability issues are potentially of serious concern, especially when response rates are low. The researcher usually tries to determine if there is a difference between the characteristics of those who did respond and the characteristics of those who did not. For example, depending on the type of information available, it may be possible to determine the ages, sex distribution or occupational characteristics of nonrespondents.

If a questionnaire is being used as an outcome instrument, the examination of its measurement properties must be extensive. We have described the validity issues involved in measuring change (see Chapter 6) and developing scales. The professional literature abounds with examples of the process of establishing validity for many of the currently used health status and functional scales, demonstrating the comprehensive approach that is necessary.

Those who are interested in pursuing the survey approach are encouraged to consult researchers who have had experience with questionnaires, as well as several informative texts listed at the end of this chapter.

REFERENCES

1. Giles LG, Muller R. Chronic spinal pain: A randomized clinical trial comparing medication, acupuncture, and spinal manipulation. *Spine* 2003;28:1490–502; discussion 1502–1503.
2. Peretti-Watel P, Bendiane MK, Obadia Y, Lapiana JM, Galinier A, Pegliasco H, et al. Disclosure of prognosis to terminally ill patients: Attitudes and practices among French physicians. *J Palliat Med* 2005;8:280–290.
3. Calancie B, Molano MR, Broton JG. Epidemiology and demography of acute spinal cord injury in a large urban setting. *J Spinal Cord Med* 2005;28:92–96.
4. Valuri G, Stevenson M, Finch C, Hamer P, Elliott B. The validity of a four week self-recall of sports injuries. *Inj Prev* 2005;11:135–137.
5. Shumway-Cook A, Patla A, Stewart AL, Ferrucci L, Ciol MA, Guralnik JM. Assessing environmentally determined mobility disability: Self-report versus observed community mobility. *J Am Geriatr Soc* 2005;53:700–704.
6. Giles WH, Croft JB, Keenan NL, Lane MJ, Wheeler FC. The validity of self-reported hypertension and correlates of hypertension awareness among blacks and whites within the stroke belt. *Am J Prev Med* 1995;11:163–169.
7. Wills TA, Cleary SD. The validity of self-reports of smoking: analyses by race/ethnicity in a school sample of urban adolescents. *Am J Public Health* 1997;87:56–61.
8. Willemsen MC, Brug J, Uges DR, Vos de Wael ML. Validity and reliability of self-reported exposure to environmental tobacco smoke in work offices. *J Occup Environ Med* 1997;39:1111–1114.
9. Reneman MF, Jorritsma W, Schellekens JM, Goeken LN. Concurrent validity of questionnaire and performance-based disability measurements in patients with chronic nonspecific low back pain. *J Occup Rehabil* 2002;12:119–129.
10. Reuben DB, Siu AL, Kimpau S. The predictive validity of self-report and performance-based measures of function and health. *J Gerontol* 1992;47:M106–110.
11. Couch KJ, Deitz JC, Kanny EM. The role of play in pediatric occupational therapy. *Am J Occup Ther* 1998;52:111–117.
12. Rozier CK, Raymond MJ, Goldstein MS, Hamilton BL. Gender and physical therapy career success factors. *Phys Ther* 1998;78:690–704.
13. Antonak RF, Livneh H. *The Measurement of Attitudes toward People with Disabilities: Methods, Psychometrics and Scales.* Springfield, IL: C Thomas, 1988.
14. McDowell I, Newell C. *Measuring Health: A Guide to Rating Scales and Questionnaires* (2nd ed.). New York: Oxford University Press, 1996.
15. Kantz ME, Harris WJ, Levitsky K, Ware JE, Jr., Davies AR. Methods for assessing condition-specific and generic functional status outcomes after total knee replacement. *Med Care* 1992;30:MS240–252.
16. Dodds TA, Martin DP, Stolov WC, Deyo RA. A validation of the Functional Independence Measurement and its performance among rehabilitation inpatients. *Arch Phys Med Rehabil* 1993;74:531–536.
17. Katz JN, Larson MG, Phillips CB, Fossel AH, Liang MH. Comparative measurement sensitivity of short and longer health status instruments. *Med Care* 1992;30:917–925.
18. Phillips BS. *Social Research: Strategy and Tactics* (2nd ed.). New York: MacMillan, 1971.
19. Likert R. A technique for the measurement of attitudes. *Arch Psychol* 1932;140:5–55.
20. Osgood CE, Suci GJ, Tannenbaum RH. *The Measurement of Meaning.* Urbana, IL: University of Illinois Press, 1957.
21. Heise DR. Semantic differential profiles for 1,000 most frequent English words. *Psychol Monogr* 1965;79:31 (Whole No. 601).

22. de Boer AG, van Lanschot JJ, Stalmeier PF, van Sandick JW, Hulscher JB, de Haes JC, et al. Is a single-item visual analogue scale as valid, reliable and responsive as multi-item scales in measuring quality of life? *Qual Life Res* 2004;13:311–320.

23. Massy-Westropp N, Ahern M, Krishnan J. A visual analogue scale for assessment of the impact of rheumatoid arthritis in the hand: Validity and repeatability. *J Hand Ther* 2005;18:30–33.

24. Villanueva I, del Mar Guzman M, Javier Toyos F, Ariza-Ariza R, Navarro F. Relative efficiency and validity properties of a visual analogue vs. a categorical scaled version of the Western Ontario and McMaster Universities Osteoarthritis (WOMAC) Index: Spanish versions. *Osteoarthritis Cartilage* 2004;12:225–231.

25. Todd KH, Funk KG, Funk JP, Bonacci R. Clinical significance of reported changes in pain severity. *Ann Emerg Med* 1996;27:485–489.

26. Duncan GH, Bushnell MC, Lavigne GJ. Comparison of verbal and visual analogue scales for measuring the intensity and unpleasantness of experimental pain. *Pain* 1989; 37:295–303.

27. Dexter F, Chestnut DH. Analysis of statistical tests to compare visual analog scale measurements among groups. *Anesthesiology* 1995;82:896–902.

28. Huskisson EC. Measurement of pain. *J Rheumatol* 1982;9:768–769.

29. Fernandez E, Nygren TE, Thorn BE. An "open-transformed scale" for correcting ceiling effects and enhancing retest reliability: The example of pain. *Percept Psychophys* 1991; 49:572–578.

30. Dixon JS, Bird HA. Reproducability along a 10 cm vertical visual analogue scale. *Ann Rheum Dis* 1981;40:87–89.

31. Sim J, Waterfield J. Validity, reliability and responsiveness in the assessment of pain. *Physiother Theory Pract* 1997;13:23–38.

32. Streiner DL, Norman GR. *Health Measurement Scales: A Practical Guide to Their Development and Use (3rd ed)*. New York: Oxford University Press, 2003.

33. Thomee R, Grimby G, Wright BD, Linacre JM. Rasch analysis of visual analog scale measurements before and after treatment of patellofemoral pain syndrome in women. *Scand J Rehabil Med* 1995; 27: 145–151.

34. Rosow I, Breslau N. A Guttman health scale for the aged. *J Gerontol* 1966;21:556–559.

35. Dickson HG, Kohler F. The multi-dimensionality of the FIM motor items precludes an interval scaling using Rasch analysis. *Scand J Rehabil Med* 1996;28:159–162.

36. Heinemann AW, Harvey RL, McGuire JR, Ingberman D, Lovell L, Semik P, et al. Measurement properties of the NIH Stroke Scale during acute rehabilitation. *Stroke* 1997; 28:1174–1180.

37. Rasch G. *Probablistic Models for Some Intelligence and Attainment Tests*. Chicago: University of Chicago, 1980.

38. Wright BD, Masters G. *Rating Scale Analysis: Rasch Measurements*. Chicago: MESA, 1982.

39. Linacre JM. Rasch analysis of rank-ordered data. *J Appl Meas* 2006; 7:129–139.

40. Andrich D. *Rasch Models for Measurement*. Beverly Hills: Sage Publications, 1988.

41. McHorney CA, Monahan PD. Postscript: Applications of Rasch analysis in health care. *Med Care* 2004; 42 (1 Supplement): 173–178.

42. UDS Data Management Service. Guide for the *Use of the Uniform Data Set for Medical Rehabilitation Including the Functional Independence Measure*. Buffalo, NY: Buffalo General Hospital, Uniform Data System for Medical Rehabilitation, 1990.

43. Wright BD, Linacre JM. *BIGSTEPS: A Rasch-Model Computer Program*. Chicago: MESA, 1988.

44. Heinemann AW, Linacre JM, Wright BD, Hamilton BB, Granger C. Relationships between impairment and physical disability as measured by the Functional Independence Measure. *Arch Phys Med Rehabil* 1993;74:566–573.

45. Wright BD, Linacre JM. Observations are always ordinal; measurements, however, must be interval. *Arch Phys Med Rehabil* 1989;70:857–860.

46. Linacre JM, Heinemann AW, Wright BD, Granger C, Hamilton B. The Functional Independence Measure as a Measure of Disability. Research Report 91–01. Chicago: Rehabilitation Services Evaluation Unit, Rehabilitation Institute of Chicago, 1991.

47. Wright BD, Stone MH. *Best Test Design.* Chicago: MESA, 1979.

48. Silverstein B, Fisher WP, Kilgore KM, Harley JP, Harvey RF. Applying psychometric criteria to functional assessment in medical rehabilitation: II. Defining interval measures. *Arch Phys Med Rehabil* 1992;73:507–518.

49. Hsueh IP, Wang WC, Sheu CF, Hsieh CL. Rasch analysis of combining two indices to assess comprehensive ADL function in stroke patients. *Stroke* 2004;35:721–726.

50. Helliwell P, Reay N, Gilworth G, Redmond A, Slade A, Tennant A, et al. Development of a foot impact scale for rheumatoid arthritis. *Arthritis Rheum* 2005;53:418–422.

51. Finlayson M, Mallinson T, Barbosa VM. Activities of daily living (ADL) and instrumental activities of daily living (IADL) items were stable over time in a longitudinal study on aging. *J Clin Epidemiol* 2005;58:338–349.

52. Ryd JL, Rheault W. Rasch analysis of the Dizziness Handicap Inventory. *J Rehabil Outcomes Meas* 1998;2:17–24.

53. Haley SM, McHorney CA, Ware JE, Jr. Evaluation of the MOS SF-36 physical functioning scale (PF-10): I. Unidimensionality and reproducibility of the Rasch item scale. *J Clin Epidemiol* 1994;47:671–684.

54. Stephenson W. *The Study of Behavior: Q Technique and Its Methodology.* Chicago: University of Chicago Press, 1975.

55. Biddle WB, Riesenberg LA, Darcy PA. Medical students' perceptions of desirable characteristics of primary care teaching sites. *Fam Med* 1996;28:629–633.

56. Trotter MJ, Fordyce WE. A process for physical therapist student selection. The Q-technique. *Phys Ther* 1975;55:151–156.

57. Kovach CR, Krejci JW. Facilitating change in dementia care. Staff perceptions. *J Nurs Adm* 1998;28:17–27.

58. Moore C. *Group Techniques for Idea Building.* Beverly Hills, CA: Sage Publications, 1987.

59. Delbecq AL, Van De Ven A, Gustafson DH. *Group Techniques for Program Planning.* Middleton, WI: Green Briar Press, 1986.

60. Lopopolo RB, Schafer DS, Nosse LJ. Leadership, administration, management, and professionalism (LAMP) in physical therapy: A Delphi study. *Phys Ther* 2004;84:137–150.

61. Cabral D, Katz JN, Weinblatt ME, Ting G, Avorn J, Solomon DH. Development and assessment of indicators of rheumatoid arthritis severity: Results of a Delphi panel. *Arthritis Rheum* 2005;53:61–66.

62. Saliba D, Solomon D, Rubenstein L, Young R, Schnelle J, Roth C, et al. Quality indicators for the management of medical conditions in nursing home residents. *J Am Med Dir Assoc* 2004;5:297–309.

63. Wyrwich KW, Nelson HS, Tierney WM, Babu AN, Kroenke K, Wolinsky FD. Clinically important differences in health-related quality of life for patients with asthma: An expert consensus panel report. *Ann Allergy Asthma Immunol* 2003;91:148–153.

64. Davis S, Piercy F, Meszaros PS, Huebner A, Shettler L, Matheson J. Female adolescent smoking: a Delphi study on best prevention practices. *J Drug Educ* 2004;34:295–311.

CHAPTER 16

Systematic Reviews and Meta-Analysis

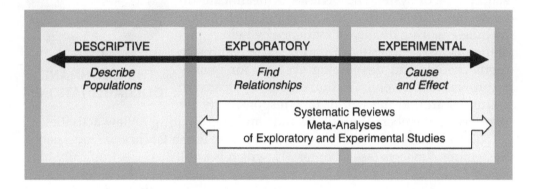

The processes of making clinical decisions are complex indeed. In seeking the evidence on which to base clinical practice, clinicians and researchers are faced with a myriad of published papers and web-based sites often offering unclear or conflicting information regarding the choice of intervention approaches, expectations of outcomes or use of measurement tools.

Given these challenges, the emergence of the **systematic review** has been timely, providing a structured approach to analyzing available information to aid in making important clinical decisions. Although the term systematic review has been used for more than 30 years, its current use has become standardized through the efforts of an international organization called the Cochrane Collaboration (see Box 16.1). Systematic review refers to a rigorous process of searching, appraising and summarizing existing information on a selected topic. Reviews are most commonly focused on the effectiveness of interventions, but may also address the accuracy of diagnostic tools or identification of prognostic factors.

The key word "systematic" differentiates this process from the classical "review" article. Traditional narrative literature reviews have been and continue to be a good source of information, particularly on the background of a specific topic. The traditional review, however, does not include a detailed description of the methods and criteria used to select and evaluate articles that are included. Authors may approach their topics with a bias from their clinical perspective that may not represent the breadth of information. The procedures for conducting a systematic review, on the other hand, are

BOX 16.1 The Cochrane Collaboration

The impetus for developing the current procedures for systematic review can be traced to a 1979 letter written by Archie Cochrane (1908–1988), a British physician, who suggested that a critical summary of randomized clinical trials was needed in medical specialties to provide a reliable source of evidence for medical care.[1]

In 1993, The Cochrane Collaboration was initiated in his honor, creating an international not-for-profit organization, dedicated to promotion of clinical trials evidence and development and dissemination of systematic reviews of healthcare interventions.[2] The principles of the Collaboration include ensuring quality of evidence by being open and responsive to criticism, applying advances in methodology, and developing systems for quality improvement.[3] Twelve Cochrane Centres, located in countries around the world, take responsibility for supporting members through training and coordinating review activities.

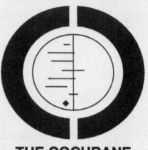

THE COCHRANE
COLLABORATION®

The primary product of the Collaboration is the Cochrane Database of Systematic Reviews (see Chapter 31), which is published electronically four times a year as part of The Cochrane Library. These systematic reviews are prepared and regularly updated by 51 Review Groups that are made up of individuals interested in particular topic areas.[4] Examples of topics include movement disorders, wounds, stroke, neuromuscular disease, back problems, developmental and learning problems, bone and joint trauma, and HIV/AIDS. Rigorous standards have been developed to ensure that these reviews provide accurate and thorough appraisals of the literature. The *Cochrane Handbook for Systematic Reviews of Interventions* is a detailed reference for writing systematic reviews that can be accessed online.[5]

formulated to be inclusive of the body of research evidence at the time the review is undertaken.

When selected studies provide common estimates of the same variables, the separate samples in each study can be viewed as part of one larger target population, allowing for synthesis of results. This **meta-analysis** process combines the studies using a quantitative index to develop a single overall estimate of the intervention effect. This approach can provide important results when several smaller studies are not sufficient to demonstrate meaningful outcomes.

Thorough systematic reviews and meta-analyses can provide evidence to inform practitioners in their decisions to maintain, alter or discard methods of clinical practice. With a well-done systematic review, the clinical and research communities can have confidence that up to the time of publication, the information is current and comprehensive.

The terms systematic review and meta-analysis are often used interchangeably, but they do have different objectives. While both present a critical appraisal of studies, only the meta-analysis includes a statistical synthesis of data. The purpose of this chapter is to describe the process of conducting systematic reviews and meta-analyses, as shown in Figure 16.1.

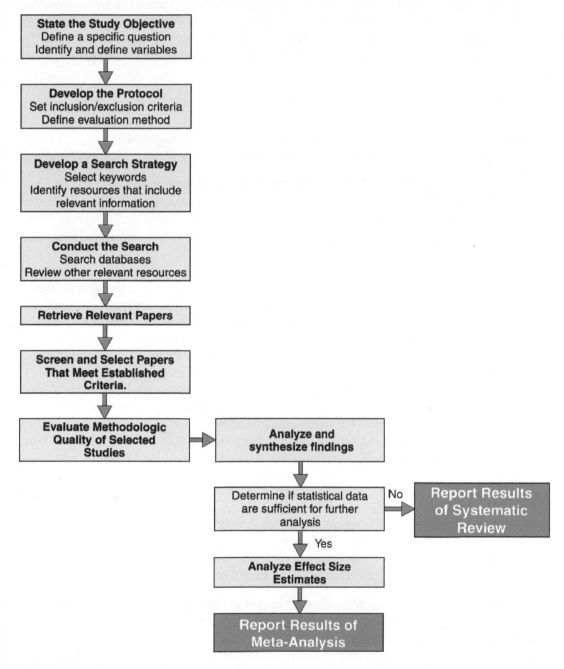

FIGURE 16.1   Summary of the systematic review process, showing the distinction in end products for systematic reviews and meta-analyses.

STUDY OBJECTIVE: ASKING THE QUESTION

The protocol for a systematic review specifies all aspects of the review process and is analogous to the protocol written for a primary research study (see Chapter 32). As with any research endeavor, a systematic review begins with a well-defined, circumscribed question or purpose statement. The question will serve as the foundation for locating relevant references for the review. When asking a question about intervention, the researcher must delineate the treatment, outcome measures and population characteristics. For example, Pang et al[6] were interested in the effect of exercise training for improving aerobic capacity in individuals with stroke. They asked three specific questions for their review:

1. Does aerobic exercise training improve aerobic capacity in individuals recovering from stroke?
2. How much improvement in aerobic capacity can be obtained?
3. What are the specific exercise protocols used to induce an aerobic training effect?

A question about diagnostic tools must specify the test, reference standard and outcomes (see Chapter 27). For instance, Garcia Peña et al[7] conducted a systematic review to determine the accuracy of a protocol for diagnosing appendicitis in children and adolescents using ultrasonography and computed tomography, using surgeons' estimated likelihood of appendicitis as the reference standard.

Questions about prognosis include the prognostic factors and outcomes of interest. As an example, Langer-Gould et al[8] reviewed studies to identify clinical and demographic factors associated with long-term physical or cognitive disability in patients with multiple sclerosis. Systematic reviews can also focus on risk assessment. For instance, Caldwell et al[9] examined randomized controlled trials that compared celecoxib with a placebo, and analyzed the risk of serious cardiovascular events based on that data.

Systematic reviews can also address qualitative research, to explore the experiences of patients outside of the standard quantitative outcome measures.[10] There is at least one Cochrane Review Group dedicated to fostering the application of qualitative research in systematic reviews.[11] This group has worked to develop methods for critical analysis of qualitative studies as well as an appreciation for the role of qualitative studies in evidence-based practice. For example, Noyes and Popay[12] studied the experiences of patients, care providers and policy makers in the treatment of tuberculosis. They asked two questions:

1. What does qualitative research tell us about the facilitators and barriers to accessing and complying with tuberculosis treatment?
2. What does qualitative research tell us about the diverse results and effect sizes of the randomized controlled trials included in the Cochrane review?

They retrieved 58 studies and were able to identify themes related to socio-economic circumstances, material resources, the experience of stigma around tuberculosis, social supports and incentives that influenced the provision of care.

For practicality, we will focus the remainder of this discussion on quantitative measures related to interventions, but the reader should be aware that systematic reviews serve important roles in understanding many types of research questions.

Background and Research Rationale

Just like other research articles, a systematic review will include a review of literature to support the research question. The background or introductory section of the paper typically includes epidemiologic data to demonstrate the prevalence of the condition and its health impact. Variations in treatment options and outcomes of interest are described. Information on etiology, pathophysiology, effect of interventions, and conflicting ideas about patient management provides a rationale for the review question. The background may also include findings of previous systematic reviews, describing why an updated review is important.

SELECTION CRITERIA

In primary studies, researchers specify characteristics of subjects that will determine who will be chosen to participate in the study. For a systematic review, the "subjects" of the review are the studies themselves. Therefore, selection criteria specify inclusion and exclusion requirements for studies to be used for the review. These requirements are usually based on types of studies, participants, interventions and outcomes. The author of the review must specify definitions that will guide this selection process.

Types of Studies

By definition a systematic review is a critical summary of published papers and, when available, selected unpublished papers on a defined topic. Researchers must decide what types of studies to include in the review. Many authors restrict systematic reviews of interventions to the "gold standard" of randomized controlled studies (RCTs) published in peer-reviewed journals. When the literature is replete with RCTs on a particular topic, this may be an effective strategy. When published work is less robust, however, the researcher may find that cohort and case-control studies and case series are valuable for understanding the scope of knowledge about an intervention. These designs are most relevant for reviews related to diagnosis and prognosis.

When possible, reviews should include primary research studies as well as conference proceedings, abstracts, theses and dissertations. It is important to balance the desire for higher levels of evidence with the need to find the "best evidence available." Reviews that are done as part of the Cochrane Collaboration focus primarily on RCTs. Most of the systematic reviews conducted by the Agency for Healthcare Research and Quality (AHRQ) Evidence-based Practice Centers include nonrandomized studies.[13,14]

Levels of Evidence

A useful hierarchy has been developed to categorize studies by "levels of evidence,"[15] as shown in Table 16.1. Levels are described for studies of interventions, diagnosis and prognosis, defined according to the strength of the design used. Although the highest level of evidence for intervention is the RCT, the table shows that cohort studies and clinical prediction rules are the most effective designs for prognosis and diagnosis studies. The lowest level of evidence describes the contribution of expert opinion or basic research that does not have direct clinical application.

TABLE 16.1   LEVELS OF EVIDENCE

Level		Intervention	Prognosis	Diagnosis
1	a	Systematic review of randomized controlled trials (RCT)	Systematic review of cohort studies; clinical prediction rule[a] validated in different populations	Systematic review of Level 1 diagnostic studies; clinical prediction rule[a] validated at several clinical sites
	b	Individual RCT (with narrow confidence interval)	Individual cohort study with ≥ 80% follow-up; clinical prediction rule[a] validated in a single population	Validating cohort with good reference standards;[b] Clinical prediction rule[a] validated within one center
	c			Absolute SpPins and SnNouts[c]
2	a	Systematic review of cohort studies	Systematic review of retrospective cohort studies or untreated control groups in RCTs	Systematic review of Level 2 diagnostic studies
	b	Individual cohort study (or low quality RCT, e.g. with <80% follow-up)	Retrospective cohort study or follow-up of untreated control patients in RCT; derivation of clinical prediction rule[a]	Exploratory cohort study with good reference standards;[b] clinical prediction rule[a] after derivation
3	a	Systematic review of case-control studies		Systematic review of Level 3b studies
	b	Individual case-control study		Non-consecutive study or with inconsistent reference standard
4		Case-series or poor quality cohort and case-control studies[d]	Case-series and poor quality prognostic cohort studies[d]	Case-control study, poor or non-independent reference standard
5		Expert opinion or bench research	Expert opinion or bench research	Expert opinion or bench research

[a]Clinical prediction rules are described in Chapter 27.

[b]Good reference standards are independent of the test, and are applied blindly or objectively to all patients. Poor reference standards are haphazardly applied, but still independent of the test.

[c]An "Absolute SpPin" is a diagnostic finding whose *S*pecificity is so high that a *P*ositive result rules *in* the diagnosis. An "Absolute SnNout" is a diagnostic finding whose *S*ensitivity is so high that a *N*egative result rules *out* the diagnosis. See Chapter 27 for detailed definitions.

[d]Poor quality cohort or case-control studies are those that fail to define comparison groups, measure exposures and outcomes in the same way for all subjects, identify known confounders, or incorporate sufficiently long follow-up of patients.

Adapted from Oxford Centre for Evidence-based Medicine Levels of Evidence (May 2001). Available at <http://www.cebm.net/levels_of_evidence.asp> Accessed April 15, 2007.

Subcategories at each level delineate systematic reviews versus individual studies. Because systematic reviews provide a composite and critical understanding of the literature on a particular topic, they are considered a higher form of evidence than individual studies. Each of the levels can also be given a minus sign (−) to denote studies where evidence is weaker, such as having wide confidence intervals, or systematic reviews with inconsistent findings.[15]

An overall grade can be given to systematic reviews based on the types of studies included:[15]

a. Consistent level 1 studies
b. Consistent level 2 or 3 studies OR extrapolations from level 1 studies
c. Level 4 studies OR extrapolations from level 2 or 3 studies
d. Level 5 evidence OR troublingly inconsistent or inconclusive studies of any level

Types of Participants

The population of interest must be specified to identify the types of subjects or patients recruited in the chosen studies. Characteristics may include age range, gender, or specific diagnostic categories. These characteristics may be defined narrowly or within wide ranges. For example, in their study of aerobic capacity, Pang et al[6] defined acuity and chronicity of stroke according to time since onset. Because study populations can be so variable, systematic reviews have to set reasonable ranges for subject characteristics.

Types of Interventions

Selection criteria must indicate definitions of interventions and comparison treatment if relevant. Because studies are rarely consistent in the application of interventions, these definitions are generally broad enough to allow a reasonable match. For instance, in the study of aerobic capacity and stroke, the authors defined aerobic exercise as

> . . . a structured exercise program that involves the use of large muscle groups for extended periods of time in activities that are rhythmic in nature, including but not limited to walking, stepping, running, swimming, cycling and rowing.[6, p.99]

Therefore, they included studies that used cycle ergometers or treadmills, as well as water-based and land-based exercises with walking, functional strengthening and balance activities. Factors such as duration of treatment or length of follow-up may also be stipulated.

Types of Outcome Measures

The choice of outcome measures will also be essential in the specification of selection criteria. Outcomes include measurements or endpoints, including improvement in condition or reduction of symptoms. Reviewers may specify particular instruments, such as a health status questionnaire or a diagnostic test. Included studies will often have a variety of outcomes that must involve at least one specified measure. For example, in the study of stroke and aerobic capacity, the authors specified interest in outcomes of peak oxygen consumption and peak workload during a graded exercise test, as well as walking velocity and walking endurance.[6] However, the actual tools used to measure these outcomes may be different across studies. Clear definitions will facilitate decisions about how to search for the information that will be included in the project.

SEARCH STRATEGY

A major component of the review process is description of the **search strategy.** The goal is to find a comprehensive list of relevant documents that should be considered. The first task, of course, is to decide where to look and to develop a list of appropriate search terms. Chapter 31 provides a description of several search engines and databases as well as effective search strategies. Online tutorials have also been prepared to help researchers become more familiar with this process.[16–18] The researcher must develop a thorough search strategy to be sure that all relevant materials have been found. In most cases more than one database should be used to provide the widest search possible. Many researchers will limit reviews to articles in a particular language as a matter of practicality, although this clearly reduces the scope of available studies.

The report of a systematic review must indicate which databases were used and the specific search terms entered. Authors may provide a detailed list of the search strategy as a useful reference (see Chapter 31). In addition to online resources, hand searching through pertinent journals and reference lists of published papers can help to ensure that the search is complete. When the number of citations identified is large, the researcher should look through titles and abstracts as a first pass to identify papers that are clearly not germane to the review.

Reviewing Systematic Reviews

Reviews that were limited to RCTs can be replicated using broader selection criteria including case-control or case series studies. For this purpose, examination of the list of excluded studies in the published review may yield appropriate papers. For example, Green et al[19] conducted a systematic review of physical therapy interventions for shoulder pain. Having set criteria that limited studies to randomized allocation to treatment groups, this review excluded 38 studies out of 64 potential references. Therefore, several of the 38 excluded papers may be useful for a new study.

The Grey Literature

Because of the potential for bias when search strategies are limited to databases of peer-reviewed scholarly journals, the systematic review process should also include examination of the "grey" literature. **Grey literature** refers to unpublished studies or studies that are available through sources other than the customary journals.[20] Examples include working papers, theses, and fact sheets disseminated by condition-specific associations, such as the Arthritis Foundation or the Muscular Dystrophy Association, or the government. Studies of systematic reviews have shown that a difference in conclusions could result from the inclusion or exclusion of grey literature,[21] potentially affecting the estimate of intervention effectiveness.[22]

Conducting the Search

The challenge of conducting a search is to retrieve all of the relevant papers and exclude the irrelevant ones. The selection of papers, reports and reviews depends on the criteria established in the protocol. Even with a careful search strategy, however, not all identified papers will meet the pre-established criteria. For example, for a systematic review of treatments for developmental stuttering, Bothe et al[23] initially located 162 articles through a search, but having set robust criteria, they ended up including only 39 papers in their final analysis! A systematic review should include a list of excluded studies with specific reasons for their exclusion.

Publication Bias

Systematic reviews are obviously influenced by the literature that is available. **Publication bias** is an issue that really "belongs" to the research community, specifically primary researchers and journal editors.[24-26] Researchers may fail to submit the results of studies where the results are not statistically significant or editors may decline to publish such studies. In other words, there has been a bias against negative or inconclusive results. Because the value of systematic review is to broaden the evidence for *or* against a proposed outcome, evidence of no effect must be part of the picture.

EVALUATING METHODOLOGIC QUALITY

Once the selection process is complete, the studies are ready to be critically reviewed. As a rule, a minimum of two primary reviewers will independently assess content and rate the quality and applicability of each selected paper or information source. Therefore, the reviewers will need to discuss the details of the process, including how the papers will be assessed. It is often useful for reviewers to evaluate a few sample papers in a training process. When disagreement occur, they should be resolved by consensus or by resolution from a third party.

Reviewers will go through each study to describe its parameters, and record information on a data extraction form. This process allows the reviewers to gather the same information on each study, so that comparisons can be readily made. These forms generally record elements that are important for assessing quality of design and data analysis. A sample data extraction form is shown in Figure 16.2.

Types of Study Bias

Because studies typically differ in their design, quality and validity, results of some trials may be more meaningful than others. Therefore, it is important to consider study quality.[27] Four types of bias related to internal validity have been identified that can have an influence on the outcome of a systematic review.[5] **Selection bias** is one of the most important factors that can distort treatment effects because of the way comparison groups are formed.[28] Random allocation and concealment of allocation are essential elements of a clinical trial to assure that bias is not introduced. **Performance bias** refers to differences in the provision of care to experimental and control groups in a study. The

Data Extraction Form

Study Title _____

Authors _____

Journal _____ **Year** _____ **Vol** _____ **Pages** _____

Study Type _____

Include ☐   **Exclude** ☐

Reason for exclusion: _____

METHODS/TRIAL QUALITY

Participants • Age (Mean, range) • Other sample characteristics • Subject inclusion/exclusion criteria	
Method of subject selection	
Method of group assignment (randomization) Was allocation concealed?	
Study design	
Blinding • Participants • Investigators • Outcome assessors	
Type of intervention • Intervention(s) • Control condition(s) • Duration and other protocol information	
Intention-to-treat analysis	

FIGURE 16.2 Sample data extraction form for systematic reviews. (Adapted from <http://www
.cochrane-renal.org/docs/data_extraction_form.doc> Accessed July 19, 2007.)

most effective way to prevent this bias is through blinding of those who receive and give care. **Attrition bias** is related to the differential loss of subjects across comparison groups. This becomes especially relevant for studies with follow-up periods, and is addressed through intention to treat analysis. The fourth type is **detection bias**, which occurs if outcome assessment differs across comparison groups.

Outcome assessments	
Compliance	
Match of intervention and controls	
Baseline similarly between groups	

RESULTS

	Experimental Group(s)	Control Group(s)
Observed n		
Excluded subjects		
Lost to follow-up		
Primary Outcome • Mean, standard deviation • Proportion • Other effect size index		
Secondary Outcomes		
Statistical analyses • Description of groups • Comparison of groups		

FIGURE 16.2 (cont.)

The use of quality assessment tools is an essential component of systematic reviews to determine if these forms of bias affect the value of included papers for answering the research question. Even with randomized trials, articles often neglect to provide important information on specific elements of the trial. Assessment of study validity may be used first as a threshold for deciding which studies to include in the review. As part of the review, the quality assessment will provide possible explanations for differences in study results.

Rating Scales

Several rating scales have been developed. The criteria used and resultant ratings must be described in a systematic review so that readers can evaluate the validity of the reviewer's conclusions. Published checklists have varied numbers of items, with some based on "yes/no" answers for each item, while others allow for "unclear" responses. Most scales result in a total score based on summing the "yes" responses for each study. There is no gold standard for this process, and most scoring systems have not been validated. Nonetheless, these various scales generally focus on similar concepts as relevant to assessing the quality of a study.

We will describe three commonly used scales, although several others can be found in the literature.[29-34] The CONSORT statement[34] and the STARD statement,[35] which are checklists of items that should be included in the report of a randomized trial or diagnostic study, can also be used for this purpose (see Chapters 9 and 27).

The Jadad Scale

One of the original tools for evaluating quality is the **Jadad scale**, the *Instrument to Measure the Likelihood of Bias*, which is composed of three questions (see Table 16.2).[36] This scale focuses on randomization, blinding and attrition to determine quality of a study. The maximum total score is 5. While simple and quick, the Jadad scale is limited in its scope and does not consider many important design issues.

The PEDro Scale

The **Physiotherapy Evidence Database (PEDro) scale** has become widely used in rehabilitation and medical literature. Developed by physiotherapists at the University of Sydney, it is based on a description of the study's structure.[37] In addition to items related to randomization, blinding and attrition, the scale also includes analysis of design and statistics (see Table 16.3). Each criterion is graded 1 for "yes" and 0 for "no" or "unclear," with a maximum total score of 10. The PEDro scale has reasonable reliability,[38,39] and has been shown to be a more comprehensive measure of methodological quality than the Jadad scale.[40]

TABLE 16.2   JADAD SCALE: *INSTRUMENT TO MEASURE THE LIKELIHOOD OF BIAS*

1. Was the study described as randomized?	Yes (1 pt)	No (0 pt)
2. Was the study described as double blind?	Yes (1 pt)	No (0 pt)
3. Was there a description of withdrawals and dropouts?	Yes (1 pt)	No (0 pt)

Add 1 point:
For question 1 if the randomization method was described and it was appropriate.
For question 2 if the method of double blinding was described and it was appropriate.

Deduct 1 point:
For question 1 if the method of randomization was not appropriate.
For question 2 if the method of double blinding was not appropriate.

Reference: Jadad AR, et al. Assessing the quality of reports of randomized clinical trials: Is blinding necessary? *Control Clin Trials* 1996;17:1–12.

TABLE 16.3   PEDro SCALE[a]

1. Eligibility criteria were specified.[b]	no/yes[c]
2. Subjects were randomly allocated to groups (in a crossover study, subjects were randomly allocated an order in which treatments were received).	no/yes
3. Allocation was concealed.	no/yes
4. The groups were similar at baseline regarding the most important prognostic indicators.	no/yes
5. There was blinding of all subjects.	no/yes
6. There was blinding of all therapists who administered the therapy.	no/yes
7. There was blinding of all assessors who measured at least one key outcome.	no/yes
8. Measures of at least one key outcome were obtained from more than 85 percent of the subjects initially allocated to groups.	no/yes
9. All subjects for whom outcome measures were available received the treatment or control condition as allocated or, where this was not the case, data for at least one key outcome was analyzed by "intention to treat."	no/yes
10. The results of between-group statistical comparisons are reported for at least one key outcome.	no/yes
11. The study provides both point measures and measures of variability for at least one key outcome.	no/yes

[a]Available at <http://www.pedro.fhs.usyd.edu.au/scale> Accessed on April 16, 2007. This website includes detailed explanations for each criterion.

[b]This first item refers to external validity, but is not included in the total PEDro score.

[c]Each item is given 1 point for a yes answer. The maximum total score is 10.

The QUADAS Scale

Whiting et al[41] have validated a scale to review studies of diagnostic test accuracy, shown in Table 16.4. The **Quality Assessment of Diagnostic Accuracy Studies (QUADAS)** is a 14-item scale, which has been shown to have good rater reliability.[42] Items are rated "yes," "no," or "unclear," and the total score is expressed as a percentage of items that are given a "yes" rating.

Presentation of Methodologic Quality

Systematic reviews will usually include tabular results of the quality assessment as a consensus score between the two reviewers. Table 16.5 is an example of such a table using the PEDro score for a systematic review of hand splinting for adults following stroke.[43] Each study in the review is identified and scores are shown for each criterion as well as a total score. Some reviewers choose a cutoff score to delineate a high versus low quality study. Others may include the level of evidence that each study achieves. This type of presentation allows the reader to quickly see the overall quality of the studies included in the review.

Data Synthesis

Once the articles of interest have been critically reviewed, the researcher must then determine if and how the results of the studies can be synthesized. The reviewers will

---

TABLE 16.4 **QUALITY ASSESSMENT OF DIAGNOSTIC ACCURACY STUDIES: QUADAS**

1. Was the spectrum of patients representative of the patients who will receive the test in practice?[a]
2. Were selection criteria clearly described?
3. Is the reference standard likely to correctly classify the target condition?
4. Is the time period between reference standard and index test short enough to be reasonably sure that the target condition did not change between the two tests?
5. Did the whole sample or a random selection of the sample, receive verification using a reference standard of diagnosis?
6. Did patients receive the same reference standard regardless of the index test result?
7. Was the reference standard independent of the index test (i.e. the index test did not form part of the reference standard)?
8. Was the execution of the index test described in sufficient detail to permit replication of the test?
9. Was the execution of the reference standard described in sufficient detail to permit its replication?
10. Were the index test results interpreted without knowledge of the results of the reference standard?
11. Were the reference standard results interpreted without knowledge of the results of the index test?
12. Were the same clinical data available when test results were interpreted as would be available when the test is used in practice?
13. Were uninterpretable/ intermediate test results reported?
14. Were withdrawals from the study explained?

---

[a]Each item is graded as Yes, No or Unclear.

Reference: Whiting R, Rutjes AW, Reitsma JB, Bossuyt PM, Kleijnen J. The development of QUADAS: A tool for the quality assessment of studies of diagnostic accuracy included in systematic reviews. *BMC Med Res Methodol* 2003;3:25.

TABLE 16.5 **METHODOLOGICAL RATING OF RANDOMIZED CONTROLLED TRIALS**

Study	PEDro Criterion Score[a]											Total	Quality	Level[b]
	1	2	3	4	5	6	7	8	9	10	11			
McPherson et al., 1982	Y	Y	N	N	N	N	N	Y	N	Y	Y	4	LOW	1b
Rose et al., 1987	Y	Y	N	N	N	N	N	N	N	Y	N	2	LOW	1b
Poole et al., 1990	N	Y	N	Y	N	N	Y	Y	N	Y	Y	6	HIGH	2b
Langlois et al., 1991	Y	Y	N	N	N	N	N	N	N	Y	Y	3	LOW	1b
Lannin et al., 2003	Y	Y	Y	Y	N	N	Y	Y	Y	Y	Y	8	HIGH	1b

[a]For this example, a score of 5 has been arbitrarily assigned as the cutoff for high versus low quality. The items for the PEDro scale are shown in Table 16.6.

[b]Levels of evidence are defined in Table 16.1.

Adapted from Lannin NA, Herbert RD. Is hand splinting effective for adults following stroke? A systematic review and methodological critique of published research. *Clin Rehabil* 2003;17:807–816, Table 4, p. 813. Used with permission.

determine the degree of heterogeneity or homogeneity in the included studies. Heterogeneity refers to dissimilarity in specific aspects of the studies:[44]

- Composition of treatment groups, including different inclusion and exclusion criteria, different baseline levels, or differences in timing or dose of intervention
- Design of the study, including length of follow-up and proportion of subjects who dropped out
- Management of patients, including how treatments are regulated and the presence of complications or co-morbid conditions

If papers have published conflicting or inconclusive findings, it will be difficult to interpret the results of the systematic review. We know that studies with small sample sizes or small effect sizes may show no significant effect of the intervention, leaving the possibility of a Type II error (see Chapter 18). We also know that the choice of measurement scale or tool may affect the sensitivity or responsiveness of measurement. Other study characteristics, such as criteria for subject selection or operational definitions, may have an impact on the ability to generalize findings.

Once again, a tabular presentation is helpful to understand the variations across studies and their overall findings. Table 16.6 illustrates one possible format for a systematic review of outcomes of cardiovascular exercise programs for people with Down Syndrome.[45] Notice that the table includes information on sample size and characteristics of subjects, as well as a description of the intervention and outcome measures. This table also shows the PEDro score for each study, which allows the reader to analyze the findings of the study in relation to its quality.

Discussion and Conclusions

The final section of the systematic review will be a discussion of findings and the reviewer's overall conclusions based on the quality of evidence that was obtained. This can be a complex process if studies have varying methods and results, as is often the case. The reviewer has the responsibility to integrate the findings to clarify the state of knowledge in a clinical context. By comparing studies in terms of their quality and procedures, the discussion will put the results in context. Suggestions for future research should be proposed.

META-ANALYSIS

Meta-analysis is an extension of the systematic review that incorporates a statistical combination of several studies that have related research hypotheses. Meta-analysis can be done for systematic reviews of clinical trials, evaluation of diagnostic tests or epidemiologic studies. The first meta-analysis was actually done in 1904 by Karl Pearson, who combined data from several sources to compare infection and mortality rates among British soldiers who had and had not volunteered for typhoid fever inoculations.[46] He recognized that the sample size of any single study is likely to be too small to obtain a conclusive result. Gene Glass, an educational researcher, is credited with coining the term "meta-analysis" to mean

> . . . the statistical analysis of a large collection of analysis results from individual studies for the purpose of integrating the findings.[47, p.3]

TABLE 16.6 SUMMARY OF FINDINGS FROM FOUR STUDIES IN A SYSTEMATIC REVIEW

Author	PEDro Score	n	Mean Age ± SD (y)	Sex	Severity of Intellectual Disability	Previous Exercise Participation	Program Details	Training Intensity	Body Structure/ Function Outcomes
Rimmer et al	6	52	39.4 ± 6.4	29 W, 23 M	Mild to moderate	Sedentary for at least 1y prior to the program	30min aerobic machine-based (eg, treadmill, stationary bicycle) exercise program, 15min PRE; 3/wk for 12wk	50%–70% Vo$_2$peak	Vo$_2$peak; time to exhaustion; bench press and leg press 1-RM; grip strength; body weight and BMI
Tsimaras et al	5	25	24.6 ± 3.3	25 M	IQ 45–60	Not reported	10-min warm-up, 30min jog/walking program; 3/wk for 12wk	65%–75% max HR assessed at start of program	Vo$_2$peak, Vepeak, time to exhaustion
Varela et al	6	16	21.4 ± 3.0	16 M	Mean IQ 38.8	Not reported	10-min warm-up, 25-min rowing program, 10-min cool down; 3/wk for 16wk	55%–70% Vo$_2$peak	Vo$_2$peak, Vepeak, time to exhaustion, distance traveled, work level reached; body weight, body fat percentage
Millar et al	6	14	17.7 ± 2.9	3 W, 11 M	IQ 30–70	Not reported	10-min warm-up, 30-min brisk walking/jogging, 10-min cool down program; 3/wk for 10wk	65%–75% max HR	Vo$_2$peak, Vepeak, time to exhaustion

Abbreviations: 1-RM, 1 repetition maximum; BMI, body mass index; HR, heart rate; IQ, intelligence quotient; max, maximum; M, men; ND, no data; PRE, progressive resistance exercise; SD, standard deviation; Vepeak, peak ventilation; W, women.

Adapted from Dodd KJ, Shields N. A systematic review of the outcomes of cardiovascular exercise programs for people with Down syndrome. *Arch Phys Med Rehabil* 2005;86:2051–2058. Table 1, p. 2054. Used with permission.

Systematic Review or Meta-Analysis?

As the researcher approaches the synthesis of data in a systematic review, the question of statistical analysis must be addressed. When studies meet criteria for homogeneity, the synthesis of results may go beyond the descriptive systematic analysis to include a meta-analysis. Meta-analysis can be a powerful tool for synthesizing information across multiple studies, but it can also be misleading if the studies are not appropriately combined. When measurements are inconsistent or comparisons do not make sense, systematic review may have to be sufficient to qualitatively synthesize the information.

The major advantages of meta-analysis are to (1) increase power by increasing sample size, (2) improve estimates of effect size, (3) resolve uncertainty when conflicting results occur, and (4) improve the generalizability of findings.[48] Individual studies may have nonsignificant findings because of small sample size (see Chapter 18). Therefore, combining samples from several studies has the potential effect of increasing the ability to detect important differences.

Because we are faced with massive amounts of information from primary studies, the ability to apply statistical methods to calculate combined estimates of effects can provide more confidence in the outcome. Meta-analytical methods increase the likelihood of finding the true effects of a treatment or the strength of a relationship. Readers who are not familiar with statistical methods will find it helpful to review procedures in later chapters to better understand processes described here.

Evaluating Heterogeneity

The degree to which studies in a systematic review are similar is based on the heterogeneity of the treatment effect across the studies. This heterogeneity can be due to two main reasons. Either it is a random effect due to chance differences between studies, or study samples may be drawn from truly different populations.[49] The statistic used most often to test for heterogeneity is chi-square (see Chapter 25). A nonsignificant test indicates that there is a common treatment effect across studies, and therefore the observed differences are what would be expected by chance. A large chi-square value indicates that a common treatment effect is unlikely.

Effect Size

The concept of **effect size** is central to meta-analysis. Effect size is an estimate of the magnitude of difference between groups or the effect of the intervention. Effect sizes can be obtained for continuous data such as means or correlations, or binary data such as relative risk and odds ratios. Estimates from individual studies are combined to reflect the overall size of the effect of the independent variable. The larger the difference, the greater the "effect" of the intervention (see Chapter 27). Meta-analysis does not pool subjects into a single sample; rather each study adds to the estimate of the population parameter (the measured variable) by contributing its sample effect size index. The result is usually a more precise overall estimate.[50]

The statistical methods of analyzing and summarizing the outcome of studies depend on the kind of data used to document the outcome.[51] An **effect size index** is created for the data in each study that allows comparison across studies, based on means for quantitative variables, proportions or frequencies for categorical data, or correlation values for measures of association.

For the comparison of means in a two-group comparative study with continuous scale data, the effect size index is given the symbol d. Because measures in various studies can use different units, this index normalizes the data into a common metric. The index is based on the mean difference between groups divided by the pooled standard deviation of the two groups (see Appendix C). For a study based on proportions, such as relative risk or odds ratio, the effect size index is the ratio itself.

Weighting Effect Size

The process of meta-analysis requires that the individual effect sizes for each study be combined to form a common estimate of the effect. But because sample sizes vary across studies, the contribution to the overall effect is not equal. A study with a larger sample will contribute a more precise estimate of effect than one with fewer subjects. Therefore, adjustments in the calculation of the effect size are used to weight the contribution of each individual study. The methods for calculating weights are specific to the index used, and can be carried out using various software programs, several of which are in the public domain. The Cochrane Collaboration supports the use of *RevMan* software.[52]

Forest Plots

The results of a meta-analysis are usually reported by presenting data in a plot that illustrates results of individual studies and a cumulative summary. To illustrate this process, we will consider a meta-analysis by Panpanich et al[53] to study the effect of the antibiotic azithromycin compared to other antibiotic agents for the treatment of acute lower respiratory tract infections. They found 14 trials that met their inclusion criteria. Through pooled analysis they showed a relative risk (RR) of 0.96 for clinical failure associated with the azithromycin.*

The plot shown in Table 16.7 is called a **forest plot,** showing results of the review. The outcome of each study is shown by a small square icon, representing the relevant outcome for the study, in this case relative risk. Each horizontal line represents the confidence interval around that estimate. The size of the square corresponds to the weight of the study, which is related to sample size. The confidence interval for the total combined value is indicated by a diamond shape at the bottom of the plot. The center line of the plot indicates no difference in risk between groups. For this example, relative risk values that are to the left of the center line represent a result in favor of the azithromycin. The plot allows us to visually understand the inconsistency in findings and large variance in several studies for this review.

Sensitivity Analysis

Because there are so many differences in study designs and methods of data synthesis, there is always a question regarding the sensitivity of results of a systematic review;

---

*See Chapter 28 for a discussion of relative risk (RR). A relative risk of 1.0 indicates no excess risk associated with the treatment. In this example, an RR of 0.96 is close to 1.0, and indicates no substantial difference in clinical failure with either treatment. An RR of less than 1.0 indicates a reduction in risk associated with the intervention.

TABLE 16.7 EXAMPLE OF A FOREST PLOT

Review: Azithromycin for acute lower respiratory tract infections
Comparison: 01 Azithromycin versus amoxillin or amoxycillin-clavulanate
Outcome: 01 Clinical failure

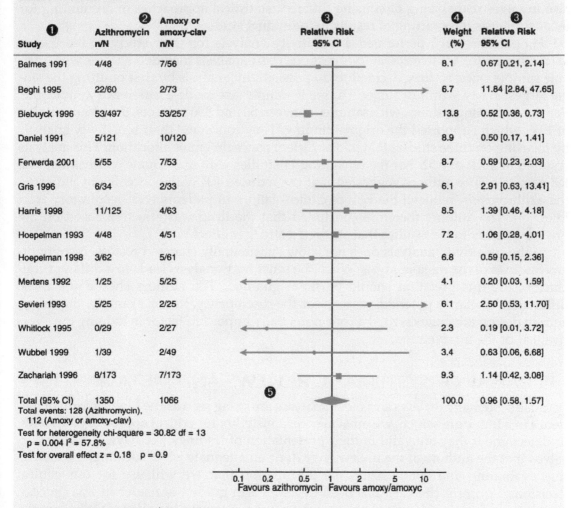

Study	Azithromycin n/N	Amoxy or amoxy-clav n/N	Relative Risk 95% CI	Weight (%)	Relative Risk 95% CI
Balmes 1991	4/48	7/56		8.1	0.67 [0.21, 2.14]
Beghi 1995	22/60	2/73		6.7	11.84 [2.84, 47.65]
Biebuyck 1996	53/497	53/257		13.8	0.52 [0.36, 0.73]
Daniel 1991	5/121	10/120		8.9	0.50 [0.17, 1.41]
Ferwerda 2001	5/55	7/53		8.7	0.69 [0.23, 2.03]
Gris 1996	6/34	2/33		6.1	2.91 [0.63, 13.41]
Harris 1998	11/125	4/63		8.5	1.39 [0.46, 4.18]
Hoepelman 1993	4/48	4/51		7.2	1.06 [0.28, 4.01]
Hoepelman 1998	3/62	5/61		6.8	0.59 [0.15, 2.36]
Mertens 1992	1/25	5/25		4.1	0.20 [0.03, 1.59]
Sevieri 1993	5/25	2/25		6.1	2.50 [0.53, 11.70]
Whitlock 1995	0/29	2/27		2.3	0.19 [0.01, 3.72]
Wubbel 1999	1/39	2/49		3.4	0.63 [0.06, 6.68]
Zachariah 1996	8/173	7/173		9.3	1.14 [0.42, 3.08]
Total (95% CI)	1350	1066		100.0	0.96 [0.58, 1.57]

Total events: 128 (Azithromycin),
   112 (Amoxy or amoxy-clav)
Test for heterogeneity chi-square = 30.82 df = 13
   p = 0.004 I^2 = 57.8%
Test for overall effect z = 0.18   p = 0.9

0.1   0.2   0.5   1   2   5   10
Favours azithromycin   Favours amoxy/amoxyc

❶ List of studies by first author

❷ Number of subjects in experimental and control groups (n = number of adverse events, N = number of subjects in group). For example, for the study by Balmes (1991), the total sample was 104 subjects; 11 subjects had adverse outcomes.

❸ Relative risk (RR) of clinical failure associated with use of azithromycin. Square icon indicates RR, with larger squares representing larger sample sizes. Confidence intervals are shown by the horizontal line and in parentheses. An arrow at the end of the horizontal line indicates a value that goes beyond the scale on the plot.

❹ Weight for RR based on sample size.

❺ Overall RR measure for all studies combined. Larger icon representative of total for all sample sizes.

From Panpanich R, Lerttrakarnnon P, Laopaiboon M. Azithromycin for acute lower respiratory tract infections. *Cochrane Database Syst Rev* 2004; CD001954. Used with permission.

that is, would the conclusion of the review be different if the method of analysis was changed?[5] **Sensitivity analysis** is a technique that assesses if findings change when key assumptions or decisions differ. For systematic reviews these key assumptions include the criteria for inclusion and exclusion of studies. For meta-analysis this process also involves reanalyzing data using different statistical approaches or accounting for inconsistencies in reporting of results in individual studies.

Panpanich et al[53] performed a sensitivity analysis for their study of the use of azithromycin for acute respiratory infection. Their analysis included studies with variable sample sizes, so they decided to do a sensitivity analysis by first omitting the single largest study with 770 subjects to see if sample size made a difference in outcome. For the remaining studies, with samples between 50 and 350 subjects, they found an RR of 1.06, which supported the original finding. They continued their sensitivity analysis by focusing on three studies that had sufficient concealment of allocation. This analysis resulted in a RR of 0.52. For the remaining 11 studies with inadequate concealment the RR was 1.14. The authors suggested that the reduced RR with concealment indicated the azithromycin reduced the risk of clinical failure in patients with respiratory tract infection. The authors therefore concluded that the drug was effective based on the greater validity in the studies that showed a stronger effect.

If the sensitivity analysis does not show substantially changed results, it strengthens findings of the meta-analysis. When the sensitivity analysis leads to a different conclusion, the interpretation should be more guarded. The authors should use these differences to clarify potential reasons for the discrepancy. In our example, the difference in design attributes is used as one potentially important factor in judging the effectiveness of the intervention.

APPRAISAL OF SYSTEMATIC REVIEWS AND META-ANALYSES

Because systematic reviews and meta-analyses are being seen as the highest form of evidence in a literature search, we must take responsibility for critical appraisal of reviews, to determine if they are valid in their presentation of findings. We have to assure ourselves that the authors of the review have done an adequate job of locating, summarizing, evaluating and synthesizing the information that we will use for our clinical decisions. A useful checklist has been developed to guide the reader in this process, based on three areas of concern: (1) Are the results of the study valid? (2) What are the results? and (3) Will the results help me in caring for my patients?[54] This checklist is shown in Table 16.8.

FIND OUT MORE

The scope of this text naturally limits the detail we can provide on systematic reviews and meta-analysis. For those interested in further information we recommend three important references. We have already cited the *Cochrane Handbook for Systematic Reviews of Interventions,*[5] which is a comprehensive guide for writing systematic reviews and meta-analyses. This handbook is updated frequently and supports the Cochrane Review process. The Centres for Reviews and Dissemination[55] and the EBM Toolbox provided by the Oxford Centre for Evidence Based Medicine[56] provide valuable online resources as well.

TABLE 16.8 CRITICAL APPRAISAL OF SYSTEMATIC REVIEWS AND META-ANALYSES

	Yes	No	Can't Tell
ARE THE RESULTS OF THE STUDY VALID?			
Was the review question clear?			
• Did the question specify the population studied?			
• Did the question specify the interventions used?			
• Did the question specify the outcomes that were measured?			
Were the inclusion and exclusion criteria for selection of studies specified and appropriate?			
• Was a comprehensive search strategy explained?			
• Were bibliographic databases identified?			
• Does it appear that the retrieved references include the important, relevant studies?			
Did the reviewers appraise the validity of the included studies?			
• Was the scale for measurement of methodological quality described adequately?			
• Were assessments reliable, i.e., did the reviewers explain the seriousness of disagreements and how they were handled?			
• Was there a wide variation in validity of the included studies?			
If results of studies were combined in a meta-analysis, was it reasonable to do so?			
• Were the studies measuring the same magnitude of effect?			
• Were results of all included studies adequately reported?			
• Were the results similar from study to study?			
WHAT ARE THE RESULTS?			
What are the overall results of the review?			
• Did the reviewers clearly express the "bottom line" conclusions?			
• Did the reviewers include specific effect size measures?			
How precise are the results?			
• Did the reviewers report point estimates and confidence intervals from included studies?			
WILL THE RESULTS HELP ME IN THE CARE OF MY PATIENT?			
Can the results be applied to my patient?			
• Are the patients in the included studies similar enough to my patient?			
• Were subgroup analyses included to help understand the influence of various patient characteristics?			
• Are the settings of the included studies similar enough to mine?			
Were all important outcome measures included?			
Are the benefits of the intervention worth the harm and costs?			

Adapted from Oxman AD, Cook DJ, Guyatt G. Users' guide to the medical literature: VI. How to use an overview. *JAMA* 1994; 272:1367–1371.

A Guide for the Future

The value of conducting and reading systematic reviews or meta-analyses cannot be overestimated. Reviews that are conducted with a rigorously defined process, such as those described by contributors to the Cochrane Collaboration[57] and the Centre for Evidence Based Medicine[58] are essential to a clinician's ability to sort through evidence in an efficient way. With a well-done systematic review, the clinical and research communities can have confidence that up to the time of publication, the information is current and comprehensive.

Another important application of systematic reviews is to avoid repeating studies of interventions that have already been clearly determined to be effective. Scientific and ethical justification for new clinical trials, as well as interpretation of their findings, should be based on defensible assessments of relevant previous research.[59] With evidence that there has been unnecessary replication of clinical trials, the editorial policy of *Lancet* now requires that authors demonstrate that they have looked at existing systematic reviews of the topic of their present study or have conducted a systematic review themselves to justify what new information would be added by yet another study.[60] There may always be questions about whether all the available information has been included and whether bias has been totally eliminated. It, then, becomes the reader's ("consumer's") responsibility to evaluate those possibilities (see Chapter 33) and to judge the applicability of findings to clinical practice.

Systematic reviews will also clarify areas of practice that require further primary research. Most reviews identify continued uncertainty about the effectiveness of interventions, and therefore are a rich source of ideas for further research. In a review of 2,535 reviews from the Cochrane Library, Clarke et al[61] found that 82.0% of them made suggestions about specific interventions that needed further evaluation. The majority of reviews also suggested outcome measures that were most appropriate for specific conditions.

A final caution, however. Systematic reviews and meta-analyses are an important tool to help us integrate information from many studies. But they are only tools. They help us understand what the literature has to tell us, if anything. It is most important to recognize that the results of a systematic review are only as good as the decisions that were made in developing the review—which studies were included, how they were analyzed, and the degree to which the information is up to date. To be useful as clinical references for evidence-based practice, systematic reviews should be updated regularly as new data become available. For instance, the review groups for the Cochrane Collaboration are responsible for updates on a regular two-year schedule.[5] Sometimes the update will include more recent studies, or it may indicate that no further research has been done since the original review was published. Both types of information are important for clinicians.

Synthesis of data from individual studies requires rigorous quantitative methods, and also requires that the data from individual studies are reported well.[49] Systematic reviews and meta-analyses represent only one component of evidence-based practice and cannot replace sound clinical decision making.

REFERENCES

1. Cochrane AL. 1931–1971: A critical review, with particular reference to the medical professions. *Medicines for the Year 2000.* London: Office of Health Economics, 1979:1–11.
2. Shiffman RN, Shekelle P, Overhage JM, Slutsky J, Grimshaw JM, Deshpande AM. Standardized reporting of clinical practice guidelines: A proposal from the conference on guideline standardization. *Ann Int Med* 2003; 139:493–498.
3. Cochrane Collaboration Strategic Plan 2003. Available at <http://www.cochrane.org/admin/stratp03.doc> Accessed April 20, 2007.
4. Cochrane Review Groups (CRGs). Available at <http://www.cochrane.org/contact/entities.htm> Accessed April 20, 2007.
5. Higgins JPT, Green S, (eds). *Cochrane Handbook of Systematic Reviews of Interventions 4.2.6* [updated September 2006]. Available at <http://www.cochrane.org/resources/handbook> Accessed January 30, 2006.
6. Pang MY, Eng JJ, Dawson AS, Gylfadottir S. The use of aerobic exercise training in improving aerobic capacity in individuals with stroke: A meta-analysis. *Clin Rehabil* 2006;20:97–111.
7. Garcia Peña BM, Mandl KD, Kraus SJ, Fischer AC, Fleisher GR, Lund DP, et al. Ultrasonography and limited computed tomography in the diagnosis and management of appendicitis in children. *JAMA* 1999;282:1041–1046.
8. Langer-Gould A, Popat RA, Huang SM, Cobb K, Fontoura P, Gould MK, et al. Clinical and demographic predictors of long-term disability in patients with relapsing-remitting multiple sclerosis: A systematic review. *Arch Neurol* 2006;63:1686–16891.
9. Caldwell B, Aldington S, Weatherall M, Shirtcliffe P, Beasley R. Risk of cardiovascular events and celecoxib: A systematic review and meta-analysis. *J R Soc Med* 2006;99: 132–140.
10. Dixon-Woods M, Fitzpatrick R. Qualitative research in systematic reviews has established a place for itself. *BMJ* 2001;323:765–766.
11. The Cochrane Qualitative Research Methods Group (CQRMG). Available at <http://www.joannabriggs.edu.au/cqrmg/> Accessed April 26, 2007.
12. Noyes J, Popay J. Directly observed therapy and tuberculosis: How can a systematic review of qualitative research contribute to improving services? A qualitative metasynthesis. *J Adv Nurs* 2007;57:227–243.
13. Norris SL, Atkins D. Challenges in using nonrandomized studies in systematic reviews of treatment interventions. *Ann Intern Med* 2005;142:1112–1119.
14. Agency for Healthcare Research and Quality (AHRQ). Department of Health and Human Services. Available at <http://www.ahrq.gov/clinic/epcix.htm> Accessed May 31, 2006.
15. Centre for Evidence-Based Medicine. Oxford Centre for Evidence Based Medicine. Available at <www.cebm.net> Accessed April 16, 2007.
16. PubMed tutorial. Available at <http://www.nlm.nih.gov/bsd/disted/pubmed.html> Accessed April 17, 2007.
17. OVID Tutorial: Training and Documentation. Available at <http://www.ovid.com/site/help/ovid-tutorial.jsp> Accessed April 17, 2007.
18. PEDro tutorial: Reading clinical trials in physiotherapy. Available at <http://www.pedro.fhs.usyd.edu.au/tutorial.html> Accessed April 17, 2007.
19. Green S, Buchbinder R, Hetrick S. Physiotherapy interventions for shoulder pain. *Cochrane Database Syst Rev* 2003:CD004258.
20. Weintraub I. The role of greyliterature in the sciences. Available at <http://library.brooklyn.cuny.edu/access/greyliter.htm> Accessed May 25, 2006.

21. Conn VS, Valentine JC, Cooper HM, Rantz MJ. Grey literature in meta-analyses. *Nurs Res* 2003;52:256–261.
22. McAuley L, Pham B, Tugwell P, Moher D. Does the inclusion of grey literature influence estimates of intervention effectiveness reported in meta-analyses? *Lancet* 2000;356: 1228–1231.
23. Bothe AK, Davidow JH, Bramlett RE, Ingham RJ. Stuttering treatment research 1970–2005: I. Systematic review incorporating trial quality assessment of behavioral, cognitive, and related approaches. *Am J Speech Lang Pathol* 2006;15:321–341.
24. Pickar JH. Do journals have a publication bias? *Maturitas* 2007;57(1):16–19.
25. Williamson PR, Gamble C. Application and investigation of a bound for outcome reporting bias. *Trials* 2007;8:9.
26. Hojat M, Gonnella JS, Caelleigh AS. Impartial judgment by the "gatekeepers" of science: Fallibility and accountability in the peer review process. *Adv Health Sci Educ Theory Pract* 2003;8:75–96.
27. Moher D, Jadad AR, Tugwell P. Assessing the quality of randomized controlled trials. Current issues and future directions. *Int J Technol Assess Health Care* 1996;12:195–208.
28. Kunz R, Oxman AD. The unpredictability paradox: Review of empirical comparisons of randomised and non-randomised clinical trials. *BMJ* 1998;317:1185–1190.
29. MacDermid JC. An introduction to evidence-based practice for hand therapists. *J Hand Ther* 2004;17:105–117.
30. Voskuil DW, Monninkhof EM, Elias SG, Vlems FA, van Leeuwen FE. Physical activity and endometrial cancer risk: A systematic review of current evidence. *Cancer Epidemiol Biomarkers Prev* 2007;16:639–648.
31. Downs SH, Black N. The feasibility of creating a checklist for the assessment of the methodological quality both of randomised and non-randomised studies of health care interventions. *J Epidemiol Community Health* 1998;52:377–384.
32. van Tulder MW, Assendelft WJ, Koes BW, Bouter LM. Method guidelines for systematic reviews in the Cochrane Collaboration Back Review Group for Spinal Disorders. *Spine* 1997;22:2323–2330.
33. Kwakkel G, Wagenaar RC, Koelman TW, Lankhorst GJ, Koetsier JC. Effects of intensity of rehabilitation after stroke. A research synthesis. *Stroke* 1997;28:1550–1556.
34. CONSORT Website. Available at <http://www.consort-statement.org/> Accessed August 19, 2005.
35. The STARD Initiative—Toward complete and accurate reports of studies on diagnostic accuracy. Available at <http://www.consort-statement.org/stardstatement.htm> Accessed October 16, 2006.
36. Jadad AR, Moore RA, Carroll D, Jenkinson C, Reynolds DJ, Gavaghan DJ, et al. Assessing the quality of reports of randomized clinical trials: Is blinding necessary? *Control Clin Trials* 1996;17:1–12.
37. Physiotherapy Evidence Database (PEDro). Available at <http://www.pedro.fhs.usyd .edu.au/index.html> Accessed June 26, 2006.
38. Maher CG, Sherrington C, Herbert RD, Moseley AM, Elkins M. Reliability of the PEDro scale for rating quality of randomized controlled trials. *Phys Ther* 2003;83:713–721.
39. Tooth L, Bennett S, McCluskey A, Hoffmann T, McKenna K, Lovarini M. Appraising the quality of randomized controlled trials: Inter-rater reliability for the OTseeker evidence database. *J Eval Clin Pract* 2005;11:547–555.
40. Bhogal SK, Teasell RW, Foley NC, Speechly MR. The PEDro scale provides a more comprehensive measure of methodological quality than the Jadad scale in stroke rehabilitation literature. *J Clin Epidemiol* 2005;58:668–673.

41. Whiting P, Rutjes AW, Dinnes J, Reitsma J, Bossuyt PM, Kleijnen J. Development and validation of methods for assessing the quality of diagnostic accuracy studies. *Health Technol Assess* 2004;8:iii, 1–234.

42. Whiting PF, Weswood ME, Rutjes AW, Reitsma JB, Bossuyt PN, Kleijnen J. Evaluation of QUADAS, a tool for the quality assessment of diagnostic accuracy studies. *BMC Med Res Methodol* 2006;6:9.

43. Lannin NA, Herbert RD. Is hand splinting effective for adults following stroke? A systematic review and methodologic critique of published research. *Clin Rehabil* 2003;17: 807–816.

44. Simon S. Do the pieces fit together? Systematic reviews and meta-analyses. In: Simon SD (Ed.), *Statistical Evidence in Medical Trials: What Do the Data Really Tell Us?* New York: Oxford University Press, 2006, pp. 101–136.

45. Dodd KJ, Shields N. A systematic review of the outcomes of cardiovascular exercise programs for people with Down syndrome. *Arch Phys Med Rehabil* 2005;86:2051–2058.

46. Pearson K. Report on certain enteric fever inoculation statistics. *BMJ* 1904;3:1243–1246.

47. Glass GV. Primary, secondary and meta-analysis of research. *Educ Res* 1976;5:3–8.

48. Sacks HS, Berrier J, Reitman D, Ancona-Berk VA, Chalmers TC. Meta-analyses of randomized controlled trials. *N Engl J Med* 1987;316:450–455.

49. Lau J, Ioannidis JP, Schmid CH. Quantitative synthesis in systematic reviews. *Ann Int Med* 1997;127:820–826.

50. Cohn LD, Becker BJ. How meta-analysis increases statistical power. *Psychol Methods* 2003;8:243–253.

51. Lipsey MW, Wilson DB. *Practical Meta-Analysis.* Thousand Oaks, CA: Sage Publications, 2001, Chapter 3.

52. The Information Management System. Cochrane Collaboration. Available at <www .cc-ims.net> Accessed May 7, 2007.

53. Panpanich R, Lerttrakarnnon P, Laopaiboon M. Azithromycin for acute lower respiratory tract infections. *Cochrane Database Syst Rev* 2004:Issue 4. Art. No.: CD001954. DOI: 10.1002/14651858.CD001954.pub2.

54. Oxman AD, Cook DJ, Guyatt G. Users' guide to the medical literature: VI. How to use an overview. *JAMA* 1994;272:1367–1371.

55. Centre for Reviews and Dissemination. Available at <http://www.york.ac.uk/inst/ crd/index.htm> Accessed May 3, 2007.

56. Centre for Evidence-Based Medicine. The EBM toolbox. Available at <http://www .cebm.net/toolbox.asp> Accessed May 3, 2007.

57. Cochrane Collaboration. Available at <htttp://www.cochrane.org> Accessed on April 10, 2007.

58. Oxford Centre for Evidence Based Medicine. Available at <http://www.cebm.net/ toolbox.asp> Accessed March 13, 2006.

59. Clarke M, Hopewell S, Chalmers I. Reports of clinical trials should begin and end with up-to-date systematic reviews of other relevant evidence: A status report. *J R Soc Med* 2007;100:187–190.

60. Young KM. Where's the evidence?: "Evidence-based practice" is not a reality for most nurses. *Am J Nurs* 2003;103:11.

61. Clarke L, Clarke M, Clarke T. How useful are Cochrane reviews in identifying research needs? *J Health Serv Res Policy* 2007;12:101–103.

PART IV

Data Analysis

CHAPTER 17
Descriptive Statistics

In the investigation of most clinical research questions, some form of quantitative data will be collected. Initially these data exist in *raw form,* which means that they are nothing more than a compilation of numbers representing empirical observations from a group of individuals. For these data to be useful as measures of group performance, they must be organized, summarized, and analyzed, so that their meaning can be communicated. These are the functions of the branch of mathematics called statistics. **Descriptive statistics** are used to characterize the shape, central tendency, and variability within a set of data, often with the intent to describe a population. Measures of population characteristics are called **parameters**. A descriptive index computed from sample data is called a **statistic**. When researchers generalize sample data to populations, they use statistics to estimate population parameters. In this chapter we introduce the basic elements of statistical analysis for describing quantitative data.

FREQUENCY DISTRIBUTIONS

Because the numerical data collected during a study exist in unanalyzed, unsorted form, a structure is needed that allows us to recognize trends or averages. Table 17.1A presents a set of hypothetical scores of 48 therapists on a test of attitudes toward working with geriatric clients. For this example, a maximum score of 20 indicates an overall positive attitude; zero indicates a strong negative bias. The total set of scores for a particular variable is called a **distribution**. The total number of scores in the distribution is given the symbol n. In this sample, $n = 48$.

Although visual inspection of a distribution allows us to see all the scores, this list is long and unwieldy, and inadequate for describing this group of therapists or comparing them with any other group. We can begin to summarize the data by presenting them in a **frequency distribution**. A frequency distribution is a table of rank ordered scores that shows the number of times each value occurred, or its *frequency* (f). The first two columns in Table 17.1B show the frequency distribution for the attitude scores. Now we can tell more readily how the scores are distributed. We can see the lowest and highest scores, where the scores tend to cluster, and which scores occurred most often. The sum of the numbers in the frequency column (f) equals n, the number of subjects or scores in the distribution.

Sometimes frequencies are more meaningfully expressed as percentages of the total distribution. We can look at the percentage represented by each score in the distribution, or at the *cumulative percentage* obtained by adding the percentage value for each score to all percentages that fall below that score. For example, it may be useful to know

TABLE 17.1   DISTRIBUTION OF ATTITUDE SCORES (N = 48)

A. RAW DATA

	Score		Score		Score
1	9	17	16	33	19
2	13	18	18	34	10
3	15	19	15	35	12
4	16	20	15	36	15
5	20	21	11	37	17
6	17	22	20	38	13
7	15	23	19	39	16
8	14	24	15	40	15
9	10	25	11	41	14
10	15	26	14	42	16
11	17	27	18	43	12
12	13	28	14	44	15
13	19	29	17	45	16
14	12	30	11	46	18
15	16	31	16	47	19
16	12	32	17	48	14

B. FREQUENCY DISTRIBUTION

Attitude Score

	Frequency	Percent	Cumulative Percent
9	1	2.1	2.1
10	2	4.2	6.3
11	3	6.3	12.5
12	4	8.3	20.8
13	3	6.3	27.1
14	5	10.4	37.5
15	9	18.8	56.3
16	7	14.6	70.8
17	5	10.4	81.3
18	3	6.3	87.5
19	4	8.3	95.8
20	2	4.2	100.0
Total	48	100.0	

that 18.8% of the sample had a score of 15 or that 56.3% of the sample had scores of 15 and below. Percentages are useful for describing distributions because they are independent of sample size. For example, suppose we tested another sample with 150 therapists, and found that 84 individuals obtained a score of 15. Although there are more people in this second sample with this score than in the first sample, they both represent the same percentage of the total sample (56%). Therefore, the samples may be more similar than frequencies would indicate.

Grouped Frequency Distributions

When clinical data are collected, researchers will often find that very few subjects, if any, obtain the exact same score. Consider a hypothetical sample of 30 patients for whom we obtained measurements of shoulder abduction range of motion, shown in Table 17.2A. Obviously, creating a frequency distribution is a useless process if almost every score has a frequency of one. In this situation, a *grouped frequency distribution* can be constructed by grouping the scores into *classes*, or intervals, where each class represents a unique range of scores within the distribution. Frequencies are then assigned to each interval.

Table 17.2B shows a grouped frequency distribution for the range of motion data. The classes represent ranges of 10 degrees. The classes are *mutually exclusive* (no overlap) and *exhaustive* within the range of scores obtained. The choice of the number of classes to be used and the range within each class is an arbitrary decision. It depends on the overall range of scores, the number of observations, and how much detail is relevant for the intended audience. Although information is inherently lost in grouped data, this approach is often the only feasible way to present comprehensible data when

TABLE 17.2   SHOULDER ABDUCTION RANGE OF MOTION: GROUPED FREQUENCY DISTRIBUTION AND STEM-AND-LEAF PLOT

A. RAW DATA

	Score		Score
1	60	16	94
2	68	17	95
3	72	18	95
4	77	19	96
5	77	20	98
6	80	21	100
7	82	22	102
8	84	23	105
9	85	24	108
10	86	25	110
11	90	26	112
12	91	27	115
13	92	28	125
14	93	29	130
15	94	30	132

B. GROUPED FREQUENCY DISTRIBUTION

	Frequency	Percent
60–69	2	6.7
70–79	3	10.0
80–89	5	16.7
90–99	10	33.3
100–109	4	13.3
110–119	3	10.0
120–129	1	3.3
130–139	2	6.7
Total	30	100.0

C. STEM-AND-LEAF PLOT

Frequency	Stem	&	Leaf
2.00	6	.	08
3.00	7	.	277
5.00	8	.	02456
10.00	9	.	0123445568
4.00	10	.	0258
3.00	11	.	025
1.00	12	.	5
2.00	13	.	02

large amounts of information are collected for continuous data. The groupings should be clustered to reveal the important features of the data. The researcher must recognize that the choice of the number of classes and the range within each class can influence the interpretation of how a variable is distributed.

Graphing Frequency Distributions

Graphic representation of data often communicates information about trends and general characteristics of distributions more clearly than a tabular frequency distribution. The most common methods of graphing frequency distributions are the stem-and-leaf plot, histogram, and frequency polygon.

The **stem-and-leaf plot** is a refined grouped frequency distribution that is most useful for presenting the pattern of distribution of a continuous variable. The pattern is derived by separating each score into two parts. The *leaf* consists of the last or rightmost single digit of each score, and the *stem* consists of the remaining leftmost digits. Table 17.2C illustrates a stem-and-leaf plot for the shoulder range of motion data. The scores have leftmost digits of 6 through 13. These values become the stem. The last digit in each score becomes the leaf. To read the stem-and-leaf plot, we look across each row, attaching each single leaf digit to the stem. Therefore, the first row represents the scores 60 and 68; the second row, 72, 77 and 77; the third row, 80, 82, 84, 85 and 86; and so on.

This display provides a concise summary of the data, while maintaining the integrity of the original data. If we compare this plot with the grouped frequency distribution, it is clear how much more information is provided by the stem-and-leaf plot in a small space, and how it provides elements of both tabular and graphic displays.

A **histogram** is a bar graph, composed of a series of columns, each representing one score or class interval. Figure 17.1A is a histogram showing the distribution of attitude scores given in Table 17.1. The frequency for each score is plotted on the Y-axis

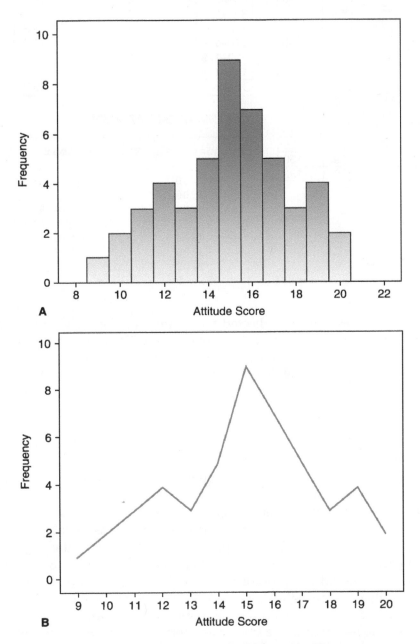

FIGURE 17.1   Graphic plots of data from Table 17.1. (A) Histogram, (B) Frequency polygon.

(vertical), and the measured variable, in this case attitude score, is on the X-axis (horizontal). The bars are centered over the scores.

A **frequency polygon** is a line plot, where each point on the line represents frequency or percentage. Figure 17.1B illustrates a frequency polygon for the attitude data. When grouped data are used, the dots in the graph are located at the midpoint of each class interval to represent the frequency in that class.

Shapes of Distributions

When graphs of frequency distributions are drawn, the distributions can be characterized by their shape. Although real data seldom achieve smooth curves, minor discrepancies are often ignored in an effort to describe overall the shape of a distribution.

Some distributions are symmetrical; that is, each half is a mirror image of the other. Curves A and B in Figure 17.2 are symmetrical. When scores are equal throughout the distribution, the shape is described as *uniform*, or rectangular, as shown in Curve A. Curve B represents a special case of the symmetrical distribution called the **normal distribution**. In statistical terminology, "normal" refers to a specific type of bell-shaped distribution where most of the scores fall in the middle of the scale and progressively fewer fall at the extremes. The unique characteristics of this distribution curve are discussed in greater detail later in this chapter.

A **skewed distribution** is asymmetrical. The degree to which the distribution deviates from symmetry is its *skewness*. Curve C in Figure 17.2 is *positively skewed*, or skewed to the right, because most of the scores cluster at the low end and only a few scores at the high end have caused the tail of the curve to point toward the right. If we were to plot a distribution for annual family income in the United States, for example, it would be positively skewed, because most families have low to moderate incomes. When the

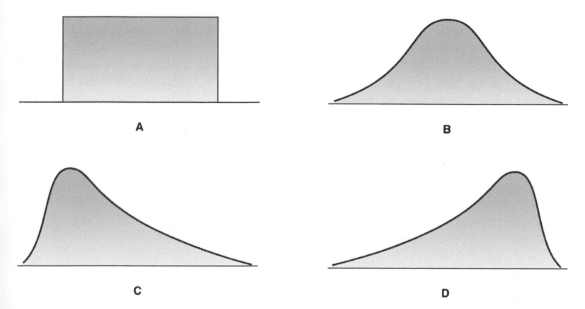

FIGURE 17.2 Common shapes of frequency distributions: (A) Symmetrical rectangular, (B) Normal curve, (C) Skewed to the right, (D) Skewed to the left.

curve "tails off" to the left, the distribution is *negatively skewed*, or skewed to the left, as in Curve D. We might see a negatively skewed distribution if we plotted exam scores for an easy test, on which relatively few students achieved a low score.

MEASURES OF CENTRAL TENDENCY

Although frequency distributions enable us to order data and identify group patterns, they do not provide a practical quantitative summary of a group's characteristics. Numerical indices are needed to describe the "typical" nature of the data and to reflect different concepts of the "center" of a distribution. These indices are called measures of **central tendency**, or averages. The term *average* can denote three different measures of central tendency: the mode, the median, and the mean.

The Mode

The **mode** is the score that occurs most frequently in a distribution. It is most easily determined by inspection of a frequency distribution. The frequency distribution in Table 17.1 shows that the mode for the attitude data is 15 because it occurs nine times, more than any other score. When class intervals are used, the mode is taken as the midpoint of the interval with the largest frequency. When more than one score occurs with the highest frequency, a distribution is considered *bimodal* (with two modes) or *multimodal* (with more than two modes). Many distributions of continuous variables do not have a mode.

The mode has only limited application as a measure of central tendency for continuous data, but can be useful in the assessment of categorical variables. For example, it may be of interest to determine the diagnostic category seen most often in a clinic.

The Median

The **median** of a series of observations is that value above which there are as many scores as below it; that is, it divides a rank-ordered distribution into two equal halves. When a distribution contains an odd number of scores, such as 4, 5, 6, 7, 8, the middle score, 6, is the median. With an even number of scores, the midpoint between the two middle scores is the median, so that for the series 4, 5, 6, 7, 8, 9, the median lies halfway between 6 and 7. Therefore, the median equals 6.5. For the distribution of attitude scores given in Table 17.2, with $n = 48$, the median will lie midway between the 24th and 25th scores. As both of these are 15, the median is 15.

The advantage of the median as a measure of central tendency is that it is unaffected by the value of extreme scores. It is an index of average *position* in a distribution, not amount. It is therefore a useful measure in describing skewed distributions. For instance, the average cost of a house is usually cited in terms of the median, because the distribution tends to be skewed to the right.

The Mean

The **mean** is the sum of a set of scores divided by the number of scores, n. This is the value most people refer to as the "average." The symbol used to represent the mean of a population is the Greek letter mu, μ, and the mean of a sample is represented by $\overline{X}$.

The bar above the X indicates that the value is an average score. The formula for calculation of the sample mean from raw data is

$$\overline{X} = \frac{\sum X}{n} \qquad\qquad (17.1)$$

where the Greek letter Σ (sigma) stands for "the sum of." This is read, "the mean equals the sum of X divided by n," where X represents each individual score in the distribution. For example, we can apply this formula to the ROM scores shown in Table 17.2. In this distribution of thirty scores, the sum of scores is 2,848. Therefore, $\overline{X} = 2,848/30 = 94.9$.

Comparing Measures of Central Tendency

Determining which measure of central tendency is most appropriate for describing a distribution depends on several factors. Foremost is the intended application of the data. The scale of measurement of the variable is another important consideration. All three measures of central tendency can be applied to variables on the interval or ratio scales, although the mean is most useful. For data on the nominal scale, only the mode is meaningful. If data are ordinal, both the median and mode can be applied.

It is necessary to consider how the summary measure will be used statistically. Of the three measures of central tendency, the mean is considered the most stable; that is, if we were to repeatedly draw random samples from a population, the means of those samples would fluctuate less than the mode or median. Only the mean can be subjected to arithmetic manipulations, making it the most reasonable estimate of population characteristics. For this reason, the mean is used more often than the median or mode for statistical analysis of ratio or interval data.

We can also consider the utility of the three measures of central tendency for describing distributions of different shapes. With uniform and normal distributions, any of the three averages can be applied with validity. With skewed distributions, however, the mean is limited as a descriptive measure because, unlike the median and mode, it is affected by the quantitative value of every score in a distribution and can be biased by extreme scores. For instance, in the previous example of ROM scores (*see* Table 17.2), if the first subject obtained a score of 20 instead of 60, the mean would decrease from 94.9 to 93.6. The median and mode would be unaffected by this change.

The curves in Figure 17.3 illustrate how measures of central tendency are affected by skewness. The median will typically fall between the mode and the mean in a skewed curve, and the mean will be pulled toward the tail. Because of these properties, the choice of which index to report with skewed distributions depends on what facet of information is appropriate to the analysis. It is often reasonable to report all three values, to present a complete picture of a distribution's characteristics.

MEASURES OF VARIABILITY

The shape and central tendency of a distribution are useful but incomplete descriptors of a sample. To illustrate this point, consider the following dilemma: You are responsible for planning the musical entertainment for a party of seven individuals, but you

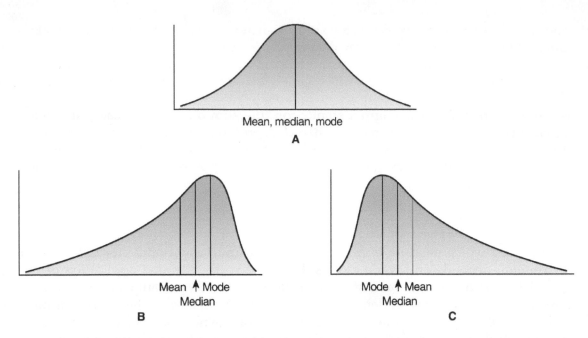

FIGURE 17.3   Relationship of mean, median, and mode in unimodal symmetrical (A) and skewed (B, C) distributions. The mean is pulled toward the tail of skewed curves.

don't know what kind of music to choose—so you decide to use their average age as a guide. The guests' ages are 3, 3, 13, 14, 59, 70, and 78 years. If you based your decision on the mode of 3 years, you would bring in characters from Sesame Street. Using the median of 14 years, you might hire a heavy metal band. And according to the mean age of 34.3 years, you might decide to play soft rock, although nobody in the group is actually in that age range. And the Tommy Dorsey fans are completely overlooked! What we are ignoring is the spread of ages within this group.

Consider now a more serious example, using the hypothetical exam scores reported in Table 17.3, obtained from two different groups of students. If we were to describe these two distributions using measures of central tendency only, they would appear

TABLE 17.3   TEST SCORES OBTAINED FROM TWO GROUPS OF STUDENTS

GROUP A

	Score
1	78
2	80
3	82
4	85
5	85
6	85
7	86
8	88

Statistics

	Group A
N	8
Mean	83.63
Median	85.00
Mode	85

GROUP B

	Score
1	65
2	69
3	78
4	85
5	85
6	93
7	96
8	98

Statistics

	Group B
N	8
Mean	83.63
Median	85.00
Mode	85

identical; however, a careful glance reveals that the scores for Group B are more widely scattered than those for Group A. This difference in **variability**, or dispersion of scores, is an essential element in data analysis. The description of a sample is not complete unless we can characterize the differences that exist *among* the scores as well as the central tendency of the data. In this section we describe five commonly used statistical measures of variability: range, percentiles, variance, standard deviation and coefficient of variation.

Range

The simplest measure of variability is the **range**, which is the difference between the highest and lowest values in a distribution. For the test scores reported in Table 17.3, the range for Group A is 88 − 78 = 10, and for Group B, 98 − 65 = 33.* These values suggest that the first group was more homogeneous. Although the range is a relatively simple statistical measure, its applicability is limited because it is determined using only the two extreme scores in the distribution. It reflects nothing about the dispersion of scores between the two extremes. One aberrant extreme score can greatly increase the range, even though the variability within the rest of the data set is unchanged. In addition, the range of scores tends to increase with larger samples, making it an ineffective value for comparing distributions with different numbers of scores. Therefore, although it is easily computed, the range is usually employed only as a rough descriptive measure, and is typically reported in conjunction with other indices of variability.

Percentiles and Quartiles

Percentiles are used to describe a score's position within a distribution. Percentiles divide data into 100 equal portions. A particular score is located in one of these portions, which represents its position relative to all other scores. For example, if a student taking a college entrance examination scores in the 92nd percentile (P_{92}), that individual's score was higher than 92% of those who took the test. Percentiles are helpful for converting actual scores into comparative scores or for providing a reference point for interpreting a particular score. For instance, a child who scores in the 20th percentile for weight in his age group can be evaluated relative to his peer group, rather than considering only the absolute value of his weight.

Quartiles divide a distribution into four equal parts, or quarters. Therefore, three quartiles exist for any data set. Quartiles Q_1, Q_2, and Q_3 correspond to percentiles at 25%, 50%, and 75% of the distribution (P_{25}, P_{50}, P_{75}). The score at the 50th percentile or Q_2 is the median. The distance between the first and third quartiles, $Q_3 − Q_1$, is called the **interquartile range**, which represents the boundaries of the middle 50% of the distribution. A **box plot** graph, also called a box-and-whisker plot, (Figure 17.4) is a useful way to demonstrate visually the spread of scores in a distribution, including the median and interquartile range.[1] Box plots may be drawn with the "whiskers" representing highest and lowest scores. The whiskers may also be drawn to represent the

---

*Research reports will usually report range by providing the actual minimum and maximum scores, rather than their difference.

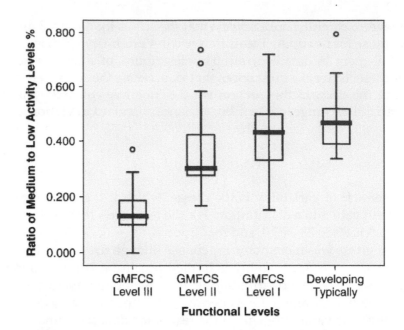

FIGURE 17.4   These box plots show four distributions of scores of functional level based on the Gross Motor Function Classification System (GMFCS). The distributions compare the ratio of medium to low activity levels (%) among children who were developing normally and children with cerebral palsy at functional levels I, II and III. The upper and lower margins of the box indicate the interquartile range $(Q_3 - Q_1)$, demarcating the 25th and 75th percentiles. The center line sits at the median score (50th percentile). The outer bars (whiskers) indicate the range of scores at each end of the distribution, with circles indicating outliers beyond 3 standard deviations from the mean. (From Bjornson KF et al. Ambulatory physical activity performance in youth with cerebral palsy and youth who are developing typically. *Phys Ther* 2007;87:248–257, Figure 4, p. 255. Used with permission of the American Physical Therapy Association.)

90th and 10th percentiles, as shown in Figure 17.4, and outliers beyond those values may be indicated as circles outside the whiskers.

Quartiles are often used in clinical research as a basis for differentiating subgroups within a sample. For example, researchers studied the relationship between bone density and walking habits in 239 postmenopausal women.[2] The sample was grouped into quartiles based on year-round distance walked, and these four groups were compared on bone density and several anthropometric variables. Quartiles provided the structure for creating comparison groups where no obvious criteria were available.

Variance

Measures of range have limited application as indices of variability because they are not influenced by every score in a distribution and they are sensitive to extreme scores. To more completely describe a distribution we need an index that reflects the variation within a full set of scores. This value should be small if scores are close together and large if they are spread out. It should also be objective so that we can compare samples of different sizes and determine if one is more variable than another.

We can begin to examine variability by looking at the deviation of each score from the mean; that is, we subtract the mean from each score in the distribution to obtain a *deviation score*, $X - \overline{X}$. Obviously, samples with larger deviation scores will be more variable around the mean. For instance, consider the distribution of test scores from Group B in Table 17.3. The deviation scores for this sample are shown in Table 17.4A. The mean of the distribution is 83.63. For the score $X = 65$, the deviation score will be $65 - 83.63 = -18.63$. Note that the first three deviation scores are negative values because these scores are smaller than the mean.

TABLE 17.4   GROUP B TEST SCORES (FROM TABLE 17.3) AND DEVIATION SCORES USED TO COMPUTE VARIANCE (s^2) AND STANDARD DEVIATION (s)

A. DATA

X	$(X - \overline{X})$	$(X - \overline{X})^2$	X^2
65	−18.63	347.08	4225
69	−14.63	214.04	4761
78	−5.63	31.69	6084
85	1.38	1.90	7225
85	1.38	1.90	7225
93	9.38	87.98	8649
96	12.38	153.26	9216
98	14.38	206.78	9604
$\Sigma X = 669$	$\Sigma(X - \overline{X}) = 0.00$	$\Sigma(X - \overline{X})^2 = 1044.63$	$\Sigma X^2 = 56{,}989$
$\overline{X} = 83.63$			

B. CALCULATIONS

$$s^2 = \frac{\Sigma(X - \overline{X})^2}{n - 1} = \frac{1044.63}{8 - 1} = 149.23 \qquad s = \sqrt{\frac{\Sigma(X - \overline{X})^2}{n - 1}} = \sqrt{149.23} = 12.22$$

C. COMPUTATIONAL FORMULAE

$$s^2 = \frac{\Sigma X^2 - \frac{(\Sigma X)^2}{n}}{n - 1} \qquad s^2 = \frac{(56{,}989) - \frac{(669)^2}{8}}{8 - 1} = \frac{1043.39}{7} = 149.13$$

$$s = \sqrt{\frac{\Sigma X^2 - \frac{(\Sigma X)^2}{n}}{n - 1}} \qquad s = \sqrt{\frac{(56{,}989) - \frac{(669)^2}{8}}{8 - 1}} = \sqrt{149.13} = 12.21$$

The numerator in these formulae is the computational expression for sum of squares.

D. OUTPUT (Data from Table 17.3)

Descriptive Statistics

	N	Minimum	Maximum	Mean	Std. Deviation
Group A	8	78	88	83.63	3.335
Group B	8	65	98	83.63	12.212

As a measure of variability, the deviation score has intuitive appeal, as these scores will obviously be larger as scores become more heterogeneous and farther from the mean. It might seem reasonable, then, to take the average of these values, or the mean deviation, as an index of dispersion within the sample. This is a useless exercise, however, because the sum of the deviation scores will always equal zero, $\Sigma(X - \overline{X}) = 0$, as illustrated in the second column in Table 17.4A. If we think of the mean as a central balance point for a distribution, then it makes sense that the scores will be equally dispersed above and below that central point.

This dilemma is solved by squaring each deviation score to get rid of the minus signs, as shown in the third column of Table 17.4A. The sum of the squared deviation scores, $\Sigma(X - \overline{X})^2$, is called the **sum of squares (SS)**. As variability increases, the sum of squares will be larger.

We now have a number we can use to describe the sample's variability. In this case, $\Sigma(X - \overline{X})^2 = 1044.63$. As an index of relative variability, however, the sum of squares is limited because it can be influenced by the sample size; that is, as n increases, the sum will also tend to increase simply because there are more scores. To eliminate this problem, the sum of squares is divided by n, to obtain the mean of the squared deviation scores (shortened to **mean square, MS**). This value is a true measure of variability and is called the **variance**.

For population data, the variance is symbolized by σ^2 (lowercase Greek sigma squared). When the population mean is known, deviation scores are obtained by $X - \mu$. Therefore, the population variance is defined by

$$\sigma^2 = \frac{SS}{N} = \frac{\Sigma(X - \mu)^2}{N} \tag{17.2}$$

With sample data, deviation scores are obtained using $\overline{X}$, not μ. Because sample data do not include all the observations in a population, the sample mean is only an estimate of the population mean. This substitution results in a sample variance slightly smaller than the true population variance. To compensate for this bias, the sum of squares is divided by $n - 1$ to calculate the sample variance, given the symbol s^2:

$$s^2 = \frac{SS}{n - 1} = \frac{\Sigma(X - \overline{X})^2}{n - 1} \tag{17.3}$$

This corrected statistic is considered an *unbiased estimate* of the parameter σ^2. For the data in Table 17.4, $SS = 1044.63$ and $n = 8$. Therefore,

$$s^2 = \frac{1044.63}{8 - 1} = 149.23$$

When means are not whole numbers, calculation of deviation scores can be biased by rounding. Computational formulae provide more accurate answers. See Table 17.4C for calculations using the computational formula for variance.

Standard Deviation

The limitation of variance as a descriptive measure of a sample's variability is that it was calculated using the squares of the deviation scores. It is generally not useful to describe sample variability in terms of squared units, such as degrees squared or pounds squared. Therefore, to bring the index back into the original units of measurement, we take the positive square root of the variance. This value is called the **standard deviation**, symbolized by *s*. The formula for standard deviation is

$$s = \sqrt{s^2} = \sqrt{\frac{SS}{n-1}} = \sqrt{\frac{\sum(X - \overline{X})^2}{n-1}} \tag{17.5}$$

For the preceding example,

$$s = \sqrt{\frac{1044.63}{8-1}} = \sqrt{149.23} = 12.22$$

See Table 17.4C for the corresponding computational formula.

The standard deviation of sample data is usually reported along with the mean so that the data are characterized according to both central tendency and variability. A mean may be expressed as $\overline{X} = 83.63 \pm 12.22$, which tells us that the average of the deviations on either side of the mean is 12.22. An *error bar graph* shows these values for both groups, illustrating the difference in their variability to indicate the mean and standard deviation (see Figure 17.5).

The standard deviation can be used as a basis for comparing samples. The results shown in Table 17.4D show the standard deviations for both Groups A and B (from Table 17.3). The *error bar graph* in Figure 17.5 illustrates the comparison of means and

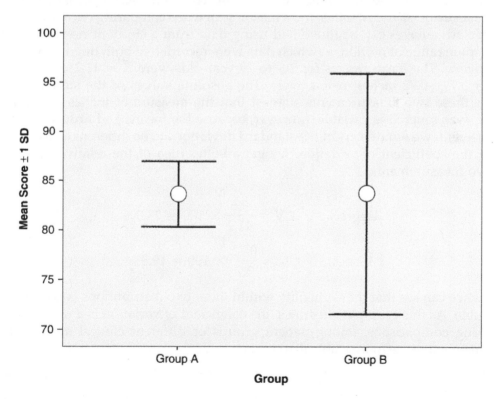

FIGURE 17.5   Example of an error bar graph showing the mean and error bar indicating one standard deviation above and below the mean. The error bars indicate that the Group A is less variable than Group B, even though they have the same mean.

standard deviations for these two groups. Because the standard deviation for Group A is smaller, we know that the Group B scores were more spread out around the mean. In clinical studies it may be relevant to describe the degree of variability among subjects as a way of estimating the generalizability of responses. Variance and standard deviation are fundamental components of any analysis of data. We explore the application of these concepts to many statistical procedures throughout the coming chapters.

Coefficient of Variation

The **coefficient of variation (CV)** is another measure of variability that can be used to describe data measured on the interval or ratio scale. It is the ratio of the standard deviation to the mean, expressed as a percentage:

$$CV = \frac{s}{\overline{X}} \times 100 \qquad (17.5)$$

There are two major advantages to this index. First, it is independent of units of measurement because units will mathematically cancel out. Therefore, it is a practical statistic for comparing distributions recorded in different units. Second, the coefficient of variation expresses the standard deviation as a proportion of the mean, thereby accounting for differences in the magnitude of the mean. The coefficient of variation is, therefore, a measure of *relative variation*, most meaningful when comparing two distributions.[†]

These advantages can be illustrated using data from a study of normal values of lumbar spine range of motion, in which data were recorded in both degrees and inches of excursion.[3] The mean ranges for 20- to 29-year-olds were $\overline{X} = 41.2 \pm 9.6$ degrees, and $\overline{X} = 3.7 \pm 0.72$ inches, respectively. The absolute values of the standard deviations for these two measurements suggest that the measure of inches, using a tape measure, was much less variable; however, because the means and units are substantially different, we would expect the standard deviations to be different as well. By calculating the coefficient of variation, we get a better idea of the relative variation of these two measurements:

$$\text{Degrees:} \quad CV = \frac{9.6}{41.2} \times 100 = 23.3\%$$

$$\text{Inches:} \quad CV = \frac{0.72}{3.7} \times 100 = 19.5\%$$

Now we can see that the variability within these two distributions is actually fairly comparable. As this example illustrates, the coefficient of variation is a useful measure for making comparisons among patient groups or different clinical assessments to determine if some are more stable than others.

[†]The coefficient of variation cannot be used when a variable mean is a negative number. Because *CV* is expressed as a percentage, it cannot be interpreted as a negative value.

THE NORMAL DISTRIBUTION

Earlier in this chapter we discussed the symmetrical distribution known as the **normal distribution**. This distribution represents an important statistical concept because so many biological, psychological and social phenomena manifest themselves in populations according to this shape. If we were to graph the population frequency distribution of variables such as height or intelligence, the graph would resemble the bell-shaped curve. Unfortunately, in the real world we can only estimate such data from samples and, therefore, cannot expect data to fit the normal curve exactly. For practical purposes, then, the normal curve represents a theoretical concept only, with well defined properties that allow us to make statistical estimates about populations using sample data.

The fact that the normal curve is important to statistical theory should not imply, however, that data are not useful or valid if they are not normally distributed. Many sociological variables, such as socioeconomic class, income, ethnic background and age, are skewed. Such data can be handled using statistics appropriate to nonnormal distributions (see Chapter 22).

Proportions of the Normal Curve

The statistical appeal of the normal distribution is that its characteristics are constant and, therefore, predictable. As shown in Figure 17.6, the curve is smooth, symmetrical and bell-shaped, with most of the scores clustered around the mean. The mean, median and mode have the same value. The vertical axis of the curve represents the frequency of data. The frequency of scores decreases steadily as scores move in a negative or positive direction away from the mean, with relatively rare observations at the extremes. Theoretically, there are no boundaries to the curve; that is, scores potentially exist with infinite magnitude

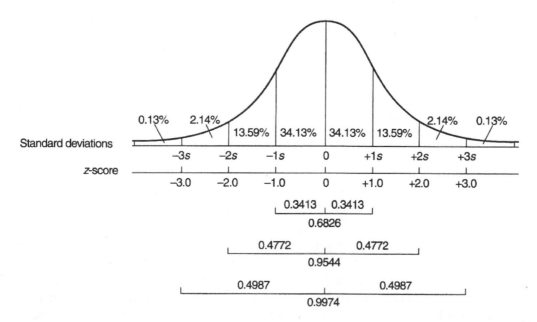

FIGURE 17.6 Areas under the normal curve, showing standard deviations and corresponding z-scores.

above and below the mean. Therefore, the tails of the curve approach but never quite touch the baseline.

Because of these standard properties, we can also determine the proportional areas under the curve represented by the standard deviations in a normal distribution. Statisticians have shown that 34.13% of the area under the normal curve is bounded by the mean and the score one standard deviation above or below the mean. Therefore, 68.26% of the total distribution (the majority) will have scores within ±1 standard deviation (±1s) from the mean. Similarly, ±2s from the mean will encompass 95.45%, and ±3s will cover 99.74% of the total area under the curve. At ±3s we have accounted for virtually the entire distribution. Because we can never discount extreme values at either end, we never account for the full 100%. This information can be used as a basis for interpreting standard deviations. For example, if we are given $\overline{X} = 65 \pm 6.06$, we can estimate that approximately 68% of the individuals in the sample have scores between 58.94 and 71.06.

Standardized Scores

Statistical data are meaningful only when they are applied in some quantitative context. For example, if a patient has a pulse rate of 58 beats/min, the implication of that value is evident only if we know where that score falls in relation to a distribution of normal pulse rates. If we know that $\overline{X} = 68$ and $s = 10$ for a given sample, then we know that an individual score of 58 is one standard deviation below the mean. This gives us a clearer interpretation of the score. When we express scores in terms of standard deviation units, we are using **standardized scores**, also called **z-scores**. For this example, a score of 58 can be expressed as a z-score of −1.0, the minus sign indicating that it is one standard deviation unit below the mean. A score of 88 is similarly transformed to a z-score of +2.0, or two standard deviations above the mean.

A z-score is computed by dividing the deviation of an individual score from the mean by the standard deviation:

$$z = \frac{X - \overline{X}}{s} \qquad (17.6)$$

Using the example of pulse rates, for an individual score of 85 beats/minute, with $\overline{X} = 68$ and $s = 10$,

$$z = \frac{85 - 68}{10} = \frac{17}{10} = 1.7$$

Thus, 85 beats/minute is 1.7 standard deviations above the mean.

The Standardized Normal Curve

The normal distribution can also be described in terms of standardized scores. Theoretically, there are an infinite number of normal distributions, corresponding to every combination of means and standard deviations. The mean of a normal distribution of z-scores will always equal zero (no deviation from the mean), and the standard deviation will always be 1.0. As shown in Figure 17.6, the area under the standardized normal curve between $z = 0$ and $z = +1.0$ is approximately 34%, the same as that defined by the area between the mean ($z = 0$) and one standard deviation. The total area within $z = \pm1.00$ is 68.26%. Similarly, the total area within $z = \pm2.00$ is 95.45%. Using this model, we can determine the proportional area under the curve bounded by any two points in a normal distribution. These values are given in Appendix Table A.1.

Determining Areas Under the Normal Curve

We can illustrate this process using hypothetical values for pulse rates, with $\overline{X} = 68$ and $s = 10$. Suppose we want to determine what percentage of our sample has a pulse rate above 80 beats/minute. First, we determine the z-score for 80 beats/minute:

$$z = \frac{80 - 68}{10} = \frac{12}{10} = 1.2$$

Therefore, 80 beats/minute is slightly more than one standard deviation above the mean.

We want to determine the proportion of our total sample that is represented by all scores above 80, or above $z = 1.2$. This is the shaded area above 80 in Figure 17.7. We can now refer to Table A.1. This table is arranged in three columns, one containing z-scores and the other two representing areas either from 0 to z or above z (in one tail of the curve). For this example, we are interested in the area above z, or above 1.2. If we look to the right of $z = 1.20$ in Table A.1, we find that the area above z equals .1151. Therefore, scores above 80 beats/minute represent 11.51% of the total distribution.

We might also be interested in determining the area above 50 beats/minute. First we determine the z-score for 50 beats/minute:

$$z = \frac{50 - 68}{10} = \frac{-18}{10} = -1.8$$

Therefore, 50 beats/minute is slightly less than two standard deviations below the mean.

Now we want to determine the proportion of our total sample that is represented by all scores above 50, or above $z = -1.8$. We already know that the scores above the

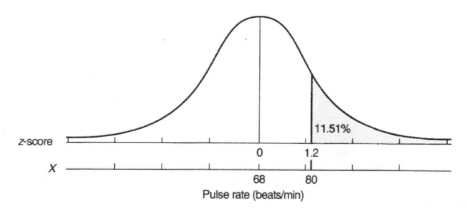

FIGURE 17.7 Distribution of pulse rates with $\overline{X} = 68$ and $s = 10$ showing the area under the normal curve above 80 beats/minute, or $z = 1.2$. The shaded area in the tail of the curve represents 11.51% of the curve (from Table A.1).

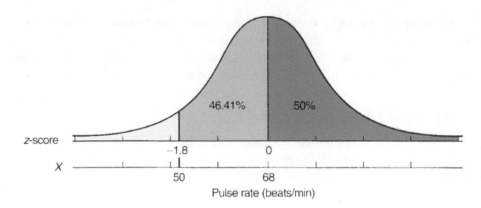

FIGURE 17.8 Distribution of pulse rates with $\overline{X}$ = 68 and s = 10, showing the area under the normal curve above 50 beats/minute, or z = −1.8. The light green area represents z = 0 to −1.8 = .4641 (from Table A.1). Together, the green areas represent 96.41% of the total area under the curve.

mean (above z = 0) represent 50% of the curve, as shown by the dark green area in Figure 17.8. Therefore, we are now concerned with the light green area between 68 and 50, which is equal to the area from z = 0 to z = −1.8. Together these two shaded areas represent the total area above 50. Table A.1 uses only absolute values of z. Because it includes standardized units for a symmetrical curve, the proportional area from 0 to z = +1.8 is the same as the area from 0 to z = −1.8. The area between z = 0 and z = −1.8 is .4641. Therefore, the total area under the curve for all scores above 80 beats/minute will be .50 + .4641 = .9641, or 96.41%.

Standardized scores are very useful for interpreting an individual's standing relative to a normalized group. For example, many standardized tests, such as psychological, developmental and intelligence tests, use z-scores to demonstrate that an individual's score is above or below the "norm" (the standardized mean) or to show what proportion of the subjects in a distribution fall within a certain range of scores.

Skewness

The validity of estimates using the standard normal curve depends on the closeness with which a sample approximates the normal distribution. Many clinical samples are too small to provide an adequate approximation and are more accurately described as skewed. Most computer programs for descriptive statistics can compute measures of skewness. A value close to zero indicates a normal (or near-normal) distribution. As values become increasingly positive or negative, they indicate the extent to which the data are skewed.

Because many statistical procedures are based on assumptions related to the normal distribution, researchers should evaluate the shape of the data as part of their initial analysis. Alternative statistical operations can be used with skewed data, or data may be transformed to better reflect the characteristics of a normal distribution (see Appendix D). Unfortunately, many researchers do not test for skewness as part of their initial analysis, running the risk of invalid statistical conclusions.[4] Skewness should be reported to help readers understand the shape of a distribution, and to evaluate the appropriate use of statistical procedures.[5]

COMMENTARY

Description Is an Essential Beginning

Descriptive statistics are the building blocks for data analysis. They serve an obvious function in that they summarize important features of quantitative data. Every study will include a description of subjects and responses using one or more measures of central tendency and variance, as a way of understanding the study sample, and establishing the framework for further analysis.

Descriptive measures are limited in their interpretation because they do not attempt to infer anything that goes beyond the data themselves. Therefore, if we collect information about the average performance of a group of patients, we are using a descriptive process; however, if we use this information to predict future performance of these patients or to make generalizations about the effectiveness of the treatment they received, we are going beyond the scope of descriptive data. We must remain cognizant of the limitations of descriptive information for generalization. Interpretations that go beyond sample data are based on inferential statistics. It is also essential to understand, however, the assumptions underlying most inferential procedures, which are based on descriptive characteristics of a distribution, including central tendency, variance, and the degree to which the distribution approaches the normal curve.

Although descriptive values cannot be used alone for generalizations, they do provide essential information about structure and patterns in data. While most inferential statistical analyses are used to test specific preset hypotheses (an approach called **confirmatory data analysis**), descriptive measures are also used to gain insight into data as part of an approach called **exploratory data analysis (EDA)**.[6,7] Graphic representations of data, such as box plots, stem-and-leaf plots, and histograms, are used to scrutinize the data, to reveal the shape of distributions, and to examine the variability in different subgroups of a sample. The visual analysis of graphics provides the opportunity to inspect and interpret data, often allowing the researcher to see patterns that might not have otherwise been clear. Graphs are more powerful than summary statistics, for example, to find gaps in scores within a certain range, or to identify a particular score that is "somewhere in left field," or to show that there is a "pile-up" of scores at one point in the distribution.[8] This type of analysis can be used to generate hypotheses, or to suggest alternative questions of the data. Other, more complex, statistical procedures can also be used to explore data structures, such as factor analysis and multivariate regression (see Chapter 29).

The take-home message, however, is the importance of descriptive statistics as the basis for sound statistical reasoning.[5] Descriptive analyses are necessary to demonstrate that statistical tests are used appropriately, and that their interpretations are valid.[4]

REFERENCES

1. Williamson DF, Parker RA, Kendrick JS. The box plot: A simple visual method to interpret data. *Ann Int Med* 1989;110:916–921.
2. Krall EA, Dawson-Hughes B. Walking is related to bone density and rates of bone loss. *Am J Med* 1994;96:20–26.
3. Fitzgerald GK, Wynveen KJ, Rheault W, Rothschild B. Objective assessment with establishment of normal values for lumbar spinal range of motion. *Phys Ther* 1983;63:1776–1781.
4. Findley TW. Research in physical medicine and rehabilitation. IX. Primary data analysis. *Am J Phys Med Rehabil* 1991;70:S84–S93.
5. Gonzales VA, Ottenbacher KJ. Measures of central tendency in rehabilitation research: What do they mean? *Am J Phys Med Rehabil* 2001;80:141–146.
6. NIST/SEMATECH e-Handbook of Statistical Methods. <http://www.itl.nist.gov/div898/handbook/> Accessed on March 13, 2006.
7. Tukey JW. *Exploratory Data Analysis*. Boston: Addison-Wesley, 1977.
8. Cohen J. Things I have learned (so far). *Amer Psychologist* 1990;45:1304–1312.

CHAPTER 18
Statistical Inference

In the previous chapter we presented statistics that can be used to summarize and describe data. Descriptive procedures are not sufficient, however, for testing theories about the effects of treatments or for generalizing relationships from samples to populations. For these purposes, researchers use a process of statistical *inference*. The process of drawing inferences is familiar to everybody. When we decide to read a book by a certain author after having enjoyed other books by that same author, we are inferring something about the probable quality of the new book. When a specific treatment approach produces beneficial effects for a particular patient, a clinician might decide to use that approach for other patients with similar conditions. The difference between these subjective inferences and statistical inference is that the researcher uses objective criteria to make such decisions.

Inferential statistics involve a decision making process that allows us to estimate population characteristics from sample data. The success of this process requires that we make certain assumptions about how well the sample represents the larger population. These assumptions are based on two important concepts of statistical reasoning: **probability** and **sampling error**. The purpose of this chapter is to introduce these fundamental concepts and to demonstrate the principles of their application for drawing valid conclusions from research data.

PROBABILITY

Probability is a complex but essential concept for understanding inferential statistics. We all have some notion of what probability means, as evidenced by the use of terms such as "likely," "probably" or "a good chance." We use probability as a means of prediction: "There is a 50% chance of rain tomorrow," or "This operation has a 75% chance of success." Statistically, we can view probability as a system of rules for analyzing a complete set of possible outcomes, or a *sample space*. For instance, a sample space could represent the two sides of a coin or the six faces on a die. An event is a single observable happening or outcome, such as the appearance of tails on the flip of a coin or a 3 on the toss of a die. A sample space could be a set of IQ scores for all students in a given school system. An event might be the random selection of one student's IQ score of 110. In other words, each score in the sample space is a potential event.

Probability is the likelihood that any one event will occur, given all the possible outcomes. We use a lowercase p to signify probability, expressed as a ratio or decimal. For example, given the two possible outcomes for the flip of a coin, the likelihood of getting tails on any single flip will be 1 of 2, or 1/2, or .5. Therefore, we say that the probability of getting tails is 50%, or $p = .50$. Suppose we want to know the probability of getting a

3 when a die is thrown. The sample space is the set of six faces of the die, or six possible outcomes. Therefore, the probability that we will roll a 3 is 1 of 6, or 1/6, or $p = .167$. Conversely, the probability that we will not roll a 3 is 5 of 6, or 5/6, or $p = .833$. What is the probability that we will roll a 3 or higher? There are now four possible events—3, 4, 5 and 6—that meet this criterion. Therefore, the probability is 4 of 6, 2/3 or $p = .667$, that we will roll a 3 or higher on any single roll of one die. Now, if we were to throw two dice, what is the probability of rolling a 7? (see Box 18.1)

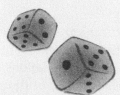

BOX 18.1 The Rules of Chance

If two dice are tossed, what is the probability of throwing a seven? If we look at all the possible combinations (shown below), with six sides on each die, we will have $6 \times 6 = 36$ possible outcomes. We can see from the chart that there are six possible ways to make a 7. Therefore, the probability of throwing a 7 on one toss of two dice is $6/36 = 1/6$ or $p = .167$.

For those who are interested in games of chance, consider the following probabilities.

What is the probability of throwing an 11 on one toss of two dice? There are two ways to make 11. Therefore, the probability of throwing an 11 is $2/36 = 1/18$ or $p = .055$.

Now, what is the probability that you would throw a 7 or 11 (a "natural" in craps) on one toss of two dice? There are nine possible outcomes that meet this criterion, or $9/36 = 1/4$ or $p = .25$.

Try throwing two dice 36 times. How often should each of the sums from 2 through 12 come up? According to the laws of chance, the probability of each sum appearing should follow the grid below, i.e., six 7s, five 6s, and so on. How close did you come?

DIE #1

	⚀	⚁	⚂	⚃	⚄	⚅
⚀	2	3	4	5	6	7
⚁	3	4	5	6	7	8
⚂	4	5	6	7	8	9
⚃	5	6	7	8	9	10
⚄	6	7	8	9	10	11
⚅	7	8	9	10	11	12

DIE #2

For an event that is certain to occur, $p = 1.00$. For instance, if we toss a die, the probability of rolling a 3 or not rolling a 3 is 1.00 ($p = .167 + .833$). These two events are *mutually exclusive* and *complementary* events because they cannot occur together and because they represent all possible outcomes. Therefore, the sum of their probabilities will always equal 1.00. We can also show that the probability of an impossible event is zero. For instance, the probability of rolling a 7 with one die is 0 out of 6, or $p = 0.00$. In the real world, the probability for most events falls somewhere between 0 and 1. Scientists will generally admit that nothing is a "sure bet" and nothing is impossible!

Applying Probability to a Distribution of Scores

This concept can now be applied to a distribution of scores. Suppose we had access to data for height of all adult men alive today. This distribution of millions of scores would approximate the normal curve. Suppose, too, that the mean height was 69 in., with a standard deviation of 3 in. Now, what if we select one man at random from this population? What is the probability that the man will be between 66 and 72 in. tall, or within ±1 standard deviation of the mean? We know this range represents 68.26% of the population as shown by the center blue area in Figure 18.1. This means that approximately 68 of 100 men can be expected to be between 66 and 72 in. tall. Therefore, there is a 68% probability ($p = .68$) that any one man we select will fall within this range. Similarly, the probability of selecting a man 78 in. or taller (scores beyond +3 standard deviations) is .0013, as this area represents 0.13% of the total distribution, as shown by the gray area in the tail of Figure 18.1.

It is important to understand that probability is predictive in that it reflects what *should* happen over the long run, not necessarily what will happen for any given trial or event. When a surgeon advises that an operation has a 75% probability of success, it means that in the long run, for all such cases, 75% can be expected to be successful. For

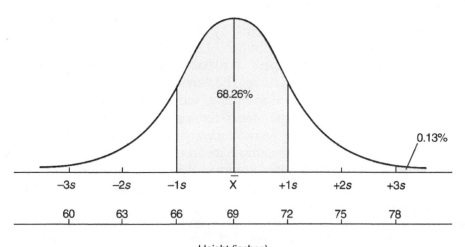

FIGURE 18.1 Hypothetical distribution of heights for adult males, with $\overline{X} = 69$ and $s = 3$. Center area represents ±1s, or 68.26% of the population. Gray area to the right represents ≥3s, or 0.13% of the population.

any single patient the surgery will not be 75% successful; it will either be a success or not. Therefore, once an event occurs, it is no longer "probable." It either happened as predicted or not. Probability applies to the proportion of time we can *expect* a given outcome to occur in the idealized "long run."

We use probability in research as a guideline for making decisions about how well sample data estimate the characteristics of a population. We also use probabilities to determine if observed treatment differences are likely to be representative of population differences or if they could have occurred *by chance*. We try to estimate what would happen to others in the population on the basis of our limited sample. To understand these applications of probability, we must first understand the statistical relationship between samples and populations.

SAMPLING ERROR

The estimation of population characteristics from sample data is based on the assumption that samples are random and valid representatives of the population. Even when truly random samples are used, however, we cannot be sure that one sample's characteristics will be identical to those of the population, simply because fewer cases are included in the sample. For example, if we had access to birth records for all live births in the United States for the past year, we might find that the population parameters for birth weight were $\mu = 120$ ounces and $\sigma = 5$. Now suppose we randomly select a sample of 10 babies, and find that $\overline{X} = 115$ ounces and $s = 30$. Because selection was unbiased, this sample should be a good representative of the population; however, the sample mean and standard deviation are somewhat different from the population values and, therefore, do not provide accurate estimates.

What would account for this difference? Random selection implies that all members of a population have an equal opportunity of being chosen but, obviously, this does not guarantee proportional representation of all parts of the population. We could obtain a sample with many lighter babies just by chance. It is highly unlikely that a sample of 10 would match the overall distribution of population characteristics.

If we choose a second random sample of 10 babies, the odds are that we will obtain a different mean and standard deviation. The laws of chance tell us that through a process of infinitely repeated random sampling, we should expect to see such differences among the sample means. The tendency for sample values to differ from population values is called **sampling error**. Sampling error of the mean for any single sample is equal to the difference between the sample mean and the population mean ($\overline{X} - \mu$). The greater the sampling error, the less accurate $\overline{X}$ is as an estimate of μ. In practice, sampling error is unpredictable because it occurs strictly by chance, by virtue of who happens to get picked for any one sample.

Theoretically, if we were to randomly draw an infinite number of samples from a population, each with $n = 10$, the means of these samples would exhibit varying degrees of sampling error. We would expect, by chance, that most of the sample means would be close to the population mean. If we plotted the sample means, we would find that the distribution would take the shape of a normal curve, and that the mean of all the sample means would be equal to the population mean. This distribution of sample means is called a **sampling distribution of means**. A sampling distribution will consistently take the shape of the normal curve.*

Obviously, a sampling distribution is a theoretical concept only, because one does not go through such a sampling process in practice. Clinical researchers work with only one sample from which inferences are made about a population; however, because of the predictable properties of the normal curve, we can use the concept of the sampling distribution to formulate a basis for drawing inferences from sample data.

Standard Error of the Mean

Because a sampling distribution is a normal curve, we can also establish its variability. The standard deviation of a theoretical sampling distribution of means is called the **standard error of the mean ($\sigma_{\overline{X}}$).** This value is considered an estimate of the population standard deviation, σ. The curve in Figure 18.2A represents a hypothetical sampling distribution formed by repeated sampling of birth weights, with samples of $n = 10$. The means of such small samples tend to vary, and in fact, we see a wide curve with great variability. The sampling distribution in the curve in Figure 18.2B was constructed from the same population, but with samples of $n = 50$. These sample means form a narrower distribution curve with less variability and, therefore, a smaller standard deviation. As sample size increases, samples become more representative of the population, and their means are more likely to be closer to the population mean; that is, their sampling error will be smaller. Therefore, the standard deviation of the sampling distribution is an indicator of the degree of sampling error, reflecting how accurately the various sample means estimate the population mean.

Because we do not actually construct a sampling distribution, we need some useful way to estimate the standard error of the mean from sample data. This estimate, $s_{\overline{X}}$, is based on the standard deviation and size of the sample:

$$s_{\overline{X}} = \frac{s}{\sqrt{n}}$$

(18.1)

Using our example of birth weights, for a single sample of 10 babies, we found a mean of 115 with a standard deviation of 30 (see Figure 18.2A). Therefore, $s_{\overline{X}} = 30/\sqrt{10} = 9.5$. With a sample of $n = 50$, $s_{\overline{X}} = 30/\sqrt{50} = 4.2$. As illustrated in Figure 18.2, as n increases, the standard error of the mean decreases. With larger samples the sampling distribution is expected to be less variable, and therefore, a statistic based on a large sample is considered a better estimate of a population parameter than one based on a smaller sample.

A sample mean, together with its standard error, helps us imagine what the sampling distribution curve would look like. For example, for a sample of $n = 50$, with $\overline{X} = 115$ and $s_{\overline{X}} = 4.2$, the theoretical sampling distribution might look like the curve

---

*This phenomenon is explained by the *central limit theorem*, which demonstrates that even for skewed distributions, the sampling distribution of means will approach the normal curve as n increases. Therefore, we can use sampling distributions and the probabilities associated with the normal curve to predict population characteristics for any distribution.

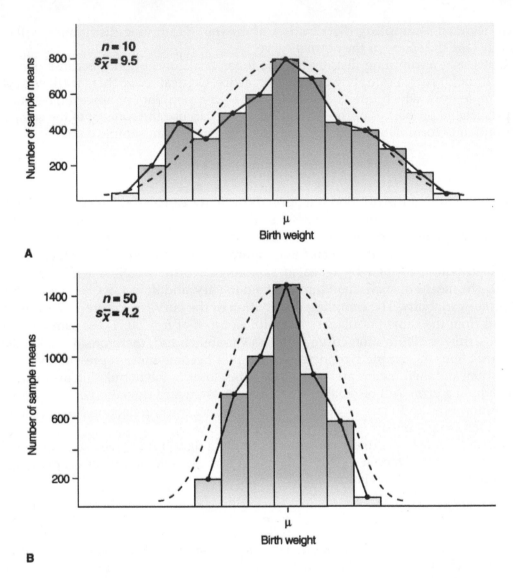

FIGURE 18.2 Hypothetical sampling distributions for birth weight. Curve A is drawn for samples with $n = 10$. Curve B is drawn for samples with $n = 50$.

shown in Figure 18.2B. If we use this curve as an estimate of the population distribution, we can determine the probability of drawing a single sample with a certain mean. Based on our knowledge of the normal curve, the chances are 95.45 out of 100 that any single random sample we might draw from this population would have a mean between 106.6 and 123.4 ($\pm 2s_{\bar{X}}$). Therefore, the probability is 95.45% that a sample mean will lie within this range. We can also say that there is less than a 5% chance that any sample mean drawn from this population will be less than 106.6 or above 123.4. We should note that the standard error cannot be a direct measure of variance in the population, because it is a function of sample size.

CONFIDENCE INTERVALS

For many research applications, sample data are used to estimate unknown population parameters. For example, we can sample medical records to determine length of hospital stay for patients with certain diagnoses or we could study normative values for tests of motor function. The purpose of these types of analyses is to estimate how the population behaves and to use this information for decision making or as a foundation for further research.

We can use our knowledge of sampling distributions to estimate population parameters in two ways. A **point estimate** is a single value obtained by direct calculation from sample data, such as using $\overline{X}$ to estimate μ. We know, however, that any single sample value will most likely contain some degree of error as a population estimate. Therefore, it is often more meaningful to use an **interval estimate**, by which we specify an interval within which we believe the population parameter will lie. Such an estimate takes into consideration not only the value of a single sample statistic, but the relative accuracy of that statistic as well.

For example, Fitzgerald et al[1] estimated the population mean for lumbar spinal extension for 30- to 39-year-olds. Based on a random sample of 42 individuals, they determined that $\overline{X} = 40.0$ degrees and $s = 8.8$ degrees. Therefore, the point estimate of μ is the sample mean, 40.0 degrees. How can we tell how accurate this estimate is? Perhaps we would be more comfortable giving a range of values within which we are fairly sure the population mean will fall. For instance, we might guess that the population mean is likely to be within 5 degrees of the sample mean, to fall within the interval 35 to 45 degrees. We must be more precise than guessing allows, however, in proposing such an interval, so that we can be "confident" that the interval is an accurate estimate.

A **confidence interval (CI)** is a range of scores with specific boundaries, or *confidence limits*, that should contain the population mean. The boundaries of the confidence interval are based on the sample mean and its standard error. The wider the interval we propose, the more confident we will be that the true population mean will fall within it. This degree of confidence is expressed as a probability percentage, such as 95% confidence.

To illustrate the procedure for constructing a 95% confidence interval, consider the example of lumbar spine extension, with $\overline{X} = 40.0$, $s = 8.8$, $n = 42$, and $s_{\overline{X}} = 8.8/\sqrt{42} = 1.36$. The sampling distribution estimated from this sample is shown in Figure 18.3. We know that 95.45% of the total distribution will fall within $\pm 2s_{\overline{X}}$ from the mean, or within the boundaries of $z = \pm 2$. Therefore, to determine the proportion of the curve within 95%, we need to determine points just slightly less than $z = \pm 2$. By referring to Table A.1 in the Appendix, we can determine that 0.95 of the total curve (0.475 on either side of the mean) is bounded by a z-score of ± 1.96, just less than 2 standard error units above and below the mean. Therefore, as shown in Figure 18.3, 95% of the total sampling distribution will fall between $-1.96s_{\overline{X}}$ and $+1.96s_{\overline{X}}$. We are 95% sure that the population mean will fall within this interval. This is called the *95% confidence interval*.

We obtain the boundaries of a confidence interval using the formula

$$CI = \overline{X} \pm (z)s_{\overline{X}}$$ (18.2)

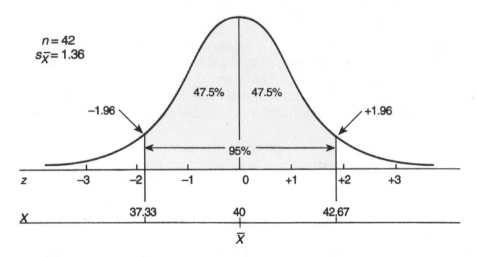

FIGURE 18.3 95% Confidence interval for sampling distribution of lumbar extension range of motion for 30–39 year olds.

For 95% confidence intervals, $z = \pm 1.96$.
 For our data, therefore,

$$95\% \text{ CI} = 40.0 \pm (1.96)(1.36)$$

$$= 40.0 \pm 2.67$$

$$95\% \text{ CI} = 37.33, 42.67$$

We are 95% confident that the population mean of lumbar extension for 30 to 39-year-olds will fall between 37.33 and 42.67 degrees.

How can we interpret this statement? Because of sampling error, one sample we select may have a mean of 50 degrees, with 95% confidence limits between 40 and 60 degrees. Another sample could have a mean of 52 degrees, with 95% confidence limits between 42 and 62 degrees. The 95% confidence limits indicate that if we were to draw 100 random samples, each with $n = 42$, we could construct 100 confidence intervals around the sample means, 95 of which could be expected to contain the true population mean, as illustrated in Figure 18.4. Five of the 100 intervals would not contain the population mean. This would occur just by chance, because the scores chosen for those five samples would be too extreme and not good representatives of the population. In reality, however, we construct only one confidence interval based on the data from only one sample. Theoretically, then, we cannot know if that one sample would produce one of the 95 correct intervals or one of the 5 incorrect ones. Therefore, there is a 5% chance that the population mean is not included in the obtained interval, that is, a 5% chance the interval is one of the incorrect ones.

To be more confident of the accuracy of an interval, we could construct a 99% confidence interval, allowing only a 1% risk that the interval we propose will not contain

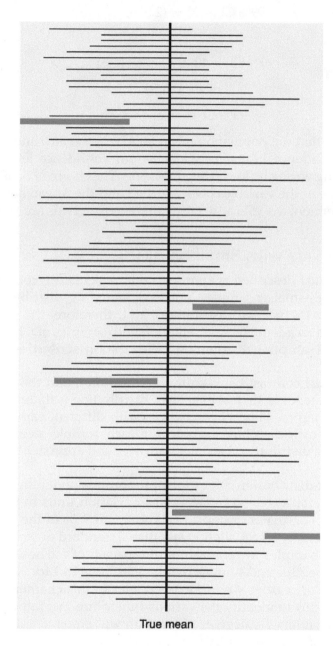

True mean

FIGURE 18.4   95% Confidence intervals for 100 random samples, showing how the intervals overlap with the true population mean. In 5 of the 100 samples (highlighted), the confidence interval does not contain the population mean.

the true population mean. Using Table A.1, we can determine that 99% of the area under the curve (0.495 on either side of the mean) is bounded by $z = \pm2.576$. Therefore,

$$99\% \text{ CI} = \overline{X} \pm (2.576)s_{\overline{X}}$$

For our data,

$$99\% \text{ CI} = 40 \pm (2.576)(1.36)$$

$$= 40 \pm 3.50$$

$$99\% \text{ CI} = 36.5, 43.5$$

We are 99% confident that the population mean falls between 36.5 and 43.5 degrees.

Note that the confidence limits get wider as our confidence level increases. We reduce the risk of being wrong by sacrificing precision. The choice of confidence interval depends on the nature of the variables being studied and the researcher's desired level of accuracy. By convention, the 95% and 99% confidence intervals are used most often.

Confidence Intervals with Small Samples

The process we have just described is appropriate for calculating confidence intervals for large samples. With smaller samples, however, sampling distributions tend to be more spread out than the normal distribution, and, therefore, the standard normal curve is not considered an adequate representation with samples of n less than 30. Thus, an alternate theoretical sampling distribution, called the **t-distribution**, is used to evaluate smaller samples.[†]

The major statistical contrast between the t-distribution and the standard normal distribution is the difference in their shape. The t-distribution is flatter and wider at the tails than the normal curve. This shape changes with different sample sizes, so that there are actually many t-distributions, one for each sample size. As sample size increases, the sampling distribution becomes narrower and approaches the shape of the normal curve.

The spread of the t-distribution changes the proportions under the curve; that is, we cannot estimate the percentages within standard deviation units in the same proportions as in the normal curve. For example, we know that 95% of the normal sampling distribution falls within $z = \pm1.96$, slightly less than 2 standard deviation units. To find this area with smaller samples, we use values of t instead of z. These values are given in Table A.2 in the Appendix, and summarized here in Table 18.1 for 90%, 95%, and 99% confidence intervals. For reasons we will explain later in this chapter, statisticians use **degrees of freedom (df)** to identify the various t-distributions, rather than n. For the creation of confidence intervals, degrees of freedom will equal $n - 1$. Therefore, for a sample of $n = 6$, $df = 5$; with $n = 10$, $df = 9$; and so on.

By referring to Table 18.1, we find that for $n = 6$ ($df = 5$), 95% of the total area falls within $t = \pm2.571$. With a sample of $n = 10$ ($df = 9$), 95% of the area falls within $t = \pm2.262$. With $n = 30$, this area is bounded by $t = \pm2.042$. As n increases, the value of t approaches $z = 1.96$.

[†]Because the t-distribution approaches z as the sample size increases, it can also be used with larger samples.

TABLE 18.1   VALUES OF *t* FOR 90%, 95% AND 99% CONFIDENCE INTERVALS

df	90%	95%	99%
5	2.015	2.571	4.032
6	1.943	2.447	3.707
7	1.895	2.365	3.499
8	1.860	2.306	3.355
9	1.833	2.262	3.250
10	1.812	2.228	3.169
11	1.796	2.201	3.106
12	1.782	2.179	3.055
13	1.771	2.160	3.012
14	1.761	2.145	2.977
15	1.753	2.131	2.947
16	1.746	2.120	2.921
17	1.740	2.110	2.898
18	1.734	2.101	2.878
19	1.729	2.093	2.861
20	1.725	2.086	2.845
30	1.697	2.042	2.750
40	1.684	2.021	2.704
60	1.671	2.000	2.660
120	1.658	1.980	2.617
∞	1.645	1.960	2.576

We use these values to create confidence intervals using the formula

$$CI = \overline{X} \pm (t)s_{\overline{X}} \tag{18.3}$$

Therefore, to create a 95% confidence interval for a sample with $n = 18$, $\overline{X} = 5.0$, and $s_{\overline{X}} = 2.0$, we locate $t = 2.110$ for 17 *df*. Thus,

$$95\% \ CI = 5.0 \pm (2.110)(2.0)$$

$$= 5.0 \pm 4.22$$

$$95\% \ CI = 0.78, 9.22$$

This means that we are 95% confident that the population mean falls between 0.78 and 9.22. If our sample size increases to $n = 31$ ($df = 30$, $t = 2.042$), our confidence interval changes:

$$95\% \ CI = 5.0 \pm (2.042)(2.0)$$

$$= 5.0 \pm 4.084$$

$$95\% \ CI = .916, 9.084$$

Note that the interval is narrower when more scores are used. We have become more precise in our estimate by using a larger sample.

HYPOTHESIS TESTING

The estimation of population parameters is only one part of statistical inference. More often inference is used to answer questions concerning comparisons or relationships, such as, "Is one treatment more effective than another?" or "Is there a relationship between the length of time a treatment is applied and the degree of improvement observed?" These types of questions usually involve the comparison of means, proportions, correlations or some other statistic.

Consider a study in which a hypothesis was proposed that a single intervention session of soft tissue mobilization would be effective for increasing external rotation in patients with musculoskeletal shoulder problems.[2] Experimental and control groups were formed through random assignment. Range of motion (ROM) measurements were taken and the improvement from pretest to posttest was calculated for each subject. The researchers found that the mean improvement in external rotation was 16.4 degrees for the treatment group and 1 degree for the control group. On the basis of the difference between these means, should the researcher conclude that the research hypothesis has been supported?

According to the concept of sampling error, we would expect to see some differences between groups even when a treatment is not at all effective, because of chance differences in subject characteristics. Therefore, we need some mechanism for deciding if an observed effect reflects chance only or if we can argue with confidence that the differences represent "real" effects. We do this through a process of *hypothesis testing*.

Statistical Hypotheses

Before we can interpret observed differences, we must consider two possible explanations for the observed outcome. The first possible explanation is that the difference between the groups occurred by chance, as a result of sampling error. This is the **null hypothesis (H_0)**, which states that the group means are not different. No matter how the research hypothesis is stated, the researcher's goal will always be to statistically test the null hypothesis. The second explanation is that there is a true difference between the groups, and the treatment was effective. This is expressed as the **alternative hypothesis (H_1)**.

The Null Hypothesis

Statistical hypotheses are formally stated in terms of the population parameter, μ, even though the actual statistical tests will be based on sample data. Therefore, the null hypothesis can be stated formally as

$$H_0: \mu_A = \mu_B \quad \text{or} \quad H_0: \mu_A - \mu_B = 0$$

which predicts that the mean of Population A is not different from the mean of Population B, or that there will be no treatment effect. For the example of joint mobilization and shoulder ROM, under H_0 the mean change in external rotation would be the same for those who do (μ_A) and those who do not (μ_B) receive mobilization. Because of the nature of chance differences, however, we must realize that even when there is no true treatment effect, groups will probably not have equal means. Therefore, the null hypothesis really indicates that observed differences are sufficiently small to be considered functionally equivalent to zero.[3] So rather than saying the means are equal, it is more accurate to say they are not significantly different; that is, any observed difference between groups would probably be the result of chance.

"Disproving" the Null Hypothesis

We can never actually "prove" or "accept" the null hypothesis. The purpose of an experiment is to give the data a chance of *disproving* it. In essence, we are using a decision making process based on the concept of negative inference. No one experiment can establish that a null hypothesis is true; that is, it would take an infinite number of unsuccessful experiments to prove that a treatment has no effect. We can, however, discredit the null hypothesis by any one trial that shows that the treatment is effective. Therefore, the purpose of testing the statistical hypothesis is to decide whether or not H_0 is *false*.

There is often confusion about the appropriate way to express the outcome of a statistical decision. We can only legitimately say that we *reject* or *do not reject* the null hypothesis. When we do not reject H_0, we mean that the null hypothesis is consistent with our findings. The word "retained" has also been used to denote this outcome.[3]

This is analogous to the use of "guilty" and "not guilty" in a court of law. A jury can reach a guilty verdict if evidence is sufficient (beyond a reasonable doubt) that the defendant committed the crime. Otherwise, the verdict is not guilty. The jury cannot find the defendant "innocent." A "not guilty" verdict is expected if the evidence is not sufficient to establish guilt. But we know that doesn't necessarily mean the defendant is innocent!

We start, therefore, with the assumption that there is no treatment effect in a research study (the null hypothesis). Then we ask if the data are consistent with this assumption. If the answer is yes, then we must acknowledge the possibility that no effect exists. If the answer is no, then we have discredited that assumption. Therefore, there probably is an effect. It is important to remember that finding no effect does not necessarily mean there is no effect.

The Alternative Hypothesis

The second explanation for the observed findings is that the treatment is effective; that is, the observed difference is too large to be considered a result of chance alone. This is the alternative hypothesis (H_1), stated as

$$H_1: \mu_A \neq \mu_B \quad \text{or} \quad H_1: \mu_A - \mu_B \neq 0$$

These statements predict that the observed difference between the two population means is not due to chance. We say, then, that the observed difference is "real," or that the likelihood that the difference is due to chance is very small. When we reject the null we can *accept* the alternative hypothesis; that is, we say that the alternative hypothesis is consistent with our findings.

In most cases, the researcher hopes that the data will support the alternative hypothesis, and that H_0 will be rejected; that is, the alternative hypothesis represents the research hypothesis. There may be situations, however, where the researcher does not expect a difference, such as trying to show that a new experimental treatment is as effective as a standard treatment. In such a case, the research hypothesis will be the same as the null hypothesis, and the researcher hopes to reject the alternative hypothesis.

Directional and Nondirectional Hypotheses

The preceding alternative hypotheses state that a difference will exist between Populations A and B. These are considered **nondirectional** hypotheses, because they do not specify which group mean is expected to be larger. Alternative hypotheses can also be expressed in **directional** form, indicating the expected direction of difference between sample means. We could state

$$H_1: \mu_A > \mu_B \quad (H_1: \mu_A - \mu_B > 0)$$

or

$$H_1: \mu_A < \mu_B \quad (H_1: \mu_A - \mu_B < 0)$$

These hypotheses predict that the mean of Population A is either greater or smaller than the mean of Population B. For instance, we might predict that the experimental group receiving mobilization will show a greater improvement than the control group.

Errors in Hypothesis Testing

Hypothesis testing will always result in one of two decisions: Either reject or do not reject the null hypothesis. By rejecting the null hypothesis, the researcher concludes that it is *unlikely* that chance alone is operating to produce observed differences. This is called a **significant effect**, that is, one that is *probably not due to chance*. When the null hypothesis is not rejected, the researcher concludes that the observed difference is probably due to chance and is *not significant*.

The decision to reject or not reject the null hypothesis is based on the results of objective statistical procedures; however, this objectivity does not guarantee that a correct decision will be made. Because such decisions are based on sample data only, it is possible that the true relationship between experimental populations is not accurately reflected in the statistical outcome.

Any one decision can be either correct or incorrect. Therefore, we can classify four possible decision outcomes, shown in Figure 18.5. If we do not reject H_0 when it is in

		TRUTH	
		H_0 is true	H_0 is false
DECISION	Reject H_0	Type I Error α	Correct
	Do Not Reject H_0	Correct	Type II Error β

FIGURE 18.5   Potential errors in hypothesis testing.

fact true (observed differences are really due to chance), we have made a correct decision. If we reject H_0 when it is false (differences are real), we have also made a correct decision. If, however, we decide to reject H_0 when it is true, we have made an error, called a **Type I error**. In this case, we have concluded that a real difference exists, when in fact, the differences are due to chance. Having committed this type of statistical error, we might decide to use a treatment that is not really effective. Conversely, if we do not reject H_0 when it is false, we have committed a **Type II error**. Here we would conclude that differences are due to chance, when in fact, the samples represent different populations. In this situation, we might ignore an effective treatment or abandon a potentially fruitful line of research.

In any statistical analysis we may draw a correct conclusion, or we may commit one of these two types of errors. If we reject the null hypothesis, and decide that treatment groups are different, we may be correct or we may be making a Type I error (but not Type II). If we do not reject the null hypothesis, and decide that no differences exist, we may be correct or we may be making a Type II error (but not Type I). The seriousness of one type of error over the other is relative. Historically, statisticians and researchers have focused attention on Type I error as the primary basis of hypothesis testing; however, the consequences of failing to recognize an effective treatment may be equally important. Although we never know for sure if we are committing one or the other type of error, we can take steps to decrease the probability of committing one or both.

TYPE I ERROR: LEVEL OF SIGNIFICANCE

When looking at the results of an experiment, we know that observed differences may be due to treatment effects or due to chance. On one level then, how can we ever make a decision regarding the null hypothesis, if we can never be certain if it is true or false? Well, we must be willing to take some risk in making a mistake if we reject the null hypothesis when it is true. We must be able to set some criterion for this risk, a dividing line that allows us to say that a mistake in rejecting H_0 (a Type I error) is "unlikely."

Therefore, we want to determine the probability of committing a Type I error, and must set a standard for rejecting the null hypothesis. This standard is called the **level of significance**, denoted as **alpha (α)**. The level of significance represents a criterion for judging if an observed difference can be considered sampling error or real. The larger an observed difference is, the less likely it occurred by chance.

The probability that an observed difference did occur by chance is determined by statistical tests (which are covered in the coming chapters). This probability is denoted as p. For example, we might find that an analysis comparing two means yields $p = .18$. This means that there is an 18% probability that the difference between the means occurred by chance alone. Therefore, if we decide to reject H_0, and conclude that the tested groups are different from each other, we have an 18% chance of being wrong, that is, an 18% chance of committing a Type I error.

The question facing the researcher is how to decide if this probability is acceptable. We know there is some chance that any observed difference will be the result of sampling error. But how much of a chance is small enough that we would be willing to accept the risk of being wrong? Is an 18% chance of being wrong acceptable? Think of it this way: The weather report says that there is a 75% chance of rain today. Will you take your umbrella? If you decide *not* to take it, and it rains, you were wrong in your decision. Now let's say that the report is for a 5% chance of rain. Are you more likely to leave your umbrella home? If you do, are you less likely to be wrong? What is the maximal risk you are willing to take that you will be wrong—that you will get wet?

For research purposes, the selected alpha level defines the *maximal acceptable risk* of making a Type I error if we reject H_0. Typically, researchers set this standard at 5%, which is considered a small risk. This means that we would be willing to accept a 5% chance of *incorrectly rejecting* H_0, but no more. Therefore, for a given analysis, if p is equal to or less than .05, we would be willing to reject the null hypothesis; that is, the difference would be considered significant. If p is greater than .05, we would not reject the null hypothesis. For the earlier example with $p = .18$, if we set $\alpha = .05$, we would not reject the null hypothesis. At $p = .18$, the probability that the observed difference is due to chance is too great. If a statistical test demonstrates that two means are different at $p = .04$, we could reject H_0, with only a small acceptable risk (4%) of committing a Type I error.

Choosing a Level of Significance

How does a researcher decide on a level of significance as the criterion for statistical testing? The conventional designation of .05 is really an arbitrary standard. A researcher may choose other criterion levels depending on how critical a Type I error would be. For example, suppose we were involved in the study of a drug to reduce spasticity, comparing control and experimental groups. This drug could be very beneficial to patients with upper motor neuron involvement; however, the drug has potentially serious side effects and is very expensive to produce. In such a situation we would want to be very confident that observed results were real, and not due to chance. If we reject the null hypothesis and recommend the drug, we would want the probability of our committing a Type I error to be very small. We do not want to encourage the use of the drug unless it is clearly and markedly beneficial. We can minimize the risk of statistical error by lowering the level of significance to .025 or .01. If we use $\alpha = .01$ as our criterion for rejecting H_0, we would have only 1 out of 100 chances of making a Type I error. This would mean that we could have greater confidence in our decision to reject the null hypothesis.

Although researchers usually choose .05 as a convenient standard, there are situations, as just described, where lower levels of significance are appropriate. In the absence of compelling justification, however, it is not necessary to make the level of significance more rigorous than $\alpha = .05$. It is generally considered unacceptable to designate values of alpha higher than .05.

Researchers should specify the minimal level of significance required for rejecting the null hypothesis prior to data collection. The decision to use .05 or .01, or any other value, should be based on the concern for Type I error, not on what the data look like. If a researcher chooses $\alpha = .01$ as the criterion, and statistical testing shows significance at $p = .04$, the researcher would not reject H_0. If $\alpha = .05$ had been chosen as the criterion, the opposite conclusion would be reached. It is not appropriate to decide on the criterion level after the statistical probabilities have been determined. That's like setting the rules of a game after it has been played so you can win! Because data are influenced by sampling error, it is important that the determination of the level of significance remains an unbiased process.

Interpreting Probability Values

Researchers must be aware of the appropriate interpretation of p values: The p value is the probability of finding an effect as big as the one observed when the null hypothesis is true. Therefore, with $p = .02$, even if there is no true difference, you would expect to observe this size effect 2% of the time. Said another way, if we performed 100 similar experiments, two of them would result in a difference this large, even though no true difference exists.

It is tempting, then, to reverse this definition, to assume that there is a 98% probability that a real difference exists. This is not the case, however. The p value is based on the assumption that the null hypothesis is true, although it cannot be used to prove it. The p value will only tell us how rarely we would expect a difference this large in the population just by chance. It is the researcher's responsibility to determine if this result is sufficiently unlikely that the null hypothesis should be rejected.

We must also be careful to avoid using the magnitude of p as an indication of the degree of validity of the research hypothesis. It is inadvisable to use terms such as "highly significant" or "more significant" because they imply that the value of p is a measure of treatment effect, which it is not. The level of significance can be considered a point along a continuum that demarcates the line between chance and reality. Once the level of significance is chosen, it represents a decision rule. The decision is dichotomous: either yes or no, significant or not significant. Once the decision is made, the magnitude of p reflects only the relative degree of confidence that can be placed in that decision. That said, researchers will still caution that a nonsignificant p value is not necessarily the end of the story, especially if it is close to α. A lack of statistical significance does not necessarily imply a lack of practical importance and vice versa (see Commentary). The pragmatic difference in clinical effect with $p = .04$ or $p = .06$ may truly be negligible. We must, therefore, also consider the possibility of Type II error.

TYPE II ERROR: STATISTICAL POWER

We have thus far established the logic behind classical statistical inference, based on the probability associated with rejecting a true null hypothesis, or Type I error. But what happens when we find no significant difference between groups and we do not reject the null hypothesis? Does this necessarily mean that there is no real difference?

If we do not reject the null hypothesis when it is indeed false, we have committed a Type II error; that is, we have found no significant difference when a difference really does exist. Unfortunately when results are not significant, researchers often assume that the experimental treatment was not effective. Researchers and journal editors are often unable or unwilling to publish reports that end in nonsignificant outcomes.[4-7] A nonsignificant outcome may, however, simply mean that the available evidence is not strong enough to reject the null hypothesis. The implications of this issue can be far reaching. For instance, the literature may demonstrate conflicting results, with some studies showing a treatment is effective and others failing to do so. Researchers may try to explain these apparent discrepancies by unknowingly proposing flawed theoretical models, or important research directions may be abandoned prematurely. We may be losing a great deal of valuable information or moving critically off course by ignoring the possibilities of Type II error.

The probability of making a Type II error is denoted by **beta (β)**, which is the *probability of failing to reject a false null hypothesis*. If $\beta = .20$, there is a 20% chance that we will make a Type II error, or that we will not reject H_0 when it is really false. The fact that samples are really different does not guarantee that a statistically significant finding will result. The value of β represents the likelihood that we will be unable to statistically identify real differences.

The complement of β error, $1 - \beta$, is the statistical **power** of a test. *Power is the probability that a test will lead to rejection of the null hypothesis*, or the probability of attaining statistical significance. If $\beta = .20$, power $= .80$. Therefore, for a statistical test at 80% power, the probability is 80% that we would correctly demonstrate a statistical difference and reject H_0 if actual differences exist. The more powerful a test, the less likely one is to make a Type II error. Power can be thought of as sensitivity. The more sensitive a test, the more likely it will detect important clinical differences that truly exist. Where $\alpha = .05$ has become the conventional standard for Type I error, it has been suggested that $\beta = .20$, with corresponding power of 80%, represents a reasonable protection against Type II error.[8]

The Determinants of Statistical Power

The statistical power of a test is a function of four factors: the significance criterion (α), the variance in the data (s^2), sample size (n), and a factor that reflects the magnitude of the observed differences, called the **effect size (ES).**

The Significance Criterion

Although there is no direct mathematical relationship between α and β, there is trade-off between them. Lowering the level of significance reduces the chance of Type I error by requiring stronger evidence for a statistical test to demonstrate significant differences. This also means that the chance of missing a true effect is increased. As the probability of committing a Type I error decreases, the probability of committing a Type II error increases. By making the standard for rejecting H_0 more rigorous (lowering α), we make it harder for sample results to meet this standard.

Variance

The power of a statistical test is increased as the variance within a set of data is reduced. The ability to detect differences between groups is enhanced when the groups are distinctly different. When the variability within groups is large, differences between groups will be less obvious. Variance can be reduced, and power increased, by experimental design, such as using repeated measures or homogeneous blocks of subjects, by controlling for sources of random measurement error, or by increasing the size of the sample.

Sample Size

The influence of sample size on power of a test is critical. The larger the sample, the greater the statistical power. Smaller samples are less likely to be good representations of population characteristics, and, therefore, true differences between groups are less likely to be recognized. When very small samples are used, as is often the case in clinical research, power is substantially reduced.

Effect Size

Power is also influenced by the size of the "effect" of the experimental variable. When comparing groups, this effect will be the difference between sample means, or an estimate of the effect of the independent variable. In studies where relationships are of interest, this effect will be the degree of correlation or association between variables. This is the essence of most research questions: "How large an effect will my treatment have?" or "How strong is the relationship between two variables?" Treatments that result in large changes or correlations are more likely to produce significant outcomes than those with small or negligible effects.

Therefore, **effect size** is a measure of the *degree to which the null hypothesis is false.*[8] For instance, if we hypothesize that no difference exists between strength scores for two groups, we are hypothesizing that the effect size is zero. If we find an actual difference of 20 foot-pounds, the effect size is 20. The larger the effect size, the greater the effective difference between the groups.

Power Analysis

We can analyze power for two purposes. One is to estimate the sample size in recruiting a sample during planning stages of a study. The second purpose is to determine the probability that a Type II error was committed when a study results in a nonsignificant finding. Procedures for power analysis are described in Appendix C for *t*-tests, analysis of variance, correlation, regression and chi-square tests. Some computer programs include analyses of effect size and power for various tests.

Determining Sample Size: A Priori Analysis

One of the first questions researchers ask when planning a study is, "How many subjects are needed?" An easy answer is as many subjects as possible; however, this is not helpful when one is trying to place realistic limits on time and resources for data collection. Researchers may arbitrarily suggest that a sample size of 30 or 50 is "reasonable." Unfortunately, these estimates may be inadequate for many research designs or for studies with small effect sizes. By specifying a level of significance and desired power in the planning stages of a study, a researcher can estimate how many subjects would be needed to detect a significant difference for an expected effect size. This is called *a priori* power analysis.

The smaller the effect size, the larger the required sample. When the sample size estimate is beyond realistic limits, a researcher may try to redesign the study by controlling variability in the sample, choosing a different dependent variable or increasing effect size, or the researcher may decide not to conduct the study given that significant results are so unlikely. Many clinical variables may produce small to medium effect sizes because of the inherent variability among patients and the lack of standardization and sensitivity in clinical measures. Therefore, sample size becomes extremely important in designing a study that has a reasonable chance of success.

The major challenge in *a priori* power analysis is obviously the unknown effect size. The researcher must make an educated guess, which may be based on previous research findings from the literature. Alternatively, the estimate may reflect an effect that would be considered clinically meaningful.

Power analysis should be incorporated into the planning stages of every experimental or correlational study. The lack of such planning often results in a high probability of Type II error and needlessly wasted efforts.[9]

Measuring Type II Error: Post Hoc Analysis

When a study is completed and results are not significant, the researcher will want to determine the likelihood that a Type II error has been committed. By knowing the observed effect size, the level of significance used, and the sample size, the researcher can determine the degree of power that was achieved in the analysis. If power is low, the researcher might draw only tentative conclusions about the lack of significant treatment effect, and consider replicating the study with a larger sample to increase the power of the test.

For the consumer of research, it is often useful to evaluate the power of nonsignificant tests reported in the literature. In some cases, the clinical significance of a study will be greater than suggested by the statistical outcome because of the lack of power. For example, many meta-analyses have demonstrated important treatment effects even when individual clinical trials did not produce significant outcomes because they used small samples.[10]

CONCEPTS OF STATISTICAL TESTING

Statistical procedures are used to test hypotheses through the calculation of a test statistic, or test ratio. Different statistics are used to test differences between means, correlations and proportions. The test statistic is used to determine if a significant effect is attained, by establishing the probability that such a difference would occur if H_0 were true.

We will illustrate this concept using a one-sample test. Let us assume we want to determine whether the mean IQ of 3-year-old children who were born prematurely is different from the mean IQ of the general population of 3-year-old children, which is known to be 100. The null hypothesis, $H_0: \mu = 100$, states that the mean of the population of premature children is 100; that is, the premature children are from the general population. The alternative hypothesis, $H_1: \mu \neq 100$, states that the premature children come from a population with a mean IQ different from 100, that is, different from the overall population. This is a nondirectional hypothesis. We draw a random sample of $n = 150$ premature children, with mean $\overline{X} = 105$ and standard deviation $s = 33$. The difference between this sample mean and the known population mean may be the result of chance, or it may indicate that premature children should not be considered part of the overall population. The researcher must determine the probability that one would observe a difference as large as 5 points by chance if the population mean for premature children is truly 100.

We begin by assuming that the null hypothesis is true; that is, the observed difference of 5 points is due to chance. We then ask, How often would we expect to see a difference of 5 points or more if H_0 were true? The answer to this question is based on the defined properties of the normal sampling distribution and our desired level of significance, $\alpha = .05$.

The z-Ratio

Recall from Chapter 17 that we can determine the area beyond any point in a normal distribution using values of z, or standard deviation units. For an individual sample score, X, a z-score represents the distance between that score and the sample mean, $\overline{X}$, divided by the standard deviation of the distribution (refer back to Equation 17.6). When z is applied to a sampling distribution of means, the ratio reflects the distance between an individual sample mean, $\overline{X}$, and the population mean, μ, divided by the standard error of the mean:

$$z = \frac{\overline{X} - \mu}{s_{\overline{X}}}$$

(18.5)

For our example, with $\overline{X} = 105, s = 35, n = 150$ and $\mu = 100$, we calculate $s_{\overline{X}} = 35/\sqrt{150} = 2.86$. Therefore,

$$z = \frac{105 - 100}{2.86} = \frac{5.0}{2.86} = 1.75$$

This tells us that the sample mean for premature children is 1.75 standard error units above the population mean of 100. We must now ask, Is this a significant difference? That is, is the difference large enough that we would consider the mean IQ of premature children to be different from 100?

Let us assume we could plot the sampling distribution of means of IQ for the general population, which takes the form of the normal curve. We know that 95% of the area under the curve is bounded by $z = \pm1.96$, as shown in Figure 18.6. Therefore, there is a 95% chance that any one sample chosen from this population would have a mean within those boundaries. Said another way, it is *highly likely* that any one sample chosen from this general population would have a mean IQ within this range. Conversely, there is only a 5% chance that any chosen sample mean would fall above or below those points. This means that it is *unlikely* that a sample chosen from this general population would have a mean with a z-score greater than ±1.96. Any value that has only a 5% chance of occurring is considered "unlikely," based on a .05 level of significance. In other words, if our sample yields a mean with a z-ratio beyond ±1.96, it is unlikely that that sample is from the general population (H_1). If the sample mean of IQ for premature children falls within $z = \pm1.96$, then there is a 95% chance that the sample does come from a population with $\mu = 100$ (H_0).

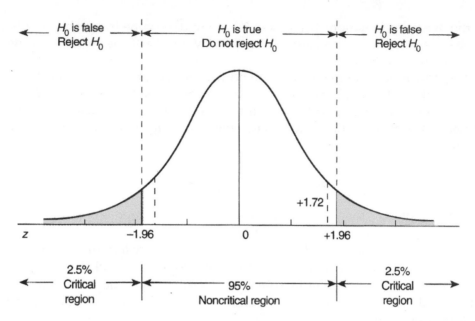

FIGURE 18.6 Standard normal distribution of z-scores showing critical values for a two-tailed test (nondirectional) at α_2 = .05 and the calculated z-score for IQ.

The Critical Region

The tails of the curve depicted in Figure 18.6, representing the area above and below $z = \pm1.96$, encompass the **critical region**, or the region of rejection. The value of z that defines these areas is the **critical value**. When we calculate z for our study sample, it must be *equal to or greater than* the absolute critical value if H_0 is to be rejected. If a calculated z-ratio falls within the critical region ($z \geq \pm1.96$), the ratio is *significant*. If the ratio is less than the critical value ($z < \pm1.96$), it represents a difference that is not significant, or likely due to chance.

In our example, $z = 1.75$ for the mean IQ of premature children. This value is less than the critical value of 1.96 and falls within the central *noncritical region* of the curve. Therefore, it is likely that this sample does come from a population with $\mu = 100$, or the general population. In other words, the observed difference between the means of the general population and the sample of premature children is not large enough to be considered significant at $\alpha = .05$. The difference between the sample mean and population means is probably due to chance. We do not reject the null hypothesis.

Directional versus Nondirectional Tests

The process we have just described is considered *nondirectional* because we did not predict the direction of the difference between the sample means. Consequently, the critical region was established in both tails, so that a large enough positive or negative z-ratio would lead to rejection of the null hypothesis. This is considered a **two-tailed test**. For convenience, we can designate our level of significance as $\alpha_2 = .05$, to indicate a two-tailed probability with $\alpha/2$ in each tail.

The critical value, against which the calculated z-ratio is compared, is determined according to the specified level of significance. If $\alpha_2 = .05$, then a total of 5% of the curve must be in the two tails of the curve. Therefore, using Appendix Table A.1, we see that for $\alpha_2 = .01$ (.005 in each tail), the critical value of $z = \pm 2.576$. Similarly, for $\alpha_2 = .10$ (.05 in each tail), $z = \pm 1.645$.

In situations where a researcher has sufficient reason to propose an alternative hypothesis that specifies which mean will be larger, a *directional* test can be performed. For example, we could hypothesize that the mean IQ of premature children is greater than 100. This is a directional hypothesis. In this case, it is not necessary to locate the critical region in both tails, because we do not expect a negative ratio. We are only interested in the positive tail of the curve. Therefore, we would perform a **one-tailed test.** We can specify the level of significance as $\alpha_1 = .05$ because the full 5% will be located in one tail of the curve. The critical value will now represent that point at which the area in the positive tail equals 5% of the total curve. Using Table A.1, we find that this area starts at $z = 1.645$, as shown in Figure 18.7. We are hypothesizing that there is only a 5% chance that any sample chosen from the general population would have a mean IQ above $z = 1.645$. The value of the calculated z-ratio must be greater than or equal to 1.645 to be considered significant. Based on our example, $z = 1.75$ would now fall in the critical region, and, therefore, be considered significant. With a one-tailed test, we would reject the null hypothesis.

One-Tailed or Two-Tailed?

You have undoubtedly noted that the z-ratio in this example is considered significant with a one-tailed test, but not with a two-tailed test. This happens because the critical region for the one-tailed test is larger. Therefore, the one-tailed test is more powerful;

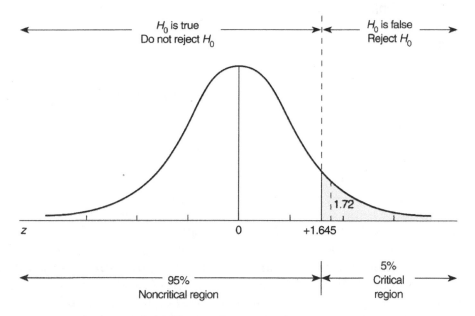

FIGURE 18.7   Standard normal distribution of z-scores showing critical values for a one-tailed test (directional) at $\alpha_1 = .05$ and the calculated z-score for IQ.

that is, one is less likely to commit a Type II error using the one-tailed test. One would think, then, that researchers would routinely use one-tailed tests, making it easier to attain significance. This situation has sparked many debates about the appropriate use of directional and nondirectional alternative hypotheses. Some statisticians favor exclusive use of two-tailed (nondirectional) tests, based on a conservative and traditional approach to data analysis.[11] With this argument, one-tailed tests should only be used when it is impossible for the difference to go in the opposite direction. A test of IQ, for instance, would not fit this criterion. Others have argued that the rationale behind most research questions supports one-sided tests, especially in studies where a control or placebo group is involved.[12] These proponents argue that the ethics of research would demand that a study be based on a sound theoretical rationale that would identify an expected direction of difference.

We think the middle ground on this issue is most reasonable: Researchers are obliged to justify whether the research hypothesis is directional or nondirectional, and use the appropriate statistical approach. This means that the decision to use a one- or two-tailed test is a reasoned, not an arbitrary, one and certainly not made after data are collected and analyzed. With sufficient manipulation of statistics, almost any result can be given statistical significance. The interpretation of statistical outcomes is, however, based on the search for truth about clinical phenomena, not contrived outcomes. Therefore, if a researcher decides on the directionality of a test after the experimental results are known, the theoretical probabilities associated with the test cannot be considered an accurate representation of the data. It is also important to realize that if a directional hypothesis is proposed, and results go in the direction opposite to that expected, H_0 cannot be rejected because it is not possible to accept the alternative. Therefore, a one-tailed test should be applied only when a sound rationale can be provided. The choice of a one- or two-tailed test should always be specified prior to data analysis and should be reported with published data.

Degrees of Freedom

The last concept we introduce here is that of **degrees of freedom (df)**. We can think of degrees of freedom geometrically, indicating the available directions of movement within a given space. A point on a line is free to move in one dimension only, and has one degree of freedom. A point in a three-dimensional space, such as a cube, has three degrees of freedom. Therefore, degrees of freedom refer to those components that are *free to vary* within a defined system.

In statistical terminology, degrees of freedom refer to the number of components that are free to vary within a set of data. For example, suppose we took five measurements with a sum of 30 and a mean of 6. Theoretically, any set of five numbers could be specified to equal a sum of 30; however, once four of the scores are known, the fifth is automatically determined. If we measured 8, 9, 10 and 11, the fifth score would have to be -8 to get a total of 30. Therefore, this set of data has four degrees of freedom. Four values are free to vary, given the restrictions imposed on the data, in this case a sum of 30 with a mean of 6. In this situation, the degrees of freedom will equal one less than the number of scores, or $n - 1$. As we present statistical tests in the coming chapters, we will describe the rules for determining the degrees of freedom associated with specific procedures.

PARAMETRIC VERSUS NONPARAMETRIC STATISTICS

Statistics that are used to estimate population parameters are called **parametric statistics**. The validity of parametric tests is dependent on certain assumptions about the nature of data. The primary assumption is that samples are randomly drawn from parent populations with normal distributions. Therefore, the sample should be a useful representation of population "parameters." With small samples, or with distributions that have not been previously described, it may be unreasonable to accept this assumption. Tests of "goodness of fit" can be performed to determine how well data match the normal distribution. A second assumption is that variances in the samples being compared are roughly equal, or homogeneous. A test for *homogeneity of variance* can substantiate this assumption. A third assumption is that data are measured on the interval or ratio scales. Therefore, scores can be subjected to arithmetic manipulations to calculate means and standard deviations.

When statistical conditions do not meet these requirements, **nonparametric tests** can be used. Nonparametric tests make fewer assumptions about population data, and can be used when normality and homogeneity of variance criteria are not satisfied. They can be used effectively, therefore, with very small samples. In addition, they have been specifically developed to operate on data at the nominal and ordinal scales. Alternatively, data can be transformed to another scale of measurement, such as a logarithmic scale, to create distributions that more closely satisfy the necessary assumptions for parametric tests (see Appendix D).

Statisticians do not agree on absolute rules for using parametric or nonparametric procedures. The classical school insists that if all the assumptions behind parametric tests are not met, nonparametric tests should be used; however, parametric tests are generally considered robust enough to withstand even major violations of these assumptions without seriously affecting the validity of statistical outcomes,[13,14] including their use with ordinal data.[15,16] Many researchers prefer to use parametric procedures because they are generally considered more powerful. As this is not the appropriate forum to settle this debate, we take a moderate position and suggest that nonparametric tests are most useful when ordinal or nominal data are collected and when samples are small and normality cannot be assumed. When their application is justified, parametric tests are preferred because they are more powerful and more versatile with complex research designs. This issue is discussed further in Chapter 22.

An algorithm for choosing parametric and nonparametric statistical tests for given research designs can be found in Appendix B.

COMMENTARY

Statistical Significance versus Clinical Significance

The emphasis placed on significance testing in clinical research must be tempered with an understanding that statistical tests are tools for analyzing data and should never be used as a substitute for knowledgeable interpretation of outcomes. A big difference exists between **statistical significance** and **clinical significance.** Statistical tests are not sensitive to units of measurement, nor can they be responsive to the practical or clinical implications of the data. Suppose we compared a mobilization procedure to no treatment and found a significant difference between groups with means of 90 and 95 degrees shoulder range of motion. Knowing the inherent error in range of motion testing, could we reasonably conclude that 5 degrees represents a clinically important difference? A mean difference that is small can be statistically significant just because enough subjects were used in the experiment to make the test powerful. But the difference may be very unimportant. Conversely, when a test does not result in a statistically significant outcome, but the effect size is clinically meaningful, we should be aware of the possibility of Type II error, and not automatically assume that the treatment is not effective. The word *significant* should not be used in research literature to mean important, conclusive, distinctive, or marked. Its use should be reserved for the reporting of statistical results.

Several considerations are important in interpreting the results of statistical tests.[3]

1. **Think about what the numbers mean.**   Look at plots of the data and consider measures of variability. Use confidence intervals to establish reasonable ranges for the treatment effect. The researcher must have a thorough knowledge of the phenomenon being studied and a reasonable understanding of the measurements used.

2. **Don't confuse significance level with size of treatment effect.**   Remember that the probabilities associated with the null hypothesis only tell us how likely it is that the treatment caused the effect. Probability does not represent the size of the treatment effect.

3. **Is the effect meaningful?**   When the null hypothesis is rejected, look at the size of the treatment effect. Effect size indices can help to assess the magnitude of the effect (see Chapter 27 and Appendix C). The effect size can be an important benchmark to understand responses obtained with various instruments, such as health status measures, and for interpreting change in responses over time.[17] When the null hypothesis is not rejected, we must consider the effect size over statistical significance to avoid discarding potentially important discoveries, especially with new treatment approaches.[10] The researcher must determine when the observed difference is large enough to warrant corrective action or a change in practice, with or without a significant test. Rosnow and Rosenthal[18] cautioned against the dogma of the yes-no decision based on $p = .05$. They wrote,

   > ... surely, God loves the .06 nearly as much as the .05. Can there be any doubt that God views the strength of evidence for or against the null as a fairly continuous function of the magnitude of p?

   This concept is of great importance to clinical researchers, who should use statistics as a form of input to, but not the sole criterion for, clinical decisions.

4. **Interpret results in the context of other studies.**   The development of a body of knowledge is an incremental process. Each study contributes to an

understanding of theory, expanding our thinking and interpretation. Sometimes studies will show similar or conflicting results; sometimes outcomes will show differences, while others show no differences. We must be able to reflect on the collective impact of this information, and critically assess its meaningfulness. This requires that researchers recognize the need for replication and meta-analytic approaches (see Chapter 16).

As we search for the answers to research questions, we are constantly aware of the need to consider the validity of our designs, measurements and theoretical constructs. In addition to these elements, however, we must also consider the validity of analysis procedures, or **statistical conclusion validity** (see Chapter 9). We can start with a well designed study, but our outcomes will not be meaningful unless we choose appropriate statistical tests and interpret them accurately. For example, we would want to know that we had sufficient power, that we have not violated the assumptions of the statistical procedure, and that our measurements are reliable.

This is an issue that must be addressed in the planning stages of a study. All too often statistical consultants are handed the results of a study and asked to help analyze the data. This requires retrospective definition of assumptions, often a frustrating task. It is impossible to correct deficiencies in design or data collection after the fact. A statistician should be consulted in the design phase of a study, to set the proper operational definitions, to determine appropriate procedures and to assure that the research question can be answered. There is no greater disappointment than the realization that months of hard work are fruitless because the data cannot be analyzed to generate the desired interpretation.

Because statistics are essential for interpreting clinical research, we must be educated consumers as we read reports of research and as participants in a study. We do not have to be statisticians to have a working knowledge that will allow us to be critical in the use of statistical information for clinical decision making. Read on!

REFERENCES

1. Fitzgerald GK, Wynveen KJ, Rheault W, Rothschild B. Objective assessment with establishment of normal values for lumbar spinal range of motion. *Phys Ther* 1983;63: 1776–1781.
2. Godges JJ, Mattson-Bell M, Thorpe D, Shah D. The immediate effects of soft tissue mobilization with proprioceptive neuromuscular facilitation on glenohumeral external rotation and overhead reach. *J Orthop Sports Phys Ther* 2003;33:713–718.
3. Keppel G. *Design and Analysis: A Researcher's Handbook* (4th ed.). Englewood Cliffs, NJ: Prentice Hall, 2004.
4. Ioannidis JP. Effect of the statistical significance of results on the time to completion and publication of randomized efficacy trials. *JAMA* 1998;279:281–286.
5. Chan AW, Altman DG. Identifying outcome reporting bias in randomised trials on PubMed: Review of publications and survey of authors. *BMJ* 2005;330:753.
6. Chan AW, Krleza-Jeric K, Schmid I, Altman DG. Outcome reporting bias in randomized trials funded by the Canadian Institutes of Health Research. *CMAJ* 2004;171:735–740.
7. Krzyzanowska MK, Pintilie M, Tannock IF. Factors associated with failure to publish large randomized trials presented at an oncology meeting. *JAMA* 2003;290:495–501.

8. Cohen J. *Statistical Power Analysis for the Behavioral Sciences* (2nd ed.). Hillsdale, NJ: Lawrence Erlbaum, 1988.

9. Bernstein J, McGuire K, Freedman KB. Statistical sampling and hypothesis testing in orthopaedic research. *Clin Orthop Relat Res* 2003:55–62.

10. Altman DG, Bland JM. Absence of evidence is not evidence of absence. *BMJ* 1995;311: 485.

11. Dubey SD. Some thoughts on the one-sided and two-sided tests. *J Biopharm Stat* 1991;1: 139–150.

12. Peace KE. One-sided or two-sided p values: Which most appropriately address the question of drug efficacy? *J Biopharm Stat* 1991;1:133–138.

13. Kerlinger FN. *Foundations of Behavioral Research* (3rd ed.). New York: Holt, Rinehart & Winston, 1985.

14. Nunally J, Bernstein IH. *Psychometric Theory* (3rd ed.). New York: McGraw-Hill, 1994.

15. Wang ST, Yu ML, Wang CJ, Huang CC. Bridging the gap between the pros and cons in treating ordinal scales as interval scales from an analysis point of view. *Nurs Res* 1999;48:226–229.

16. Gaito J. Measurement scales and statistics: Resurgence of an old misconception. *Psychol Bull* 1980;87:564–567.

17. Kazis LE, Anderson JJ, Meenan RF. Effect sizes for interpreting changes in health status. *Med Care* 1989;27:S178–S189.

18. Rosnow RL, Rosenthal R. Statistical procedures and the justification of knowledge in psychological Science. *Am Psychologist* 1989; 44:1276–1284.

CHAPTER 19

Comparing Two Means: The t-Test

The simplest experimental comparison involves the use of two independent groups created by random assignment. This design allows the researcher to assume that all individual differences are evenly distributed between the groups, so that the groups are equivalent at the start of the experiment. Statistically, the groups are considered random samples of the same population, and therefore, any observed differences among them should be the result of sampling error or chance. After the application of a treatment variable to one group, the researcher wants to determine if the groups are still from the same population, or if their means can be considered significantly different.

Comparisons can also be made using a repeated measures design. A researcher may be interested in looking at the difference between two conditions or performances by the same group of subjects. In this case, the subjects serve as their own control, and the researcher wants to determine if the conditions are significantly different.

The purpose of this chapter is to introduce procedures for evaluating the comparison between two means using the *t*-test and confidence intervals. These procedures can be applied to differences between two independent samples or between scores obtained with repeated measures. These procedures are based on parametric operations and, therefore, are subject to all assumptions underlying parametric statistics.

THE CONCEPTUAL BASIS FOR COMPARING GROUP MEANS

The concept of statistical significance for comparing means is based on the relationship between two sample characteristics: the mean and the variance. The difference between group means indicates the degree of separation *between* groups (the effect size). Variance measures tell us how variable the scores are *within* each group. Both of these characteristics represent sources of variability that are used to describe the extent of treatment effects.

Suppose we wanted to compare two randomly assigned groups, one experimental and one control, to determine if treatment made a difference in their performance. Theoretically, if the experimental treatment was effective, and all other factors were equal and constant, all subjects within the treatment group would achieve the same score, and all subjects within the control group would also achieve the same score, but scores would be different between groups. As illustrated in Figure 19.1A, everyone in the treatment group performed better than everyone in the control group. Consider all the

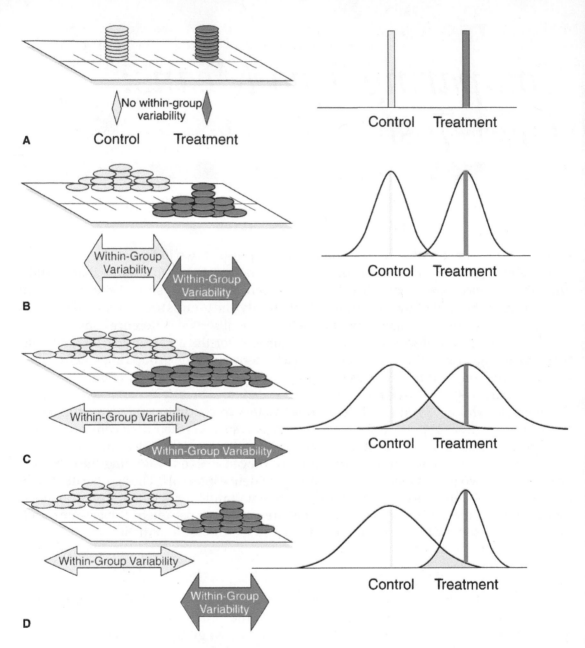

FIGURE 19.1 Four sets of hypothetical distributions with the same means, but different variances. In (**A**) all subjects in each group received the same score, but the groups were different from each other. There is no variance within groups. In (**B**) the subjects' scores were more spread out, but the control and treatment conditions are still clearly different. There is some variance within groups, but the variance between groups is greater. In (**C**) the subjects are much more variable. There is greater variance within groups, and therefore, the groups are not distinctly different. In (**D**) the variances of the two groups are not equal.

scores in this sample for both groups combined. If we were asked to *explain* why these scores were different, we would say that all differences were due to the effect of treatment. There is a difference *between the groups*, but no variance *within the groups*.

Error Variance

Now let's consider the more realistic situation where subjects within a group do not all respond the same way. As shown in Figure 19.1B, the scores in the treatment and control groups are variable, but we still tend to see higher scores among those who received treatment. If we look at the entire set of scores, and we were asked again to explain why scores are different, we would say that some of the differences can be *explained* by the treatment effect; that is, most of the higher scores were in the treatment group. However, the scores are also influenced by personal characteristics, inconsistencies in measurement, and behavioral and environmental factors. These factors create variance within the groups, variance that is *unexplained*, due to all the other unknown factors influencing the response.

This unexplained portion is called **error variance**. The concept of statistical "error" does not mean mistakes or miscalculation. It refers to all sources of variability within a set of data that cannot be explained by the independent variable. Any given score is a composite of the treatment effect and error variance. Random assignment allows us to assume that these error components are unsystematic chance variations, and therefore, are independent of the treatment effect.[1]

The distribution in Figure 19.1B is represented by a pair of curves. This graphic shows means that are far apart, with few overlapping scores (the gray area) at one extreme of each curve. The curves show that the individuals in the treatment and control groups behaved very differently, whereas subjects within each group performed within a narrow range (error variance is small). In such a comparison, the null hypothesis would probably be rejected, as the treatment effect has clearly differentiated the groups.

Contrast this with the distributions in Figure 19.1C, which show the same means, but greater variability within the groups, as evidenced by the wider spread of the curves. Factors other than the treatment variable are causing subjects to respond very differently from each other. Here we find a great deal of overlap, indicating that many subjects from both groups had the same score, regardless of whether or not they received the experimental treatment. These curves reflect a greater degree of error variance; that is, the treatment does not help to explain most of the differences among scores. In this case, it is less likely that the treatment is differentiating the groups, and the null hypothesis would probably not be rejected. Any group differences observed here are probably due to chance variation.

The Statistical Ratio

The subjective judgments we have made about the distributions in Figure 19.1 are not adequate, however, for making research decisions about the effectiveness of treatment. We know groups can look different just by chance. So how do we objectively determine if observed differences between groups are true population differences or only chance differences? In other words, how do we decide if we should reject the null hypothesis? We make this decision on the basis of its *probability of being true*. This is what a test of statistical significance is designed to do.

The significance of the difference between group means is judged by a ratio derived as follows:

$$\text{Ratio} = \frac{\text{Difference } between \text{ group means}}{\text{Variability } within \text{ groups}}$$

The numerator represents the separation between the groups, which is a function of all sources of variance, including treatment effects and error. The denominator reflects the variability within groups as a result of error alone. Therefore, when H_0 is false, that is, when a treatment effect does exist ($\mu_1 \neq \mu_2$), the ratio is conceptually represented as

$$\frac{\text{Treatment effect} + \text{error}}{\text{Error}}$$

When H_0 is true, that is, when no real treatment effect exists ($\mu_1 = \mu_2$), the ratio reduces to

$$\frac{\text{Error}}{\text{Error}}$$

As the treatment effect increases, the absolute value of this ratio gets larger. As the error variance increases, the ratio gets smaller, approaching 1.0. If we want to demonstrate that two groups are significantly different, this ratio should be as large as possible. Thus, we would want the separation between the group means to be large and the variability within groups to be small. We emphasize the variance *between* and *within* groups as essential elements of significance testing which will be used repeatedly as we continue our discussion. Most statistical tests are based on this relationship.

Statistical Hypotheses

The null hypothesis for a two-level design states that the two population means are equal:

$$H_0: \mu_1 = \mu_2$$

The alternative hypothesis can be stated in a nondirectional format,

$$H_1: \mu_1 \neq \mu_2$$

or a directional format,

$$H_1: \mu_1 > \mu_2 \qquad \text{or} \qquad H_1: \mu_1 < \mu_2.$$

Nondirectional hypotheses are tested using a two-tailed test of significance. Directional hypotheses are tested using a one-tailed test. Even though we are actually comparing sample means, our hypotheses are written in terms of population parameters.

Equality of Variances

Most parametric statistics require the assumption of equal variances among groups, or **homogeneity of variance**. While there is an expectation that error variance will exist within each group, the assumption is that the degree of variance will be roughly equivalent. Look at the scenarios in Figure 19.1 B and C. In one case (B) the variances are small, and in the other (C) they are larger; however, in both cases they are similar across groups. If we consider the spread of scores in Figure 19.1D, we can see that the treatment group is much less variable than the control group. In this situation, the two groups have different variances, and the assumption of homogeneity of variance is not met.

Most statistical procedures that compare means include a test that will determine if the difference in the variance components is significant. We can expect some difference in variances just by chance. With random assignment, larger samples will have a better chance of showing equal variances than small samples. Therefore, the test for homogeneity of variance will clarify if the observed difference in variances is large enough to be meaningful. When variances are significantly different (they are not equal), adjustments can be made in the test for means that will account for these differences.*

THE *t*-TEST FOR INDEPENDENT SAMPLES

The *t*-test is the statistical procedure used to compare two means.[†] The **independent** or **unpaired *t*-test** is used when the means of two independent groups of subjects are compared. Such groups are usually created through random assignment, although samples of convenience or intact groups may be used.[‡] Groups are considered independent because each is composed of an independent set of subjects, with no inherent relationship derived from repeated measures or matching.

The *t* Statistic: Equal Variances

The test statistic for the unpaired *t*-test is calculated using the formula

$$t = \frac{\overline{X}_1 - \overline{X}_2}{s_{\overline{X}_1 - \overline{X}_2}} \tag{19.1}$$

The numerator of this ratio represents the difference between the independent group means, or the effect size. The term in the denominator is called the **standard error of**

---

*This can sometimes be confusing when the test of homogeneity of variance is performed in conjunction with a test for differences between means. Two different tests are actually being done. First the test for homogeneity of variance determines if the variances are significantly different. Then the test for means will determine if the means are significantly different. If the first test shows that variances are not equal, an adjustment will be made in the test for means.

[†]Recall from the discussion in Chapter 18 that the *t*-distribution is an analog of the standard normal distribution, developed to represent smaller sampling distributions. The *t*-distribution was originally developed by W.S. Gossett in 1908, who wrote under the pseudonym of "Student." Therefore, the *t*-test is often referred to as Student's *t*-test.

[‡]When intact groups are used, regression procedures may be the more appropriate form of analysis because groups cannot be randomly assigned to treatment conditions. See Chapters 24 and 29 for a discussion of regression procedures.

the difference between the means,[§] representing the variability within the two samples. Equation (19.1) can be used in situations where $n_1 = n_2$, or when $n_1 \neq n_2$ if variances are equal. An alternative formula for t, to be described shortly, is used when the assumption of equality of variance is not met.

We estimate $s_{\overline{X}_1 - \overline{X}_2}$ using a **pooled variance estimate**, given the symbol s_p^2:

$$s_p^2 = \frac{s_1^2(n_1 - 1) + s_2^2(n_2 - 1)}{n_1 + n_2 - 2} \tag{19.2}$$

where s_1^2 and s_2^2 are the group variances, and n_1 and n_2 are the respective sample sizes. This estimate provides a *weighted average* of s_1^2 and s_2^2.[**] The pooled variance estimate is based on the assumption that both samples come from the same population and that they have equal variances (any difference between variances is due to chance). Therefore, the pooled variance should estimate the population variance.

The standard error of the difference between the means is then given by[††]

$$s_{\overline{X}_1 - \overline{X}_2} = \sqrt{\frac{s_p^2}{n_1} + \frac{s_p^2}{n_2}} = \sqrt{s_p^2 \left(\frac{1}{n_1} + \frac{1}{n_2} \right)} \tag{19.3}$$

Degrees of Freedom

The number of degrees of freedom associated with the independent t-test is the total of the degrees of freedom for both groups. Therefore, $df = (n_1 - 1) + (n_2 - 1) = (n_1 + n_2 - 2)$. This can also be written $df = N - 2$, where N is the combined sample size.

Example

Suppose we are interested in testing the hypothesis that a newly designed splint will improve hand function of patients with rheumatoid arthritis, as measured by pinch strength in pounds (Figure 19.2). We propose a directional alternative hypothesis because we are interested only in documenting an improvement in function with the splint. Results that show no change or a negative change would not be significant.

We assemble a random sample of 20 subjects with rheumatoid arthritis, with similar degrees of deformity in the hand and wrist. The subjects are randomly assigned to an experimental group ($n_1 = 10$) or a control group ($n_2 = 10$). The experimental subjects wear the splint for 1 week, in addition to participating in their regularly scheduled activities. The control subjects engage in their regular activities with no splint. Pinch strength

---

[§]In Chapter 18 we introduced the concept of standard error as an estimate of population variability based on a sampling distribution of means. In this case we are estimating the variability in a sampling distribution of *differences between means*.

[**]With two samples of equal size, this equation is reduced to $s_p^2 = \dfrac{s_1^2 + s_2^2}{2}$.

[††]With equal sample sizes $s_{\overline{X}_1 - \overline{X}_2} = \sqrt{\dfrac{2s_p^2}{n}}$, where n is the number of subjects in each group.

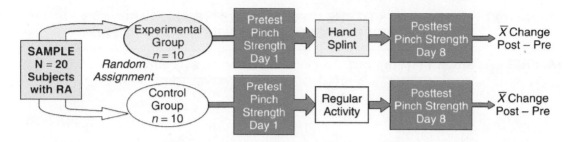

FIGURE 19.2   A pretest-posttest control group design, with two groups of patients with rheumatoid arthritis (RA) formed through random assignment. One group is treated with a hand splint; the other participates in regular activities. The difference between the posttest and pretest pinch strength (change score) is used to compare the two groups with the unpaired *t*-test.

is measured on day 1 and day 8 for both groups, and the change between the pretest and posttest measurements is used for analysis. Therefore, this study is structured as a pretest–posttest control group design, testing $H_0: \mu_1 = \mu_2$ against $H_1: \mu_1 > \mu_2$.

Hypothetical data are reported in Table 19.1A. The mean improvement in strength was 10.11 pounds for the splinted group and 5.45 pounds for the control group.

To calculate the *t*-ratio for this comparison, we first determine the value of the denominator, $s_{\bar{X}_1 - \bar{X}_2} = 1.714$, as shown in Table 19.1B. We substitute this value in Equation (19.1), and arrive at a *calculated t-ratio* of 2.718.

Critical Values of t

Now we must determine if the calculated *t*-ratio is sufficiently large to be considered significant. We do this by comparing the calculated *t* value with a **critical value** at a specified level of significance. The larger the ratio, the more likely the difference is *not* due to chance. Table A.2 in the Appendix is a table of critical values associated with *t*-distributions for samples of various sizes. At the top of the table, levels of significance are identified for one-tailed (α_1) and two-tailed (α_2) tests. Because we proposed a directional alternative hypothesis in this example, we will perform a one-tailed test at $\alpha_1 = .05$.

The column along the left side of Table A.2, labeled *df*, identifies the degrees of freedom associated with different-size samples. In this study there are $10 + 10 - 2 = 18\ df$. We look across the row for 18 *df* to the column labeled $\alpha_1 = .05$ and find the critical value 1.734. We use the summary form

$$_{(\alpha_1 = .05)}t_{(18)} = 1.734$$

to indicate the critical value of *t* associated with $\alpha_1 = .05$ and 18 *df*.

Figure 19.3 illustrates the critical value of *t* for 18 *df*, demarcating .05 in the tail of the curve for a 1-tailed test. The null hypothesis states that the difference between means will be zero, and therefore, the *t*-ratio will also equal zero. The probability that a calculated *t*-ratio will be as large or larger than 1.734 is 5% or less.

For a *t*-ratio to represent a significant difference, the absolute value of the calculated ratio must be *greater than or equal to* the critical value. In this example, the calculated

TABLE 19.1 COMPUTATION OF THE UNPAIRED t-TEST (EQUAL VARIANCES): CHANGE IN PINCH STRENGTH FOLLOWING HAND SPLINTING

A. DATA

Group 1 (splint)	Group 2 (Control)
$\overline{X}_1 = 10.11$	$\overline{X}_2 = 5.45$
$n_1 = 10$	$n_2 = 10$
$s_1^2 = 13.81$	$s_2^2 = 15.58$

B. COMPUTATIONS

$$s_p^2 = \frac{s_1^2(n_1 - 1) + s_2^2(n_2 - 1)}{n_1 + n_2 - 2} = \frac{13.81(10 - 1) + 15.58(10 - 1)}{10 + 10 - 2} = 14.695$$

$$s_{\overline{X}_1 - \overline{X}_2} = \sqrt{\frac{s_p^2}{n_1} + \frac{s_p^2}{n_2}} = \sqrt{\frac{(14.695)}{10} + \frac{14.695}{10}} = 1.714 \qquad t = \frac{\overline{X}_1 - \overline{X}_2}{s_{\overline{X}_1 - \overline{X}_2}} = \frac{10.11 - 5.45}{1.7143} = 2.718$$

C. HYPOTHESIS TEST

$H_0: \mu_1 = \mu_2 \qquad H_1: \mu_1 > \mu_2 \qquad {}_{(\alpha_1 = .05)}t_{(18)} = 1.734$ (Table A.2)

Reject H_0

D. OUTPUT

Group Statistics

	GROUP	N	Mean	Std. Deviation	Std. Error Mean
STRENGTH	1	10	10.1100	3.7159	1.1751
	2	10	5.4500	3.9472	1.2482

Independent Samples Test

	Levene's Test for Equality of Variances		t-test for Equality of Means					95% Confidence Interval of the Mean	
	F	Sig.	t	df	Sig. (2-tailed)	Mean Difference	Std. Error Difference	Lower	Upper
Equal variances assumed	.685	❶.419	2.718	18	❷ .014	❸ 4.6600	❹ 1.7143	❺1.0584	8.2616
Equal variances not assumed			2.718	17.935	.014	4.6600	1.7143	1.0575	8.2625

❶ Levene's test compares the variances of the two groups (see s^2 in section A). This difference is not significant ($p = .419$). Therefore, we will use the t-test for equal variances.

❷ The two-tailed significance is .014. Because this analysis was based on a one-tailed test (directional alternative hypothesis), we use half of the two-tailed value. Therefore, $p = .007$. This is a significant test, and we reject H_0.

❸ The difference between the means of group 1 and 2 (the numerator of the t-test).

❹ The standard error of the difference between the means (denominator of the t-test).

❺ 95% confidence interval does not contain zero, confirming that the difference between the means is significant.

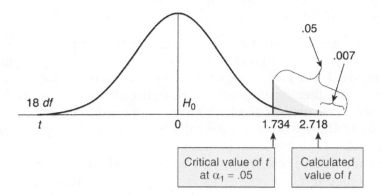

FIGURE 19.3 Curve representing a *t* distribution for 18 *df*, showing the critical value of 1.734 for a one-tailed test at .05. The null hypothesis (H_0) states that the *t* ratio will equal zero. The calculated value for this example is $t = 2.718$ (from Table 19.1). This value demarcates an area in the tail of the curve of .007. Because this probability is less than .05, we consider the test to be significant.

value $t = 2.718$ is greater than the critical value 1.734. Therefore, the group means are considered significantly different at $\alpha_1 = .05$ (see Table 19.1C). We reject H_0 and accept H_1, and conclude that patients wearing the hand splint improved more than those in the control group.

One- Versus Two-Tailed Tests

Note that each column in Appendix Table A.2 represents both a one- and a two-tailed probability. Note, too, that each two-tailed probability is twice its corresponding one-tailed probability. For instance, the critical value of *t* at $\alpha_1 = .05$ for 18 *df* is 1.734. This is also the critical value for *t* at $\alpha_2 = .10$. The critical value for $\alpha_1 = .01$ is the same as that for $\alpha_2 = .02$. Some statistical tables and computer packages provide values for only a one- or two-tailed test. If this occurs, it is a simple matter to convert the probability values. The probability reported for a one-tailed test is doubled to get a two-tailed test. Conversely, the probability reported for a two-tailed test is halved to get a one-tailed test. Please be clear that it is the probabilities that are doubled or halved, not the critical values.

The astute reader will also note that the same calculated value of *t* may be significant for a one-tailed test but not for a two-tailed test; that is, critical values are lower for one-tailed tests at a given alpha level. In other words, the one-tailed test is more powerful. This occurs because one-tailed tests require proof in only one direction, and the full 5% probability can fall in one tail of the curve rather than being split between both sides. This concept is clarified in Chapter 18 (see Figures 18.6 and 18.7). Because of the different critical values associated with one- or two-tailed tests at the same probability level, the type of *t*-test used should always be specified in advance of data analysis and should be stated in a research report.

The Sign of t

Critical values of t are absolute values, so that negative or positive ratios are tested against the same criteria. The sign of t can be ignored when a nondirectional hypothesis has been proposed. The critical region for a two-tailed test is located in both tails of the t-distribution, and therefore a positive or negative value can be considered significant. The sign will be an artifact of which group happened to be designated Group 1. If the groups were arbitrarily reversed, the ratio would carry the opposite sign, with no change in outcome.

The sign is of concern, however, when a directional alternative hypothesis is proposed. In a one-tailed test, the researcher is predicting that one specific mean will be larger than the other, and the sign must be in the predicted direction for the alternative hypothesis to be accepted. For the current example, the ratio is positive, because the mean improvement for the experimental group $(\overline{X}_1)$ was larger than the mean improvement for the control group $(\overline{X}_2)$, as predicted $(H_1: \mu_1 > \mu_2)$.

If the difference is in the opposite direction to that predicted, the researcher cannot reverse the alternative hypothesis, and H_0 cannot be rejected. It is important, therefore, to be sure of direction when performing a one-tailed test.

Computer Output

Table 19.1D shows the output for an unpaired t-test for the example of strength and hand splints. There are several pieces of information to consider.

First, the output provides a summary of the descriptive statistics associated with each group. This information is useful as a first pass, to confirm that the correct number of subjects were included, and to see how far apart the means and variances are. Standard deviations are reported, and these can be squared to obtain variance values.

Next, notice that there are actually two lines of output for the independent samples test, labeled according to the assumption of equal variances. We must determine which of these to use. Computer packages automatically run the t-test for equal and unequal variances, and the researcher must choose which one should be used for analysis. The columns labeled Levene's Test for Equality of Variances will tell us whether the variances are significantly different. Refer to the probability associated with Levene's test (Table 19.1D❶), which is $p = .419$. This value is greater than .05, and we will conclude that the variances are not significantly different (they are equal). Therefore, we will use the first line of data for "Equal variances assumed."

For the data in Table 19.1, we performed a one-tailed test. The computer output reports only a 2-tailed significance (Table 19.1D❷). Therefore, to get the one-tailed probability we divide .014 by 2; therefore, $p = .007$ for this test. Because this value is less than .05, we reject the null hypothesis.

Confidence Intervals

Recall from Chapter 18 that a confidence interval specifies an interval or range of scores within which the population mean is likely to fall. We can also use this approach to set a confidence interval to estimate the *difference between group means* that exists in the population as follows:

$$95\% \text{ CI} = (\overline{X}_1 - \overline{X}_2) \pm (t)s_{\overline{X}_1 - \overline{X}_2} \tag{19.4}$$

where $s_{\overline{X}_1 - \overline{X}_2}$ is calculated using Equation (19.3). We will be 95% confident that the true *difference between population means* will fall within this interval.

Consider again the data shown in Table 19.1 for changes in pinch strength, with a difference between means of 4.66. The unpaired *t*-test is significant at $\alpha_1 = .05$, and H_0 is rejected. Now let us examine how we can use a confidence interval to arrive at the same conclusion.

We create the 95% confidence interval using $(\alpha_2 = .05)$ $t_{(18)} = 2.101$ (from Table A.2). Even though we had proposed a directional hypothesis for this study, by definition, confidence intervals only look at two-tailed test values. The standard error of the difference between means is 1.714, calculated using the pooled variance estimate as shown in Table 19.1B. We substitute these values in Equation (19.4) to determine the 95% confidence limits:

$$95\% \text{ CI} = (10.11 - 5.45) \pm 2.101(1.714)$$

$$= 4.66 \pm 3.60$$

$$= 1.06, 8.26$$

We are 95% confident that the true mean difference, $\mu_1 - \mu_2$, lies between 1.06 and 8.26.

The Null Value. The null hypothesis states that the difference between two means will be zero. If we look carefully at the 95% confidence interval for these data, we see that the null value, zero, is not contained within it. As we are 95% confident that the true mean difference lies somewhere within this interval, it is unlikely that the true mean difference is zero. Therefore, we can reasonably reject H_0. This confirms the results of the *t*-test for these same data. Confidence intervals are reported in Table 19.1D❺.

The *t* Statistic: Unequal Variances

Studies have shown that the validity of the unpaired *t*-test is not seriously compromised by violation of the assumption of equality of variance when $n_1 = n_2$;[2] however, when sample sizes are unequal, differences in variance can affect the accuracy of the *t*-ratio. If a test for equality of variance shows that variances are significantly different, the *t*-ratio must be adjusted.

Consider the previous example, in which we examined the effect of a hand splint on pinch strength. Table 19.2 shows alternative data for this comparison, with unequal sample sizes ($n_1 = 15$, $n_2 = 10$). The variances in this analysis are significantly different (Levene's test, $p = .038$, Table 19.2D❶). In this instance, we will use the second line of data in the output, "Equal variances not assumed."

TABLE 19.2 **COMPUTATION OF THE UNPAIRED t-TEST (UNEQUAL VARIANCES): CHANGE IN PINCH STRENGTH FOLLOWING HAND SPLINTING**

A. DATA

Group 1 (splint)	Group 2 (Control)
$\overline{X}_1 = 10.80$	$\overline{X}_2 = 5.65$
$n_1 = 15$	$n_2 = 10$
$s_1^2 = 25.17$	$s_2^2 = 4.89$

B. COMPUTATIONS

$$t = \frac{\overline{X}_1 - \overline{X}_2}{\sqrt{\dfrac{s_1^2}{n_1} + \dfrac{s_2^2}{n_2}}} = \frac{10.80 - 5.65}{\sqrt{\dfrac{25.17}{15} + \dfrac{4.89}{10}}} = \frac{5.15}{1.472} = 3.498 \tag{19.4}$$

C. HYPOTHESIS TEST $H_0: \mu_1 = \mu_2$ $H_1: \mu_1 > \mu_2$ $_{(\alpha_1 = .05)}t_{(20.6)} \cong 1.723$ (Table A.2)
Reject H_0

D. OUTPUT

Group Statistics

	GROUP	N	Mean	Std. Deviation	Std. Error Mean
STRENGTH	1	15	10.8000	5.0171	1.2954
	2	10	5.6500	2.2117	.6994

Independent Samples Test

	Levene's Test for Equality of Variances		t-test for Equality of Means							
									95% Confidence Interval of the Mean	
	F	Sig.	t	df	Sig. (2-tailed)	Mean Difference	Std. Error Difference	Lower	Upper
Equal variances assumed	4.866	.038 ❶	3.039	23	.006	5.150	1.6949	1.6439	8.6561
Equal variances not assumed			3.498	20.625 ❷	.002 ❸	5.150 ❹	1.4722 ❺	2.0851	8.2149 ❻

❶ Levene's test is significant ($p = .038$), indicating that the variance of group 1 is significantly different from the variance of group 2. Therefore, we will use the t-test for unequal variances.

❷ With 25 subjects, the adjusted total degrees of freedom for the test of unequal variances is 20.625.

❸ The two-tailed probability for the t-test is .002. This analysis was based on a one-tailed test (directional alternative hypothesis). The one-tailed probability level is half of the two-tailed value. Therefore, $p = .001$. This is significant, and we reject H_0.

❹ Difference between the means of group 1 and 2 (numerator of the t-test).

❺ Standard error of the difference (denominator of the t-test).

❻ The 95% confidence interval does not contain zero, confirming that the difference between means is significant.

When the larger sample also has the larger variance, as in this example ($n_1 > n_2$ and $s_1^2 > s_2^2$), the *t*-test becomes less powerful; that is, fewer significant differences will be found. Therefore, this issue is moot if significant differences are obtained, but is of concern in cases where H_0 is not rejected.

This problem is of a different import when the smaller sample has the larger variance ($n_1 < n_2$ and $s_1^2 > s_2^2$), especially when one variance is more than twice the other. In this case, the probability of a Type I error is increased. This discrepancy increases as the relative sample sizes and variance differences become more disparate.[3] Obviously, this issue is of concern only when a significant difference is obtained.

When sample size and variances are unequal, the *t*-ratio is modified so that it is no longer based on a pooled variance estimate, but instead uses the *separate variances* of the two groups (see Table 19.2B):

$$t = \frac{\overline{X}_1 - \overline{X}_2}{\sqrt{\dfrac{s_1^2}{n_1} + \dfrac{s_2^2}{n_2}}} \qquad 19.5$$

The degrees of freedom associated with the *t*-test for unequal variances are also adjusted downward, so that the critical value for *t* is also modified. In this example, 20.6 degrees of freedom are used to determine the critical value of *t* (see Table 19.2D❷).[‡‡] The output shows that the test is significant at $p = .001$ (Table 19.2D❸).

THE *t*-TEST FOR PAIRED SAMPLES

Researchers often use repeated measures or matched designs to improve the degree of control over extraneous variables in a study. In these designs subjects may be matched on relevant variables, such as age and intelligence, or any other variable that is potentially correlated with the dependent variable. Sometimes twins or siblings are used as matched pairs. More commonly, however, clinical researchers will use subjects as their own controls, exposing each subject to both experimental conditions and then comparing their responses across these conditions.

In these types of studies, data are considered *paired* or correlated, because each measurement has a matched value for each subject. To determine if these values are significantly different from each other, a **paired *t*-test** is performed. This test analyzes *difference scores* (*d*) within each pair, so that subjects are compared only with themselves or with their match. Statistically, this has the effect of reducing the total error variance in the data because most of the extraneous factors that influence data will be the same across both treatment conditions. Therefore, tests of significance involving paired comparisons tend to be more powerful than unpaired tests.

[‡‡] The adjusted degrees of freedom are determined according to:

$$df = \frac{(s_1^2/n_1 + s_2^2/n_2)^2}{(s_1^2/n_1)^2\left(\dfrac{1}{n_1 - 1}\right) + (s_2^2/n_2)^2\left(\dfrac{1}{n_2 - 1}\right)}$$

The *t* Statistic: Paired Data

The test statistic for paired data is based on the ratio

$$t = \frac{\bar{d}}{s_{\bar{d}}} \tag{19.6}$$

where $\bar{d}$ is the mean of the difference scores, and $s_{\bar{d}}$ represents the **standard error of the difference scores**. This ratio also reflects the relationship of *between-* and *within-group* variance components. The numerator is a measure of the differences between pairs of scores, and the denominator is a measure of the variability within the difference scores.

The paired *t*-test is based on the assumption that samples are randomly drawn from normally distributed populations with equal variances; however, because the number of scores in both treatment conditions must be the same, it is unnecessary to test this assumption with correlated samples.

Degrees of Freedom

The total *df* associated with a paired *t*-test are $n - 1$, where n is the number of pairs of scores.

Example

Suppose we set up a study to test the effect of using a lumbar support pillow on angular position of the pelvis in relaxed sitting (Figure 19.4). We hypothesize that pelvic tilt will change with use of a support pillow (a nondirectional hypothesis). We test eight subjects, each one sitting relaxed in a straight-back chair with and without the pillow (in random order). The angle of the pelvic tilt is measured using a flexible ruler, with measurements transformed to degrees.

Because each subject is measured under both experimental conditions, this is a repeated measures design, testing the hypothesis $H_0: \mu_1 = \mu_2$ against $H_1: \mu_1 \neq \mu_2$,

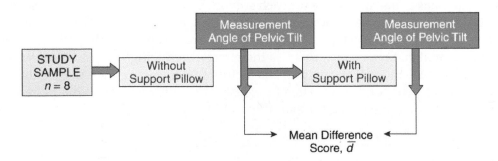

FIGURE 19.4   A repeated measures design. Measurements of pelvic tilt are taken under two conditions in each subject. The difference score for conditions with and without the support pillow are used to calculate the paired *t*-test.

where means represent repeated conditions. These hypotheses may also be expressed in terms of difference scores: $H_0: \bar{d} = 0$ and $H_0: \bar{d} \neq 0$.

Hypothetical data are reported in Table 19.3A. A difference score, d, is calculated for each pair of scores. By substituting values in Equation (19.6), we obtain $t = -1.532$ (see Table 19.3B and D).

The absolute value of the calculated ratio is compared with a critical value, in this case for a two-tailed test with $n - 1 = 7\ df$: Using Table A.2, we find

$$_{(\alpha_2 = .05)}t_{(7)} = 2.365.$$

Because the calculated value is less than the critical value, these conditions are not considered significantly different. The output in Table 19.3D❹ shows that t is significant at $p = .169$. Because this is higher than .05, H_0 is not rejected (see Table 19.3C).

Confidence Intervals

For the paired t-test, a confidence interval is obtained using the formula:

$$95\%\ CI = \bar{d} \pm t(s_{\bar{d}})$$

Therefore,

$$95\%\ CI = -3.375 \pm 2.365(2.203)$$

$$= -3.375 \pm 5.210$$

$$= -8.58, 1.84$$

We are 95% confident that the true difference in pelvic angle between the pillow and nonpillow conditions is between -8.58 and 1.84 degrees (see Table 19.3D❺). However, because zero is contained within this interval, these means are not significantly different.

INAPPROPRIATE USE OF MULTIPLE *t*-TESTS

The t-test is one of the most commonly applied statistical tests. Unfortunately, it is also one of the most misused.[4] The sole purpose of the t-test is to compare two means. Therefore, when more than two means are analyzed within a single sample, the t-test is inappropriate. For instance, if we wanted to compare three types of exercise, it would be incorrect to use the t-test because the analysis involves three comparisons within one sample.

The problem with using multiple t-tests within one set of data is that the more comparisons one makes, the more likely one is to commit a Type I error, that is, to find a significant difference when none exists. Remember that α is the probability of committing a Type I error for any single comparison. At $\alpha = .05$, there is a 5% chance we will be in error if we say that group means are different. Although it is true that $\alpha = .05$ for each individual comparison, the potential *cumulative error* in a set of comparisons is actually

TABLE 19.3 **COMPUTATION OF THE PAIRED t-TEST: ANGLE OF PELVIS WITH AND WITHOUT A LUMBAR SUPPORT PILLOW**

A. DATA

Subject	X_1 (without pillow)	X_2 (with pillow)	d
1	108	112	-4
2	102	96	6
3	98	105	-7
4	112	110	2
5	100	106	-6
6	85	98	-13
7	92	90	2
8	95	102	-7
	$\Sigma X_1 = 819$	$\Sigma X_2 = 792$	$\Sigma d = -27$
	$\overline{X}_1 = 102.375$	$\overline{X}_2 = 99.00$	$\overline{d} = -3.375$
			$s_d = 6.232$

B. COMPUTATIONS

$$s_{\overline{d}} = \frac{s_d}{\sqrt{n}} = \frac{6.232}{\sqrt{8}} = 2.203 \qquad t = \frac{\overline{d}}{s_{\overline{d}}} = \frac{-3.375}{2.203} = -1.532$$

C. HYPOTHESIS TEST

$H_0: \mu_1 = \mu_2 \qquad H_0: \mu_1 \neq \mu_2 \qquad {}_{(\alpha_2 = .05)}t_{(7)} = 2.365 \text{ (Table A.2)}$
Do not reject H_0

D. OUTPUT

Paired Samples Statistics

		Mean	N	Std. Deviation	Std. Error Mean
Pair 1	PILLOW	99.0000	8	8.63548	3.05310
	NONE	102.3750	8	7.40536	2.61819

Paired Samples Correlations

	N	Corr	Sig.
Pair 1 PILLOW & NONE	8	❶ .708	.049

Paired Samples Test

	Paired Differences							
				95% Confidence Interval of the Difference				
	Mean	Std. Deviation	Std. Error Mean	Lower	Upper	t	df	Sig. (2-tailed)
Pair 1 NONE-PILLOW	❷ -3.37500	❸ 6.23212	2.20339	❺ -8.5818	1.83518	-1.532	7	❹ .169

❶ The analysis includes the correlation of pillow and non-pillow scores and significance of that correlation.
❷ Mean of the difference scores, $\overline{d}$ (numerator of the t-test).
❸ Standard error of the difference scores, $s_{\overline{d}}$ (denominator of the t-test)
❹ Because we proposed a non-directional alternative hypothesis, this two-tailed value is used. This test is not significant.
❺ 95% confidence interval of the difference scores contains zero, indicating no significant difference.

greater than .05. Consider the interpretation that, for $\alpha = .05$, if we were to repeat a study 100 times when *no difference really existed*, we could expect to find a significant difference five times, as a random event, just by chance. Five percent of our conclusions could be in error. For any one comparison, however, we cannot know if a significant finding represents one of the potentially correct or incorrect decisions. Theoretically, any one test could be in error.

Consider a different random event, such as a strike of lightning.[5] Suppose you had to cross a wide open field during a lightning storm. There may be only a small risk of getting struck (perhaps 5 percent?)—but would you prefer to cross the field just once, or several times? Would you consider the risk greater if you crossed the field several times? This same logic applies to repeated *t*-tests. The more we repeat comparisons within a sample, the greater are our chances that one or more of those comparisons will result in a random event, a significant difference even when one does not exist.

This problem can be avoided by using the more appropriate *analysis of variance (ANOVA)*, which is a logical extension of the *t*-test specifically designed to compare more than two means. As an adjunct to the analysis of variance, *multiple comparison procedures* have been developed that control the Type I error rate, allowing valid interpretations of several comparisons at the desired α level. These procedures are discussed in Chapters 20 and 21.

COMMENTARY

The Significance of Significance

Researchers in many disciplines, epidemiologists and biostatisticians foremost among them, have become disenchanted with the overemphasis placed on reporting *p* values in research literature.[4] In an effort to make hypothesis testing more meaningful, investigators in these disciplines have relied on the confidence interval as a more practical estimate of a population's characteristics.[6] As we have shown, the outcomes of hypothesis testing using either confidence intervals or *t*-tests will be the same; however, the confidence interval gives the researcher information not provided by the *t*-test. Rather than just indicating if two means are significantly different, the confidence interval essentially estimates true effect size; that is, it estimates how large a difference can be expected in the population. This information can then be used for evaluating the results of assessments and for framing practice decisions.

Confidence intervals may be more clinically useful than relying on probability values when the magnitude of differences is relevant to clinical decision making and prediction of normal or abnormal responses. Like *p* values, however, confidence intervals do not tell us about the importance of the observed effect. That remains a matter of clinical judgment.

REFERENCES

1. Keppel G. *Design and Analysis: A Researcher's Handbook* (4th ed.). Englewood Cliffs, NJ: Prentice Hall, 2004.

2. Glass GV, Peckham PD, Sanders JR. Consequences of failure to meet assumptions underlying the fixed effects analysis of variance and covariance. *Rev Educ Res* 1972;42: 237–288.
3. Scheffe HA. *The Analysis of Variance*. New York: Wiley, 1959.
4. Ottenbacher K. A "tempest" over *t*-tests. *Am J Occup Ther* 1983;37:700–702.
5. Dallal GE. Multiple comparison procedures. Available at: <http://www.tufts.edu/ ~gdallal/mc.htm> Accessed February 20, 2006.
6. May K. A note on the use of confidence intervals. *Understanding Statistics* 2003;2:133–135.

CHAPTER 20

Comparing More than Two Means: Analysis of Variance

As knowledge and clinical theory have developed, clinical researchers have proposed more complex research questions, necessitating the use of elaborate multilevel and multifactor experimental designs. The **analysis of variance (ANOVA)** is a powerful analytic tool for analyzing such designs, where three or more conditions or groups are compared. The analysis of variance is used to determine if the observed differences among a set of means are greater than would be expected by chance alone. The ANOVA is based on the F statistic, which is similar to t in that it is a ratio of between-groups treatment effects to within-group variability. The test can be applied to independent groups or repeated measures designs.*

The purpose of this chapter is to describe the application of the analysis of variance for a variety of experimental research designs. An introduction to the basic concepts underlying analysis of variance is most easily addressed in the context of a single-factor experiment (one independent variable) with independent groups. We then follow with discussions of more complex models, including factorial designs and repeated measures designs.

ANALYSIS OF VARIANCE FOR INDEPENDENT SAMPLES: ONE-WAY CLASSIFICATION

In a single-factor experiment, the one-way analysis of variance is applied when three or more independent group means are compared. The descriptor "one-way" indicates that the design involves one independent variable, or factor, with three or more levels.

---

*As with all parametric tests, the ANOVA is based on the assumption that samples are drawn randomly from normally distributed populations with equal variances. Tests for homogeneity of variance can be performed to validate the latter assumption. With samples of equal size, the analysis of variance is considered "robust" in that reasonable departures from the assumptions of normality and homogeneity will not seriously affect the validity of inferences drawn from the data.[1] With unequal sample sizes, gross violations of homogeneity of variance can increase the chance of Type I error. In such cases, a nonparametric analysis of variance can be applied (see Chapter 22), or data can be transformed to a different scale that improves homogeneity of variance within the sample distribution (see Appendix D).

Although the ANOVA can be applied to two-group comparisons, the t-test is generally considered more efficient for that purpose.[†]

Statistical Hypotheses

The null hypothesis for a one-way multilevel study states that there is no significant difference among the group means, represented by

$$H_0: \mu_1 = \mu_2 = \mu_3 = \ldots = \mu_k$$

where k is the number of groups or levels of the independent variable. The alternative hypothesis (H_1) states that *at least two means* will differ.

Sums of Squares

In the last chapter we established that mean differences can be evaluated using a statistical ratio that relates the treatment effect to experimental error. The analysis of variance uses the same process, except that the ratio must now account for the relationships among several means. The F-test (named for Sir Ronald Fisher, who developed the test) is used to determine how much of the total observed variability in scores can be explained by differences among several treatment means and how much is attributable to unexplained differences among subjects. To analyze this variability with several groups, we must refer to the concept of **sum of squares (SS)**, introduced in Chapter 17. The sum of squares is calculated by subtracting the sample mean from each score $(X - \overline{X})$, squaring those values, and taking their sum $(SS = \Sigma(X - \overline{X})^2)$. The larger the sum of squares, the greater the variability of scores within a sample.

Example

To illustrate how this concept is applied to analysis of variance, consider a hypothetical study of the effect of using different modalities for 10 days to gain pain-free range of motion (ROM) in patients with tendonitis. Through random assignment, we create four independent groups: one to get ultrasound (US), a second to get ice, a third to get massage, and a fourth group to serve as a control (see Figure 20.1). We use a lowercase n to indicate the number of subjects in each group ($n = 11$) and an uppercase N to represent the total number of subjects in the study ($N = 44$). The independent variable, type of modality, has four levels ($k = 4$). Therefore, this is a single-factor, multilevel design. The dependent variable is elbow ROM, measured in degrees. Hypothetical data for this study are reported in Table 20.1A.

[†]The results of a t-test and analysis of variance with two groups will be the same. The t-test is actually a special case of the analysis of variance, with the relationship $F = t^2$.

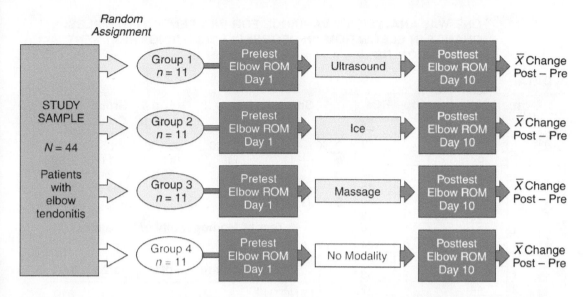

FIGURE 20.1 One-way multi-group design to study change in elbow ROM following treatment with different modalities in patients with tendonitis.

Total Sum of Squares

To estimate the total variability in these data, consider the set of 44 scores as one total sample, ignoring group assignment. We can calculate a mean for this total sample, called the **grand mean,** $\overline{X}_G$, around which all 44 scores will vary. For the data in Table 20.1, the sum of all 44 scores is 1,638, and $\overline{X}_G = 37.23$. The sum of squares for this total sample ($\Sigma(X - \overline{X}_G)^2$) represents the deviations of each individual score from the grand mean. This *total sum of squares* (SS_t) reflects the *total variability* that exists within this set of 44 scores. This variability is illustrated in Figure 20.2A, showing the entire distribution of scores above and below the grand mean.

Partitioning Sum of Squares

As we have described before, total variability in a set of data can be attributed to two sources: a treatment effect (*between* the groups), and unexplained sources of variance, or **error variance**, among the subjects (*within* the groups). As its name implies, the analysis of variance partitions the total variance within a set of data (SS_t) into these two components. The *between-groups sum of squares* (SS_b) reflects the spread of group means around the grand mean. The larger this effect, the greater the separation between the groups. The within-groups or *error sum of squares* (SS_e) reflects the spread of scores within each group around the group mean, or the differences among subjects. In Figure 20.2B, we can see that the means for groups 1 and 2 are close together, and both appear separated from groups 3 and 4. The spread of scores in group 4 appears to be less than in the other groups.

Because hand calculations are complex, computer programs will most often be used to obtain results for an ANOVA. For those who like to see the math, computational

TABLE 20.1 **ONE-WAY ANALYSIS OF VARIANCE FOR INDEPENDENT SAMPLES: CHANGE IN ELBOW ROM (IN DEGREES) FOLLOWING TREATMENT FOR TENDONITIS ($k = 4$, $N = 44$)**

A. DATA

	Grp	ROM
1	1	23
2	1	54
3	1	52
4	1	33
5	1	48
6	1	52
7	1	58
8	1	31
9	1	43
10	1	47
11	1	45
12	2	44
13	2	52
14	2	53
15	2	52
16	2	33
17	2	46
18	2	56
19	2	42
20	2	43
21	2	29
22	2	48

	Grp	ROM
23	3	47
24	3	49
25	3	29
26	3	33
27	3	45
28	3	29
29	3	43
30	3	19
31	3	34
32	3	27
33	3	33
34	4	19
35	4	14
36	4	23
37	4	14
38	4	36
39	4	29
40	4	37
41	4	22
42	4	19
43	4	18
44	4	35

	Group 1 US	Group 2 Ice	Group 3 Massage	Group 4 Control	Total
$\sum X$	486.00	498.00	388.00	266.00	1,638.00
n	11	11	11	11	44
$\overline{X}$	44.18	45.27	35.27	24.18	37.23

B. OUTPUT

Test of Homogeneity of Variances

	Levene Statistic	df1	df2	❶ Sig.
LENGTH	.321	3	40	.810

ANOVA

LENGTH	Sum of Squares	df	Mean Square	F	❷ Sig.
Between Groups	3158.09	3	1052.70	11.89	.000
❸ Within Groups	3541.64	40	88.54		
Total	6699.73	43			

❶ As with the *t*-test, the Levene statistic indicates that there is no significant difference ($p = .810$) between the variances across the four groups.

❷ The probabilities associated with the *F* test do not distinguish between one and two-tailed tests. Because the probability is less than .05, we reject H_0 and conclude that there is a significant difference among groups.

❸ In different programs, the source of variance "Within Groups" may also be called "Error" or "Residual" variance.

formulae for calculating total, between-groups and error sums of squares are shown in Table 20.2.

The *F* Statistic

Degrees of Freedom

The total degrees of freedom (df_t) within a set of data will always be one less than the total number of observations, in this case $N - 1$. In our example, $N = 44$ and $df_t = 43$. The number of degrees of freedom associated with the between-groups variability (df_b)

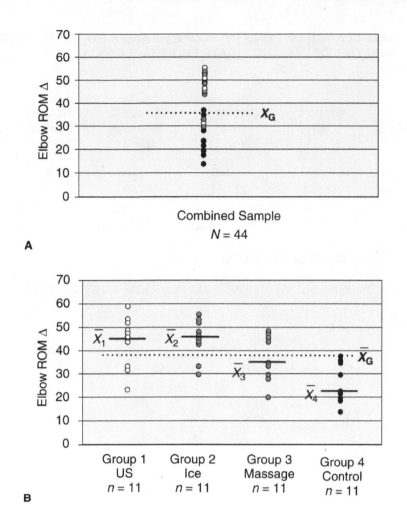

FIGURE 20.2 Scores from tendonitis study (Table 20.1). **A.** The total variance in the sample is reflected in the distribution of scores from all four groups around the grand mean $(\overline{X}_G)$. **B.** The between-groups variance is determined by the distribution of the four group means. The error variance reflects the variability of scores within each of the groups around the group mean.

is one less than the number of groups $(k - 1)$, in this case $df_b = 3$. There are $n - 1$ degrees of freedom within each group, so that the number of degrees of freedom for the within-groups error variance (df_e) for all groups combined will be $(n_1 - 1) + (n_2 - 1) + \ldots + (n_k - 1)$, or $N - k$. For the data in Table 20.1, $df_e = 44 - 4 = 40$. The degrees of freedom for the separate variance components are additive, so that $(k - 1) + (N - k) = (N - 1)$.

Mean Squares

The concepts of between-groups and within-groups variability are once again used to define a statistical ratio. These sources of variability are defined as between-groups and error sums of squares. We convert the sums of squares to a variance estimate, or

TABLE 20.2   CALCULATION OF SUMS OF SQUARES AND F STATISTIC FOR ONE-WAY ANALYSIS OF VARIANCE (DATA FROM TABLE 20.1)

A. DATA

	Group 1 US $N = 11$	Group 2 Ice $N = 11$	Group 3 Massage $N = 11$	Group 4 Control $N = 11$
ΣX	486	498	388	266
ΣX^2	22,654	23,252	14,590	7,182
$\bar{X}$	44.18	45.27	35.27	24.18
s	10.87	8.40	9.50	8.66

B. COMPUTATION OF SUMS OF SQUARES

$$\Sigma X = 486 + 498 + 388 + 266 = 1{,}638 \qquad \Sigma X^2 = 22{,}654 + 23{,}252 + 14{,}590 + 7{,}182 = 67{,}678$$

$$SS_t = \sum X^2 - \frac{(\sum X)^2}{N} = 67{,}678 - \frac{(1638)^2}{44} = 6{,}699.73 \tag{20.1}$$

$$SS_b = \sum \frac{(\sum X_i)^2}{n} - \frac{(\sum X)^2}{N} = \left[\frac{(486)^2}{11} + \frac{(498)^2}{11} + \frac{(388)^2}{11} + \frac{(266)^2}{11}\right] - \frac{(1{,}638)^2}{44} = 3{,}158.09 \tag{20.2\,a}$$

$$SS_e = \sum X^2 - \sum \frac{(\sum X_i)^2}{n} = 67{,}678 - \left[\frac{(486)^2}{11} + \frac{(498)^2}{11} + \frac{(388)^2}{11} + \frac{(266)^2}{11}\right] = 3{,}541.64 \tag{20.3}$$

C. COMPUTATION OF F STATISTIC

$$df_b = k - 1 = 4 - 1 = 3 \qquad MS_b = \frac{SS_b}{df_b} = \frac{3158.09}{3} = 1{,}052.70$$

$$F = \frac{MS_b}{MS_e} = \frac{1052.70}{88.54} = 11.89$$

$$df_e = N - k = 44 - 4 = 40 \qquad MS_e = \frac{SS_e}{df_e} = \frac{3541.64}{40} = 88.54$$

D. HYPOTHESIS TEST

$$H_0: \mu_1 = \mu_2 = \mu_3 \quad H_1: \mu_1 \neq \mu_2 \neq \mu_3 \qquad (\alpha = .05) F_{(3,40)} = 2.84$$

Reject H_0

[a]The term $\dfrac{(\sum X_i)^2}{n}$ in equation 20.2 represents the square of the sum of scores within each individual group divided by the number of subjects in that group.

mean square (MS), by dividing each sum of squares by its respective degrees of free-dom. A mean square can be calculated for the between- and error-variance compo-nents as follows:

$$MS_b = \frac{SS_b}{df_b}$$ (20.4a)

$$MS_e = \frac{SS_e}{df_e}$$ (20.4b)

The F-Ratio

Mean square values are used to calculate the **F statistic** as a ratio of the between-groups variance to the error variance:

$$F = \frac{MS_b}{MS_e}$$ (20.5)

When H_0 is true and no treatment effect exists, the total variance in a sample is due to error, and MS_e is equal to or larger than MS_b, yielding an F-ratio of approximately 1.0 or less. When H_0 is false and the treatment effect is significant, the between-groups variance is large, yielding an F-ratio greater than 1.0. The larger the F-ratio, the greater the difference between the group means relative to the variability within the groups. In our example, $F = 11.89$, as shown in Table 20.2C.

Critical Values of F

Like t, the calculated F-ratio is compared to a critical value to determine its significance. Table A.3 in the Appendix contains critical values of F at $\alpha = .05$. Because mean squares are based on squared values, the F-ratio cannot be a negative number, and therefore, we do not distinguish tails for an F test.

The critical value of F for the desired α is located in the table by the degrees of free-dom associated with the between-groups and error variances, with df_b across the top of the table and df_e along the side. For our example, $df_b = 3$ and $df_e = 40$ (always given in that order). Therefore, from Table A.3,

$$_{(.05)}F_{(3,40)} = 2.84$$

We compare this critical value with our calculated value, $F = 11.89$. The calculated value must be *greater than or equal to* the critical value to achieve statistical significance. In this case, we can reject H_0.

A significant F-ratio does not indicate that each group is different from all other groups. Actually, it only tells us that there is a significant difference between at least two of the means (largest versus smallest). At this point, a separate test must be done to determine exactly where the significant differences lie. Various **multiple comparison tests** are described for this analysis in the next chapter. When the F-ratio is smaller than the critical value, H_0 is not rejected and no further analyses are appropriate.

The ANOVA Summary Table

Computer-generated output will present the results of an analysis of variance in a summary table that provides sums of squares and mean square data for determination of the *F* ratio. The table presents data for the between-groups and error sources of variance, as shown in Table 20.1B. The probability level associated with the *F*-ratio is given in the last column of the summary table. This table may be included in the results section of a research report. Terminology used in the table will vary among computer programs and research reports. Rather than listing "between groups" as a source of variance, some programs list the name of the independent variable. The error variance may be called the within-groups variance, residual or between-subjects variance.

In reporting the results of an ANOVA, some researchers may simply indicate if the *F* ratio has achieved significance, indicating $p < .05$, although most reports will include the exact probability obtained by computer analysis. Some authors do not include summary tables in their research reports, choosing instead to report *F*-ratios in the body of the text. When this is done, the calculated value of *F* is given, along with the associated degrees of freedom and probability. For example, for the data in Table 20.1, we would say:

> There was a significant difference among the four experimental groups ($F = 11.89$, $df = 3,40, p < .001$).

ANALYSIS OF VARIANCE: TWO-WAY CLASSIFICATION

Because of the complexity of human behavior and physiological function, many clinical investigations are designed to study the simultaneous effects of two or more independent variables. This approach is often more economical than testing each variable separately and provides a stronger basis for generalization of results to clinical practice.

Example

As an example, let us assume we wanted to compare the effect of prolonged versus quick stretch for improving ankle range of motion against a control (Factor A). At the same time we are interested in determining if the position of the knee during stretch (flexed or extended) will affect the outcome (Factor B). Instead of looking at each of these factors separately, we can examine their combined influence using a two-way factorial design. This design involves two independent variables: type of stretch (with three levels) and knee position (with two levels). Within the 3 × 2 framework, there are six treatment combinations. As shown in Figure 20.3, we can arrange the design in a table with six cells, so that rows correspond to type of stretch and columns to positions. Each cell represents a unique combination of levels for A and B. We could allocate 10 subjects per cell, for a total of 60 subjects. The design of factorial experiments was discussed in Chapter 10.

The appropriate statistical analysis for this design is a **two-way analysis of variance**. The descriptor "two-way" indicates a two-dimensional analysis, involving two independent variables. In this example, each variable is an independent factor (not

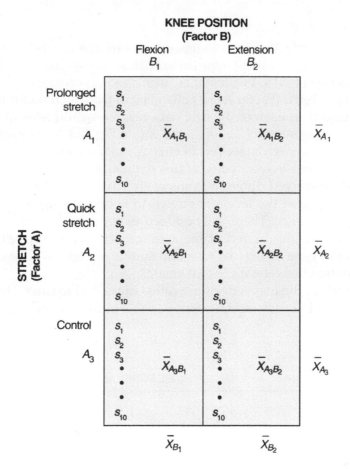

FIGURE 20.3   Two-way (3 × 2) factorial design testing the effects of (**A**) stretch ($k = 3$) and (**B**) knee position ($k = 2$) on ankle range of motion. Sixty subjects are randomly assigned to each of six experimental conditions ($n = 10$). The marginal means for each independent variable are obtained by pooling data across the second variable.

repeated). The two-way ANOVA is an extension of the one-way analysis. It, too, partitions the total variance in the set of scores into between-groups and error components. The between-groups variance explains the independent variable effects, and the error variance accounts for all sources of variation unexplained by treatment; however, because the design incorporates two independent variables, the between-groups component must be further partitioned to account for the separate and combined effect of each independent variable. Therefore, we can ask three questions of these data:

1. What is the effect of variable A, independent of variable B?
2. What is the effect of variable B, independent of variable A?
3. What is the joint effect or interaction of variables A and B?

These components are called main effects and interaction effects, each explaining part of the total treatment effect.

Main Effects

In a two-way design, the effect of each independent variable can be examined separately, essentially creating two single-factor experiments. These effects are called **main effects**, illustrated in Figure 20.4. For instance, using the preceding example, we can study the main effect of stretch (Factor A) by collapsing or pooling data for the two knee positions. With 10 subjects in each of the original cells, we would now obtain a mean for 20 scores at each level of stretch ($\overline{X}_{A_1}$, $\overline{X}_{A_2}$, and $\overline{X}_{A_3}$ in Fig 20.4A). These three means represent the average between-groups effect of stretch, independent of the effect of knee position. The sum of squares associated with this main effect accounts for the separation among groups that received different forms of stretch.

Similarly, we can collapse the levels of stretch to obtain two means for the main effect of knee position (Factor B). There will be 30 scores per cell ($\overline{X}_{B_1}$ and $\overline{X}_{B_2}$), as shown in Figure 20.4B. These two means reflect the average between-groups effect of knee position, independent of type of stretch. A second sum of squares will be calculated to account for the separation between these two groups.

The means for levels of the main effects are called **marginal means**. They represent the average separate effect of each independent variable in the analysis. Comparison of

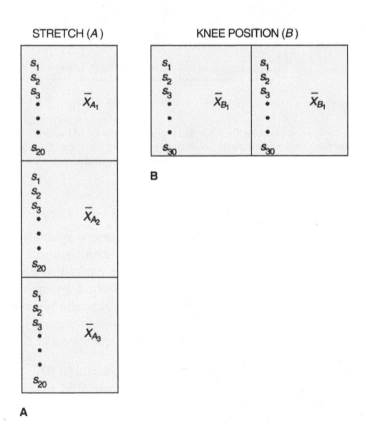

FIGURE 20.4   Diagrams of main effects for stretch treatment and knee position in a two-way factorial design.

the marginal means within each factor indicates how much of the variability in all 60 scores can be attributed to the overall effect of stretch alone or knee position alone.

Interaction Effects

In addition to the analysis of main effects, the factorial experiment has the added advantage of being able to look at combinations of levels of each independent variable. Statistically, these are referred to as **interaction effects**. Interaction is present when the effects of one variable are not constant across different levels of the second variable, that is, when various combinations of levels cause differential effects.

To illustrate this concept, consider the hypothetical means given for the six treatment groups in Figure 20.5. Each mean represents a unique combination of stretch and knee position. We can plot these means to more clearly illustrate these relationships. In Figure 20.5A, we have represented range of motion, the dependent variable, along the Y-axis. The three stretch groups are represented along the X-axis. The means for range of motion for each knee position are plotted at each level of stretch, with lines connecting the means. Note that in this example, the lines are parallel, which means that the pattern of response at each knee position is consistent across all levels of stretch. We can reverse the plot, as shown in Figure 20.5B, with knee position on the X-axis, demonstrating a constant pattern for each level of stretch across both

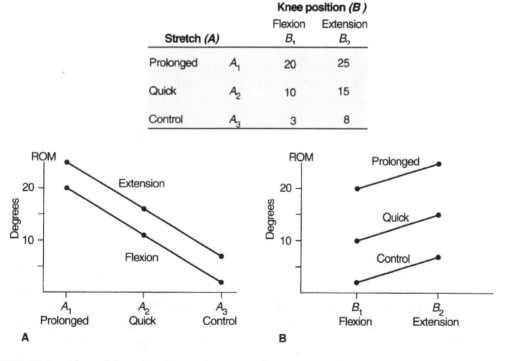

Stretch (A)		Knee position (B)	
		Flexion B_1	Extension B_2
Prolonged	A_1	20	25
Quick	A_2	10	15
Control	A_3	3	8

FIGURE 20.5 Plots of data showing no interaction between stretch treatment and knee position. Parallel lines indicate that responses on one variable are constant across the second variable.

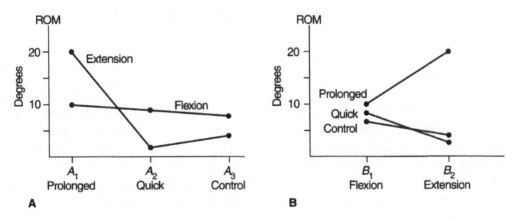

		Knee position (B)	
		Flexion	Extension
Stretch (A)		B_1	B_2
Prolonged	A_1	10.3	19.6
Quick	A_2	9.1	3.1
Control	A_3	8.0	3.6

FIGURE 20.6 Plots of data showing interaction between stretch treatment and knee position. Lines that are not parallel or that cross indicate that responses on one variable will vary depending on the level of the second variable. In this example, prolonged stretch with knee extension consistently produces a greater response than other combinations of the two variables.

knee positions. These graphs are called interaction plots, in this case demonstrating a situation where there is no interaction; that is, prolonged stretch (A_1) will generate the highest response under both knee conditions and knee extension scores are higher across all levels of stretch.

Now consider a different set of results for the same study, given in Figure 20.6. The interaction plots for these data show lines that are not parallel; that is, the pattern of the baseline variable across all levels of the second variable is not constant. For example, in Figure 20.6A, the plot for knee flexion indicates little difference across levels of stretch. On the other hand, the line for knee extension shows a distinct difference for prolonged stretch. In Figure 20.6B, we see that the three flexion measures are fairly close (between 8 and 10 degrees), and two of the extension measures are also close (between 3 and 4 degrees), but the effect of prolonged stretch with knee extension is quite different. When lines are not parallel or when they cross, interaction is present. In this example, it is not the use of prolonged stretch alone that makes the treatment more effective. It is the combination of prolonged stretch with knee extension. Therefore, there is an interaction between the two independent variables. The analysis of variance will account for this difference among the interaction means as a third component of the between-groups sum of squares.

Statistical Hypotheses

When two independent variables are examined in a single experiment, three statistical hypotheses are usually proposed, one for each main effect and one for the interaction effect. For example, for a 3×2 factorial design, the following null hypotheses would be proposed:

1. $H_0: \mu_{A_1} = \mu_{A_2} = \mu_{A_3}$
2. $H_0: \mu_{B_1} = \mu_{B_2}$
3. $H_0: \mu_{A_1B_1} = \mu_{A_1B_2} = \mu_{A_2B_1} = \mu_{A_2B_2} = \mu_{A_3B_1} = \mu_{A_3B_2}$

An alternative hypothesis can be proposed for each null hypothesis. These hypotheses may be general statements of difference, or they may specify differences between specific means. An *F*-ratio is calculated to test each null hypothesis.

Presentation of Data for a Two-Way ANOVA

We have chosen not to include a mathematical example for a two-way analysis of variance, as we expect that all such analyses will be done by a computer. Those interested in details of the computations should refer to advanced statistical texts. We will examine the format for presentation of results of a two-way ANOVA, as shown in Table 20.3.

Note that there are three between-groups sources of variance listed, two main effects and the interaction effect. These are usually listed in the summary table according to the name of the independent variable. Thus, for our example, type of "stretch" and "knee position" are listed as main effects. The interaction between two variables is signified by ×, such as Stretch × Knee Position, read "stretch by knee position." The error term represents the unexplained variability between subjects within all combinations of stretch and knee position.

TABLE 20.3 SUMMARY TABLE FOR A TWO-WAY ANALYSIS OF VARIANCE: EFFECT OF STRETCH AND KNEE POSITION ON ANKLE RANGE OF MOTION ($N = 60$) (DATA TAKEN FROM FIGURE 20.6)

	Sum of Squares	df	Mean Square	F	Sig.
STRETCH	1080.729	2	540.364	41.843	.000❶
POSITION	2.017	1	2.017	.156	.694
STRETCH × POSITION	707.722	2	353.861	27.401	.000
Error ❷	697.362	54	12.914		
Total	2487.830	59	42.167		

❶ Computer programs will generate *p* values with a specified level of precision, that is, to a set number of decimal places. Therefore, a *p* value of .000 does not indicate zero probability. It simply means that the probability is <.001, but the precision of the output does not allow the exact value to be printed.

❷ Error variance may also be called residual variance.

Note: Some elements of data generated by SPSS, which are not essential to understanding the output, are not included in this table.

Degrees of Freedom

The number of degrees of freedom associated with each main effect is one less than the number of levels of that independent variable $(k - 1)$. To clarify this notation, we use $(A - 1)$ degrees of freedom for Factor A, and $(B - 1)$ for Factor B, where the letters A and B represent the number of levels of each factor. Therefore, for stretch with three levels, $df = 2$. For knee position with two levels, $df = 1$. The number of degrees of freedom for the interaction between these variables is the product of their respective degrees of freedom, $(A - 1)(B - 1)$. Therefore, the interaction effect in this example has $2 \times 1 = 2$ degrees of freedom.

The total degrees of freedom associated with an experiment will always be one less than the total number of observations, $N - 1$. In this study, with $n = 10$ per group ($N = 60$), $df_t = 59$. The error degrees of freedom can be determined by using $(A)(B)(n - 1)$ with equal-size groups or by subtracting the combined between-groups degrees of freedom from the total degrees of freedom. For this example, $df_e = (3)(2)(9) = 59 - 2 - 1 - 2 = 54$.

The F Statistic and Critical Values

Calculation of F is based on the ratio of between-groups to error mean squares. Mean square values are determined by dividing the sum of squares for each effect by its associated degrees of freedom. Each between-groups effect generates an F-ratio, based on its own mean square divided by the mean square for the common error term, MS_e. For example, for the data shown in Table 20.3, the F-ratios for the main effects of stretch (A) and knee position (B)[§] are obtained by

$$F_A = \frac{MS_A}{MS_e} = \frac{540.364}{12.914} = 41.843 \qquad F_B = \frac{MS_B}{MS_e} = \frac{2.017}{12.914} = 0.156$$

Similarly, the F-ratio for the interaction term, $A \times B$, is calculated according to

$$F_{A \times B} = \frac{MS_{A \times B}}{MS_e} = \frac{353.861}{12.914} = 27.401$$

Each F-ratio is compared with a critical value from Appendix Table A.3. The degrees of freedom associated with the specific between-groups effect (main effect or interaction) are located across the top and the degrees of freedom associated with the error term are listed along the side. The critical values for each effect shown in Table 20.3 are:

$$\text{Stretch} \qquad (.05)F_{(2,54)} = 3.17$$

$$\text{Knee Position} \qquad (.05)F_{(1,54)} = 4.02$$

$$\text{Stretch} \times \text{Knee Position} \qquad (.05)F_{(2,54)} = 3.17$$

[§]The use of the subscript B to denote Factor B should not be confused with the use of subscript b to denote "between-groups" in previous examples. In this example, both A and B represent between-groups sources of variance for the two independent variables.

Therefore, this ANOVA demonstrates a significant main effect for type of stretch and a significant interaction effect between stretch and knee position.

The ANOVA Summary Table

The information contained in an ANOVA table provides a convenient summary of a study's design and results. For example, from Table 20.3 we can tell that there are two independent variables, stretch and knee position, with three and two levels, respectively (by looking at degrees of freedom); that there are 60 subjects in the study ($df_t = N - 1 = 59$); and that the outcome was dependent on which type of stretch was used in a particular knee position.

Interpreting Interaction and Main Effects

Simple Effects

In most cases, researchers develop factorial designs with the expectation of specific patterns of interaction between the independent variables; that is, they hypothesize that certain combinations of treatments will be most effective. If this were not the case, the researcher could just as easily design separate one-way studies. Clinical interpretation of interaction is often facilitated by dividing the factorial design into several smaller "single-factor" experiments, each represented by the rows and columns in the design, as shown in Figure 20.7. These separate effects are called **simple effects**. Interaction is defined as a significant difference between simple effects.[2] Each line in an interaction

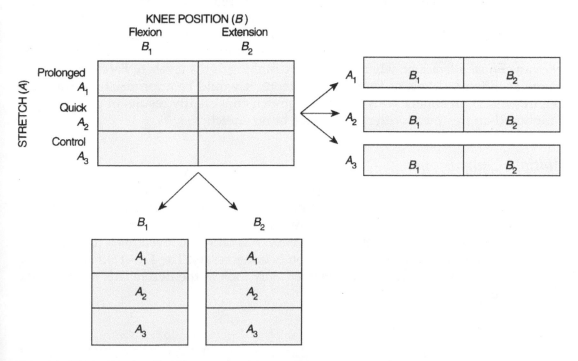

FIGURE 20.7 Simple effects for a 3 × 2 factorial design.

plot (see Figures 20.5 and 20.6) represents a simple effect. Simple effects are distinguished from main effects, which are based on averaged values across a second variable. An analysis of simple effects will reveal differential patterns within each of the independent variables. Such an analysis can be carried out on row effects, column effects or both. With simple effects, the researcher can inspect the data to determine which levels of either variable contribute most to the observed differences. The analysis of simple effects is similar to carrying out several single-factor analyses of variance, with between-groups effects extracted from the larger factorial design.**

Main Effects

When there is no interaction effect in an experiment, the main effects are easily interpreted by referring to the outcome of the F-test for each independent variable. In that case, the analysis is essentially reduced to a one-way design, and combinations of treatments are ignored. If an interaction effect is present and main effects are not significant, interpretation is also straightforward; however, when an interaction effect is present, significant main effects are more difficult to interpret. For example, look again at the interaction plots in Figure 20.5. With no interaction present, it is easy to see that range of motion was consistently higher with the knee in extension and with prolonged stretch.

In Figure 20.6, where there is a significant interaction, the separate effects of knee position and type of stretch must be examined more carefully. In Figure 20.6A, with type of stretch (Factor A) along the baseline, we can see that the level of response at different knee positions changes at different levels of stretch. Therefore, we cannot draw any general conclusions about the main effect of knee position. This is called a *disordinal interaction* and the main effect of knee position is ignored in the interpretation of results. In Figure 20.6B, however, where knee position is plotted on the baseline, we can see that although prolonged stretch with knee extension shows the largest difference, it is also true that prolonged stretch is consistently above all other levels of stretch. This illustrates an *ordinal interaction*, where the relative ranking of the levels of Factor A does not change at different levels of Factor B. Therefore, it would be appropriate to conclude that, in general, treatment with prolonged stretch consistently results in greater range of motion than treatment with quick stretch or no stretch.

Multiple Comparisons

Multiple comparison tests are also used to compare means for each significant effect following an analysis of variance. For significant main effects, the marginal means are compared. For example, we would compare $\overline{X}_{A_1}$, $\overline{X}_{A_2}$ and $\overline{X}_{A_3}$ (see Figure 20.4) to examine the main effect of stretch. When a main effect has only two levels, as with knee position in this example, a multiple comparison is unnecessary. The F-test functions like a t-test. Therefore, if F is significant, one need only look at the two means to determine which is greater.

**See Keppel[2] and Green[3] for detailed discussion of statistical procedures for analyzing simple effects.

For significant interaction effects, the individual group means are compared. For example, we could determine which of the six combinations of stretch and knee position would produce the greatest changes in ankle range of motion. Based on the data shown in Figure 20.6, we might expect to find that prolonged stretch with knee extension (A_1B_2) elicits a more effective response than the other five combinations.[††]

ANALYSIS OF VARIANCE: THREE-WAY CLASSIFICATION

A multifactor analysis of variance can be performed with any number of independent variables, although we rarely see analyses beyond three dimensions. For example, we could expand the preceding study to look at the effects of stretch, knee position, and three forms of exercise for increasing ankle range of motion.

The analysis of a three-way design is a direct extension of the two-way ANOVA. With three independent variables, A, B and C, the total variability in the data is divided into seven parts: three main effects (one for each independent variable), three double interactions testing each pair of independent variables in combination ($A \times B$, $A \times C$, and $B \times C$) and a triple interaction ($A \times B \times C$) testing all possible combinations of the three variables.[‡‡] A sum of squares is calculated for each of these effects, to account for their contribution to the total variance in the sample. As in other analyses, each main effect has $k - 1$ degrees of freedom, and degrees of freedom for the interaction terms are the product of the degrees of freedom for each effect in the interaction. The total degrees of freedom will be $N - 1$, and the error term will have $(A)(B)(C)(n - 1)$ degrees of freedom. An F-ratio is calculated for each main effect and each interaction effect, using the mean square for the error term in the denominator.

The advantage of higher order factorial designs is the ability to examine how combinations of several variables influence behavior. Because treatment variables rarely exist in isolation, this approach can greatly enhance the construct validity and generalization of research results to practice. Unfortunately, such designs can also become overly complex, requiring large numbers of treatment groups and subjects. In addition, because the statistical analysis breaks down the total variance into so many components, interaction tests for the ANOVA will generally have lower power.

REPEATED MEASURES ANALYSIS OF VARIANCE

Up to now we have discussed the analysis of variance only as it is applied to completely randomized designs. These designs, where subjects are randomly assigned to treatment groups, are also called *between-subjects designs* because all sources of variance represent differences between subjects (within a group and between groups). Clinical investigators, however, often use repeated factors to evaluate the performance of each subject under several experimental conditions. The repeated measures design is logically applied to study variables where practice or carryover effects are minimal and where

---

[††]See Tables 21.6 and 21.7 in the next chapter for results of multiple comparison tests for the two-way analysis of variance shown in Table 20.3.
[‡‡]These interactions are illustrated in Figure 10.6 in Chapter 10.

differences in an individual's performance across treatment levels are of interest. This type of study can involve one or more independent variables.

In a repeated measures design, all subjects are tested under k treatment conditions. The analysis of variance is modified to account for the correlation among successive measurements on the same individual. For this reason, such designs are also called *within-subjects designs*. The statistical hypotheses proposed for repeated measures designs are the same as those for independent samples, except that the means represent treatment conditions rather than groups.

The statistical advantage of using repeated measures is that individual differences are controlled. When independent groups are compared, it is likely that groups will differ on extraneous variables and that these differences will be superimposed on treatment effects; that is, both treatment differences and error variance will account for observed differences between groups. With repeated measures designs, however, we have only one group, and differences between treatment conditions should primarily reflect treatment effects. Therefore, error variance in a repeated measures analysis will be smaller than in a randomized experiment. Statistically, this has the effect of reducing the size of the error term in the analysis of variance, which means that the F-ratio will be larger. Therefore, the test is more powerful than when independent samples are used.

Single-Factor Repeated Measures Designs

Example

The simplest repeated measures design involves one independent variable, where all levels of treatment are administered to all subjects. To illustrate this approach, let us consider a single-factor experiment designed to look at differences in isometric elbow flexor strength with the forearm in three positions: pronation, neutral and supination. The independent variable, forearm position, has three levels ($k = 3$). Logically, this question warrants a repeated measures design, where each subject's strength is tested in each position (see Figure 20.8).

In a repeated measures design, we are interested in a comparison across treatment conditions *within each subject*. It is not of interest to look at averaged group performance at each condition. Therefore, statistically, each subject is considered a unique block in the design. We can represent the design diagrammatically as shown in Figure 20.9, with

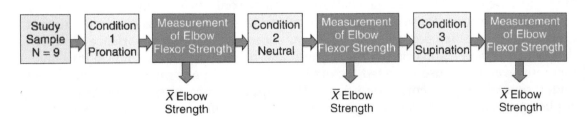

FIGURE 20.8 One-way repeated measures design for comparison of elbow flexor strength in three forearm positions. Although the diagram shows a consistent sequence, the order of elbow positions can be randomly or systematically varied.

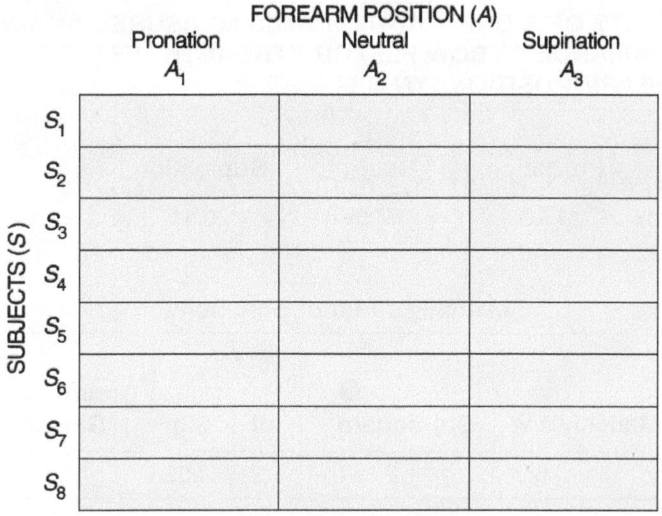

FOREARM POSITION (*A*)

		Pronation A_1	Neutral A_2	Supination A_3
	S_1			
	S_2			
SUBJECTS (*S*)	S_3			
	S_4			
	S_5			
	S_6			
	S_7			
	S_8			

FIGURE 20.9 Conceptual format of a one-way repeated measures design, showing how "subjects" becomes a factor in the analysis.

rows corresponding to subjects ($n = 9$), and columns representing experimental conditions. Note that this diagram resembles a two-way factorial design, with forearm position as one independent variable and "subjects" as the other. Using this interpretation, each cell in the design has a sample size of $n = 1$. Each individual subject is considered a separate level of the independent variable *subjects*.

Using the format of a two-way analysis, the **repeated measures analysis of variance** will look at the main effect of forearm position, the main effect of subjects, and the interaction between these two factors. Because each cell in the design has only one score, there can be no variability within a cell. Therefore, the error term for this analysis is actually the interaction between subjects and treatment; that is, interaction reflects the inconsistency of subjects across the levels of treatment. This interaction represents the variance that is unexplained by the treatment variable and will serve as the denominator for the *F*-ratio.

Degrees of Freedom

The total degrees of freedom associated with a repeated measures design will equal one less than the total number of observations made, or $nk - 1$. In our example, $df_t = (9)(3) - 1 = 26$.

As in other analyses, the number of degrees of freedom associated with the main effects will be $k - 1$ for the independent variable, and $n - 1$ for subjects. The degrees of freedom for the error term are determined as they are for an interaction, so that $df_e = (k - 1)(n - 1)$. Table 20.4C shows these values in a summary table for the current example.

TABLE 20.4 RESULTS OF A ONE-WAY REPEATED MEASURES ANALYSIS OF VARIANCE: ELBOW FLEXOR STRENGTH TESTED IN THREE FOREARM POSITIONS ($N = 9$)

A. DATA

	Pronation	Neutral	Supination
Mean Scores	17.3	27.56	29.11

B. OUTPUT

Mauchly's Test of Sphericity

Within Subjects Effect	Mauchly's W	Chi-Square ❶	df	Sig.	Epsilon ❷ Greenhouse-Geisser	Huynh-Feldt
POSITION	.664	2.861	2	.239	.749	.883

Tests of Within-Subjects Effects

Measure: STRENGTH
Sphericity Assumed

Source	Sum of Squares	df	Mean Square	F	Sig.	
POSITION	736.889	2	368.444	50.338	.000	❸
Error	117.111	16	7.319			

Tests of Between-Subjects Effects

Measure: STRENGTH

	Source	Sum of Squares	df	Mean Square	F	Sig.
❹	Error	2604.000	8	325.500		

NOTE: Portions of the output from this SPSS analysis, which do not influence interpretation of data, have been omitted for clarity.

C. SUMMARY TABLE FOR RESEARCH REPORT

Source	SS	df	MS	F	p
Subjects ❹	2604.00	8	325.50		
Position	736.89	2	368.44	50.34	❸ .000
Error	117.11	16	7.32		

❶ Mauchly's Test of Sphericity is used to determine if adjustments are needed to degrees of freedom for the repeated measure. Many statistics are converted to familiar values to determine their associated probabilities. In this case, Mauchly's W is converted to chi-square for this purpose.

❷ Two versions of epsilon are used for the adjustment of *p*. In this instance, they are not applied because the sphericity test is not significant.

❸ The repeated measure of Forearm Position is significant ($p < .001$).

❹ The effect of "subjects" as a source of variance is presented as "Between-Subjects Effects." The error term in this analysis is the Subjects effect. No *F* value is generated for this effect, but could be calculated by dividing sum of squares by mean square ($F = 8.00$).

The F Statistic

The sums of squares for the treatment effect and the error effect are divided by their associated degrees of freedom to obtain the mean squares. These mean square values are then used to calculate the F-ratio for treatment according to

$$F_A = \frac{MS_A}{MS_{A \times S}} \tag{20.6}$$

where MS_A is the mean square for the treatment variable, and $MS_{A \times S}$ is the mean square for the interaction of treatment and subjects, or the error term. For the data in Table 20.4,

$$F = \frac{368.44}{7.32} = 50.34$$

We can calculate an F-ratio for the effect of subjects, using $F_S = MS_S / MS_{A \times S}$; however, this is not a meaningful test. We expect subjects to differ from each other, and it is generally of no experimental interest to establish that they are different. The F-ratio for subjects is not given in most computer printouts (Table 20.4❹), and this effect is generally ignored in the interpretation of data.[§§]

The critical value for the F-ratio for treatment is located in Appendix Table A.3, using the degrees of freedom for treatment (df_b) and the degrees of freedom for the error term (df_e). Therefore, the critical value for this effect will be $_{(.05)}F_{A_{(2,16)}} = 3.63$. The calculated F-ratio exceeds this critical value and, therefore, is significant. The null hypothesis for treatment effects is rejected. The summary table shows that this difference is significant at $p < .001$ (Table 20.4❺). We conclude that elbow flexor strength does differ across forearm positions. It will be appropriate at this point to perform a multiple comparison test on the three means to determine which forearm positions are significantly different from the others.[***]

Variance Assumptions with Repeated Measures Designs

We have previously discussed the fact that the analysis of variance is based on an assumption about the homogeneity of variances among treatment groups. This assumption is also made with repeated measures designs; however, with repeated measures we cannot examine variances of different groups because only one group is involved. Instead, the variances of interest reflect difference scores across treatment conditions within a subject. For example, with three repeated treatment conditions, A_1, A_2, A_3, we will have three difference scores: $A_1 - A_2, A_1 - A_3$, and $A_2 - A_3$. When used in this way with repeated measures, the homogeneity of variance assumption is

---

[§§]The one-way repeated measures ANOVA is used to generate MS values for calculation of models 2 and 3 of the ICC reliability coefficient (see Chapter 26). For interpretation of the ICC, it is useful to determine that the between-subjects effect is significant. These computations are easily done by hand if they are not generated in the computer analysis.

[***]See Table 21.7 in the next chapter for the multiple comparison for the repeated measures analysis of variance shown in Table 20.4.

called the **assumption of sphericity**, which states that the variances within each of these sets of difference scores will be relatively equal and correlated with each other.

We have also established that reasonable departures from the variance assumption would not seriously affect the validity of the analysis of variance, except in situations where sample sizes were grossly unequal. One might think, then, that violations of the variance assumption would be unimportant for repeated measures, where treatment conditions must have equal sample sizes. This is not the case, however. Because the repeated measures test examines correlated scores across treatment conditions, it is especially sensitive to variance differences, biasing the test in the direction of Type I error. In other words, the repeated measures test is considered too liberal when variances are not correlated, increasing the chances of finding significant differences above the selected α level.

To address this concern, most computer programs will run a repeated measures ANOVA in two different ways, using multivariate and univariate statistics. Multivariate tests are preferable in that they do not require the assumption of sphericity. Several multivariate tests are usually run simultaneously, with unfamiliar names such as *Piallai's Trace, Wilks' Lambda, Hotelling's Trace* and *Roy's Largest Root*. Because these tests are all based on different procedures, they are usually converted to a common reference, an *F*-ratio. These tests examine all possible sets of difference scores, and determine if there is a significant difference among them. If they are significant, multiple comparison tests should follow. Because researchers are generally less familiar with these multivariate tests, they do not tend to be reported, but they appear prominently in computer output.

The second approach, used more often in clinical research, involves the standard repeated measures *F*-test, but with an adjustment to the value of *p* to account for possible violations of sphericity. A test called **Mauchly's Test of Sphericity** (Table 20.4B) is performed first to determine if the adjustment is needed.[†††] If the sphericity test is significant, correction is achieved by decreasing the degrees of freedom used to determine the critical value of *F*, thereby making the critical value larger. If the critical value is larger, then the calculated value of *F* must be larger to achieve significance. This compensates for bias toward Type I error by making it harder to demonstrate significant differences. Note that there is no difference in how the ANOVA is run, and the generated *F*-ratio with its associated degrees of freedom for the ANOVA remains unchanged. Only the probability associated with that *F* will change. This adjustment is only relevant, however, when the *F*-ratio is significant.

The degrees of freedom for the *F*-ratio are adjusted by multiplying them by a correction factor given the symbol **epsilon** (Table 20.4❷). Two different versions of epsilon are used: the **Greenhouse-Geisser correction**[4] and the **Huynh-Feldt correction**.[5] The Greenhouse-Geisser correction is usually considered first. If it results in a significant *F*, agreeing with the original analysis, then the probability associated with the Greenhouse-Geisser correction is used. When it does not result in a significant outcome, disagreeing with the original analysis, then the Huynh-Feldt correction is applied.

[†††]The power of Mauchly's test will vary with sample size.[3] With small samples it loses power. With large samples it may be significant even though the impact of violating the sphericity assumption is minor.

These correction factors are shown in Table 20.4❷ for the one-way repeated measures analysis for the comparison of elbow flexor strength across three forearm positions. Because the test for sphericity is not significant ($p = .239$), we are not concerned about this adjustment. If the test for sphericity had been significant, however, the probabilities generated in the computer analysis for the ANOVA table would be the corrected ones.

Multifactor Repeated Measures Designs

The concepts of repeated measures analysis can also be applied to multifactor experiments. Such designs can include all repeated factors or a combination of repeated and independent factors. When all factors are repeated, the design is referred to as a repeated measures or within-subjects design. When a single experiment involves at least one independent factor and one repeated factor, the design is called a **mixed design**. We present the general concepts behind these types of analyses and describe the format for presentation of results. We base our examples on a two-factor design, although these concepts can be easily expanded to accommodate more complicated designs.

Within-Subjects Designs

With two repeated factors, the design is an extension of the single-factor repeated measures design. Suppose we redesigned our previous example to study isometric elbow flexor strength with the forearm in three positions and with the elbow at two different angles. We would then be able to see if the position of the elbow had any influence on strength when combined with different forearm positions. In this 3×2 repeated measures design, if $n = 8$, each subject would be tested six times, for a total of 48 measurements.

With two repeated factors, variance is partitioned to include a main effect for ·subjects and for each treatment variable, as well as for subject by treatment interactions (forearm $\times$ subjects, elbow $\times$ subjects, and forearm $\times$ elbow $\times$ subjects). These interactions represent the random or chance variations among subjects for each treatment effect. The mean squares for these interaction terms are used to calculate an error term for each repeated main effect, as shown in Table 20.5. The assignment of degrees of freedom for each of these variance components follows the rules used for the regular two-way analysis of variance: for each main effect $df = k - 1$; for each interaction effect $df = (A - 1)(B - 1)$.

Each treatment effect in this study (forearm, elbow, and forearm $\times$ elbow) is tested by the ratio $F = MS/MS_e$, where the error term is the interaction of that particular treatment effect with subjects. As shown in Table 20.5, each repeated factor is essentially being tested as it would be in a single-factor experiment, with its own error term. By separating out an error component for each treatment effect, we have created a more powerful test than we would have with one common error term; that is, the error component is smaller for each separate treatment effect than it would be with a combined error term. Therefore, F-ratios tend to be larger. In this example, only the main effect of forearm position is significant ($p = .013$).

Once again, researchers will generally ignore ratios for the effect of subjects (Table 20.5❷). The effect of subjects is only important insofar as it is used to determine the

TABLE 20.5   SUMMARY TABLE FOR A TWO-FACTOR REPEATED MEASURES ANALYSIS OF VARIANCE: ELBOW FLEXOR STRENGTH WITH VARIATIONS IN THREE FOREARM POSITIONS AND TWO ELBOW POSITIONS ($N = 8$)

Tests of Within-Subjects Effects

Measure: STRENGTH
Sphericity Assumed

Source	Sum of Squares	df	Mean Square	F	Sig.
ELBOW	368.521	1	368.521	1.112	.327
Error(ELBOW) ❶	2319.979	7	331.426		
FOREARM	1145.167	2	572.583	6.074	.013
Error(FOREARM)	1319.833	14	94.274		
ELBOW * FOREARM	27.167	2	13.583	.120	.888
Error(ELBOW*FOREARM)	1587.833	14	113.417		

Tests of Between-Subjects Effects ❷

Measure: STRENGTH

Source	Sum of Squares	df	Mean Square	F	Sig.
Intercept	37688.021	1	37688.021	268.521	.000
Error	982.479	7	140.354		

❶ Each repeated measures effect is tested against its own error term, whicn is the interaction between that effect and the effect of subjects

❷ The between-subjects effect is often eliminated from the summary table in a research report. It does not provide important information to the interpretation of the main or interaction effects, but is used in the determination of the error term for each effect.

Note: Some portions of the SPSS computer printout have been omitted for clarity.

error terms for the treatment effects. This effect will often be omitted from the summary table.

Mixed Designs

In a two-factor analysis, where only one factor is repeated, the overall format for the analysis of variance is a combination of between-subjects (independent factors) and within-subjects (repeated factors) analyses. In a mixed design, the independent factor is analyzed as it would be in a regular one-way analysis of variance, pooling all data for the repeated factor. The repeated factor is analyzed using techniques for a repeated measures analysis (see Table 20.6).

TABLE 20.6   SUMMARY TABLE FOR TWO-WAY (3 × 3) ANALYSIS OF VARIANCE WITH ONE REPEATED FACTOR (MIXED DESIGN): ELBOW FLEXOR STRENGTH WITH VARIATIONS OF ICE AND FOREARM POSITION (N = 24)

A. DATA

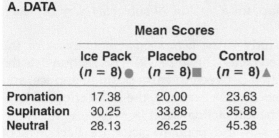

Mean Scores

	Ice Pack (n = 8)●	Placebo (n = 8)■	Control (n = 8)▲
Pronation	17.38	20.00	23.63
Supination	30.25	33.88	35.88
Neutral	28.13	26.25	45.38

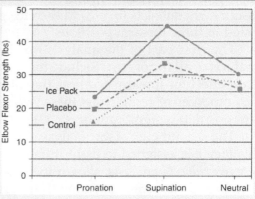

B. OUTPUT

Tests of Within-Subjects Effects

Measure: STRENGTH
Sphericity Assumed

	Source	Sum of Squares	df	Mean Square	F	Sig.
❶	FOREARM	2686.778	2	1343.389	32.801	.000
	FOREARM * ICE	750.389	4	187.597	4.580	.004
	Error(FOREARM)	1720.167	42	40.956		

Tests of Between-Subjects Effects

Measure: STRENGTH

	Source	Sum of Squares	df	Mean Square	F	Sig.
❷	ICE	1315.528	2	657.764	3.432	.051
	Error	4025.083	21	191.671		

C. SUMMARY TABLE FOR RESEARCH REPORT

Source of Variance	df	SS	MS	F	p
Between subjects ❷					
Ice	2	1315.53	657.76	3.432	.051
Error	21	4025.08	191.67		
Within subjects ❶					
Forearm	2	2686.78	1343.39	32.80	.000
Ice × Forearm	4	750.39	187.60	4.58	.004
Error	42	1720.17	40.96		

❶ The within-subjects effects includes the repeated measure and the interaction of the repeated measure with the independent measure.

❷ The between-groups effect is computed for the independent measure, ice. This section is a equivalent to a one-way analysis of variance.

Note: This analysis is run in SPSS using the General Linear Model (GLM). Portions of the printout have been omitted for clarity.

For example, suppose we wanted to look at the effect of ice applied to the biceps brachii on elbow flexor strength in three forearm positions. Ice is an independent factor, and forearm position is a repeated factor. Assume we have three levels of ice (ice pack, placebo and control), and three levels of forearm position, as before. We randomly assign eight subjects ($n = 8$) to each ice group, for a total of 24 subjects ($N = 24$), each tested in three forearm positions.

The first part of the analysis for this study is the *within-subjects* analysis, or the analysis of all factors that include the repeated factor (Table 20.6❶). This section lists the main effect for forearm position, the interaction between forearm position and ice, and a common error term to test these two effects. In this example, the main effect of forearm position is significant ($p < .001$), as is the interaction effect ($p = .004$).

The second part of the analysis addresses the independent factor, ice. Each level of this factor is assigned to eight different subjects. Comparison across these groups is a *between-subjects* analysis, shown in Table 20.6❷. This is actually a one-way analysis of variance for the effect of ice, with two sources of variance: the between-groups effect (ice) and the within-groups variance, or error term. In this example, there is also significant difference among the three levels of ice ($p = .051$).

COMMENTARY

Beyond Analysis of Variance

The analysis of variance provides researchers with a statistical tool that can adapt to a wide variety of design situations. We have covered only the most common applications in this chapter. Many other designs, such as nested designs, randomized blocks and studies with unequal samples, require mathematical adjustments in the analysis that are too complex for us to cover here. Fortunately, computer packages are readily available for performing analyses of variance, and are generally flexible enough to accommodate all the design variations that researchers might require in clinical research. The **general linear model (GLM)** is usually used to accommodate the variety of design options for the ANOVA.

The *t*-test and analysis of variance are based on several assumptions about the nature of data. We have reviewed these assumptions in several places in this and previous chapters. In general, these tests are robust to violations of these assumptions (with the exception of repeated measures designs), so that they can be used with confidence in most research situations; however, when clinical experiments are performed with very small samples, the data may violate these assumptions sufficiently to warrant transforming the data to a different scale of measurement that better reflects the appropriate characteristics for statistical analysis (see Appendix D), or it may be appropriate to use nonparametric statistics that do not make the same demands on the data. In Chapter 22 we describe several nonparametric tests that can be used in place of the *t*-test and the single-factor analysis of variance.

When the analysis of variance results in a significant finding, researchers are usually interested in pursuing the analysis to determine which specific levels of the independent variables are different from each other. Multiple comparison tests, designed specifically for this purpose, are described in the next chapter. At that time we look at some of the data presented here, and show how those data can be analyzed further using multiple comparison techniques.

As we continue to discuss statistical tests in subsequent chapters, many readers will find it helpful to refer to the chart provided in Appendix B, which presents an overview of statistical tests and criteria for choosing a particular test for analyzing different types of data and designs.

REFERENCES

1. Ferguson GA. *Statistical Analysis in Psychology and Education* (5th ed.). New York: McGraw-Hill, 1981.
2. Keppel G. *Design and Analysis: A Researcher's Handbook* (4th ed.). Englewood Cliffs, NJ: Prentice Hall, 2004.
3. Green SB, Salkind NJ, Akey TM. *Using SPSS for Windows and Macintosh: Analyzing and Understanding Data* (4th ed.). Upper Saddle River, NJ: Prentice Hall, 2004.
4. Geisser S, Greenhouse SW. An extension of Box's results on the use of the F distribution in multivariate analysis. *Ann Math Statist* 1958;29:885–891.
5. Huynh H, Feldt LS. Estimation of the Box correction for degrees of freedom from sample data in the randomized block and split-plot designs. *J Educ Statist* 1976;1:69–82.

CHAPTER 21

Multiple Comparison Tests

When an analysis of variance results in a significant *F*-ratio, the researcher is justified in rejecting the null hypothesis and concluding that not all *k* population means are equal; however, this outcome tells us nothing about which means are significantly different from which other means. In this chapter we describe the most commonly used statistical procedures for deciding which means are significantly different. These procedures are called ***multiple comparison tests***.

Several multiple comparison procedures are available, most given names for the individuals who developed them. Each test involves the rank ordering of means and successive contrasts of pairs of means. The pairwise differences between means are tested against a critical value to determine if the difference is large enough to be significant. The major difference between the various tests lies in the degree of protection offered against Type I and Type II error. A conservative test will protect against Type I error, requiring that means be far apart to establish significance. A more liberal test will find a significant difference with means that are closer together, thereby offering greater protection against Type II error.

Most multiple comparison procedures are classified as **post hoc** because specific comparisons of interest are decided *after* the analysis of variance is completed. These are considered **unplanned comparisons**, in that they are based on exploration of the outcome. Therefore, these tests are most useful when a general alternative hypothesis has been proposed. We will describe the three most commonly reported *post hoc* multiple comparison procedures: Tukey's honestly significant difference method, the Newman–Keuls test, and the Scheffé comparison. Other *post hoc* tests used less often include *Duncan's Multiple Range Test*[1] and *Fisher's Least Significant Difference*.[2] These tests are generally considered too liberal, resulting in too great a risk of Type I error (see Figure 21.1).

Other multiple comparison tests are classified as **a priori**, or **planned comparisons**, because specific contrasts are planned *prior* to data collection based on the research rationale. Technically, these comparisons are appropriate even when an *F*-test is not significant, as they are planned before data are collected, and therefore, the overall null hypothesis is not of interest. Although several planned comparison tests are available, we will describe one commonly used method called the Bonferroni *t*-test.*

---

*Other types of planned comparisons include *orthogonal contrasts*, which allow for comparison of specific combinations of means, and *Dunnett's test*,[3] which focuses on comparison of a control group with each of several experimental groups.

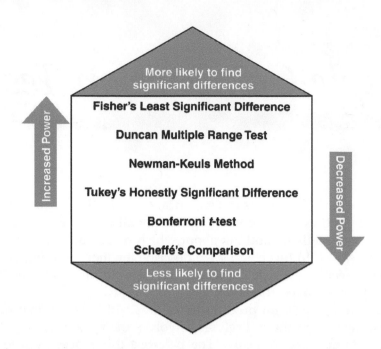

FIGURE 21.1   List of multiple comparison procedures, sorted according to power.

As some statistical computer packages do not include multiple comparison tests for the analysis of variance, it is useful to be able to perform these tests by hand. Fortunately, most multiple comparison procedures are simple enough to be carried out efficiently with a hand calculator once the analysis of variance data are obtained.

THE TYPE I ERROR RATE: PER COMPARISON VERSUS FAMILY

At the end of Chapter 19 we discussed the inappropriate use of multiple t-tests when more than two comparisons are made within a single set of data. This issue is based on the desired protection against Type I error in an experiment, which is specified by α. At $\alpha = .05$, we limit ourselves to a 5% chance that we will experience the random event of finding a significant difference when none exists. We take a 5% risk that we will be in error if we say that group means are different for any single comparison. We must differentiate this **per comparison error rate** (α_{PC}) from the situation where α is set at .05 for each of several comparisons in one experiment. Although it is true that $\alpha = .05$ for each individual comparison, the potential cumulative error for the set of comparisons is actually greater than .05. This cumulative probability has been called the **familywise error rate** (α_{FW}) and represents the probability of making at least one Type I error in a set or "family" of statistical comparisons.[†]

[†]Some statistical references use the term *experimentwise error rate* to indicate the error for all effects within an experiment, whereas *familywise error rate* is used to indicate specific sets of effects, such as main effects and interaction effects in an analysis of variance.[4]

The Type I error rate for a family of comparisons, where each individual comparison is tested at $\alpha = .05$, is equal to

$$\alpha_{FW} = 1 - (1 - \alpha)^c \qquad (21.1)$$

where c represents the total number of comparisons. The maximum number of pairwise contrasts for any set of data will be $k(k - 1)/2$. If we want to compare three means, testing each comparison at $\alpha = .05$, we will perform $c = 3(3 - 1)/2 = 3$ comparisons. Therefore,

$$\alpha_{FW} = 1 - (1 - .05)^3 = 1 - (.95)^3 = .143$$

This means that if we perform three t-tests and find three significant differences, we risk a greater than 14% chance that at least one of these significant differences occurred by chance. This exceeds the generally accepted standard of 5% risk for Type I error.

As the number of comparisons increases, so does the probability that at least one significant difference will occur by chance. For example, with α_{PC} set at .05, tests involving four, five and six means will result in the following familywise probabilities of Type I error:

(Four means: 6 comparisons) $\alpha_{FW} = 1 - (1 - .05)^6 = .26$

(Five means: 10 comparisons) $\alpha_{FW} = 1 - (1 - .05)^{10} = .40$

(Six means: 15 comparisons) $\alpha_{FW} = 1 - (1 - .05)^{15} = .54$

Clearly, the likelihood of finding significant differences among a set of means, even when H_0 is true for all comparisons, will be extremely high as the number of comparisons increases.

Several of the multiple comparison procedures we describe base their critical values on per comparison error rates; others base their Type I error rate on the entire family of comparisons. There is no consensus about preferences for one approach over the other. Use of a per comparison error rate will result in greater statistical power, but with the potential for more Type I errors. Conversely, use of the familywise error rate will produce fewer Type I errors, but will result in fewer significant differences. Researchers must determine if Type I or Type II error is of greater concern in a particular study and apply statistical tests accordingly. In most cases, one hopes to strike a balance between the two types of statistical error.

One-Tailed Versus Two-Tailed Tests

Post hoc comparisons are usually tested using two-tailed probabilities. Where specific contrasts are not specified in advance, it follows that directions of difference cannot be predicted. One-tailed tests can be performed for planned comparisons; however, unless evidence in favor of directional hypotheses is quite strong, it is generally statistically safer to perform two-tailed tests. Contrasts involving two-tailed tests will always be based on the absolute difference between means. One-tailed tests must result in a statistical ratio that supports the directional hypothesis.

STATISTICAL RATIOS FOR MULTIPLE COMPARISON TESTS

To illustrate the concept of multiple comparison tests, we will use a hypothetical study introduced in Chapter 20, comparing the effects of ultrasound (US), ice and friction massage for relieving pain in 44 patients with elbow tendonitis. The four group means, shown in Table 21.1A, represent the change in pain-free range of motion for three treatment groups and a control group. Eleven subjects were tested in each group. The plot of means shows how these group means are distributed.

The null hypothesis for this study states that no differences exist among the four group means:

$$H_0: \mu_1 = \mu_2 = \mu_3 = \mu_4$$

TABLE 21.1   DATA FOR MULTIPLE COMPARISON TESTS: CHANGE IN PAINFREE ELBOW ROM FOLLOWING TREATMENT FOR TENDONITIS ($N = 44$)

A. GROUP MEANS (in degrees)

1. Ultrasound	$\overline{X}_1 = 44.18$	$n_1 = 11$
2. Ice	$\overline{X}_2 = 45.27$	$n_2 = 11$
3. Massage	$\overline{X}_3 = 35.27$	$n_3 = 11$
4. Control	$\overline{X}_4 = 24.18$	$n_4 = 11$

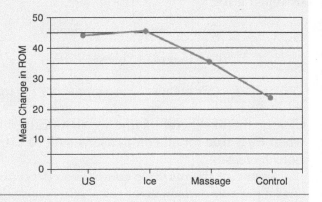

B. ANALYSIS OF VARIANCE

	Sum of Squares	df	Mean Square	F	Sig.
Between groups	3158.09	3	1052.70	11.89	.000
Within groups (Error)	3541.64	40	88.54		

C. TABLE OF MEAN DIFFERENCES

		4	3	1	2
	Means	**Control** 24.18	**Massage** 35.27	**Ultrasound** 44.18	**Ice** 45.27
4	24.18	—	11.09	20.00	21.09
3	35.27		—	8.91	10.00
1	44.18			—	1.09

The analysis of variance for these data, shown in Table 21.1B, is significant ($p < .001$), and it is now of interest to examine individual differences among means.

The process of testing differences among several means is fairly consistent for all multiple comparison procedures. In each test, means are first arranged in *ascending order of size,* and differences between pairs of means are obtained, as shown in Table 21.1C. This table shows the absolute differences between all pairs of means, using a triangular format. With $k = 4$, there will be a total of $4(4 - 1)/2 = 6$ comparisons. The entries in the body of the table are the pairwise mean differences. Values are not entered below the diagonal to avoid redundancies. Each pairwise comparison, or contrast, is tested against a **minimum significant difference (MSD)**. If the absolute difference between a pair of means is *equal to or greater than* the minimum significant difference, then the contrast is considered significant.

$$|\overline{X}_1 - \overline{X}_2| \geq \text{Minimum significant difference}$$

If the pairwise difference is smaller than the minimum significant difference, the means are not significantly different from each other.

Calculation of the minimum significant difference is based on the error mean square, MS_e, taken from the analysis of variance, and a critical value taken from a statistical table. The MS_e reflects the degree of variance within groups (between subjects). Logically, the greater the variance within groups, the less likely we will see a significant difference between means. Critical values for the MSD are used differently, depending on the number of means being compared and the type of error rate used (per comparison or familywise). The relevant critical values are located according to the degrees of freedom associated with the error term, df_e, in the analysis of variance.[‡] For the example we are using, the error mean square is 88.54, with 40 degrees of freedom (see Table 21.1B).

TUKEY'S HONESTLY SIGNIFICANT DIFFERENCE (HSD)

Tukey developed one of the simplest multiple comparison procedures, which he called the **honestly significant difference (HSD)** method.[5] Tukey's procedure sets a familywise error rate, so that α identifies the probability that one or more of the pairwise comparisons will be falsely declared significant. Therefore, this test offers generous protection against Type I error.

Tukey's HSD test is calculated using the **studentized range statistic**, given the symbol q. Critical values of q are found in Appendix Table A.6. The q statistic is influenced by the overall number of means that are being compared. At the top of Table A.6, the number or "range" of means being compared is given the symbol r.[§] Logically, as the number of sample means increases, the size of the difference between the largest and

---

[‡]It is not uncommon to find that the exact value for the error degrees of freedom is not listed in these tables. In that case, it is usually sufficient to refer to the closest value for degrees of freedom for an approximate critical value. To be conservative, the next lowest value for degrees of freedom should be used.

[§]In this case, r stands for *range.* This symbol should not be confused with the use of the r for the correlation coefficient.

smallest means will also increase, even when H_0 is true. The q statistic provides a mechanism for adjusting critical values to account for the effect of larger numbers of means.

Minimum Significant Difference

The minimum significant difference for Tukey's HSD procedure is given by

$$MSD = q\sqrt{\frac{MS_e}{n}} \qquad (21.2)$$

where MS_e is the mean square error, n is the number of subjects *in each group* (assuming equal sample sizes**), and q is taken from Appendix Table A.6, for the desired level of α, df_e, and the number of means, r. For the example we are using, $q = 3.79$ for $\alpha = .05$, $r = 4$, and $df_e = 40$. Therefore,

$$MSD = 3.79\sqrt{\frac{88.54}{11}} = 10.75$$

This minimum significant difference is compared with each pairwise mean difference in Table 21.2B. Absolute differences that are equal to or greater than this value are significant. For example, the difference between the largest and smallest means $(\overline{X}_2 - \overline{X}_4)$ is equal to 21.09. This value exceeds the minimum significant difference and is, therefore, significant. To present these results in a clear format, an asterisk denotes those differences that are significant in Table 21.2B. According to these results, the three experimental groups are different from the control, but the treatment groups are not different from each other.

A computer analysis of these data is presented in terms of *homogeneous subsets of means* (Table 21.2C). In this output, each subset (listed in the same column) represents means that are not significantly different. Means that are listed in separate columns are significantly different from one another. These results show that the mean for the control group is significantly different from the three treatment means.

NEWMAN-KEULS METHOD

The **Newman-Keuls (NK) test** (sometimes called Student-Newman-Keuls test) is similar to the Tukey method, except that it uses a per comparison error rate.[5] Therefore, α specifies the Type I error rate for each pairwise contrast, rather than for the entire set of comparisons. Overall, then, as the number of comparisons increases, the chances of committing a Type I error are greater using this procedure than using Tukey's test.

**When samples are not of equal size, the *harmonic mean* of the sample size is used in calculations of the minimum significant difference. The harmonic mean, n', is equal to $\dfrac{k}{\Sigma\left(\dfrac{1}{n}\right)}$ where k is the number of groups, and n is the sample size for each group. For example, if there are two groups, with $n_1 = 10$ and $n_2 = 5$, $n' = \dfrac{2}{\left(\dfrac{1}{10} + \dfrac{1}{5}\right)} = 6.67$. This procedure can be used with all multiple comparison tests.

TABLE 21.2   SIGNIFICANT DIFFERENCES (*) FOR TUKEY'S HSD TEST ($\alpha = .05$)

A. MINIMUM SIGNIFICANT DIFFERENCE: 10.75

B. TABLE OF MEAN DIFFERENCES

	Means	4 Control 24.18	3 Massage 35.27	1 Ultrasound 44.18	2 Ice 45.27
4	24.18	—	11.09*	20.00*	21.09*
3	35.27		—	8.91	10.00
1	44.18			—	1.09

C. OUTPUT: Homogeneous Subsets of Means

	GROUP	N	Subset for alpha = .05	
			1	2
Tukey HSD	Control	11	24.18	
	Massage	11		35.27
	US	11		44.18
	Ice	11		45.27

The Newman-Keuls method is also based on the studentized range q; however, values of q are used differently for each contrast, depending on the number of *adjacent* means, r, within an ordered **comparison interval.** To illustrate how this is applied, consider the four sample means for the tendonitis study, ranked in ascending size order: (4) Control, (3) Massage, (1) US, (2) Ice (see Figure 21.2). If we compare the two smaller means, the comparison interval for Control → Massage includes two adjacent means. Therefore, $r = 2$ for that comparison. If we compare the largest and smallest

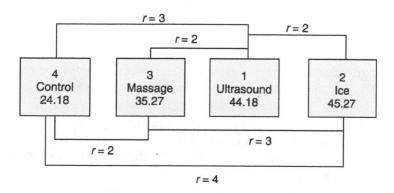

FIGURE 21.2   Comparison intervals for a set of four group means, arranged in size order. Based on data from Table 21.1.

means, the interval for Control $\rightarrow$ Ice contains four adjacent means (4-3-1-2), and so $r = 4$. Similarly, if we compare means for Massage and Ice, the comparison interval contains three adjacent means (3-1-2), so $r = 3$.

Therefore, a comparison interval represents the steps between ordered means for a given comparison. As shown in Figure 21.2, with four means we will have intervals of two, three, and four means. In contrast to Tukey's approach which uses one critical difference for all comparisons, the Newman-Keuls test will use a larger critical difference as r increases. This adjusts for the fact that larger differences are expected with a greater range of means, even when H_0 is true.

Minimum Significant Difference

The minimum significant difference for the Newman-Keuls comparison is

$$\text{MSD} = q_{(r)}\sqrt{\frac{MS_e}{n}} \tag{21.3}$$

where values of $q_{(r)}$ are obtained from Table A.6 for each comparison interval. For the example we are using, we find q for $\alpha = .05$ and $df_e = 40$ for comparison intervals of $r = 2, 3,$ and 4:

$$q_{(r=2)} = 2.86$$

$$q_{(r=3)} = 3.44$$

$$q_{(r=4)} = 3.79$$

With $MS_e = 88.54$ and $n = 11$, we find the corresponding minimum significant differences:

$$\text{MSD}\ (r = 2) = 2.86\sqrt{\frac{88.54}{11}} = 8.11$$

$$\text{MSD}\ (r = 3) = 3.44\sqrt{\frac{88.54}{11}} = 9.76$$

$$\text{MSD}\ (r = 4) = 3.79\sqrt{\frac{88.54}{11}} = 10.75$$

These minimum significant differences are compared with the appropriate mean differences in Table 21.3B. Significant differences are noted with an asterisk. For example, the difference between means for Control and Ice is 21.09, which exceeds the critical difference 10.75 for $r = 4$. Therefore, these two means are significantly different. The difference between means for Massage and Ice is 10.00, which exceeds the critical difference 9.76 for $r = 3$. These two means are also significantly different from each other. The difference between US and Ice is 1.09, which does not exceed the critical difference 8.11 for $r = 2$. These means are not significantly different. Of the six comparisons, five are significant. This test demonstrates that the three experimental groups are different from the control, and US and Ice are different from massage.

TABLE 21.3　SIGNIFICANT DIFFERENCES (*) FOR THE NEWMAN-KEULS TEST ($\alpha = .05$)

A. MINIMUM SIGNIFICANT DIFFERENCES:

Comparison Intervals:	$r = 2$	MSD = 8.11
	$r = 3$	MSD = 9.76
	$r = 4$	MSD = 10.75

B. TABLE OF MEAN DIFFERENCES

	Means	4 Control 24.18	3 Massage 35.27	1 Ultrasound 44.18	2 Ice 45.27
3	24.18	—	11.09* ($r = 2$)	20.00* ($r = 3$)	21.09* ($r = 4$)
2	35.27		—	8.91* ($r = 2$)	10.00* ($r = 3$)
1	44.18			—	1.09 ($r = 2$)

C. OUTPUT: HOMOGENEOUS SUBSETS OF MEANS

			Subset for alpha = .05		
	GROUP	N	1	2	3
Newman-Keuls	Control	11	24.18		
	Massage	11		35.27	
	US	11			44.18
	Ice	11			45.27

This result is also shown in Table 21.3C for subsets of means. Because the mean for the Control group is listed in a column by itself, it is different from all other means. The same is true for the mean for the Massage group. The means for US and Ice are listed in the same column, indicating that they are not different from each other.

The reader may note that the minimum difference for the Newman-Keuls test with $r = 4$ is the same as the minimum difference used for Tukey's test (in this case 10.75). The Tukey procedure uses this one minimum difference for all comparisons, whereas the Newman-Keuls test adjusts the minimum differences for smaller comparison intervals. Therefore, the minimum differences will be lower for some contrasts using the Newman-Keuls method. Consequently, the Newman-Keuls test can result in more significant differences (as it did here), and is the more powerful of the two comparisons; however, because the Newman-Keuls procedure does not control for the familywise error rate, it will produce a greater number of Type I errors than the Tukey method over the long run.

SCHEFFÉ COMPARISON

The **Scheffé comparison** is the most flexible and most rigorous of the post hoc multiple comparison tests.[6] It is based on the familiar F-distribution. It is a conservative test because it adopts a familywise error rate that applies to all contrasts. This provides strong protection against Type I error, but it also makes the procedure much less powerful than the other tests we have described. Scheffé has recommended that a less stringent level of significance be used, such as $\alpha = .10$, to avoid excess Type II error.[7]

Minimum Significant Difference

The minimum significant difference for the Scheffé comparison is given by

$$\text{MSD} = \sqrt{(k - 1)F}\sqrt{\frac{2MS_e}{n}} \tag{21.4}$$

where k is the total number of means involved in the set of comparisons, and F is the critical value for df_b and df_e obtained from Appendix Table A.3 (not the calculated value of F from the ANOVA). For the example we are using, $k = 4$ and $F = 2.84$ for 3 and 40 degrees of freedom at $\alpha = .05$. Therefore,

$$\text{MSD} = \sqrt{(4 - 1)(2.84)}\sqrt{\frac{2(88.54)}{11}} = 11.71$$

All differences between means must meet or exceed this value to be significant. Therefore, as denoted by asterisks in Table 21.4B, this analysis results in two significant comparisons (fewer than with the Newman-Keuls or Tukey method), demonstrating the lower power associated with the Scheffé comparison. According to this test, the Control and Massage groups are not significantly different from each other, where they were considered significantly different with the other tests.[††]

BONFERRONI t-TEST

Researchers often designate specific contrasts of interest prior to data collection. These contrasts usually relate to theoretical expectations of the data. When comparisons are planned in advance and when they are relatively limited in number,[‡‡] *a priori* tests can

---

[††]Note that the Control group is significantly different from US and Ice, but not from Massage. However, Massage is not different from US and Ice. This overlap may seem illogical. It occurs because of variance components from the different variables that are not independent of each other. This result suggests that the Scheffé comparison is not the most useful approach to understand the relationships in these data.

[‡‡]Glass defines a small number of comparisons as less than $k(k - 1)/4$.[8]

TABLE 21.4 **SIGNIFICANT DIFFERENCES (*) FOR THE SCHEFFÉ COMPARISON**
($\alpha = .05$)

A. MINIMUM SIGNIFICANT DIFFERENCE: 11.71

B. TABLE OF MEAN DIFFERENCES

		4	3	1	2
		Control	Massage	Ultrasound	Ice
	Means	24.18	35.27	44.18	45.27
4	24.18	—	11.09	20.00*	21.09*
3	35.27		—	8.91	0.00
1	44.18			—	1.09

C. OUTPUT: Homogeneous Subsets of Means

			Subset for alpha = .05	
	GROUP	N	1	2
Scheffé	Control	11	24.18	
	Massage	11	35.27	35.27
	US	11		44.18
	Ice	11		45.27

be used. The rationale for valid application of planned comparisons must be established before data are collected, so that the choice of specific hypotheses cannot be influenced by the data. Because the researcher is not necessarily interested in all possible contrasts, it is actually unnecessary to test the overall null hypothesis with the analysis of variance. Regardless of whether the ANOVA demonstrates a significant F-ratio, planned comparisons can be made.

The **Bonferroni comparison** (also called *Dunn's multiple comparison procedure*) is a planned comparison, using a familywise error rate that is the sum of the per comparison significance levels. Therefore, α_{FW} is dependent on the number of planned comparisons, *c*:

$$\alpha_{FW} \leq \alpha_1 + \alpha_2 + \ldots + \alpha_c \tag{21.5}$$

For example, with four planned comparisons, each tested at $\alpha = .01$, the probability of one or more Type I errors for the entire family of contrasts is not greater than $\alpha = .04$. Essentially, the procedure splits α evenly among the set of planned contrasts, so that each contrast is tested at α_{FW}/c. Therefore, if a researcher wants an overall probability of .05 for a set of four contrasts, each individual comparison will have to achieve significance at .05/4, or $p = .013$. This process of adjusting α, called **Bonferroni's adjustment (or correction)**, is used as a protection against Type I error.

The Bonferroni test is based on Student's t-distribution, with adjustments made for the number of contrasts being performed within a set of data. To facilitate these adjustments, a special table of critical values has been developed for Bonferroni's t (given the symbol $t(B)$).[9]

Minimum Significant Difference

The minimum significant difference for the Bonferroni test can be computed using

$$MSD = t(B)\sqrt{\frac{2MS_e}{n}} \qquad (21.6)$$

where $t(B)$ is taken from Appendix Table A.7 for α_{FW}, df_e, and c, where c is the total number of comparisons in the experiment. Continuing with the example we have been using, for six comparisons performed at $\alpha_{FW} = .05$, with $df_e = 40$, we find $t(B) = 2.77$. Therefore,

$$MSD = 2.77\sqrt{\frac{2(88.54)}{11}} = 11.11$$

All pairwise differences are compared with this one minimum significant difference, as shown in Table 21.5. In this case, three of the six comparisons are significant. According to these results, the three intervention groups are different from the control.

TABLE 21.5   SIGNIFICANT DIFFERENCES (*) FOR THE BONFERRONI t-TEST ($\alpha = .05$)

A. MINIMUM SIGNIFICANT DIFFERENCE: 11.11

B. TABLE OF MEAN DIFFERENCES

		4	2	1	2
	Means	**Control** 24.18	**Massage** 35.27	**Ultrasound** 44.18	**Ice** 45.27
4	24.18	—	11.09*	20.00*	21.09*
3	35.27		—	8.91	10.00
1	44.18			—	1.09

C. OUTPUT: Homogeneous Subsets of Means

				Subset for alpha = .05	
	GROUP	**N**		**1**	**2**
Bonferroni	Control	11		24.18	
	Massage	11			35.27
	US	11			44.18
	Ice	11			45.27

MULTIPLE COMPARISON PROCEDURES FOR FACTORIAL DESIGNS

Multiple comparison procedures are applicable to all analysis of variance designs. So far, we have described their use following an analysis with only one independent variable. When multifactor experiments are analyzed, the multiple comparison procedures can be used to compare means for main effects and interaction effects.

To illustrate this application, let us refer back to a study presented in Chapter 20, involving the comparison of stretch and knee position for increasing ankle range of motion. Stretch (Factor A) had three levels: prolonged, quick and control. Knee position (Factor B) had two levels: flexion and extension. This design is shown in Figure 21.3. Ten subjects were tested in each of the six treatment combinations. Recall that the marginal means, $\overline{X}_A$ and $\overline{X}_B$, represent main effects for each independent variable separately. The six cells of the design (A_1B_1 through A_3B_2) represent all combinations of the two independent variables, or the interaction means.

The outcome of the analysis of variance for this study is shown in Table 21.6A. The main effect of stretch is significant, as is the interaction effect. In practice, we would usually ignore the main effects because of the significant interaction, and proceed to analyze the six individual cell means. For purposes of illustration, however, we will look at the main effect of stretch using a multiple comparison procedure. If the variable of knee position had been significant, we would not have to perform a multiple comparison because it has only two levels. Therefore, a significant effect could be interpreted by simply looking at the marginal means, as with a t-test.

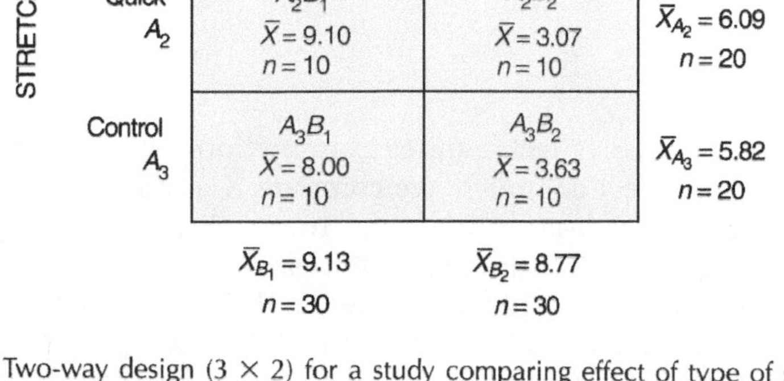

FIGURE 21.3   Two-way design (3 × 2) for a study comparing effect of type of stretch (Factor A) and knee position (Factor B) on ankle range of motion ($N = 60$). Six individual cell means are shown, as are marginal means for each independent variable.

TABLE 21.6   SIGNIFICANT DIFFERENCES (*) AMONG MARGINAL MEANS FOR MAIN EFFECT OF STRETCH USING TUKEY'S HSD TEST ($\alpha = .05$)

A. ANOVA (from Table 20.3)

	Sum of Squares	df	Mean Square	F	Sig.
Stretch	1080.73	2	540.36	41.84	.000
Position	2.02	1	2.02	.16	.694
Stretch × Position	707.72	2	353.86	27.40	.000
Error	697.36	54	12.91		
Total	2487.83	59	· 42.17		

B. MINIMUM SIGNIFICANT DIFFERENCE: 2.73

C. TABLE OF MEAN DIFFERENCES and PLOT OF MEANS

Means		A_3 Control 5.82	A_2 Quick 6.09	A_1 Prolonged 14.95
A_3	5.82	—	0.27	9.13*
A_2	6.09		—	8.86*

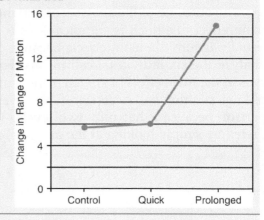

D. OUTPUT: Homogeneous Subsets of Means

	GROUP	N	Subsets for alpha = .05	
			1	2
Tukey HSD	Prolonged	20	5.82	
	Quick	20	6.09	
	Control	20		14.95

Main Effects

The analysis of a significant main effect requires examination of differences among marginal means. For the main effect of stretch, we compare $\overline{X}_{A1}$, $\overline{X}_{A2}$, and $\overline{X}_{A3}$. The application of multiple comparison tests to marginal means is the same as in previous examples, except that n must reflect the total number of subjects contributing to each mean in a contrast. Therefore, if $n = 10$ for each cell in the design, then $n = 20$ for each marginal mean for stretch (see Fig 21.3). The values of MS_e and df_e used for calculations are taken from the analysis of variance summary table. In this case, $MS_e = 12.91$ and $df_e = 54$ (we will use $df_e = 60$ for locating tabled values).

To apply Tukey's HSD to these data, we calculate the minimum significant difference:

$$\text{MSD} = q\sqrt{\frac{MS_e}{n}} = 3.40\sqrt{\frac{12.91}{20}} = 2.73$$

with q taken from Table A.6 for $\alpha = .05$, $df_e = 60$, and $r = 3$. Note that $n = 20$ represents the pooled sample size for each marginal mean. The pairwise differences between the marginal means are shown in Table 21.6C. Differences that exceed 2.73 are significant. Results in Table 21.6C and D show that prolonged stretch ($\overline{X}_{A1}$) is significantly different from quick stretch ($\overline{X}_{A2}$) and the control ($\overline{X}_{A3}$), but that the latter two means are not different from each other.

Interaction Effects

When an interaction effect is significant, multiple comparison tests are usually performed on pairwise contrasts of individual cell means. Formulas are used exactly as they were for the one-way design. In this example, we would be comparing six means.

For the means in Figure 21.3, if we choose to analyze all pairwise differences with $k = 6$, we will obtain $6(6 - 1)/2 = 15$ comparisons. To use Tukey's HSD as an example, we calculate the minimum significant difference:

$$\text{MSD} = q\sqrt{\frac{MS_e}{n}} = 4.16\sqrt{\frac{12.91}{10}} = 6.16$$

with q obtained from Table A.6 for $\alpha = .05$, $df_e = 60$, and $r = 6$. Note that $n = 10$ reflects the sample size for each of the six individual cell means.

The mean differences, shown in Table 21.7, must exceed this minimum significant difference to be considered significant. Results demonstrate that range of motion achieved with prolonged stretch with knee extension (A_1B_2) is significantly greater than with all other treatment combinations. In addition, prolonged stretch with knee flexion (A_1B_1) is greater than quick stretch and control with knee extension. These effects are illustrated in Figure 20.6 in Chapter 20.

Interpretation of pairwise differences for interactions will often be more meaningful by limiting contrasts to row or column effects, eliminating comparisons that move diagonally within the design. In other words, we would not be interested in the contrast of prolonged stretch in flexion with the other forms of stretch in extension, which are diagonal comparisons (see Figure 21.2). This type of comparison is actually confounded, because it involves different levels of both variables. We are more interested in the contrasts across A_1, across A_2, and across A_3, and three contrasts within B_1 and within B_2. This would result in a total of 9 contrasts, rather than 15. When using tests such as Bonferroni's t, where the number of comparisons is the basis for adjusting critical values, this process can significantly improve statistical power as well as clarify explanations.

MULTIPLE COMPARISONS FOR REPEATED MEASURES

The standard *post hoc* multiple comparisons procedures just described are not generally run for repeated measures analyses. Because repeated measures involve within-subject comparisons, the multiple comparison procedures do not fit logically, as they are based

TABLE 21.7 SIGNIFICANT DIFFERENCES (*) AMONG INTERACTION MEANS FOR TYPE OF STRETCH AND KNEE POSITION USING TUKEY'S HSD TEST (α = .05)

A. MINIMUM SIGNIFICANT DIFFERENCE: 6.16

B. PLOT OF MEANS

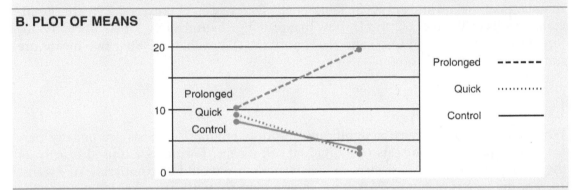

C. TABLE OF MEAN DIFFERENCES

		A_2B_2	A_3B_2	A_3B_1	A_2B_1	A_1B_1	A_1B_2
Stretch Knee		Quick Ext	Control Ext	Control Flex	Quick Flex	Prolonged Flex	Prolonged Ext
Means		3.07	3.63	8.00	9.10	10.30	19.60
A_2B_2	3.07	—	0.56	4.93	6.03	7.23*	16.53*
A_3B_2	3.63		—	4.37	5.47	6.67*	15.97*
A_3B_1	8.00			—	1.10	2.30	11.60*
A_2B_1	9.10				—	1.20	10.50*
A_1B_1	10.30					—	9.30*

on overall group differences. Therefore, the paired t-test has been used as a reasonable approach for looking at differences between pairs of means within a repeated measures design.[10,11] Each pairwise comparison is entered as a difference score, and the analysis will determine which means are significantly different. For example, let us reconsider the hypothetical study described in Chapter 20 that looked at elbow flexor strength in three forearm positions for nine subjects. The mean for pronation was 17.33, for neutral 27.56, and for supination 29.11 pounds. The results of the repeated measures analysis of variance are shown in Table 21.8A, indicating that a significant difference existed among the three forearm positions. Therefore, a *post hoc* multiple comparison test is warranted to compare the three means.

Table 21.8 presents the results of the paired t-test for three pairwise comparisons in this example. The differences for neutral-pronation and pronation-supination are significant (p = .000), but the difference for neutral-supination is not (p = .127). This analysis presents a problem, however, in terms of familywise error rate. Because several

TABLE 21.8   PAIRED *t*-TEST MULTIPLE COMPARISON OF THREE PAIRWISE CONTRASTS FOLLOWING REPEATED MEASURES ANOVA: ELBOW FLEXOR STRENGTH IN THREE FOREARM POSITIONS

A. ANOVA

	Sum of Squares	df	Mean Square	F	Sig.
Subjects	2604.00	8	325.50		
Position	736.89	2	368.44	50.34	.000
Error	117.11	16	7.319		

B. PAIRED *t*-TESTS

Paired Samples Test

	Paired Differences							
				95% Confidence Interval of the Difference				
	Mean	Std. Deviation	Std. Error Mean	Lower	Upper	t	df	Sig. (2-tailed)
Prone, Neutral	−10.22	3.76	1.25	−13.11	−7.32	−8.140	8	.000
Neutral, Supine	−1.55	2.74	.91	−3.66	.55	−1.701	8	.127
Prone, Supine	−11.77	4.71	1.57	−15.39	−8.15	−7.500	8	.000

C. TABLE OF MEAN DIFFERENCES and PLOT OF MEANS

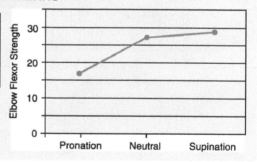

	Pronation	Neutral	Supination
Means	17.33	27.56	29.11
17.33	—	10.22*	11.78*
27.56		—	1.56

analyses are being run on the same sample, we risk inflating the value of α if each test is performed at the same .05 criterion. Therefore, this approach requires the use of the **Bonferroni adjustment,** whereby the overall value for α is divided by the number of comparisons. For instance, with three comparisons $\alpha_{FW} = .05/3 = .017$. This means that the p value for each individual comparison must be .017 or less to be considered significant. In our current example, with the two significant effects at $p = .000$, we have clearly achieved this criterion. However, if we had found a difference for any one comparison at .02, for example, where it would typically be considered significant at $\alpha = .05$, we would not consider it different for this multiple comparison.

BOX 21.1   **What's the Difference?**

An investigator is interested in comparing three treatments: experimental treatment A, experimental treatment B, and control treatment C, using three independent groups. He performs a one-way analysis of variance on the data, and finds a significant F test at $p = .05$. He therefore concludes that there is a significant difference among the three means and proceeds to perform a multiple comparison test to determine where those differences lie. But when he gets the results of the multiple comparison test, he finds that none of the means are significantly different! How can this be?

Now, in another laboratory, three different researchers are conducting three different experiments, each comparing two treatments using an unpaired t-test. One is comparing A with B, one is comparing B with C, and the third is comparing A with C. The first two of these researchers find no significant difference between their groups. The third researcher, however, does find a significant difference at $p = .05$. He is now able to report that his experimental treatment A worked.

Why should the investigator who analyzed all three treatments at once be unable to find a significant difference when the investigator who ran a single experiment can claim a successful outcome?

In the first case the investigator proposed a question that required the comparison of two treatments with respect to a control. His hypothesis is, "There will be a difference among these three groups." The comparison of the three groups is an important part of the rationale for this study, to account for the potential theoretical connections of these treatments. The ANOVA looks at the entire sample as part of this analysis, partitioning the variance across all three groups. In this case, the overall variance showed a significant effect, but this effect could not be attributed to any one specific comparison. Sometimes the variances of the individual groups are not sufficiently independent to show a significant difference, even when the overall F test does.

The investigator who studied the single comparison, on the other hand, is only concerned with the variance of two groups, and can narrow his statistical search for a difference. His hypothesis is, "There will be a difference between these two groups." And so there was!

Adapted from Dallal GE. Multiple comparison procedures. Available at: http://www.tufts.edu/~gdallal/mc.htm Accessed October 29, 2007.

TREND ANALYSIS

Multiple comparison tests are most often used in studies where the independent variable is qualitative or nominal, and where the researcher's interest focuses on determining which categories are significantly different from the others. When an independent variable is quantitative, the treatment levels no longer represent categories, but differing amounts of something, such as age, duration or intensity of a modality, dosage of a drug, or time intervals for repeated testing. When the levels of an independent variable are ordered along a continuum, the researcher is often interested in examining the shape of the response rather than just differences between levels. This approach is called a **trend analysis**.

The purpose of a trend analysis is to find the most reasonable description of continuous data based on the number of turns, or "ups and downs" seen across the levels of the independent variable. For example, if we wanted to study the changes that occur in strength as one ages, we might study 10 blocks of subjects, each representing a different age category from 8 to 80 years old. A hypothetical plot of such data is shown in Figure 21.4. A multiple comparison of means will not tell us about the directions of change across age, but a trend analysis will.

Basically, trends are classified as either linear or nonlinear. In a **linear trend**, all data rise or fall at a constant rate as the value of the independent variable increases. This trend is characterized by a straight line, as shown in Figure 21.5A. For example, we might use this function to represent the relationship between height and age in children. As a child grows older, height tends to increase proportionally.

A *nonlinear trend* demonstrates "bends" or changes in direction. A **quadratic trend**, shown in Figure 21.5B, demonstrates a single turn upward or downward, creating a concave shape to the data. This means that following an initial increase or decrease in the dependent variable, scores vary in direction or rate of change. Learning curves can be characterized as quadratic. Performance generally increases at a sharp rate through early trials and then plateaus.

Higher order nonlinear trends are more complex and are often difficult to interpret. As shown in Figure 21.5C and D, a *cubic trend* involves a second change of direction, and a *quartic trend* a third turn. As the number of levels of the independent variable increases, the number of potential trend components will also increase. There can be a maximum of $k - 1$ turns, or trend components, within any data set.

The curves in Figure 21.5 are examples of pure trends. Real data seldom conform to these patterns exactly. Even with data that represent true trends, chance factors will produce dips and variations that may distort the observed relationship. The purpose of a trend analysis is to describe the overall tendency in the data using the least number of trend components possible. Some data can be characterized by a single trend; others

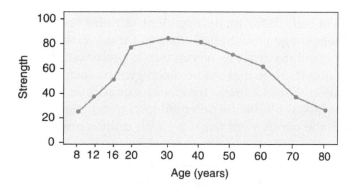

FIGURE 21.4 Hypothetical data for strength changes over 10 age ranges.

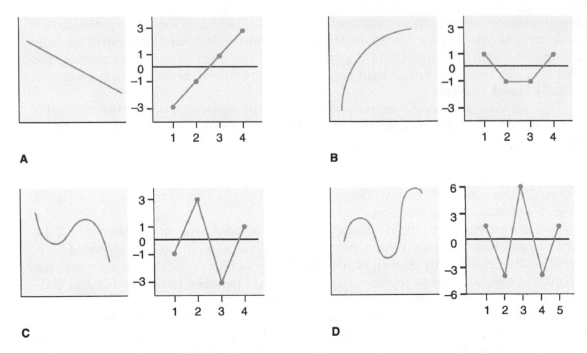

FIGURE 21.5   Examples of several types of trends: **(A)** Linear trend, **(B)** quadratic trend, **(C)** cubic trend, **(D)** quartic trend.

demonstrate more than one pattern within a single data set. The hypothetical data for strength and age illustrate this possibility (see Figure 21.4). The portion of the data from 8 to 20 years shows that individuals tend to get stronger as they grow within this age range. We can see the quadratic component within this curve after age 20. Strength appears to plateau at age 30, after which a gradual dropoff is evident.

Significance of Trend Components

Trends are tested for significance as part of an analysis of variance. The mathematical basis for analyzing trends is beyond the scope of the present discussion. Most statistical computer packages are able to run a trend analysis.[§§]

The results of trend analyses are listed as part of an ANOVA summary table. An example of this type of output for an independent samples test is given in Table 21.9, based on the hypothetical age and strength data in Figure 21.4. The top portion of the table shows how the standard analysis of variance is presented. In the bottom portion, the trend analysis is added. Note that the between-groups sum of squares for the effect of age has been partitioned into a linear trend and a quadratic trend. Because there are 10 measurement intervals, we have the potential for 9 trend components; however, testing beyond the quadratic component usually yields uninterpretable results. Therefore,

---

[§§]Some computer packages will refer to trend analyses as *orthogonal decomposition* or *orthogonal polynomial contrasts*.

TABLE 21.9   **EXAMPLE OF AN ANOVA WITH A TREND ANALYSIS FOR INDEPENDENT SAMPLES: CHANGES IN STRENGTH ACROSS 10 AGE GROUPS (N = 100)**

A. ANALYSIS OF VARIANCE

ANOVA

	Sum of Squares	df	Mean Square	F	Sig.
Age	48887.89	9	5431.98	104.00	❶ .000
Error	4700.70	90	52.23		
Total	53588.59	99			

B. TREND ANALYSIS

ANOVA

			Sum of Squares	df	Mean Square	F	Sig.
Age			48887.89	9	5431.98	104.00	❶ .000
	Linear Term	Contrast	97.42	❹ 1	97.42	1.87	❷ .175
		Deviation	48790.47	8	6098.81	116.77	❸ .000
	Quadratic Term	Contrast	46197.33	❻ 1	46197.33	884.49	❺ .000
		Deviation	2593.13	7	370.45	7.09	.000
Error			4700.70	90	52.23		
Total			53588.59	99			

❶ The difference among age groups is significant.

❷ The linear trend component is not significant (p = .175).

❸ After the linear component is accounted for, there is still some residual variance (deviation) that is significant; that is, there are other trend components that need to be accounted for in the data.

❹ Note that the total sum of squares and 9 degrees of freedom for the linear trend are based on the sum of squares and degrees of freedom associated with the between-groups effect of age.

❺ The quadratic trend is significant (p = .000). The analysis does not go beyond the quadratic effect.

❻ Note that the total sum of squares and 8 degrees of freedom for the quadratic trend are based on the residual sum of squares that remains after the linear trend is accounted for.

variance attributable to all higher order trends is included in the error term (called deviation here).

Each specific trend component is tested by an F-ratio, calculated using the mean square for that trend and the error term. In this example, only the quadratic trend is significant. When a trend component is statistically significant, subjective examination of graphic patterns of the data is usually sufficient for further interpretation.

Limitations of Trend Analysis

Two important limitations should be considered when interpreting trend analyses. First, the number and spacing of intervals between levels of the independent variable can make a difference to the visual interpretation of the curve. Obviously, with only two levels of an independent variable no trend can be established. A linear trend requires a minimum of three points, a quadratic trend a minimum of four points, and so on. With larger spans in the quantitative variable, more intervals may be necessary.

Most investigators try to use equally spaced intervals to achieve consistency in the interpretation. Others will purposefully create unequal intervals to best represent the samples of interest. For instance, trends that are established over time may involve some intervals of hours and others of days. Most computer packages that perform trend analyses will accommodate equal or unequal intervals, but distances between unequal intervals must be specified.

The second caution for interpreting trend analysis is to avoid extrapolating beyond the upper and lower limits of the selected intervals. For example, based on Figure 21.4, if we had tested only individuals between 20 and 80, we might conclude that strength declines linearly with age. Conversely, if we looked only at ages 8 through 20, we might conclude that strength increases linearly with age. By limiting the range of intervals we would have missed the quadratic function that more accurately describes the relationship between strength and age across the lifespan. Therefore, the nature of the relationship between the independent and dependent variables should be examined within and across the ranges that will allow the most complete interpretation.

COMMENTARY

Choices, Choices, Choices

There are no widely accepted criteria for choosing one multiple comparison test over another, and the selection of a particular procedure is often made either arbitrarily or on the basis of available software; however, two basic issues should guide the choice of a multiple comparison procedure.

The first issue relates to the decision to conduct either planned or unplanned contrasts. This decision rests with the researcher during the planning stages of the study, in response to theoretical expectations. With planned comparisons, the researcher asks, "Is *this* difference significant?" With *post hoc* tests the question shifts to, "*Which* differences are significant?" When the researcher is interested in exploring all possible combinations of variables, unplanned contrasts should be used.

The second issue concerns the importance of Type I or Type II error. Each multiple comparison test will control for these errors differently, depending on the use of per comparison or familywise error rates. Of the three post hoc comparisons described here, the Newman-Keuls test is the most powerful. Scheffé's comparison gives the greatest control over Type I error, but at the expense of power. Researchers often prefer Tukey's HSD because it offers both reasonable power and protection against Type I error. The power of the Newman-Keuls procedure is increased by using different comparison intervals, but use of the per comparison error rate increases the risk of Type I error.

Researchers must examine the research question to determine which multiple comparison test is most appropriate in terms of the research design. These decisions should be based on the research question, not on which test is most likely to find significant differences. The decision to run planned or unplanned comparisons and simple or complex contrasts should be made before the data are analyzed. Other than these rather straightforward criteria, when there is no overriding concern for either Type I or Type II error, there may be no obvious choice for a specific test. The researcher is obliged to consider the rationale for comparing treatment conditions or groups and to justify the basis for making these comparisons.

REFERENCES

1. Duncan DB. Multiple range and multiple F tests. *Biometrics* 1955;11:1–42.
2. Fisher RA. *The Design of Experiments* (6th ed.). New York: Hafner, 1951.
3. Dunnett CW. A multiple comparison procedure for comparing several treatments with a control. *J Am Statist Assoc* 1955;50:1096–1121.
4. Keppel G. *Design and Analysis: A Researcher's Handbook* (4th ed.). Englewood Cliffs, NJ: Prentice Hall, 2004.
5. Toothaker LE. *Multiple Comparison Procedures*. Thousand Oaks, CA: Sage Publications, 1992.
6. Scheffe HA. A method for judging all contrasts in the analysis of variance. *Biometrika* 1953;40:87–104.
7. Scheffe HA. *The Analysis of Variance*. New York: Wiley, 1959.
8. Glass GV, Hopkins KD. *Statistical Methods in Education and Psychology* (3rd ed.). Boston: Allyn and Bacon, 1996.
9. Dunn OJ. Multiple comparison among means. *J Am Statist Assoc* 1961;56:54–64.
10. Maxwell SE. Pairwise multiple comparisons in repeated measures designs. *J Educ Stat* 1980;5:269–287.
11. Green SB, Salkind NJ, Akey TM. *Using SPSS for Windows: Analyzing and Understanding Data*. Upper Saddle River, NJ: Prentice Hall, 1997.

CHAPTER 22

Nonparametric Tests for Group Comparisons

In previous chapters we have presented several statistical tests that are based on certain assumptions about the parameters of the population from which the samples were drawn. These **parametric tests** require that the assumptions of normality and homogeneity of variance are met to a reasonable degree for validity of analysis. In this chapter, we present a set of statistical procedures classified as **nonparametric**, which test hypotheses for group comparisons without normality or variance assumptions. For this reason, these methods are sometimes referred to as *distribution-free tests*.

Nonparametric methods are similar to parametric methods in that both test hypotheses and both involve the use of a statistical ratio or test statistic, with an associated probability. Similarly, the outcomes of these tests are evaluated according to a predetermined alpha level of significance. In this chapter we describe five nonparametric procedures that are the most commonly used analogs of the parametric *t*-test and *F*-test: the Mann-Whitney U-test, sign test, Wilcoxon signed-ranks test, Kruskal-Wallis one-way analysis of variance by ranks, and the Friedman two-way analysis of variance by ranks (see Table 22.1). Although these tests are easily computed with a hand-held calculator, they are also included in most statistical packages for computer analysis. We will present both the hand calculations and sample computer output.

TABLE 22.1   CORRESPONDING PARAMETRIC AND NONPARAMETRIC TESTS FOR GROUP COMPARISONS

Comparison	Parametric Test	Nonparametric Test
Two independent groups	Unpaired *t*-test	Mann-Whitney *U* test
Two related scores	Paired *t*-test	Sign test Wilcoxon signed-ranks test (T)
Three or more independent groups	One-way analysis of variance (F)	Kruskal-Wallis analysis of variance by ranks (H or χ^2)
Three or more related scores	One-way repeated measures analysis of variance (F)	Friedman two-way analysis of variance by ranks (χ_r^2)

CRITERIA FOR CHOOSING NONPARAMETRIC TESTS

Two major criteria are generally adopted for choosing a nonparametric test over a parametric procedure. The first is that assumptions of population normality and homogeneity of variance cannot be satisfied. Many clinical investigations involve variables that have not been studied sufficiently to support these assumptions. In all likelihood, most pathological conditions are represented by skewed distributions rather than symmetrical ones. In addition, small clinical samples and samples of convenience cannot automatically be considered representative of larger normal distributions.

The second criterion for choosing a nonparametric test is that data are measured on the nominal or ordinal scale. Many assessment tools have been developed around these scales. Nonparametric tests provide an objective mechanism for supporting statistical hypotheses when these levels of measurement are used.

Although nonparametric tests require fewer statistical assumptions than parametric procedures, they still put some restrictions on data. Some type of randomization procedure should be used in forming groups. This allows the researcher to make assumptions about the equality of groups before the independent variable is administered. In addition, the nonparametric tests described in this chapter apply to data that are at least at the ordinal level (see Chapter 25 for tests appropriate to nominal level data); that is, the variable of interest has an underlying continuous distribution that can be ranked, even if it cannot be measured quantitatively. For instance, strength can be measured using discrete manual muscle test grades on an ordinal scale, even though strength truly exists along a continuum. Ordinal scales are used often to measure relative changes in clinical variables such as sitting balance, function or sensation. Analysis of these types of variables represents the most appropriate use of nonparametric statistics.

The major disadvantage of nonparametric tests is that they do not accommodate complex clinical designs. There are many newer tests, however, that have been developed to allow the application of regression procedures or tests of interaction effects. These are beyond the scope of this book, but can be found in other recent texts.[1,2]

Power-Efficiency in Nonparametric Tests

Many researchers prefer to use parametric tests because they are generally more powerful. Nonparametric tests are less sensitive than parametric tests because most of them involve ranking scores rather than comparing precise metric changes. Nonparametric and parametric methods have been compared on the basis of their *power-efficiency*, which is a test's relative ability to identify significant differences for a given sample size. Generally, an increase in sample size is needed to make a nonparametric test as powerful as a parametric test. For instance, a nonparametric test may require a sample size of 50 to achieve the same degree of power as a parametric test with 30 subjects. This relationship can be expressed as a percentage that indicates the relative power-efficiency of the nonparametric test. For example, if power-efficiency is 60%, then with equal sample sizes, the nonparametric test is 60% as powerful as the parametric test. In other words, to achieve equal power with the nonparametric test, we would need 10 subjects for every 6 used with the parametric procedure.

With equal sample sizes, nonparametric tests will generally be less powerful than their parametric counterparts; however, with larger samples this discrepancy is minimized. Most of the nonparametric tests described here can achieve approximately 65% to 95% power-efficiency in comparison to their most powerful parametric analogs.[3] These figures apply to calculations based on comparisons of normal populations. With very small samples, as with six subjects or less, many nonparametric tests will be as powerful as their parametric counterparts. With larger nonnormal populations, the nonparametric statistics may actually be more powerful.[4] As power is an issue only when significant results are not obtained, a researcher need not be concerned with the relative power of nonparametric tests when the null hypothesis is rejected.

PROCEDURE FOR RANKING SCORES

Most nonparametric tests are based on rank ordering of scores. The procedure for ranking will be illustrated using the two samples shown in Table 22.2. Scores are always ranked from smallest to largest, with the rank of 1 assigned to the smallest score. Algebraic values are taken into account, so that the lowest ranks are assigned to the largest negative values, if any. The highest rank will equal n. As shown in Sample A, the rank of 1 is assigned to the smallest score (-3), the rank of 2 goes to the next smallest (0), and so on, until the rank of 8 is assigned to the highest score (16).

When two or more scores in a distribution are tied, they are each given the same rank, which is the average of the ranks they occupy. For instance, in Sample B, there are two scores with the smallest value (3). They occupy ranks 1 and 2. Therefore, they are each assigned the average of their ranks: $(1 + 2)/2 = 1.5$. The next highest value (8) receives the rank of 3, as the first two ranks are filled. The next highest value is 11, which appears three times. As we have already filled ranks 1, 2 and 3, we average the next three ranks: $(4 + 5 + 6)/3 = 5$. Each score of 11 is assigned the rank of 5. Having filled the first 6 rank positions, the last two values in the distribution are assigned ranks 7 and 8.

TABLE 22.2   EXAMPLES OF RANKED SCORES WITHOUT TIES (A) AND WITH TIES (B)

SAMPLE A ($n = 8$)	Rank	SAMPLE B ($n = 8$)	Rank
6	4	8	3
2	3	11	5
8	5	3	1.5
9	6	17	8
−3	1	11	5
0	2	3	1.5
16	8	11	5
12	7	12	7

TEST FOR TWO INDEPENDENT SAMPLES: MANN-WHITNEY U-TEST

The **Mann-Whitney U test** is one of the more powerful nonparametric procedures, designed to test the null hypothesis that two independent samples come from the same population.* This test is analogous to the parametric t-test for independent samples. Like the unpaired t-test, the U test does not require that groups be of the same size. It is, therefore, an excellent alternative to the t-test when parametric assumptions are not met.

Example

A researcher is interested in the effect of body position on a person's ability to relax, as measured by EMG biofeedback from the frontalis muscle. To study this question, 11 subjects are randomly assigned to two groups in a pretest-posttest design, with one group positioned supine, the other sitting. Results are recorded as changes in microvolt activity. The researcher hypothesizes that the positions will facilitate different levels of relaxation (a nondirectional hypothesis).

Procedure

Hypothetical data for this example are given in Table 22.3A. The first step is to combine both groups and rank all the scores in order of increasing size. The sum of the ranks assigned to each group is designated R_1 or R_2. Under the null hypothesis, we would expect the groups to be equally distributed with regard to high and low ranks, and the mean of the ranks would be equal for both groups. Any differences between the ranks should be the result of chance. The test will determine if the difference between the sums of ranks is sufficiently large to be considered significant. An alternative hypothesis can be directional or nondirectional.

The U Test Statistic

The test statistic, U, is calculated using each group as a reference, as follows:

$$U_1 = R_1 - \frac{n_1(n_1 + 1)}{2} \tag{22.1a}$$

$$U_2 = R_2 - \frac{n_2(n_2 + 1)}{2} \tag{22.1b}$$

where n_1 is the smaller sample size, n_2 is the larger sample size, and R_1 and R_2 are the sums of the ranks for the groups. Designation of n_1 or n_2 is arbitrary if groups are of equal size. Obviously, these formulas will yield different values of U. For example,

---

*Some statisticians prefer to use the Wilcoxon rank sum test to test the difference between two independent samples. This test is equivalent to the Mann-Whitney U-test.

TABLE 22.3 MANN-WHITNEY *U* TEST: CHANGE IN MICROVOLT ACTIVITY FOLLOWING RELAXATION IN TWO POSITIONS

A. DATA

Supine ($n_1 = 5$)	Rank	Sitting ($n_2 = 6$)	Rank
20	5	10	3
30	7	5	2
50	11	35	8
45	10	25	6
40	9	0	1
		15	4
	$R_1 = 42$		$R_2 = 24$

B. COMPUTATIONS

$$U_1 = R_1 - \frac{n_1(n_1 + 1)}{2} = 42 - \frac{5(5 + 1)}{2} = 27$$

$$U_2 = R_2 - \frac{n_2(n_2 + 1)}{2} = 24 - \frac{6(6 + 1)}{2} = 3 \qquad U = 3, \text{ the smaller of the values of } U_1 \text{ or } U_2$$

C. TEST FOR LARGE SAMPLES

$$z = \frac{U - \frac{n_1 n_2}{2}}{\sqrt{\frac{n_1 n_2(n_1 + n_2 + 1)}{12}}} = \frac{3 - \frac{(5)(6)}{2}}{\sqrt{\frac{(5)(6)(5 + 6 + 1)}{12}}} = \frac{-12}{\sqrt{30}} = -2.19$$

D. HYPOTHESIS TEST

Critical Value of *U*:

For $n_1 = 5$, $n_2 = 6$, at $\alpha_2 = .05$,
$U = 3$ (Table A.8)   Reject H_0.

***z* test:**

$z = -2.19 > 1.96$
(two-tailed $p = .0286$) (Table A.1) Reject H_0.

E. OUTPUT

Ranks

	GROUP	N	Mean Rank	Sum of Ranks
ACTIVITY	Supine	5	8.40	42.00
	Sitting	6	4.00	24.00
	Total	11		

Test Statistics

	ACTIVITY
Mann-Whitney U	3.000
Z	−2.191
Asymp. Sig. (2-tailed)	.028

using calculations shown in Table 22.3B, we obtain $U_1 = 27$, with Group 1 as the reference group. Using Group 2 as the reference group, we obtain $U_2 = 3$. We can show that these values are mathematically related as

$$U_1 = n_1n_2 - U_2 \tag{22.2}$$

and vice versa. For example, for the data in Table 22.3, we can demonstrate this relationship:

$$U_1 = (5)(6) - 3 = 27$$

$$U_2 = (5)(6) - 27 = 3$$

The smaller of these two values is assigned to the test statistic U. In this case, then, $U = 3$.

Critical Values of U

Critical values of U are given in Appendix Table A.8 for one- and two-tailed tests at several levels of significance. These values are compared with the *smaller value* of either U_1 or U_2. The appropriate critical values are located in the table for n_1 and n_2. The calculated value of U must be *equal to or less than* the tabled value to be significant. (*Note:* This is opposite to the way we have used critical values with parametric tests.)

For the current example, at $\alpha_2 = .05$, with $n_1 = 5$ and $n_2 = 6$, the critical value of U is 3. Because the calculated value, $U = 3$, is equal to this critical value, we can reject H_0. Our conclusion is then based on visual examination of the mean ranks, which shows that greater relaxation (higher mean rank) is attained in the supine position (Table 22.3E).

Large Samples

When sample size exceeds 25, Table A.8 cannot be used. In this situation, the value of U is converted to z and tested against the standard normal distribution:

$$z = \frac{U - \dfrac{n_1n_2}{2}}{\sqrt{\dfrac{n_1n_2(n_1 + n_2 + 1)}{12}}} \tag{22.3}$$

Even though the present example does not warrant it, we have used the data to illustrate this application in Table 22.3C. In this formula it does not matter if U_1 or U_2 is used. The absolute value of z will be the same either way.

Critical values of z (in Appendix Table A.1) are used to determine if this ratio is significant.[†] For a two-tailed test at .05 (we proposed a nondirectional hypothesis), $z = 1.96$. Our calculated value exceeds this critical value, and the null hypothesis is rejected. This outcome agrees with the results obtained using Table A.8. We can also

---

[†]For one-tailed tests at .05 and .01, the critical values are 1.645 and 2.326, respectively. For two-tailed tests, these critical values are 1.96 and 2.576, respectively. The calculated value of z must be *greater than or equal to* the critical value to be considered significant.

determine the exact probability associated with the test by finding the tail probability for z in Table A.1. For $z = 2.19$, the one-tailed probability is .0143. Because we have proposed a nondirectional hypothesis, we double this value for a two-tailed test. Therefore, $p = .0286$. These findings are shown in the computer output in Table 21.3E.

TEST FOR MORE THAN TWO INDEPENDENT SAMPLES: KRUSKAL-WALLIS ONE-WAY ANALYSIS OF VARIANCE BY RANKS

When three or more groups are compared ($k \geq 3$), a nonparametric analysis of variance is appropriate for the same reasons that an F-test is used with parametric data. The **Kruskal-Wallis one-way analysis of variance by ranks** is a nonparametric analog of the one-way analysis of variance. It is a powerful alternative to the F-test when variance and normality assumptions for parametric tests are not met. It is also the most appropriate way to handle ordinal level data when more than two groups are compared. With $k = 2$, this test is equivalent to the Mann-Whitney U-test. Multiple comparison procedures can also be applied.

Example

We want to study the effect of three modalities for relieving chronic low back pain. We randomly assign 17 subjects ($N = 17$) to receive ice ($n = 6$), hot pack ($n = 6$), or ultrasound ($n = 5$). Pain is measured on a visual analog scale from 0 mm (pain-free) to 100 mm (severe pain). Scores are recorded as the change in level of pain from pretreatment to posttreatment levels.

Procedure

Hypothetical data are reported in Table 22.4A. The procedures for the Kruskal-Wallis ANOVA are similar to those used for the Mann-Whitney U-test. The first step is to combine data for all groups and rank scores from the smallest to the largest. The smallest score receives the rank of 1, and the largest score is assigned the rank of N. Ties are assigned average ranks.

    The ranks are then summed for each group separately, as shown in Table 22.4A. If the null hypothesis is true, we would expect an equal distribution of ranks under the three conditions.

The H Statistic

The test statistic for the Kruskal-Wallis test is H, calculated according to

$$H = \frac{12}{N(N + 1)} \sum \frac{R^2}{n} - 3(N + 1) \tag{22.4}$$

where N is the number of cases in all samples combined, n is the number of cases in each individual sample, and R is the sum of ranks for each individual sample. This calculation is illustrated in Table 22.4B. For this example, $H = 7.243$.

TABLE 22.4 KRUSKAL-WALLIS ONE-WAY ANALYSIS OF VARIANCE BY RANKS: CHANGES IN LEVEL OF PAIN ($N = 14$)

A. DATA

	Group 1: Ice		Group 2: Hot Packs		Group 3: Ultrasound	
	Change score	Rank	Change score	Rank	Change score	Rank
	40	8	35	6	80	14
	60	11	25	2.5	50	10
	10	1	30	4.5	75	13
	25	2.5	40	8	70	12
	30	4.5	40	8		
R		27		29		49
n		5		5		4
$\bar{R}$		5.4		5.8		12.25

B. COMPUTATIONS

$$H = \frac{12}{N(N+1)} \sum \frac{R^2}{n} - 3(N+1)$$

$$= \frac{12}{14(14+1)} \left[\frac{(27)^2}{5} + \frac{(29)^2}{5} + \frac{(49)^2}{4} \right] - 3(14+1)$$

$$= \frac{12}{210} [914.25] - 45 = 7.243$$

C. HYPOTHESIS TEST

For $df = 2$, $\chi^2 = 5.99$ (Table A.5)   Reject H_0

D. OUTPUT

Ranks

	GROUP	N	Mean Rank
PAIN	Ice	5	5.40
	HP	5	5.80
	US	4	12.25
	Total	14	

Test Statistics

	PAIN
Chi-Square	7.340
df	2
Asymp. Sig.	.025

Note: Calculated values may vary due to rounding differences.

Critical Values

The H statistic is tested using the chi-square distribution with $k - 1$ degrees of freedom (Table A.5).[‡] With three groups we will have 2 df. Therefore, we test H against the critical value of 5.99. Our calculated value of $H = 7.243$ is significant, and we can reject H_0. The output for this analysis is shown in Table 22.4D.

Some researchers will stop here, basing their final decision on a subjective comparison of the mean ranks for each group. In this example, it is fairly clear that scores for the ultrasound group are higher than the other two groups. However, when such judgments are not sufficient, a multiple comparison procedure can be used to determine which groups are different. This will be described shortly.

Ties

A substantial number of ties can have a conservative effect on the value of H, making the test less powerful. This may be a concern when the test result is not significant and when greater than 25% of the scores are tied. A correction factor can be applied to increase the value of H under these conditions. Unless the number of ties is substantial, however, the effect of the correction will be minimal. Obviously, if H is significant without the correction, there is no point in making the adjustment. Procedures for this correction can be found in the text by Siegel and Castellan.[5]

Multiple Comparison for the Kruskal–Wallis ANOVA

When H is significant, it is usually of interest to determine which specific groups are different from each other. The Mann-Whitney U test is often used as a multiple comparison procedure; however, a Bonferroni correction should be applied to control for the increased risk of Type I error, using the same rationale that applies to multiple t-tests. Siegel and Castellan[5] present a multiple comparison procedure to protect against this increased error rate.

A multiple comparison for the Kruskal-Wallis ANOVA tests the significance of pairwise differences between conditions, based on the *mean of the ranks* for each sample: $\overline{R} = R/n$. For the data in Table 22.3, $\overline{R}_1 = 5.4$, $\overline{R}_2 = 5.8$, and $\overline{R}_3 = 12.25$. The total number of pairwise comparisons associated with an analysis will be equal to $k(k - 1)/2$. With three mean rankings ($k = 3$), we will have $3(3 - 1)/2 = 3$ comparisons.

Minimum Significant Difference

Each pairwise comparison is tested against a minimum significant difference (MSD) based on the formula

$$|\overline{R}_1 - \overline{R}_2| \geq z\sqrt{\frac{N(N + 1)}{12}\left(\frac{1}{n_1} + \frac{1}{n_2}\right)} \tag{22.5}$$

[‡]When samples are very small, with five subjects or fewer per group, alternative tables can be used to obtain critical values of H. See Siegel and Castellan.[5]

where N is the total number of subjects in all samples combined, and n_1 and n_2 are the respective sample sizes for the two groups involved in the specific pairwise comparison. Any absolute difference between mean ranks that is *equal to or larger than* the minimum significant difference is considered significant.

The value of z in Equation (22.5) is based on the total number of comparisons to be made and the desired level of significance for the overall test. We obtain z from Table 22.5. The α level selected in the table is based on the desired *familywise error rate* (α_{FW}), that is, the overall probability associated with the entire set of comparisons. Researchers may choose to keep α_{FW} at .05, which is considered a conservative practice, or they may accept higher probability levels, such as .15 or .20, when the risk of Type I error is not of great concern.[§] Typically, a larger α is chosen as k increases.[6]

Example

We can illustrate this procedure using the data in Table 22.4. To compare Groups 1 ($n_1 = 5$) and 2($n_2 = 5$), we first specify our desired familywise error rate, say $\alpha_{FW} = .15$. Next, we determine that there will be a total of three comparisons. According to Table 22.5, at $\alpha_{FW} = .15$, $z = 1.96$ for three comparisons. We can now compute the minimum significant difference for this comparison using Equation (22.5):

$$MSD = 1.96\sqrt{\frac{14(14+1)}{12}\left(\frac{1}{5}+\frac{1}{5}\right)} = 1.96\sqrt{7} = 5.19$$

TABLE 22.5 CRITICAL VALUES OF z TO BE USED IN CALCULATING MULTIPLE COMPARISONS WITH H AND χ_r^2 STATISTICS

Number of Comparisons	α_{FW} .25	.20	.15	.10	.05
1	1.150	1.282	1.440	1.645	1.960
2	1.534	1.645	1.780	1.960	2.241
3	1.732	1.834	1.960	2.128	2.394
4	1.863	1.960	2.080	2.241	2.498
5	1.960	2.054	2.170	2.326	2.576
6	2.037	2.128	2.241	2.394	2.638
7	2.100	2.189	2.300	2.450	2.690
8	2.154	2.241	2.350	2.498	2.734
9	2.200	2.287	2.394	2.539	2.773
10	2.241	2.326	2.432	2.576	2.807

[§]The actual probability associated with each individual comparison is $\alpha_{FW}/k(k-1)$. Therefore, with $k = 3$, and $\alpha_{FW} = .05$, the per comparison error rate is $.05/3(3-1) = .008$. At $\alpha_{FW} = .20$, the per comparison error rate would be $.20/3(3-1) = .03$.

We compare this minimum difference with the absolute difference between the mean ranks for Groups 1 and 2:

$$|\overline{R}_1 - \overline{R}_2| = |5.4 - 5.8| = 0.4$$

Because this difference is less than the minimum significant difference, it is not considered significant. There is no significant difference between ice and hot packs for relieving pain.

We compare Groups 1 and 3 ($n_1 = 5, n_3 = 4$) using

$$MSD = 1.96\sqrt{\frac{14(14 + 1)}{12}\left(\frac{1}{5} + \frac{1}{4}\right)} = 1.96\sqrt{7.875} = 5.50$$

The difference, $|\overline{R}_1 - \overline{R}_3| = |5.4 - 12.25| = 6.85$, is greater than this minimum significant difference, and, therefore, this represents a significant effect. Ultrasound ($\overline{R}_3$) is more effective than ice ($\overline{R}_1$).

Finally, we compare Groups 2 and 3 ($n_2 = 5, n_3 = 4$) using the minimum significant difference of 5.50 (obtained earlier for the same sample sizes):

$$|\overline{R}_2 - \overline{R}_3| = |5.8 - 12.25| = 6.45$$

This comparison is also significant. We can now conclude that ultrasound ($\overline{R}_3$) is more effective for reducing low back pain than either ice ($\overline{R}_1$) or hot packs ($\overline{R}_2$).

When all k samples are of equal size, one minimum significant difference can be used for all comparisons, using the formula

$$MSD = z\sqrt{\frac{k(N - 1)}{6}} \tag{22.6}$$

TESTS FOR TWO CORRELATED SAMPLES: SIGN TEST AND WILCOXON SIGNED-RANKS TEST

Two procedures are commonly used for testing the difference between correlated samples: the sign test and the Wilcoxon signed-ranks test. These tests are used with two-level repeated measures designs. They are analogous to the parametric t-test for correlated or paired samples.

The Sign Test

The **sign test** is one of the simplest nonparametric tests because it requires no mathematical calculations. It is used with binomial data, and does not require that measurements be quantitative. As its name implies, the data are analyzed using plus and minus signs rather than numerical values. Therefore, this test provides a mechanism for testing relative differentiations such as more–less, higher–lower, or larger–smaller. It is particularly useful when quantification is impossible or unfeasible and when subjective ratings are necessary.

Example

We are interested in the effect of knee angle on knee extensor strength. Using a manual muscle test (MMT), we will study 10 patients, six months following a total knee replacement. MMT grades are recorded from 0 (no muscle activity) to 12 (normal strength). We hypothesize that knee extensor strength will be different with the knee in 90° and 15° of flexion.

Procedure

Hypothetical data are shown in Table 22.6A. The sign test is applied to the differences between each pair of scores, based on whether the direction of difference is positive or negative. In this example, we will use the grades measured at 15 degrees as the reference and record whether the grade at 90 degrees is greater (+), the same (0), or less (−) than the reference grade, always maintaining the same direction of comparison. It does not matter which value is used as the reference, as long as the order is consistent. In the fourth column in Table 22.6A, the signs of the differences are listed. When no difference is obtained, a zero is recorded.

Under the null hypothesis, we would expect half the differences to be positive and the other half to be negative. We will reject H_0 if one sign occurs sufficiently less often. If we propose a directional alternative hypothesis, we must be sure that the direction of comparison supports the predicted direction of change. For this illustration, we have proposed a nondirectional hypothesis.

To proceed with the test, we count the number of plus signs and the number of minus signs. Ties, recorded as zeros, are discarded from the analysis, and n is reduced accordingly. In this example, 7 of the 10 subjects showed differences, with three ties. Therefore, $n = 7$. There are 6 plus signs and 1 minus sign (see Table 22.6A). We take the smaller of these two values, the *number of fewer signs*, and assign it the test statistic, x. In this case, $x = 1$, the number of minus signs.

Test Probabilities

To determine the probability of obtaining x under H_0, we refer to Appendix Table A.9. This table lists one-tailed probabilities associated with x for values up to $n = 30$, where n is the number of pairs whose differences showed direction. Two-tailed tests require doubling the probabilities given in the table.

For $x = 1$ and $n = 7$, the table shows $p = .062$. Because we have proposed a nondirectional hypothesis, we double this value for a two-tailed probability of $p = .124$. This is greater than the acceptable level of .05, and we cannot reject H_0. The probability that the difference in the number of plus and minus signs occurred by chance is too great. We conclude that there is no significant difference in knee extensor strength with the knee at 90 and 15 degrees.

The determination of the probability associated with x is based on a theoretical distribution called the *binomial probability distribution*. A binomial outcome is one that can take only two forms, in this case either positive or negative. The binomial test determines the likelihood of getting the smaller number of plus or minus signs out of the total number of differences just by chance.

TABLE 22.6 **SIGN TEST AND WILCOXON SIGNED-RANKS TEST: MMT GRADES FOR KNEE EXTENSION WITH KNEE AT TWO ANGLES**

A. DATA

Subject	Angle 90°	Angle 15°	Sign	d	Rank of d	Ranks with less frequent sign
1	8	8	0	0		
2	10	11	−	−1	−1	−1
3	7	7	0	0		
4	9	7	+	+2	+3	
5	10	8	+	+2	+3	
6	11	7	+	+4	+7	
7	10	8	+	+2	+3	
8	10	7	+	+3	+5.5	
9	8	8	0	0		
10	10	7	+	+3	+5.5	

$$T = -1$$

B. HYPOTHESIS TEST/OUTPUT FOR THE SIGN TEST

6 plus signs, 1 minus sign, $x = 1$ (number of fewer signs)

For $x = 1, n = 7, p = .124$ (Table A.9)

$$z = \frac{|D| - 1}{\sqrt{n}} = \frac{|5| - 1}{\sqrt{7}} = 1.51$$

Do not reject H_0.

Frequencies

90–15	N
Negative Differences (a)	1
Positive Differences (b)	6
Ties(c)	3
Total	10

(a) 90 < 15 (b) 90 > 15
(c) 90 = 15

Test Statistics

	90–15
Exact Sig. (2-tailed)	.125

C. HYPOTHESIS TEST/OUTPUT FOR THE SIGNED-RANKS TEST

Sum ranks with less frequent sign = −1   For $n = 7$ at $\alpha_2 = .05$, $T = 2$ (Table A. 10)   Reject H_0

$$z = \frac{T - \dfrac{n(n + 1)}{4}}{\sqrt{\dfrac{n(n + 1)(2n + 1)}{24}}} = \frac{1 - \dfrac{7(7 + 1)}{4}}{\sqrt{\dfrac{7(7 + 1)(2(7) + 1)}{24}}} = \frac{-13}{\sqrt{35}} = -2.20$$

Ranks

90–15	N	Mean Rank	Sum of Ranks
Negative Ranks	1(a)	1.00	1.00
Positive Ranks	6(b)	4.50	27.00
Ties	3(c)		
Total	10		

(a) 90 < 15; (b) 90 > 15; (c) 90 = 15.

Test Statistics

	90–15
Z	−2.217
Asymp. Sig. (2-tailed)	.027

Note: Calculated values may differ due to rounding differences.

Large Samples

With sample sizes greater than 30, x is converted to z and tested against the normal distribution according to the formula

$$z = \frac{|D| - 1}{\sqrt{n}} \tag{22.7}$$

where $|D|$ is the absolute difference between the number of plus and minus signs.

This calculation is illustrated in Table 22.6B for data with six plus signs and one minus sign, resulting in $z = 1.51$. Using the critical value of $z = 1.96$ for $\alpha_2 = .05$, this outcome does not achieve significance. The output for this analysis is also shown.

The Wilcoxon Signed-Ranks Test

The sign test evaluates differences within paired scores based solely on whether one score is larger or smaller than the other. This is often the best approach with subjective clinical variables that offer no greater precision; however, if data are able to provide information on the relative magnitude of differences, the more powerful **Wilcoxon signed-ranks test** can be used. This test examines both the direction of difference and the relative amount of difference.

Example

Consider the example presented in the previous section. In Table 22.6A, we have listed the manual muscle test grades as ordinal values, based on a scale of 0 to 12. We obtain a difference score for each subject, labeled d. When $d = 0$, the subject is dropped from the analysis, and n is reduced, as it was in the sign test.

Procedure

We proceed by ranking the difference scores, *without regard to sign*, and discarding any pairs with no difference. We then attach the sign of the difference to the obtained ranks. For instance, in our example, the rank of 1 is given to the smallest difference score (Subject 2), and then assigned -1 because it reflects a negative difference. Tied difference scores are given the mean of their ranks. Therefore, ranks 2, 3 and 4 are taken by Subjects 4, 5 and 7, who all have a difference score of 2. These scores are each assigned the average rank of 3. Subjects 8 and 10 are tied with difference scores of 3, filling ranks 5 and 6, which are averaged to rank 5.5. The final rank of 7 is assigned to Subject 6.

If the null hypothesis is true, we would expect to find an equal representation of positive and negative signs among the larger and smaller ranks; that is, the sum of the positive ranks should be equal to the sum of the negative ranks. We reject H_0 if either of these sums is too small.

The T Statistic

We determine if there are fewer positive or negative ranks, and then sum the ranks for the *less frequent sign*. This sum is assigned the test statistic, T. In this example, there are fewer ranks with negative signs, with the sum of -1. Therefore, $T = -1$. Only the absolute value of T is used to determine significance. The sign of T is of concern only when performing a one-tailed test.

Critical Values

Critical values of T are given in Appendix Table A.12 for one- and two-tailed tests, where n is the number of pairs with nonzero differences. The absolute calculated value of T must be *less than or equal to* the critical value to achieve significance. Note once again that this is opposite to the way most critical values are used. For this analysis, at $\alpha_2 = .05$, with $n = 7$, the critical value of T is 2. Therefore, our calculated value of $T = 1$ is significant (see Table 22.6C). We can reject H_0 and conclude that knee extensor strength is different with the knee at 90 and 15 degrees. Visual examination of the data tells us that strength is greater with the knee at 90 degrees.

It is interesting to note the difference between the outcome of this analysis and the outcome of the sign test on the same data. We were able to substantiate a significant difference using the Wilcoxon procedure, because it is sensitive to relative differences, not just direction. Therefore, if data achieve adequate precision, the Wilcoxon test is recommended over the sign test.

Large Samples

With sample sizes over 25, the absolute value of T can be converted to z according to

$$z = \frac{T - \dfrac{n(n+1)}{4}}{\sqrt{\dfrac{n(n+1)(2n+1)}{24}}} \tag{22.8}$$

where n is the number of paired observations. For this analysis, $z = -2.20$ (see Table 22.6C). The absolute value of z is greater than the critical value 1.96, which represents a significant difference at $\alpha_2 = .05$. According to Appendix Table A.1, the two-tailed significance associated with $z = 2.20$ is .0278. This is illustrated in the output for the z test.

TEST FOR MORE THAN TWO CORRELATED SAMPLES: FRIEDMAN TWO-WAY ANALYSIS OF VARIANCE BY RANKS

In this section we present a nonparametric test to analyze data from a single-factor repeated measures design with three or more experimental conditions. The **Friedman two-way analysis of variance by ranks** is a powerful alternative to the parametric repeated measures ANOVA when ordinal data are used or when parametric assumptions are not tenable. The test is given the designation "two-way" based on the interpretation that "subjects" is treated as an independent variable with $n = 1$ per cell of the design. It is assumed that the number of measurements in each experimental condition will be the same.

Example

We are interested in measuring the effect of changing body position on blood pressure in six patients with chronic pulmonary disease. Each patient will be placed in three positions—level, head down and head elevated—in random order. Blood pressure will be measured within 1 minute of assuming the position. We may choose to use a non-parametric form of analysis for this study because the sample is small, and because we do not have sufficient reason to assume that blood pressure for a population of patients with this disease will be normally distributed. In addition, although blood pressure measurements can be considered ratio level data, we can rationalize that the lack of reli-ability in the data warrants using a nonparametric test.

Procedure

Hypothetical data for this study are reported in Table 22.7A. Data are arranged so that rows represent subjects (n) and columns represent experimental conditions (k). In this example, $n = 6$ and $k = 3$. We begin by converting all scores to ranks; however, the ranking process for this test is different from that used with the Kruskal-Wallis ANOVA. Here the ranks are assigned across each row (within a subject). Ties are assigned average ranks within a row. The highest rank within a row will equal k.

The next step is to sum the ranks within each column. If the null hypothesis is true, we would expect the distribution of ranks to be a matter of chance, and high and low ranks should be evenly distributed across all treatment conditions. Therefore, the rank sums within each column should be equal. If the alternative hypothesis is true, at least one pair of conditions will show a difference.

The χ_r^2 Statistic

The test statistic for the Friedman ANOVA is χ_r^2 (read "chi square r"). It is computed using the formula

$$\chi_r^2 = \frac{12}{nk(k + 1)}\sum R^2 - 3n(k + 1) \tag{22.9}$$

where n is the number of subjects (rows), k is the number of treatment conditions (columns) and $\sum R^2$ is the sum of the squared ranks for each column. Calculation of χ_r^2 is illustrated in Table 22.7B. For this analysis, $\chi_r^2 = 9.25$.

Critical Values

The distribution of χ_r^2 follows the standard χ^2 distribution with $k - 1$ degrees of free-dom, where k is the number of experimental conditions (Appendix Table A.5). With 2 df, we measure our calculated value of 9.25 against 5.99 (at $\alpha = .05$). The calculated

TABLE 22.7   FRIEDMAN TWO-WAY ANALYSIS OF VARIANCE BY RANKS: BLOOD PRESSURE IN THREE POSITIONS ($n = 6$)

A. DATA

Subject	(1) Level BP	(1) Level Rank	(2) Elevated BP	(2) Elevated Rank	(3) Down BP	(3) Down Rank
1	110	1	150	2	175	3
2	100	1.5	100	1.5	110	3
3	120	1	140	3	135	2
4	110	1	130	2	155	3
5	120	1	130	2	145	3
6	130	1	155	2	170	3
R		6.5		12.5		17
$\bar{R}$		1.08		2.08		2.83
R^2		42.25		156.25		289.00

B. COMPUTATIONS

$$\chi_r^2 = \frac{12}{nk(k + 1)}\sum R^2 - 3n(k + 1)$$

$$= \frac{12}{(6)(3)(3 + 1)}[42.25 + 156.25 + 289] - 3(6)(3 + 1)$$

$$= \frac{12}{72}[487.5] - 72 = 9.25$$

C. HYPOTHESIS TEST/OUTPUT

For $k = 3$ ($df = 2$)
$\chi^2 = 5.99$ at $\alpha = .05$ (Table A.5)
Reject H_0.

Ranks

	Mean Rank
DOWN	2.83
ELEV	2.08
LEVEL	1.08

Test Statistics

N	6
Chi-Square	9.652
df	2
Asymp. Sig.	.008

Note: Calculated values may differ due to rounding differences.

value must be *equal to or larger than* the critical value to be significant. Therefore, our test is significant (see Table 22.7C).

Multiple Comparison for the Friedman ANOVA

When χ_r^2 is significant, we can test all pairwise differences using a multiple comparison procedure. Although the Wilcoxon signed-ranks test is often used for this purpose, a specific multiple comparison has been developed for the Friedman ANOVA.[5] We propose a familywise error rate as an overall level of significance for the combined set of contrasts in the experiment.

Minimum Significant Difference

The expression used to determine the minimum significant difference (MSD) for all pairwise contrasts is

$$|R_1 - R_2| \geq z\sqrt{\frac{nk(k + 1)}{6}} \qquad (22.10)$$

where R_1 and R_2 are the rank totals for each treatment condition, n is the number of subjects, and k is the number of treatment conditions. The value of z is taken from Table 22.5 for the appropriate number of comparisons ($k(k - 1)/2$) and the desired familywise α level for the combined set of comparisons. For the current example, we have a total of three comparisons, and we propose a familywise α level of .10. Therefore, $z = 2.128$.

We compute the minimum significant difference:

$$MSD = 2.128\sqrt{\frac{6(3)(3 + 1)}{6}} = 2.128\sqrt{12} = 7.37$$

For this analysis, contrasts are made between *rank totals* for each treatment condition, not mean ranks. The absolute value of differences between rank sums for each pair of treatment conditions must be *greater than or equal to* the obtained critical value. Because we are dealing with repeated measures, and all subjects are represented under each treatment, there is only one critical value for all contrasts. The three pairwise comparisons for this study are

$$|R_1 - R_2| = |6.5 - 12.5| = 6.0$$

$$|R_1 - R_3| = |6.5 - 17.0| = 10.5$$

$$|R_2 - R_3| = |12.5 - 17.0| = 4.5$$

The only difference score that exceeds the critical value of 7.37 is obtained from the second comparison between conditions 1 and 3. Therefore, there is a significant difference in blood pressure when an individual is positioned level versus head down, with higher pressures obtained in the head down position. No other contrasts are significant.

COMMENTARY

The Debate

Nonparametric procedures offer clinical researchers a powerful and easily understood statistical mechanism for analyzing changes measured with subjective tools. Because of the nature of many clinical assessments, the ability to analyze ordinal data is important. There is still some debate among statisticians and researchers concerning the appropriate application of parametric versus nonparametric statistics with ordinal data. The classical view is that only nonparametric procedures should be used with ordinal measurements; however, many researchers do apply parametric tests to ordinal data, presumably because parametric tests have greater statistical power. This practice has been justified by assuming that the ordinal intervals are consistent, even though sensitivity of measurement may be unable to document this. Therefore, the analysis would not conceptually violate the assumptions of the parametric test.[7,8] Although some assessment scales can be constructed in such a way as to define intervals as precisely as possible, it is probably unreasonable to assume that constructs such as function, manual resistance, sensation and so on, typically measured as ranks, can be measured with sufficient reliability that intervals can be considered equal. It is also likely that many of these scales are nonlinear, so that intervals at extremes of the scale will be different from those toward the center. Those who use this approach or who interpret findings of others who have used it must consider the potential for jeopardizing the validity of statistical outcomes by treating ordinal data as interval data.[9]

Nonparametric methods are also appropriate for use with interval or ratio data when distributions are skewed or when sample sizes are too small to assume representation of a normal distribution; however, nonparametric procedures can be wasteful of information when used with data on the interval or ratio scales, because precise data are reduced to ranks. Therefore, when the criterion for using nonparametric tests is based on violations of normality only, it may be useful to transform data using a logarithmic transformation to achieve a normal distribution (see Appendix D) and to apply a parametric test.

The tests that have been included in this chapter are only a sampling of available nonparametric procedures. Statisticians continue to develop and refine these tests and to expand the capabilities of nonparametric methods into areas such as regression and factorial designs. Many tests have been developed with very specific purposes, such as comparing several treatment groups with a single control or looking at differences in variables that have an inherent order. Nonparametric statistics can also be used for correlation procedures and for testing nominal scale data. These procedures are presented in Chapters 23 and 25.

REFERENCES

1. Conover WJ. *Practical Nonparametric Statistics* (3rd ed.). New York: John Wiley & Sons, 1999.
2. O'Connell AA. *Logistic Regression Models for Ordinal Response Variables.* Thousand Oaks, CA: Sage Publications, 2005.
3. Winer BJ, Michels KM, Brown DR. *Statistical Principles in Experimental Design* (3rd ed.). New York: McGraw-Hill, 1991.
4. Neave HR, Granger WJ. A Monte Carlo study comparing various two-sample tests for differences in means. *Technometrics* 1968;10:509–522.
5. Siegel S, Castellan NJ. *Nonparametric Statistics for the Behavioral Sciences* (2nd ed.). New York: McGraw-Hill, 1988.
6. Daniel WW. *Applied Nonparametric Statistics* (2nd ed.). Belmont, CA: Wadsworth Publishing, 1989.

7. Wang ST, Yu ML, Wang CJ, Huang CC. Bridging the gap between the pros and cons in treating ordinal scales as interval scales from an analysis point of view. *Nurs Res* 1999;48:226–229.
8. Gaito J. Measurement scales and statistics: Resurgence of an old misconception. *Psychol Bull* 1980;87:564–567.
9. Royeen CB, Seaver WL. Promise in nonparametrics. *Am J Occup Ther* 1986;40:191–193.

CHAPTER 23
Correlation

The statistical procedures we have described thus far have all focused on the comparison of a measured dependent variable across categories of an independent variable. These procedures are generally applied to experimental and quasi-experimental designs for the purpose of group comparisons. We will now begin to examine procedures for exploratory analyses, where the purpose of the research question is to evaluate the relationship between two measured variables. Where statistical tests of group differences address the question "Is group A different from group B?" or "Does this treatment cause this outcome?", measures of **correlation** ask, "What is the relationship between A and B?" or "Does variable A increase with variable B?"

The concept of correlation is, by and large, a familiar one. Pairs of observations, X and Y, are examined to see if they tend to "go together." For instance, we generally accept that taller people tend to weigh more than shorter people, that children resemble their parents in intelligence, and that heart rate increases with physical exertion. These variables are correlated, in that the value of one variable (X) is associated with the value of the other variable (Y). With a strong correlation, we can infer something about the second value by knowing the first. Correlation can be applied to paired observations on two different variables, such as heart rate and level of exertion, or to one variable measured on two occasions, such as intelligence of a parent and child.

Correlation coefficients are used to quantitatively describe the strength and direction of a relationship between two variables. The purpose of this chapter is to introduce several types of correlation coefficients that can be applied to a variety of exploratory research designs and types of data. The most commonly reported measure is the Pearson product-moment coefficient of correlation, for use when both X and Y are on the interval or ratio scales. We include procedures for correlating ranked data using the Spearman rho (r_S) and several correlation methods for use with data in the form of dichotomies.

SCATTER PLOTS

It is often useful to examine a statistical relationship by first creating a **scatter diagram** or **scatter plot**, as shown in Figure 23.1. In a scatter plot each point (dot) represents the intersection of a pair of related observations. With a sufficient number of data points, a scatter plot can visually clarify the strength and shape of a relationship. For instance, the points in Figure 23.1A show a pattern in which the values of Y increase in exact proportion to the values of X. This is considered a perfect positive relationship, with data points falling on a straight line. In Figure 23.1B, the data demonstrate a negative slope in a perfect negative relationship, with lower values of Y associated with higher values of X.

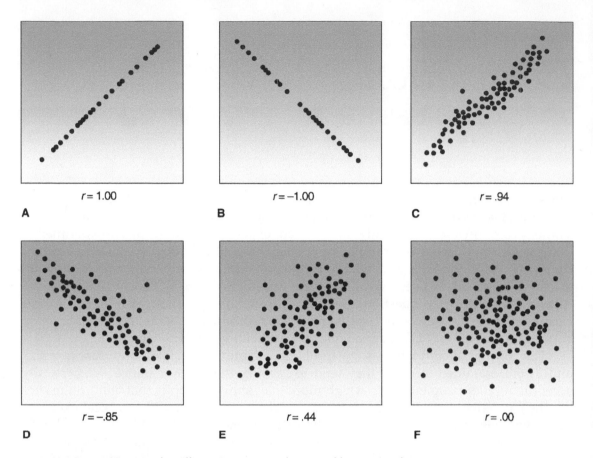

FIGURE 23.1   Scatter plots illustrating various degrees of linear correlation.

Perfect relationships are truly rare, however. Generally the association between X and Y does not follow a perfect pattern, and values of X and Y will change in varying proportions. Figure 23.1C shows a strong positive correlation; this pattern might reflect the relationship between height and weight, for example. Figure 23.1D shows a strong negative correlation; this might represent the relationship between leg length and the number of steps needed to walk a given distance. These two patterns reveal data that are clustered in relatively linear patterns. Figure 23.1E shows a weaker positive relationship, one that is harder to interpret visually than the others. We might see such a pattern if we looked at lower extremity strength and overall physical function, where a relationship exists, but individuals respond differently for a variety of reasons. Scatter plots that occur in random or circular patterns, as in Figure 23.1F, reflect no linear relationship between X and Y, or near-zero correlation. This might be the case if we studied the relationship between students' exam grades and height, for example. In this case, the value of Y is not associated with the value of X; that is, all observed variability is random.

CORRELATION COEFFICIENTS

Inspection of data in a scatter plot provides some idea about a relationship, but is not adequate for summarizing that relationship. The correlation coefficient is used to provide an index that reflects a quantitative measure of the relationship between two vari-

---

BOX 23.1 What Is a Strong Correlation?

The value of the correlation coefficient is a measure of strength of association between two variables. There are no widely accepted criteria for defining a strong versus moderate versus weak association. As a general guideline we offer the following:

0.00 to .25	Little or no relationship
.25 to .50	Fair relationship
.50 to .75	Moderate to good relationship
above .75	Good to excellent relationship

We hasten to emphasize, however, that *these values should not be used as strict cutoff points*, as they are affected by sample size, measurement error and the types of variables being studied. *Please use them as a starting point only.* We hesitate to even provide such criteria, because they are often quoted without regard to the context of the data. Sociological and behavioral scientists often use lower correlations as evidence of functionally useful relationships for the interpretation of complex abstract phenomena. Such interpretations must be based on the nature of the data, the purpose of the research and the researcher's knowledge of the subject matter.

---

ables. For most applications, a lowercase *r* is used to represent a sample correlation coefficient. Correlation coefficients can take values ranging from −1.00 for a perfect negative relationship, to 0.00 for no correlation, to +1.00 for a perfect positive relationship. The *magnitude* of the correlation coefficient indicates the *strength* of the association between X and Y. The closer the value is to ±1.00, the stronger the association (see Box 23.1). The *sign* of the correlation coefficient indicates the *direction* of the relationship. In a positive relationship, X increases as Y increases, and X decreases as Y decreases. In a negative relationship, X increases as Y decreases, and vice versa.

In reality, because of random effects, we seldom see either perfect or zero correlation. We will typically encounter values of *r* that fall between 0.00 and ±1.00. These values are expressed as decimals, usually to two places, such as $r = .75$ or $r = -.62$. The plots in Figure 23.1 represent a variety of potential outcomes for a correlation analysis between variables X and Y, showing different values of correlation coefficients. Data that cluster closer to a straight line have higher correlation coefficients.

LINEAR VERSUS CURVILINEAR RELATIONSHIPS

The pattern of a relationship between two variables is often classified as linear or nonlinear. The plots in Figures 23.1A and B are perfectly linear because the points fall on a single straight line. The plots in Figures 23.1C–E can also be considered linear, although as they begin to deviate from a straight line, their correlation decreases. The closer the points are to a straight line, the higher the value of *r*.

The coefficient *r* is a measure of **linear relationship** only. This means that the value of *r* reflects the true nature of a relationship only when scores vary in a linear fashion. When a **curvilinear relationship** is present, the linear correlation coefficient will not be able to describe it accurately.* For instance, a curvilinear shape typically characterizes the relationship between strength and age. As age increases so does strength, until a plateau is reached in adulthood, followed by a decline in elderly years. This type of relationship is illustrated in Figure 23.2.

Because *r* measures only linear functions, the correlation coefficient for a curvilinear relationship can be close to zero, even when *X* and *Y* are indeed related. For example, a systematic relationship is clearly evident between *X* and *Y* in Figure 23.2, although *r* = .18 suggests a very weak relationship. This should caution the researcher to be critical about the interpretation of correlation coefficients. By plotting a scatter diagram, researchers can observe whether the association in a set of data is linear or curvilinear, and thereby decide if *r* is an appropriate statistic for analysis.

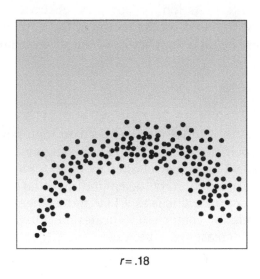

r = .18

FIGURE 23.2   Illustration of a strong curvilinear relationship, yielding a poor linear correlation.

---

*The *eta coefficient* (η), also called the correlation ratio, is an index that does not assume a linear relationship between two variables. To establish nonlinear correlation using eta, one variable must be nominal, i.e. categorical. If both variables are continuous, one must be converted to categories or groups. An ANOVA can be used to compare these groups on the continuous variable. The eta coefficient can then be computed as follows:

$$\eta = \sqrt{\frac{SS_b}{SS_t}},$$ where SS_b is the between-groups sum of squares, and SS_t is the total sum of squares from the ANOVA.

The interpretation of η is the same as *r*, although η can only range from 0.00 to +1.00 (it cannot be negative). The square of eta (η^2) is interpreted as r^2 (see Chapter 24). The value of η^2 is also an effect size index for the *t*-test and ANOVA (see Appendix C).[1,2]

THE CORRELATION MATRIX

Studies using correlation analysis often examine several variables at one time, and may include a matrix of **intercorrelations**,[†] which presents the correlation coefficients for all pairs of variables. Table 23.1 shows such an arrangement for data collected in a study of prognostic characteristics for independent ambulation in children with traumatic brain injury following inpatient rehabilitation.[3]

Note that the table is triangular; that is, values below the diagonal would be redundant of those above the diagonal and, therefore, are not included. The values on the diagonal will always be 1.00, representing the perfect correlation of each variable with itself, which is why these values are often omitted. The values off the diagonal are the correlation coefficients for each pair of variables. For example, Table 23.1 shows that the absence of lower extremity hypertonicity is associated with the ability to ambulate ($r = .49$). Hypertonicity was also associated with the degree of injury severity ($r = .44$). This correlation matrix provides the reader with a useful overview of data in a complete and concise format.

Significance of the Correlation Coefficient

Just like other sample statistics, the correlation coefficient is subject to sampling error; that is, the observed correlation is considered one of an infinite number of possible correlations that could be obtained from random samples of a population. We can subject

TABLE 23.1 INTERCORRELATIONS OF VARIABLES RELATED TO INDEPENDENT AMBULATION IN CHILDREN WITH TRAUMATIC BRAIN INJURY (N = 53)

	Variable	1	2	3	4	5	6	7
1	Ambulation	—	.49**	.40**	.25*	−.08	.33**	.37**
2	Absence of Lower Extremity Hypertonicity		—	.44**	−.01	−.13	.56**	.59**
3	Injury Severity			—	−.04	−.02	.58**	.38**
4	Absence of LE Injury				—	−.07	.02	.23*
5	Type of Brain Injury					—	−.14	−.34**
6	Cognitive Status at Admission						—	.47**
7	PEDI[‡] Functional Skills Mobility Scale Score at Admission							—

*$p \leq .03$, $df = 93$; **$p \leq .001$, $df = 93$;

‡PEDI = Pediatric Evaluation of Disability Inventory.

Adapted from: Dumas HM, Haley SM, Ludlow LH, Carey TM. Recovery of ambulation during inpatient rehabilitation: Physical therapist prognosis for children and adolescents with traumatic brain injury. *Phys Ther.* 2004; 84:232–242. Table 2, p. 237. Reprinted with permission of the American Physical Therapy Association.

[†]This terminology should not be confused with the *intraclass correlation coefficient (ICC)*, which is used in reliability studies (see Chapter 26).

the correlation coefficient to a test of significance to determine if the observed value is a random effect or if it is a good estimate of the population correlation.

The null hypothesis states that there is no relationship between X and Y in the underlying population, and therefore, the value of the correlation coefficient is zero, $H_0: r = 0$. A test of significance will determine how likely it is that an observed correlation value would have occurred by chance. Although a nondirectional alternative hypothesis can be proposed ($H_1: r \neq 0$), it is often stated with direction, predicting either a positive or a negative relationship ($H_1: r > 0$ or $H_1: r < 0$). We present specific methods for testing the significance of various correlation coefficients in the sections that follow.

The significance of a correlation coefficient does not mean that a correlation coefficient represents a strong relationship. Statistical significance only indicates that an observed value is unlikely to be the result of chance. Correlation coefficients are very sensitive to sample size, and statistical power can be relatively high even with smaller samples. Using the Pearson r, for example, with $n \geq 15$, a moderate correlation of $r = .45$ will be significant ($p < .05$). With larger samples, such as $n > 60$, even values as small as $r = .20$ will be significant. Therefore, a correlation coefficient should always be interpreted in relation to the size of the sample from which it was obtained. With a sufficient increase in sample size almost any observed correlation value will be statistically significant, even if it is so small as to be a meaningless indicator of association. For example, the data shown in Table 23.1 were obtained from a sample of 53 subjects, resulting in relatively high power. Therefore, correlations as low as .25 and .33 are still significant. Consider the case of a study of intelligence tests reported in the *New York Times* in 1986, with the headline "Children's Height Linked to Test Scores."[4] With nearly 14,000 children tested, a significant correlation was cited, but the headline missed the fact that the correlation was only .11! Although many authors report p values associated with correlation coefficients, significance is not as useful to interpretation of r as it is with t-tests or F-tests. Low correlations should not be discussed as clinically important just because they have achieved statistical significance. Such interpretations should be made only on the basis of the magnitude of the correlation coefficient and its practical significance in the context of the variables being measured.

PEARSON PRODUCT-MOMENT CORRELATION COEFFICIENT

The most commonly reported measure of correlation is the **Pearson product-moment coefficient of correlation**, developed by the English statistician Karl Pearson. The statistic is given the symbol r for sample data and ρ (rho) for a population parameter. This statistic is appropriate for use when X and Y are continuous variables with underlying normal distributions on the interval or ratio scales.

Product-moment correlation is based on the concept of **covariance**. With proportional consistency in two sets of scores, we expect that a large X is associated with a large Y, a small X with a small Y, and so on. Therefore, X and Y are said to covary; that is, they vary in similar patterns. With a strong positive relationship, then, an X score that is above the mean $\overline{X}$ should be associated with a Y score that is above the mean $\overline{Y}$. With a strong negative relationship a low X score (below $\overline{X}$) is associated with a high Y score (above $\overline{Y}$). Therefore, if we take the deviation of each score from its mean, called a *moment*, the moments for X and Y scores should be related. The product of the moments for X and Y is a reflection of the degree of consistency within the distributions, hence the name of the statistic.

Example

To illustrate the calculation of r, we use the data in Table 23.2, representing developmental scores on tests of proximal (reaching) and distal (prehensile skill) behaviors in 12 normal infants, 30 weeks of age.[5] The null hypothesis states that there is no relationship between these two behaviors and that the correlation coefficient will be equal to zero, $H_0: \rho = 0$. The alternative hypothesis states that there will be a positive relationship, $H_1: \rho > 0$.

The r Statistic

The computational formula for the Pearson r is

$$r = \frac{n \sum XY - (\sum X)(\sum Y)}{\sqrt{\left[n \sum X^2 - (\sum X)^2\right]\left[n \sum Y^2 - (\sum Y)^2\right]}} \tag{23.1}$$

where n is the number of pairs of scores.

To calculate r, we determine X^2, Y^2, and XY for each subject's scores and then substitute the sums of these terms into Equation (23.1) as shown in Table 23.2B. The calculations yield $r = .365$. This would be considered a relatively weak correlation, suggesting that there is little association between proximal and distal skills in this sample.

Test of Significance

The product-moment correlation coefficient can be subjected to a test of significance, to determine if the observed value could have occurred by chance (if it is significantly different from zero). Critical values of r are provided in Appendix Table A.4 for one- and two-tailed tests of significance with $n - 2$ degrees of freedom. The observed value of r must be *greater than or equal to* the tabled value to be significant. For this example, we locate the critical value $_{(\alpha_1 = .05)}r_{(10)} = .497$. The observed value, $r = .365$, is less than this critical value, and H_0 is not rejected. Computer output shows that $p = .121$ (see Table 12.2D). These data do not support a relationship between proximal and distal motor skills at 30 weeks of age.[‡]

[‡]See Appendix C for a power analysis for these data.

TABLE 23.2   COMPUTATION OF THE PEARSON PRODUCT-MOMENT CORRELATION COEFFICIENT: PROXIMAL VERSUS DISTAL DEVELOPMENT SCORES ($N = 12$)

A. DATA

Subject	Proximal (X)	Distal (Y)	X^2	Y^2	XY
1	17	11	289	121	187
2	10	8	100	64	80
3	14	13	196	169	182
4	21	14	441	196	294
5	16	21	256	441	336
6	21	19	441	361	399
7	22	14	484	196	308
8	18	21	324	441	378
9	18	16	324	256	288
10	16	16	256	256	256
11	18	10	324	100	180
12	20	14	400	196	280
	$\Sigma X = 211$	$\Sigma Y = 177$	$\Sigma X^2 = 3835$	$\Sigma Y^2 = 2797$	$\Sigma XY = 3168$

B. COMPUTATIONS

$$r = \frac{n\sum XY - (\sum X)(\sum Y)}{\sqrt{\left[n\sum X^2 - (\sum X)^2\right]\left[n\sum Y^2 - (\sum Y)^2\right]}} = \frac{12(3,168) - (211)(177)}{\sqrt{[12(3,835) - (211)^2][12(2,797) - (177)^2]}} = .365$$

C. HYPOTHESIS TEST

$_{(\alpha_1 = .05)}r_{(10)} = .497$ (Table A.4) $H_0: \rho = 0; H_1: \rho > 0$ Do not reject H_0

D. OUTPUT

Correlations

		Proximal	Distal
Proximal	Pearson Correlation	1	.365
	Sig. (1-tailed)		.121
	N	12	12
Distal	Pearson Correlation	.365	1
	Sig. (1-tailed)	.121	
	N	12	12

Source: Loria C. Relationship of proximal and distal function in motor development. *Phys Ther* 1980; 60:167–172.

CORRELATION OF RANKS: SPEARMAN RANK CORRELATION COEFFICIENT

The **Spearman rank correlation coefficient,** given the symbol r_S (sometimes called Spearman's rho), is a nonparametric analog of the Pearson r, to be used with ordinal data.

Example

To illustrate this procedure, we will examine the relationship between verbal and reading comprehension for a sample of 10 children with learning disability. The hypothetical scores are based on an ordinal scale (1–100), as shown in Table 23.3A. The null hypothesis states that there is no association between one's verbal and reading comprehension ability, $H_0: r_S = 0$. The alternative hypothesis states that a positive correlation is expected, $H_1: r_S > 0$.

Procedure

To calculate r_S we must first rank the observations within the X and Y distributions separately, with the rank of 1 assigned to the smallest values. Ties are given the average of their ranks (the procedure for ranking scores was described at the beginning of Chapter 22). These rankings are listed under R_X and R_Y in Table 23.3A. If there is a strong positive relationship between X and Y, we would expect these rankings to be consistent; that is, low ranks in X will correspond to low ranks in Y, and vice versa. The Spearman procedure examines the disparity between the two sets of rankings by looking at the difference between the ranks of X and Y assigned to each subject, given the value d. We then square values of d to eliminate minus signs. The sum of the squared differences, Σd^2, is an indicator of the strength of the observed relationship between X and Y, with higher sums reflecting greater disparity.

The r_S Statistic

The value of r_S is determined by the computational formula

$$r_s = 1 - \frac{6\sum d^2}{n(n^2 - 1)} \tag{23.2}$$

where Σd^2 is the sum of the squared rank differences, and n is the number of pairs. As shown in Table 23.3B, $r_S = .79$ for this example. This would be considered a relatively strong relationship.

Test of Significance

We can test the significance of r_S using critical values in Appendix Table A.13. This table uses n rather than degrees of freedom to locate critical values. The observed value of r_S must be *greater than or equal to* the tabled value to achieve significance. For this example, we find the critical value $_{(\alpha_1=.05)}r_{S(10)} = .564$. Therefore, our calculated value of $r_S = .79$ is significant. Computer output in Table 23.3D shows that $p = .003$.

TABLE 23.3 COMPUTATION OF THE SPEARMAN RANK CORRELATION COEFFICIENT (r_S): VERBAL AND READING COMPREHENSION SCORES ($N = 10$)

A. DATA

Subject	Verbal X	Reading Y	R_X	R_Y	d	d^2
1	73	71	6	5	1	1
2	59	63	3	3	0	0
3	86	92	9	10	−1	1
4	81	64	8	4	4	16
5	76	73	7	7	0	0
6	90	80	10	9	1	1
7	55	45	2	1	1	1
8	61	72	4	6	−2	4
9	41	48	1	2	−1	1
10	69	75	5	8	−3	9
						$34 = \Sigma d^2$

B. COMPUTATIONS

$$r_s = 1 - \frac{6 \sum d^2}{n(n^2 - 1)} = 1 - \frac{6(34)}{10(100 - 1)} = .79$$

C. HYPOTHESIS TEST

$(\alpha_1 = .05)^{r}s(10) = .564$ (Table A.13) $\quad H_0: r_s = 0, \quad H_1: r_s > 0$ $\qquad$ Reject H_0

D. OUTPUT

Correlations

Spearman's rho		Verbal	Reading
Verbal	Correlation Coefficient	1.000	.794(**)
	Sig. (1-tailed)	.	.003
	N	10	10
Reading	Correlation Coefficient	.794(**)	1.000
	Sig. (1-tailed)	.003	.
	N	10	10

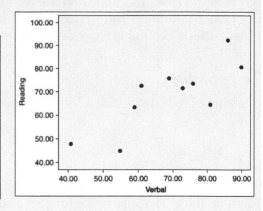

** Correlation is significant at the 0.01 level (1-tailed).

CORRELATION OF DICHOTOMIES

Measures of association are also useful with dichotomous variables. A **dichotomy** is a nominal variable that can take only two values, such as male–female, diseased–nondiseased, and yes–no responses on surveys. The integers 0 and 1 are usually assigned to represent the levels of a dichotomous variable. When either X or Y (or both) is a dichotomy, specialized correlation coefficients are used to test associations.

Phi Coefficient

The **phi coefficient,** given the symbol Φ, is used when both X and Y are dichotomous variables. The phi coefficient is a special case of the product–moment correlation coefficient, given only two values of X and Y. It can be calculated using the Pearson correlation. For example, suppose we studied the relationship between motor and verbal skills in a group of 60 adults with traumatic brain injury. We devise a set of test items for which scores are graded as Pass or Fail. We assign 1 to Pass and 0 to Fail. We use the phi coefficient to test $H_0: \Phi = 0$ against $H_1: \Phi > 0$.

Point Biserial Correlation

When one dichotomous variable (X) is correlated with one continuous variable (Y), the **point biserial correlation coefficient,** r_{pb}, can be used. It, too, is a special case of the product–moment coefficient, and can be calculated using the Pearson correlation. In this case, continuous scores on Y are classified into two series: those who scored 0 and those who scored 1 on X. For example, we could take ratings of elbow flexor spasticity (resistive force in kilograms) for patients who have had a stroke on the right (1) or left (0) sides. We can use the point biserial correlation to test $H_0: r_{pb} = 0$ against $H_1: r_{pb} \neq 0$ to determine if the degree of spasticiy is related to side of involvement.

The point biserial coefficient can be used as a measure of the degree to which the continuous variable can be used to discriminate between the two categories of the dichotomous variable. If the two categories are perfectly divided so that all high scores on Y belong to one category and all low scores belong to the other, r_{pb} would assume its maximum value. This maximum value will never reach 1.00 or -1.00 because of the inexact nature of dichotomized data. With a random distribution (no relationship), the coefficient would equal 0.00. Results for this analysis will be analogous to a t-test.

INTERPRETING CORRELATION COEFFICIENTS

Correlation Versus Comparison

The interpretation of correlation is based on the concept of *covariance.* If two distributions vary directly, so that a change in X is proportional to a change in Y, then X and Y are said to covary. With great consistency in X and Y scores, covariance is high. This is reflected in a coefficient close to 1.00. This concept must be distinguished, however, from the determination of *differences between* two distributions. To illustrate this point, suppose you were told that exam scores for courses in anatomy and physiology were highly correlated at $r = .98$. Would it be reasonable to infer, then, that a student with a 90 in anatomy would be expected to attain a score close to 90 in physiology?

Let us consider the paired distributions of exam grades listed in Table 23.4. Obviously, the scores are decidedly different. The anatomy scores range from 47 to 60 and the physiology scores from 79 to 90. The mean anatomy grade is 52.9, whereas the mean physiology grade is 82.7. But each student's scores have a proportional relationship, resulting in a high correlation coefficient. The scatterplot shows how these values result in a strong linear relationship.

TABLE 23.4   PAIRED EXAM GRADES

Student	X Anatomy	Y Physiology
1	50	80
2	56	85
3	52	83
4	57	85
5	47	77
6	48	79
7	60	90

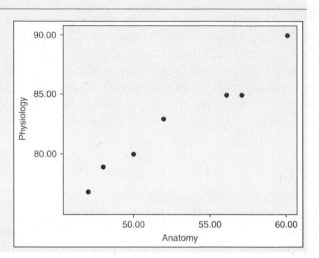

Correlation, therefore, is not going to provide information relative to the difference between sets of data, only to the relative order of scores, whatever their magnitude. A test of statistical significance for differences, like the *t*-test, is required to examine differences. It is inappropriate to make inferences about similarities or differences between distributions based on correlation coefficients.

Causation and Correlation

It is also important to distinguish the concepts of causation and correlation in research. The presence of a statistical association between two variables does not necessarily imply the presence of a causal relationship; that is, it does not suggest that X causes Y or Y causes X. In many situations a strong relationship between variables X and Y may actually be a function of some third variable, or a set of variables, that is related to both X and Y. For example, researchers have shown that weak grip strength and slowed hand reaction time are associated with falling in elderly persons.[6] Certainly, we could not infer that decreased hand function causes falls; however, weak hand musculature may be associated with general deconditioning, and slowed reaction time may be related to balance and motor recovery deficits. These associated factors are more likely to be the contributory factors to falls. Therefore, a study that examined the correlation between falls and hand function would not be able to make any valid assumptions about causative factors.

Causal factors are best established under controlled experimental conditions, with randomization of subjects into groups. When this is not possible, researchers may use correlation as a reasonable alternative, but causality must be supported by biological credibility of the association, a logical time sequence (cause precedes outcome), a dose–response relationship (the larger the causal factor, the larger the outcome) and consistency of findings across several studies. Perhaps the most notable example of this approach is the long-term research on the connection between lung cancer and smoking, following numerous studies that confirmed strong correlations, with a strong physiologic foundation, a clear temporal sequence and a consistent dose–response relationship.[7]

Willoughby offers a silly example to illustrate the temptation to infer cause-and-effect from a correlation.[8] In 1940 scholars observed a high positive correlation between vocabulary and college grades, and concluded, therefore, that an improvement in vocabulary would cause an improvement in grades. Willoughby argued that this would be the same as reasoning that a high positive correlation between a boy's height and the length of his trousers would mean that lengthening his trousers would produce taller boys! Clearly, the assumption that one variable causes another cannot be based solely on the magnitude of a correlation coefficient (see Box 23.2).

Factors Influencing Generalization of Correlation Coefficients

In most situations, a researcher looks at the degree of correlation in sample data as an estimate of the correlation that exists in the larger population. It is important, then, to consider factors that limit the interpretation and consequent generalizability of correlation values.

Range of Test Values

Generalization of correlation values should be limited to the range of values used to obtain the correlation. For example, if age and strength were correlated for subjects between 2 and 15 years old, a strong positive relationship would probably be found. It would not, however, be legitimate to extrapolate this relationship to subjects older than 15, as the sample data are not sufficient to know if the relationship holds beyond that age.

Similarly, the finding of a weak or absent correlation within one age range does not mean that no relationship exists outside that range. Even if we find no relationship between muscle strength and age for subjects aged 30 to 50, we might find a negative relationship for subjects aged 70 to 90. The nature of a relationship may vary dramatically as one varies the range of scores contributing to the correlation. Therefore, it is not safe to assume that correlation values for a total sample validly represent any subgroup of the sample, and vice versa.

Restricting the Range of Scores

The magnitude of the correlation coefficient is a function of how closely a cluster of scores resembles a straight line, based on data from a full range of X and Y values. When the range of X or Y scores is limited in the sample, the correlation coefficient will not adequately reflect the extent of their relationship. As shown in Figure 23.3, if we look only at the range of X values in the lower end of the scale, it is not possible to see the true linear relationship between the two variables. Such a correlation will be close to zero, even though the true correlation may be quite high. By limiting variation in the data, it is difficult to demonstrate covariance. Therefore, r is reduced. It is advisable to include as wide a range of values as possible for correlation analysis.

BOX 23.2 **The Evils of Pickle Eating**

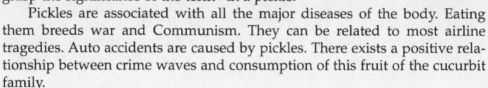

Although this classic piece may be a little dated, its point is timeless!

Pickles will kill you! Every pickle you eat brings you closer to death. It is amazing that the modern thinking man has failed to grasp the significance of the term "in a pickle."

Pickles are associated with all the major diseases of the body. Eating them breeds war and Communism. They can be related to most airline tragedies. Auto accidents are caused by pickles. There exists a positive relationship between crime waves and consumption of this fruit of the cucurbit family.

For example,

- Nearly all sick people have eaten pickles. The effects are obviously cumulative.
- 99.9% of all people who die from cancer have eaten pickles.
- 100.0% of all soldiers have eaten pickles.
- 96.8% of all Communist sympathizers have eaten pickles.
- 99.7% of the people involved in air and auto accidents ate pickles within 14 days preceding the accident.
- 93.1% of juvenile delinquents come from homes where pickles are served frequently. Evidence points to the long-term effects of pickle eating.
- Of the people born in 1839 who later dined on pickles, there has been a 100% mortality.

All pickle eaters born between 1849 and 1859 have wrinkled skin, have lost most of their teeth, have brittle bones and failing eyesight—if the ills of pickle eating have not already caused their death.

Even more convincing is the report of the noted team of medical specialists: rats force-fed with 20 pounds of pickles per day for 30 days developed bulging abdomens. Their appetites for WHOLESOME FOOD were destroyed.

In spite of all evidence, pickle growers and packers continue to spread their evil. More than 120,000 acres of fertile U.S. soil are devoted to growing pickles. Our per capita consumption is nearly four pounds.

Eat orchid petal soup. Practically no one has as many problems from eating orchid petal soup as they do with eating pickles.

Source: "Evils of Pickle Eating," by Everett D. Edington, originally printed in *Cyanograms.*

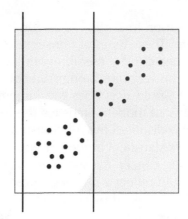

FIGURE 23.3   Illustration of the effect of restricting the range of scores for correlation. By looking only at values of *X* at the lower end of the scale, the true linear relationship between the variables is obscured.

Assumption of Independence in Correlated Values

Valid correlation also demands that correlated variables be independent of each other. For instance, it would make no statistical sense to correlate a measure of gait velocity with distance walked, as distance is a component of velocity (distance/time). Similarly, it is fruitless to correlate a subscale score on a functional assessment with the total score, as the first variable is included in the second. In each case, correlations will tend to be artificially high because part of the variance in each quantity is being correlated with itself. Researchers should always be familiar with the nature of the variables being studied to avoid spuriously high and misleading correlations.

COMMENTARY

The Stork Was Busy

The application of correlation statistics to clinical decision making must be considered carefully. All statistical analysis is limited by the clinical significance of the data being analyzed. Researchers must be equally aware of the potential danger of using statistical correlation as evidence of a clinical association simply on the basis of numbers. The utility of correlation is limited because it cannot tell us anything about the actual nature of phenomena, and almost any two variables can be correlated numerically.

For example, Snedecor and Cochran[9] cite a correlation of −.98 between the annual birth rate in Great Britain from 1875 to 1920 and the annual production of pig iron in the United States. We can view these variables as related to some general socioeconomic trends, but surely, neither one could seriously be considered a function of the other. Another classic example from many decades ago involves the high positive correlation between the number of storks seen sitting on chimneys in European towns and the number of births in these towns.[10] Further study of the "Theory of the Stork" has shown that there is correlation between deliveries outside of hospitals and the stork population in Berlin.[11] Can we infer that storks are responsible for an increased birth rate? These types of nonsense correlations help to illustrate the importance of analyzing the clinical credibility of any statistical association and understanding the nature of the variables being studied.

In a more serious vein, Gould describes the lamentable efforts of Sir Ronald Fisher (1890–1962), the father of modern statistics (he invented a little thing called the analysis of variance), who disputed the relationship between smoking and lung cancer.[12] As a smoker, Fisher's statistical argument was first that we could not know if smoking caused cancer or cancer caused smoking. Their undeniable mutual occurrence, he proposed, could reflect a precancerous state that caused a chemical irritation in the lungs that was relieved by smoking, leading to an increased use of cigarettes. More plausibly, however, he later suggested that the association was most likely due to a third factor, a genetic predisposition, which made people more susceptible to lung cancer, and at the same time created personality types that would lead to smoking. Fisher became a consultant for the tobacco companies in 1960, and was apparently instrumental in blocking law suits at that time. As this regrettable story illustrates, the often elusive nature of correlation must never allow us to lose sight of logic, and the need to continue to question and examine relationships to truthfully understand clinical phenomena. The numbers in statistics are never the final say—they just suggest a relationship. It is our job to identify the theoretical premise that supports our conclusions.

REFERENCES

1. Cohen J. *Statistical Power Analysis for the Behavioral Sciences* (2nd ed.). Hillsdale, NJ: Lawrence Erlbaum, 1988.
2. Green SB, Salkind NJ, Akey TM. *Using SPSS for Windows and Macintosh: Analyzing and Understanding Data* (4th ed.). Upper Saddle River, NJ: Prentice Hall, 2004.
3. Dumas HM, Haley SM, Ludlow LH, Carey TM. Recovery of ambulation during inpatient rehabilitation: Physical therapist prognosis for children and adolescents with traumatic brain injury. *Phys Ther* 2004;84:232–242.
4. UPI Dispatch, Science Desk. Children's height linked to test scores. *New York Times*, October 7, 1986:C4
5. Loria C. Relationship of proximal and distal function in motor development. *Phys Ther* 1980;60:167–172.
6. Nevitt MC, Cummings SR, Hudes ES. Risk factors for injurious falls: A prospective study. *J Gerontol* 1991;46:M164–170.
7. Parascandola M, Weed DL, Dasgupta A. Two Surgeon Generals' reports on smoking and cancer: A historical investigation of the practice of causal inference. *Emerg Themes Epidemiol* 2006;3:1.
8. Willoughby RR. Cum hoc ergo propter hoc. *School and Society* 1940;51:485.
9. Snedecor GW, Cochran WG. *Statistical Methods* (8th ed.). Ames, IA: Iowa State University Press, 1991.
10. Wallis WA, Roberts HV. *Statistics—A New Approach*. Glencoe, IL: Free Press, 1956.
11. Hofer T, Przyrembel H, Verleger S. New Evidence for the theory of the stork. *Paediatr Perinat Epidemiol* 2004;18:88–92.
12. Gould SJ. The smoking gun of eugenics. *Nat Hist* 1991:8–17.

CHAPTER 24
Regression

Correlation statistics are useful for describing the relative strength of a relationship between two variables; however, when a researcher wants to establish this relationship as a basis for prediction, a **regression** procedure is used (see Box 24.1). The ability to predict outcomes and characteristics is crucial to effective clinical decision making and goal setting. It also has important implications for efficiency and quality of patient care, especially in situations where resources are limited. Regression analysis provides a powerful statistical approach for explaining and predicting quantifiable clinical outcomes. For example, clinicians have looked at functional assessments in patients with extensive burns to determine which factors are predictive of quality of life outcomes.[1] Early language and nonverbal skills have been shown to be important predictors of outcome in adaptive behavior in communication and socialization for children with autism.[2] Researchers have studied patients with stroke to determine the relative contributions of specific impairments toward prediction of discharge function, rehabilitation length of stay, and discharge destination.[3] Therapists have investigated factors predictive of timely and sustained recovery following multidisciplinary rehabilitation in workmen's compensation claimants with low back pain.[4] Such analyses help us explain our empirical clinical observations and provide information that can be used to set realistic goals for our patients. The purpose of this chapter is to describe the process of regression and how it can be used to interpret clinical data.

LINEAR REGRESSION

In its simplest form, linear regression involves the examination of two variables, X and Y, that are linearly related or correlated. The variable designated X is the **independent** or **predictor variable**, and the variable designated Y is the **dependent** or **criterion variable**. For example, we could look at systolic blood pressure (Y) and age (X) in a sample of 10 women. Using regression analysis we can use these data as a basis for predicting a woman's blood pressure by knowing her age. If we plot hypothetical data for this example on a scatter plot, as shown in Figure 24.1, we can see that the data tend to fall in a linear pattern, with larger values of X associated with larger values of Y. The correlation coefficient for these data, $r = .87$, describes a fairly strong association.

If the data were perfectly correlated, all data points would fall along a straight line. This line could then be used to predict values of Y by locating the intersection of points on the line for any given value of X. With correlations less than 1.00, however, as in this example, a prediction line can only be *estimated*. If we look at the scatter diagram in

BOX 24.1 **The History of Regression**

Sometimes we get so caught up in the application of statistics that we don't stop to think about where these measures came from. Someone had to think them up! Here's some interesting background on the origin of the concept of regression.

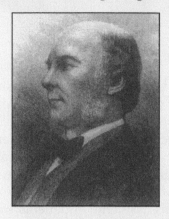 Sir Francis Galton was born near Birmingham, England in 1822. He was a tropical explorer and geographer, meteorologist, psychologist, inventor of fingerprint identification—and pioneer of statistical correlation and regression. He is best known for his study of human intelligence and his belief in eugenics. A cousin of Charles Darwin, Galton became interested in the concept of heredity, and was convinced that "genius" was almost entirely due to hereditary factors, in sharp contrast to the thinking of the day which basically held that everyone was born with equal abilities.

In 1875 Galton began experimenting with sweet pea seeds, as this was a self-fertilizing plant, and he could look at simple hereditary characteristics. He found that the offspring peas of large seeds were usually smaller than the parent, and the offspring from small seeds were usually larger than the parent—but just a little.

Galton later collected extensive data on the heights of parents and children. Because it was known that taller parents had taller children and shorter parents had shorter children, he noted that it would seem logical that the variance in height should increase over time; that is, we should see people getting taller and shorter based on their parents' heights. However, his data supported the same relationship he had found with the sweet peas. He coined the term **regression** in his report of this phenomenon, *"Regression towards mediocrity in hereditary stature."* As shown in the plate from that work, Galton reasoned that the height of the children depends on the average height of both the father and the mother, and that variance in the height of the population is reduced by "regression" towards the mean by just enough to keep it almost constant over time.

Although we tend to think of regression as an outgrowth of correlation, interestingly, Galton's work on regression was the foundation for Karl Pearson's development of correlation statistics.

See Chapter 5 for additional discussion of regression toward the mean as an issue in reliability.

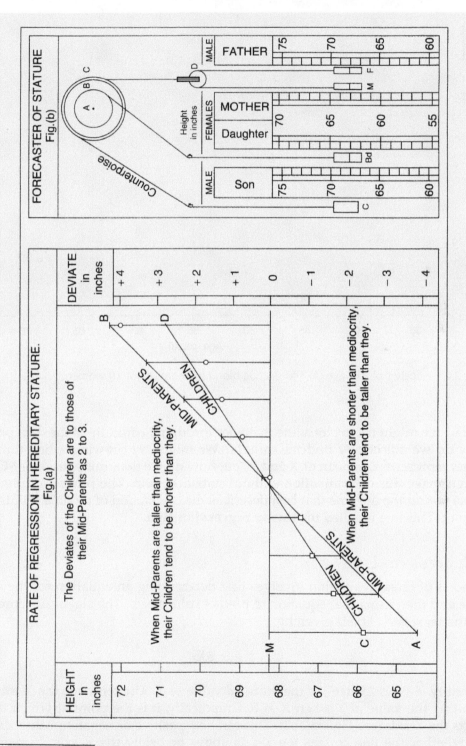

From Galton F. Regression towards mediocrity in hereditary stature. *J Anthropological Institute* 1886; 15:246–263, Plate IX.

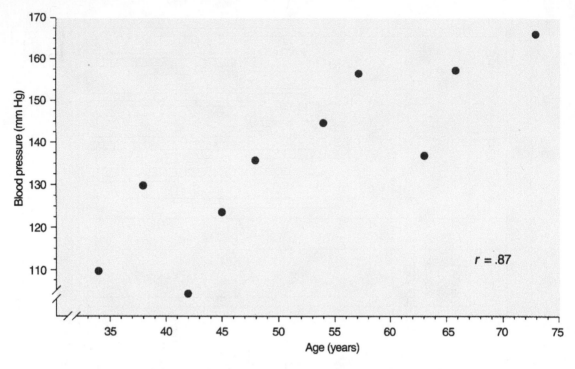

FIGURE 24.1   Scatter plot of age (*X*) and systolic blood pressure (*Y*) for 10 women.

Figure 24.1 we might try to plot a line that goes through the middle of the data points—but how do we objectively find the middle? We might try drawing a line through a point that represents the mean of *X* and *Y*, but how do we determine its slope? Clearly, we cannot make this determination without statistical help. The process of regression allows us to find the one line that best describes the orientation of all data points in the scatter plot. This line is called the **linear regression line.**

The Regression Line

The process of linear regression involves first determining an equation for the regression line and then using that equation to predict values of *Y*. The algebraic representation of the regression line is given by

$$\hat{Y} = a + bX \tag{24.1}$$

The quantity $\hat{Y}$ (said "Y-hat") is the *predicted* value of *Y*. The term *a* is the *Y*-intercept, representing the value of *Y* when *X* = 0. Graphically, it is the point at which the line intersects the *Y*-axis (see Figure 24.2). This can be a positive or negative value, depending on whether the line crosses the *Y*-axis above or below the *X*-axis. In regression analysis, *a* is called a **regression constant.** The term *b* is the *slope* of the line, which is the rate of change in *Y* for each one-unit change in *X*. In regression analysis, this term is the **regression coefficient**. When *b* is positive, *Y* increases as *X* increases. When *b* is

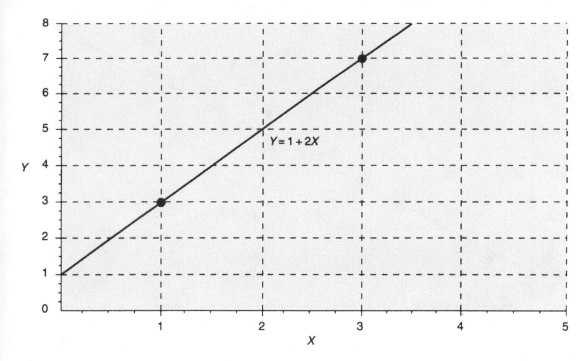

FiGURE 24.2 Graphic presentation of a linear equation.

negative, Y decreases as X increases. If $b = 0$, the slope of the line is horizontal, indicating no relationship between X and Y (Y is constant for all values of X). The positive or negative direction of the slope will correspond to a positive or negative correlation between X and Y.

We can illustrate these concepts by describing the linear equation $Y = 1 + 2X$. This equation represents a straight line that intersects the Y-axis at $Y = 1$. With a slope of 2, Y increases two units for every one-unit change in X. A line can be drawn from this equation by plotting any two points along the line and connecting them. We can arbitrarily choose any two values along the X-axis and solve for the corresponding values of Y. Thus, we can plot one point at $X = 1$, $Y = 1 + 2(1) = 3$. The second point, say at $X = 3$, is determined by $Y = 1 + 2(3) = 7$. This process is illustrated in Figure 24.2.

The Regression Model

Figure 24.3 shows the regression of blood pressure (Y) on age (X), using the hypothetical data from Figure 24.1. The values that fall on the regression line are the predicted values, $\hat{Y}$, for any given value of X; however, with $r < 1.00$, we can see that this line is only partially useful for predicting Y. Some data points are above the line, some are below, and some fall close to the line. Therefore, if we substitute any X value in the regression equation and solve for $\hat{Y}$, we will obtain a predicted value that will probably be somewhat different from the actual value of Y. We can visualize this error component in Figure 24.4. The actual Y value for each data point is some positive or negative

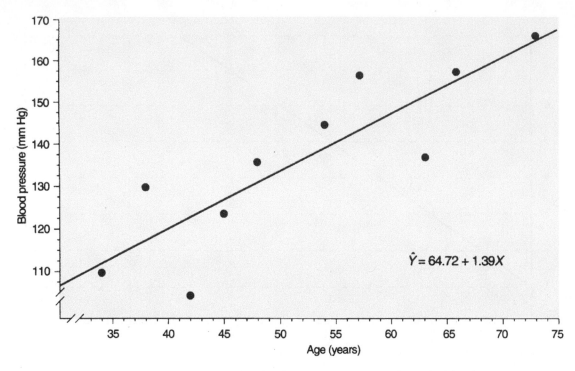

FIGURE 24.3 Least-squares regression line for the linear regression of systolic blood pressure on age.

vertical distance from $\hat{Y}$ on the regression line. These distances $(Y - \hat{Y})$ are called **residuals.** Residuals represent the degree of error in the regression line.*

The regression line, or the **line of best fit** for a set of data points, is the unique line that will minimize this error component and yield the smallest residuals. Conceptually, this involves finding the square of all the residuals (to eliminate minus signs) and summing these squares, $\Sigma(Y - \hat{Y})^2$, for every possible line that could be drawn to these data. The one line that gives the smallest sum of squares is the line of best fit. Any other line, with any other values of a and b, would yield a larger sum of the squared residuals. This method of "fitting" the regression line is called the **method of least squares**. Of course, we do not actually go through the process of finding residuals for every possible line. Formulas have been developed that allow us to calculate the line of best fit based on the sample data.

Calculation of the Regression Line and Residuals

We can illustrate the process of regression using the study for predicting systolic blood pressure (SBP) as a function of age. Table 24.1A shows hypothetical data on SBP measurements for a sample of 10 women between 34 and 73 years of age. We calculate the regression coefficient, b, and the regression constant, a, using the computa-

---

*We could more accurately represent the regression equation as $Y = a + bX \pm$ error.

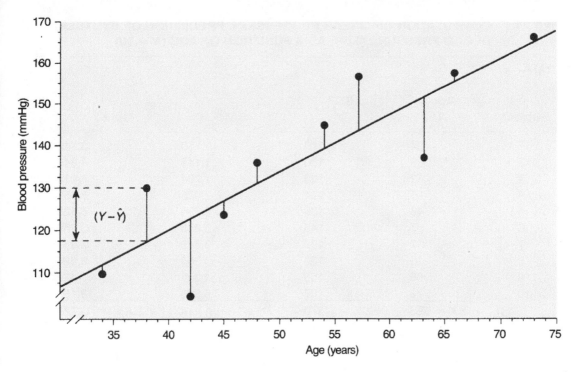

FIGURE 24.4 Deviation of scores from the least-squares regression line for the linear regression of sys-tolic blood pressure on age. Vertical distances represent $Y - \hat{Y}$.

tional formulas shown in Table 24.1B.[†] These values identify a line that intersects the Y-axis at 64.30 with a change of 1.39 units in Y for each unit change in X. Therefore, the line that best fits these data can be drawn from the regression equation $\hat{Y} = 64.30 + 1.39X$ (also see Table 24.3C). This line is superimposed on the scatter plot for these data in Figure 24.3.

We can now calculate the predicted score ($\hat{Y}$) for each subject using the regression equation, as shown in Table 24.2. For example, if we were presented with a woman who was 38 years old, we would predict that her systolic blood pressure would be $\hat{Y} = 64.30 + 1.39(38) = 117.1$. The actual blood pressure value for the 38-year-old sub-ject, however, was 130. Therefore, the residual or error component of prediction is $(Y - \hat{Y}) = 130 - 117.1 = 12.9$. Note that the data point for this subject falls above the regression line; therefore, the regression equation underestimates SBP for this subject, and we have a positive residual.

Residuals are shown under the column labeled $(Y - \hat{Y})$ in Table 24.2. For a woman aged 63, we would predict a SBP of 152.9, where the actual score was 138. Therefore, the regression equation overestimates the SBP score for this subject, and we have a negative residual of −14.9. Most of the errors of prediction in this example are relatively small,

---

[†]An alternative formula for b can be used: where $b = \left(\dfrac{s_y}{s_x}\right)$ where s_y and s_x are the standard deviations for the two variables.

TABLE 24.1 COMPUTATION OF LINEAR REGRESSION: PREDICTION OF SYSTOLIC BLOOD PRESSURE (SBP) AS A FUNCTION OF AGE ($N = 10$)

A. DATA

Subject	Age X	SBP Y	X^2	XY
1	34	110	1,156	3,740
2	38	130	1,144	4,940
3	42	105	1,764	4,410
4	45	124	2,025	5,580
5	48	136	2,304	6,528
6	57	145	3,249	8,265
7	57	157	3,249	7,949
8	63	138	3,969	8,694
9	66	158	4,356	10,428
10	73	167	5,329	12,191
	$\Sigma X = 523$	$\Sigma Y = 1,370$	$\Sigma X^2 = 28,845$	$\Sigma XY = 73,725$
	$\overline{X} = 52.3$	$\overline{Y} = 137$		

B. COMPUTATIONS

$$b = \frac{n \sum XY - (\sum X)(\sum Y)}{n \sum X^2 - (\sum X)^2} = \frac{10(73,725) - (523)(1,370)}{10(28,845) - (523)^2} = \frac{20,740}{14,921} = 1.39$$

$$a = \overline{Y} - b\overline{X} = 137 - 1.39(52.3) = 64.30$$

$$Y = 64.30 + 1.39X$$

TABLE 24.2 PREDICTED SYSTOLIC BLOOD PRESSURE (SBP) SCORES BASED ON THE REGRESSION EQUATION $\hat{Y} = 64.30 + 1.39X$

Subject	Age X	SBP Y	$\hat{Y}$	Residuals $Y - \hat{Y}$	$(Y - \hat{Y})^2$
1	34	110	112.0	−2.0	4.0
2	38	130	117.5	12.5	156.3
3	42	105	123.1	−18.1	327.6
4	45	124	127.3	−3.3	10.9
5	48	136	131.5	4.5	20.3
6	57	145	143.5	1.5	2.3
7	57	157	143.9	13.1	171.6
8	63	138	152.3	−14.3	204.5
9	66	158	156.4	1.6	2.6
10	73	167	166.2	0.8	0.6
				$\Sigma(Y - \hat{Y})^2 =$	900.7

because the correlation for these data is high ($r = .87$), and the points cluster close to the regression line. Note that the points for subjects aged 34, 66 and 73 have almost negligible residuals, as these points rest very close to the regression line (Figure 24.4).

The sum of the residuals will always be zero, as the regression line is an average for all data points. Therefore, we take the sum of the squares of these error components, $(Y - \hat{Y})^2$, as an estimate of the usefulness of the regression line for prediction. The smaller the sum of squares, the closer the data points are to the regression line and the better the prediction accuracy.

ASSUMPTIONS FOR REGRESSION ANALYSIS

In any regression procedure, we recognize that the straight line we fit to sample data is only an approximation of the true regression line that exists for the underlying population. To make inferences about population parameters from sample data, we must consider the statistical assumptions that affect the validity of the regression equation.

For any given value of X, we can assume that a random distribution of Y scores exists; that is, the observed value of Y in a sample for a given X is actually one random score from the larger distribution of possible Y scores for that X. In the example we have been using, the observed SBP for a given age is a random observation from the larger distribution of all possible blood pressure scores at that age. If we had studied several subjects at each age, we would see a range of blood pressure scores for the same value of X. Some of these Y values would be above the regression line, and some would be below it. For instance, subjects 6 and 7 were 57 years old in our sample, with different blood pressure scores. As shown in Table 24.2, subject 6 has a predicted score very close to the true score, and subject 7 has a larger residual. If we took many measurements for women at 57 years old, the mean of the distribution of Y scores would fall on the regression line.

Theoretically, we could obtain such a distribution for every value of X, as shown in Figure 24.5. Each of these distributions would have a different mean, $\overline{Y}$. If these means were connected, they would fall on a straight line that estimates the population regression line. We assume that each of these distributions is normal and that their standard deviations are equal.

These assumptions help us to understand the relevance of residual error variance to regression analysis. Conceptually, it makes sense that the regression line will contain some degree of error, as it is unlikely that any one score randomly chosen from a distribution will equal the mean. Therefore, we tend to see a scatter of points around the regression line. The least-squares line that is fitted to the sample data is an estimate of the population regression line, and $\hat{Y}$ is an estimate of the population mean for Y at each value of X.

Analysis of Residuals

One way to determine if the assumptions for regression analysis have been met is to examine a plot of residuals, as shown in Figure 24.6. By plotting the residuals (on the Y-axis) against the predicted scores (on the X-axis), we can appreciate the magnitude and distribution of the residual scores. The central horizontal axis represents the mean

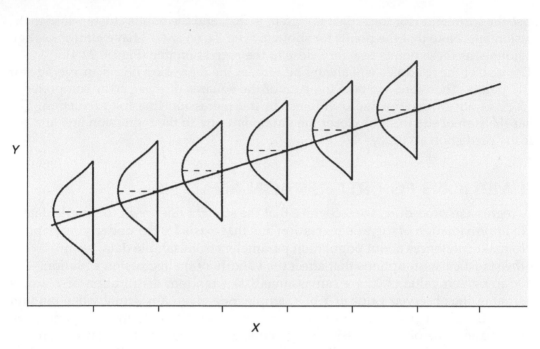

FIGURE 24.5   The linear regression model, showing theoretical normal distributions of Y around the regression line at given values of X. The mean of each distribution lies on the regression line. Therefore, $Y = \hat{Y}$ at each value of X.

of the residuals, or zero deviation from the regression line. When the linear regression model is a good fit, the residual scores will be randomly dispersed close to zero. The wider the distribution of residuals around the zero axis, the greater the error.

Several types of patterns can emerge in the residual plot. If the data meet all the basic assumptions, the pattern should resemble a horizontal band of points, as illustrated in Figure 24.6A. The horizontal orientation suggests that the residuals are evenly, but randomly, distributed around the regression line.

Figures 24.6B and C illustrate problematic residual distributions. The pattern in Figure 24.6B indicates that the variance of the residuals is not consistent, but dependent on the value of the predicted variable. Residual error increases as the predicted value gets larger; that is, the degree of accuracy in the regression model varies with the size of the predicted value. Therefore, the assumptions of normality and equality of variance are not met. The curvilinear pattern, shown in Figure 24.6C, reflects a nonlinear relationship, negating the validity of the linear model. Other deviant residual patterns may be observed, such as diagonal patterns or a run of positive or negative residuals, all indicating some problem in the interpretation of the regression model.

When data do not fall into the horizontal pattern, the researcher may choose to transform one or both sets of data to more closely satisfy the necessary assumptions. Such transformations may stabilize the variance in the data, normalize the distributions, or create a more linear relationship. Methods of data transformation are described in Appendix D. When curvilinear tendencies are observed, polynomial regression models may be used to better represent the data. This approach is discussed later in this chapter.

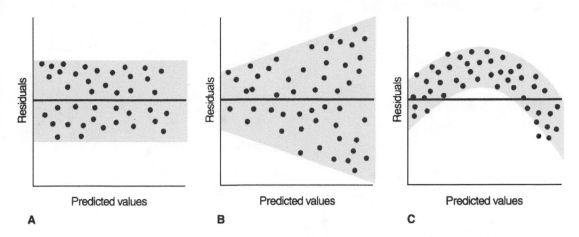

FIGURE 24.6   Patterns of residuals (*Y*-axis) plotted against predicted scores (*X*-axis). **A.** Horizontal band demonstrates that assumptions for linear regression have been met. **B.** Residuals increase as predicted values increase. **C.** Curvilinear pattern indicates nonlinear relationship.

Most computer programs for linear regression will provide options for calculating, printing and plotting residuals in a variety of formats. **Standardized residuals,** obtained by dividing each residual score by the standard deviation of the residual distribution, are often used instead of observed residuals to normalize the scale of measurement. Standardized residuals are analogous to *z*-scores, allowing the residuals to be expressed in standard deviation units. This approach is especially useful when different distributions are compared.

OUTLIERS

If a set of data points represents a distribution of related scores, the points will tend to cluster around their regression line. Sometimes, one or two deviant scores are separated from the cluster, so that they distort the statistical association. For example, the data points in Figure 24.7A show some variability, but most of the points fall within a definite linear pattern (*r* = .70). In Figure 24.7B, this distribution has one additional point, at *X, Y* = 1, 20, that does not seem to fit with the rest of the scores. Such a point is called an **outlier,** because it lies outside the obvious cluster of scores. The correlation for these data with the outlier included is quite low, *r* = .06. One extreme value has significantly altered the statistical description of the data.

What accounts for the occurrence of outliers? Researchers must consider several possibilities. The score may, indeed, be a true score, but an extreme one, because the sample is too small to generate a full range of observations. If more subjects were tested, there might be less of a discrepancy between the outlier and the rest of the scores. There may be also be circumstances peculiar to this data point that are responsible for the large deviation. For example, the score may be a function of error in measurement or recording, equipment malfunction, or some miscalculation. It may be possible to go back to the original data to find and correct this type of error. Other extraneous factors may also contribute to the aberrant score, some of which are correctable, others that are

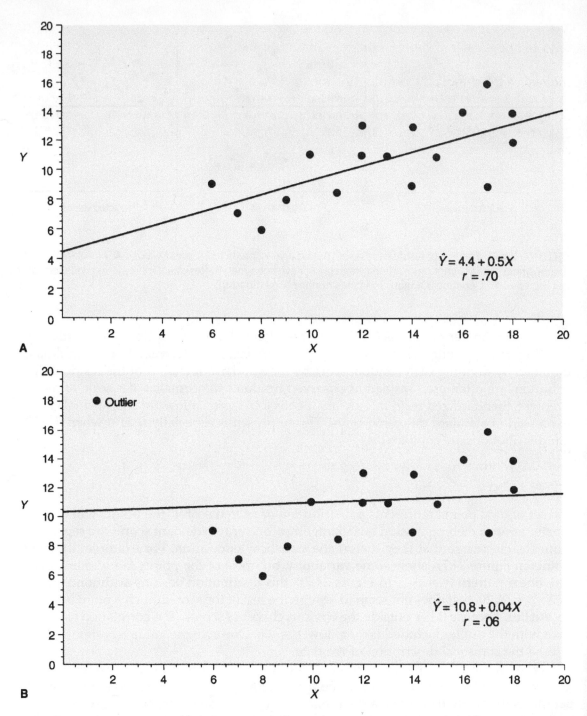

FIGURE 24.7 Regression lines for a distribution of scores (**A**) without and (**B**) with an outlier (X, Y = 1, 20). In this case, the presence of the outlier causes the regression line to underestimate the degree of association in the data.

not. For instance, the data for the point may have been collected by a different tester who is not reliable. Or the researcher may find that the subject was inappropriately included in the sample; that is, the subject may have characteristics very different from the rest of the sample, accounting for the deviant response.

Outliers should be examined because they can have serious effects on the outcome of regression. Residual plots are often helpful for identifying outliers. Some researchers consider scores beyond three standard deviations from the mean to be outliers. The researcher must determine if the deviant score should be retained or discarded in the analysis. This decision should be made only after a thorough evaluation of the experimental conditions, the data collection procedures, and the data themselves. As a general rule, there is no statistical rationale for discarding an outlier; however, if a causal factor can be identified, the point should probably be omitted, provided that the causal factor is unique to the outlier.[5] It may be helpful to perform the regression with and without the outlier, to demonstrate how inclusion of the outlier changes the conclusions drawn from the data.

ACCURACY OF PREDICTION

Once a regression line is derived, it can be used to predict Y scores based on values of X. It is important to remember that a regression line can be calculated for any set of data, even though it may not represent the data very well. The value of the correlation coefficient, r, is a rough indicator of the "goodness of fit" of the regression line. When r is close to ± 1.00, the regression line provides a strong basis for prediction. As r gets smaller, the errors of prediction will increase; however, the value of r is limited in its interpretation because it represents only the strength of an association. It will not evaluate the accuracy of prediction from the regression line. Several statistical approaches can be used for this purpose.

Coefficient of Determination (r^2)

Statisticians have shown that the square of the correlation coefficient, r^2, represents the percentage of the total variance in the Y scores that can be explained by the X scores. Therefore, r^2 is a measure of proportion, indicating the accuracy of prediction based on X. This term is called the **coefficient of determination.**

For the regression of blood pressure on age, $r = .87$ and $r^2 = .76$ (see Table 24.3). Therefore, 76% of the variance in systolic blood pressure can be accounted for by knowing the variance in age. We have 76% of the information we would need to make an accurate prediction. Obviously, some other unknown or unidentified factors must account for the remaining variance. The complement of r^2, or $1 - r^2$, reflects the proportion of variance that is not explained by the relationship between X and Y, in this case 24%. Using age as a predictor will result in a reasonable, but not thoroughly accurate, estimate of blood pressure.

Values of r^2 are more meaningful for conceptualizing the extent of an association between variables than values of r alone. For example, with a high correlation like $r = .70$, $r^2 = .49$. This means that less than 50% of the variance in Y is accounted for by knowing X, less than one might think with a correlation coefficient that seems fairly

TABLE 24.3   OUTPUT FOR REGRESSION ANALYSIS: SYSTOLIC BLOOD PRESSURE AND AGE (N = 10)

Model Summary

R	R❶ Square	Std. Error of the Estimate
.869	.756	10.741

ANOVA

Model	Sum of Squares	df	Mean Square	F	Sig.
Regression	2854.959	1	2854.959	24.744	.001
Residual	923.041	8	115.380		❷
Total	3778.000	9			

Coefficients

Model	Unstandardized Coefficients		Standardized Coefficients		
	B	Std. Error	Beta	t	Sig.
(Constant)	64.582	14.949			
Age	❸ 1.393	.280	❹ .869	4.974	❺ .001

❶ The values of R-square and SEE reflect the degree of accuracy in the regression equation.

❷ The analysis of variance of regression demonstrates that there is a significant relationship between the independent and dependent variables.

❸ The coefficients for the regression equation $\hat{Y}$ = 64.58 + 1.39(Age).

❹ The standardized coefficient is similar to a z-score, in that it is based on standardized units. The equation can be written: $\hat{Y}$ = .869(Age). No constant is necessary because the value of X is expressed in standardized units.

❺ A t-test is used to test the significance of the regression coefficient for age. This significance value will equal the probability identified in the analysis of variance of regression, as it is essentially testing the same thing.

Note: Portions of the output that are not relevant to the interpretation of results have been omitted for clarification.

strong. When strength of association is of interest, r will be properly interpreted; however, when Y is predicted from X, r^2 provides a more meaningful description of the relationship. Values of r^2 will range between 0.00 and 1.00. No negative ratios are possible as it is a squared value.

Standard Error of the Estimate (SEE)

Another way to establish the accuracy of prediction is to consider the variance of the errors on either side of the regression line, or the residuals. If the variance in the residuals is high, then the scores are widely dispersed around the regression line, indicating a large error component. The standard deviation of the distribution of errors is called the **standard error of the estimate (SEE).** For the blood pressure data, SEE = 10.61 (see Table 24.3❶).[‡]

[‡]The standard error of the estimate is defined by SEE = $\sqrt{\dfrac{\sum(Y - \hat{Y})^2}{(n - 2)}}$ where $\sum(Y - \hat{Y})^2$ is the sum of the squared residuals, and n represents the number of pairs of scores. For the data in Table 24.2, SEE = $\sqrt{\dfrac{900.7}{(10 - 2)}}$ = 10.61

The better the fit of the regression line, the less variability there will be around it and the smaller the standard error of the estimate. The SEE can be thought of as an indicator of the average error of prediction for the regression equation. Therefore, the SEE is helpful for interpreting the usefulness of a regression equation where reliance on a correlation coefficient can be misleading.

Researchers can reduce standard error, and thereby improve accuracy of prediction, by including more than one observation at each value of X within a single study. This improves the estimation of variability at each X, thereby making the regression line a better estimate of the population mean.

ANALYSIS OF VARIANCE OF REGRESSION

Up to this point, we have used regression analysis primarily as a descriptive technique. We can also draw statistical inferences about the regression equation, to document that the observed relationship between X and Y did not occur by chance. We do this by an **analysis of variance of regression.** In essence, this analysis tests the null hypothesis H_0: $b = 0$ and is analogous to testing the significance of the correlation between X and Y. If H_0 is true, the regression line is essentially horizontal, perhaps with some deviation as a result of sampling error. If H_0 is false, b is significantly different from zero.[§]

The variance components in a regression analysis are partitioned similarly to those in a regular analysis of variance. The total variance, represented by the total sum of squares (SS_t), reflects the variance explained by the regression of Y on X and the unexplained error variance. These variance components are illustrated in Figure 24.8. For a given X we can locate the observed value of Y and the predicted score $\hat{Y}$, which lies on the regression line. We can also establish the value for $\overline{Y}$, the mean of all Y scores. Without the regression line, the best we can do to predict Y is the mean of the distribution, $\overline{Y}$. For example, if we knew that the mean height for men was 5 ft 8 in., and we wanted to predict the height of any random man on the street, our best estimate would be 5 ft 8 in. But if a man's height is related to his parents' height, then we can improve this estimate if we also know the height of this man's mother and father. We know more about his height (Y) by knowing his parents' height (X). Therefore, by using the regression line we have improved our prediction by the amount $\hat{Y} - \overline{Y}$, which is the deviation of the predicted score from the mean. This distance tells us how much better we can predict Y by knowing X.

If we look at $\Sigma(\hat{Y} - \overline{Y})$ for all the data points in a distribution, we will be able to determine how much of the total variation in the sample is accounted for by knowing the regression of Y on X. The sum of the squares of these differences, $\Sigma(\hat{Y} - \overline{Y})^2$, is called the **regression sum of squares** (SS_{reg}), or that part of Y that is explained by X.

The rest of the variance is attributed to the deviation of each observed score from the regression line, $(Y - \hat{Y})$, or the residual. It is that part of Y that is not explained by X. This value is an indication of how good or poor a fit the regression line is. When the

---

[§]The slope of the regression line can also be tested using the *t*-test: $t = \dfrac{b}{(SEE/s_X\sqrt{n-1})}$, where s_X is the standard deviation of the X scores. The statistical result of this test will be the same as for the analysis of variance of regression, based on the relationship $F = t^2$.

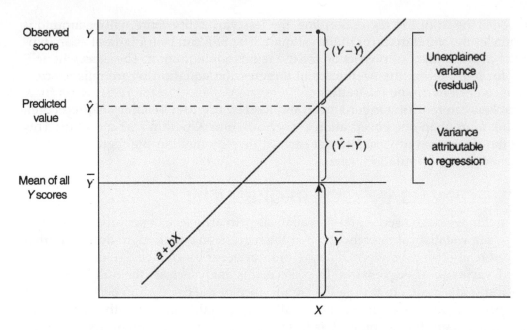

FIGURE 24.8 Illustration of the variance components in an analysis of variance for regression.

fit is good, the observed scores will fall close to the line, and the residuals will be small. This means that X is a good predictor of Y. When the fit is poor, X and Y are not strongly related, and these deviations will be large. The term $\Sigma(Y - \hat{Y})^2$ is called the **residual sum of squares** (SS_{res}), or the unexplained variance attributable to the residuals. A linear regression analysis will generate an analysis of variance table that provides these values.

The ANOVA summary table, shown in Table 24.3, represents the regression of systolic blood pressure (Y) on age (X) for a sample of 10 women (from Figure 24.3). This output follows the format of a standard analysis of variance, with a total of $N - 1$ degrees of freedom. In the linear model, one degree of freedom is always associated with the regression; therefore, $N - 2$ degrees of freedom are attributed to the residuals (the error term). The value of F is equal to MS_{reg}/MS_{res}.

In this example, the observed F-ratio for the regression is 24.74 with 1 and 8 degrees of freedom. As shown in Table 24.3❷, this test is significant at .001. This tells us that the relationship between X and Y is not likely to be the result of chance. It does not indicate how strong this relationship is. When the analysis of variance of regression results in a nonsignificant F-test, the researcher concludes that the observed relationship could have occurred by chance; that is, the regression line does not provide a reasonable basis for predicting values of Y.

RESTRICTIONS ON THE INTERPRETATION OF LINEAR REGRESSION ANALYSIS

Regression equations are derived from a set of known scores, and the accuracy of the regression line for prediction for the individuals in the test sample is reflected in the size of the residuals. The ultimate purpose of regression analysis is not, however, to predict scores we already know. The intent is to predict scores for a new sample of observations from the findings on the known data. Therefore, it is important that the reference population for the analysis be clearly specified, because predictions will not be applicable to those who do not meet population criteria. Most importantly, predictions cannot be validly made for values of X that go beyond the range of scores that were used to generate the regression line. If we determine a regression line for predicting blood pressure from age based on a sample of women 34 to 73 years, we cannot apply the equation to males or to younger subjects. We cannot know if the shape of the distribution would be altered with the addition of scores at lower age ranges. Therefore, generalization of a regression procedure is inherently limited by the range of scores used to derive the equation.

A second consideration in the interpretation of regression data is the adequacy of a linear fit. Just as with correlation, linear regression procedures are useful only if the distribution of scores demonstrates a linear association between X and Y. The lack of a significant slope does not necessarily mean that X and Y are unrelated, but may indicate that the relationship does not follow a straight line. We discuss the application of regression to curvilinear relationships in the next section.

NONLINEAR REGRESSION

There are obvious limitations inherent in linear regression for describing curvilinear relationships. Because linear regression is the most commonly used regression model, researchers should be wary about interpreting outcomes that demonstrate no relationship between X and Y. For example, look at the data plotted in Figure 24.9, showing the relationship between psychomotor ability and age for a hypothetical sample of 30 subjects aged 10 to 50 years. Using linear techniques, the correlation coefficient is low ($r = .32$). Based on this information alone, one would assume that X and Y were not

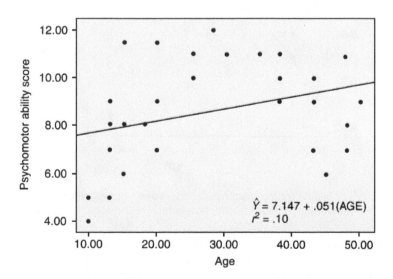

FIGURE 24.9 Linear regression of psychomotor ability (scored 0–15) on age. The regression line appears to be a poor fit.

strongly related; however, examination of the scatter plot reveals that the data form a distinctly curved pattern. The measured skill improves until age 30, when a slow decline begins. Therefore, it makes more sense to draw a curve that more accurately reflects the relationship between X and Y, as shown in Figure 24.10. We can express this curve statistically in the form of a quadratic equation:

$$\hat{Y} = a + b_1X + b_2X^2 \tag{24.2}$$

Equation 24.2 defines a parabolic curve, that is, a curve with one turn. This curve is also called a **quadratic curve.**[*] The process of deriving its equation is called **polynomial regression.** Clearly, this fitted curve is more representative of the data points than the linear regression line.

The method of calculating the regression coefficients for this equation goes beyond this text. It is advisable to use a computer to perform these more complex mathematical manipulations; however, the application of this model is similar to that of linear regression. Polynomial regression is also based on the concept of least squares, so that the vertical distance of each point from the curve is minimized. Therefore, the curve can be used for predicting Y scores in the same way as a linear regression line.

Researchers often have to decide whether a linear or polynomial regression model best fits their data. This decision is greatly facilitated by examining a scatter plot of the data. The analysis of variance for regression can be applied to determine if the linear or polynomial regression model provides a better fit for a given set of data.[††]

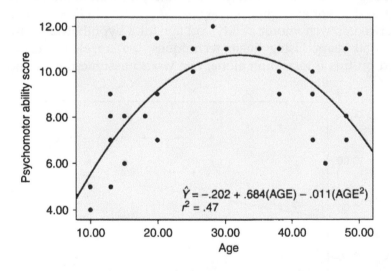

FIGURE 24.10 Curvilinear data for the hypothetical regression of psychomotor ability on age, and the least-squares curve derived through a second-order polynomial regression.

---

[*]A quadratic curve, with one turn, is considered a *polynomial of the second order*. A linear "curve," or straight line, is a polynomial of the first order. See discussion of trends in Chapter 21.

[††]It is also possible to transform nonlinear data to achieve a linear fit by transforming one or both variables, often using log values (see Appendix D).

Table 24.4 shows the analysis of variance for both a linear (A) and a quadratic (B) regression of psychomotor ability on age. The *F*-ratio for the linear regression is not significant ($p = .087$), as we might expect from looking at the data in Figure 24.9. This tells us that the linear model is not adequate for describing this relationship. In the bottom panel of Table 24.4 we see that the quadratic regression is significant ($p = .000$), indicating that the quadratic curve is a good fit for these data. The equation for the curve is

$$\hat{Y} = -.202 + .684 \, (\text{AGE}) - .011 \, (\text{AGE}^2)$$

A closer look at the analysis of variance helps us see how differently these two approaches explain the data. Note that the total sum of squares for both analyses is the same; that is, the total variability in the sample is the same, regardless of which type of regression is performed. What is different is the amount of that variance that is explained by each of the regression models. The sum of squares attributable to the regression in the linear analysis is 14.404, whereas for the quadratic regression it is 66.477. This demonstrates how a greater proportion of the total variability is explained by the curve.

ANALYSIS OF COVARIANCE

The function of experimental design is to explain the effect of an independent variable on a dependent variable while controlling for the confounding effect of extraneous factors. When extraneous factors are not controlled, the results of measurement cannot be attributed solely to the experimental treatment. Statistically, we speak of controlling the *unexplained variance* in the data, that is, the variance in scores that cannot be explained by the independent variable. All experiments will have some unexplained variance, sometimes because of the varied individual characteristics of the subjects and sometimes because of unknown or random factors that affect responses. When we cannot control these factors by purposefully eliminating them or manipulating them, we use principles of experimental design to decrease the error variance they cause.

In Chapter 9 we described several design strategies that can reduce chance variability in data, such as using homogeneous groups or matching. There are times, however, when design strategies are not capable of sufficient control. Even when random assignment is used, there is no guarantee that potentially confounding characteristics will be equally distributed, especially when dealing with small samples. The issue of concern is the ability to equate groups at the outset, so that observed differences following treatment can be attributed to the treatment and not to other unexplained factors. When the research design cannot provide adequate control, statistical control can be achieved by measuring one or more confounding variables in addition to the dependent variable, and accounting for the variability in the confounding factors in the analysis. This is the conceptual basis for **analysis of covariance (ANCOVA).**

Adjusting Group Means

The ANCOVA is actually a combination of analysis of variance and linear regression. It is used to compare groups on a dependent variable, where there is reason to suspect that groups differ on some relevant characteristic, called a **covariate,** before treatment.

TABLE 24.4   OUTPUT FOR LINEAR AND POLYNOMIAL REGRESSION OF PSYCHOMOTOR ABILITY ON AGE (N = 30) (SEE FIGURE 24.11)

A. LINEAR REGRESSION

Model Summary

R	R Square	Std. Error of the Estimate
.318	❶ .101	2.142

ANOVA

	Sum of Squares	df	Mean Square	F	Sig.
Regression	14.404	1	14.404	3.139	.087
Residual	128.463	28	4.588		❷
Total	142.867	29			

Coefficients

	Unstandardized Coefficients		Standardized Coefficients		
	B	Std. Error	Beta	t	Sig.
Age	.051	.029	.318	1.772	❷ .087
(Constant)	7.147	.892			

B. QUADRATIC REGRESSION

Model Summary

R	R Square	Std. Error of the Estimate
.682	❸ .465	1.682

ANOVA

	Sum of Squares	df	Mean Square	F	Sig.
Regression	66.477	❹ 2	33.238	11.748	.000
Residual	76.390	27	2.829		❺
Total	142.867	29			

Coefficients

	Unstandardized Coefficients		Standardized Coefficients		
	B	Std. Error	Beta	t	Sig.
Age	.684	.149	4.255	4.583	❺ .000
Age**2❻	❼ −.011	.002	−3.983	−4.290	.000
(Constant)	−.202	1.851			

---

❶ The value of R-square shows that linear prediction is quite weak.

❷ The analysis of variance of regression shows that the linear function is not significant. This is confirmed in the test of the regression coefficient for age.

❸ The value of R-square is substantially increased with the quadratic curve, indicating that the curve is better fit to the data.

❹ The variance attributable to the regression now uses 2 degrees of freedom because it involves a second-order curve.

❺ The analysis of variance of regression for the quadratic function is significant.

❻ The symbol for exponent is a double asterisk. This term is age squared.

❼ The polynomial equation for the quadratic curve is: $\hat{Y} = -.202 + .684(\text{Age}) - .011(\text{Age}^2)$.

Note: Portions of the output that are not relevant to the interpretation of results have been omitted.

The variability that can be attributed to the covariate is partitioned out, and effectively removed from the analysis of variance, allowing for a more valid explanation of the relationship between the independent and dependent variables.

Example

We can clarify this process with a hypothetical example. Suppose we wanted to compare the effect of two teaching strategies on the clinical performance of students in their first year of clinical training. We hypothesize that training with videotaped cases (Strategy 1) will be more effective than discussion and reading groups (Strategy 2). We randomly assign 12 students to two groups ($n = 6$ per group). We are concerned, however, that the students' academic performance would be a potential confounding factor in making this comparison, based on the assumption that there is a correlation between academic and clinical performance. Therefore, we would want to know if the grade point average (GPA) in the two groups had been evenly distributed. If one group happened to have a higher GPA than the other, our results could be misleading. In this example, teaching strategy is the independent variable, clinical performance is the dependent variable, and GPA is the covariate. By knowing the values of the covariate, we can determine if the groups are different on GPA, and we can use this information to adjust our interpretation of the dependent variable if necessary.

To illustrate how the ANCOVA offers this control, let us first look at a hypothetical comparison between the two teaching groups, without considering GPA. Suppose we obtain the following means for clinical performance on a standardized test (scored 0–100):

Mean clinical score	
Strategy 1	43.8 ($\pm$24.5)
Strategy 2	48.5 ($\pm$21.7)

The analysis of variance comparing these two groups is shown in Table 24.5A, demonstrating that these two means are not statistically different ($p = .734$).[‡‡] Based on this result, is it reasonable to conclude that the teaching strategies are not different? Or might we suspect that GPA may be differentially distributed between the two groups, which has biased the results? To answer these questions, we must take a closer look at the data to see how these variables are related.

Regression

Figure 24.11 shows us the distribution of GPA and clinical performance scores for Strategy 1 (●) and Strategy 2 (○) with their respective regression lines. The dependent variable, clinical performance score, is plotted along the Y-axis, and the covariate, GPA,

---

[‡‡]An unpaired *t*-test could also have been performed with the same result ($t = .349, df = 10, p = .734$); however, to adjust scores with a covariate, an analysis of variance must be used. Therefore, we have used the ANOVA here to facilitate comparison of outcomes with the ANCOVA.

TABLE 24.5 ANALYSIS OF COVARIANCE FOR COMPARISON OF CLINICAL PERFORMANCE FOLLOWING TWO TEACHING STRATEGIES (*N* = 12)

A. ANALYSIS OF VARIANCE

ANOVA

	Sum of Squares	df	Mean Square	F	Sig.
Between groups	65.333	1	65.333	.122	.734
Within groups	5360.333	10	536.033		❶
Total	5425.667	11			

B. ANALYSIS OF COVARIANCE

Tests of Between-Subjects Effects

Source	Sum of Squares	df	Mean Square	F	Sig.
GPA ❷	4977.261	1	4977.261	116.937	❷ .000
Strategy ❸	2083.733	1	2083.733	48.956	❸ .000
Error ❹	383.073	9	42.564		
Total	5425.667	11			

Estimated Marginal Means

Dependent Variable: score

	❺	Std.	95% Confidence Interval	
Strategy	Mean	Error	Lower Bound	Upper Bound
1	30.370	2.940	23.719	37.021
2	61.963	2.940	55.312	68.614

❻ Covariates appearing in the model are evaluated at the following values: GPA = 2.8417.

❶ The analysis of variance shows no significant difference between the teaching strategy groups.

❷ GPA is the covariate. This term is significant (*p* = .000), which indicates that the slope of the regression line for the covariate is significantly different from zero. This is a necessary condition for validity of the ANCOVA.

❸ The between-groups effect tests the difference between Strategy 1 and Strategy 2, based on the adjusted means, which is significant.

❹ The error term here is smaller than the error term in the ANOVA (in panel A), as it does not include the variance accounted for by the covariate.

❺ These are the adjusted means.

❻ The adjusted means are based on the regression of GPA on clinical performance (shown in Figure 24.13), using the combined mean GPA of 2.84.

Note: Portions of the output that are not relevant to interpretation have been omitted.

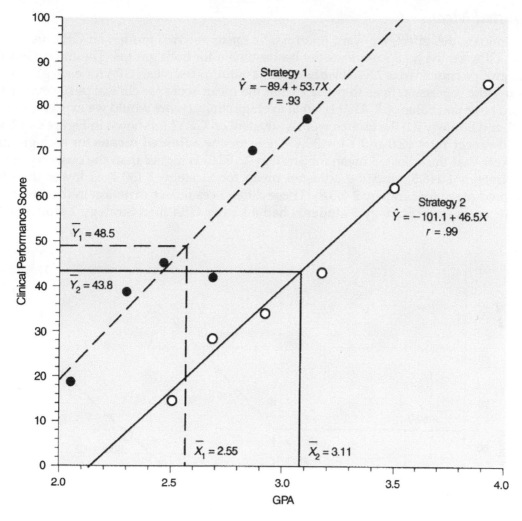

FIGURE 24.11 Regression lines defining the relationship between clinical performance score and grade point average (GPA) for two teaching strategies. GPA is the covariate for an analysis of covariance. The mean GPA for Strategy 2 is substantially lower than that for Strategy 1.

is plotted along the X-axis. We can see from this scatter plot that these variables are highly correlated for both groups ($r = .93$ and $.99$), and that the slopes of the two regression lines are fairly similar ($b = 53.7$ and 46.5).

We can also see that the regression line for Strategy 1 is higher than that for Strategy 2, indicating that Group 1 had higher values of clinical performance for any given GPA, even though the sample means for clinical score are not significantly different. There is, however, another important difference. If we look at the mean GPA for each group, we can see that the students using Strategy 1 have substantially lower GPAs than those using Strategy 2 ($\overline{X}_1 = 2.55$, $\overline{X}_2 = 3.11$). Knowing that GPA is a correlate of clinical performance, it is reasonable to believe that this difference could have confounded the statistical analysis.

Adjusted Means

To eliminate this effect, we want to *artificially equate* the two groups on GPA, using the mean GPA for the total sample as the best estimate for both groups. The mean GPA for both groups combined is 2.84. If we assign this value as the mean GPA for each group, we can use the regression lines to predict what the mean score for clinical performance (Y) would be at that value of X. That is, what average clinical score would we expect for Strategy 1 and Strategy 2 if the groups were equivalent on GPA? As shown in Figure 24.12, we would expect $\overline{Y}_1' = 62.0$ and $\overline{Y}_2' = 30.4$. These are the **adjusted means** for each group.

Note that the adjusted mean for Strategy 1 (62.0) is higher than the observed mean for Strategy 1 (48.5), and the adjusted mean for Strategy 2 (30.4) is lower than the observed mean for Strategy 2 (43.8). These differences reflect variation in the covariate; that is, on average Strategy 2 students had a higher GPA than Strategy 1 students. By

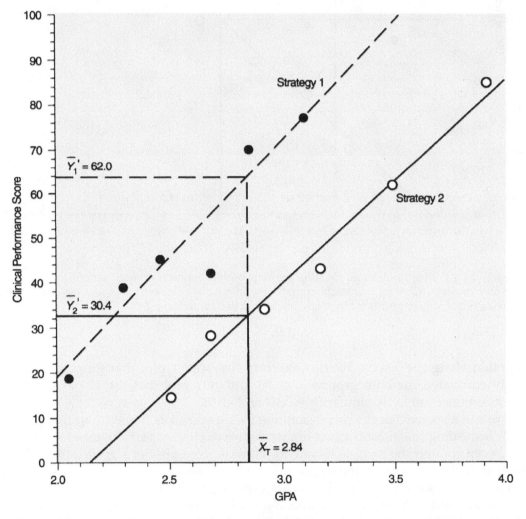

FIGURE 24.12   Adjusted means for clinical score, based on grade point average (GPA) as a covariate. Predicted values of clinical score are based on a common mean GPA for both teaching strategies.

setting a common mean GPA, we moved the average GPA up for Strategy 1 (2.55 to 2.84), increasing the corresponding clinical score; and we moved the average GPA down for Strategy 2 (3.11 to 2.84), decreasing the corresponding clinical score. Therefore, we have adjusted scores by removing the effect of GPA differences so we could compare clinical scores as if both groups had the same GPA.

This example illustrates the situation where a covariate obscures the true nature of the difference between group means. This process may also work in the opposite direction, however; that is, group means may initially appear significantly different when in fact they are not. In that case, the analysis of covariance may result in no significant difference. For example, consider a comparison of strength between men and women. We would expect to see a difference between them, with men being stronger. But this difference could be due to the weight of men versus women, rather than just gender. If we were to use weight as a covariate, we might find that the groups no longer appear different in strength.

Output

After scores are adjusted according to the regression lines, an analysis of variance is run on the adjusted values. Table 24.5B shows the results of this analysis for the teaching strategy data from Figure 24.12. Recall that the original analysis of variance showed no significant difference between these strategies (see Table 24.5A).

In the summary table for the ANCOVA, the first line of the table represents the variance attributable to the covariate, or the regression of GPA on clinical score (see Table 24.5❷). This component tests the hypothesis that the slope of the regression line is significantly different from zero. If it is not significant, the covariate is not linearly related to the dependent variable, and therefore, the adjusted mean scores will be meaningless. In this example, we can see that the covariate of GPA is significant ($p = .000$). The researcher should always examine the covariate effect first, to determine that the ANCOVA is an appropriate test. The degrees of freedom associated with this factor equal the number of covariates used in the analysis. In this case, with one covariate, we have used one degree of freedom.

The between-groups effect for Strategy is based on a comparison of the adjusted group means (see Table 24.5❺). As in a standard analysis of variance, the degrees of freedom will equal $k - 1$. Now we find that the difference between the strategy groups is significant ($p = .000$), and we can reject the null hypothesis (see Table 24.5❸). We conclude that clinical performance does differ between those exposed to videotaped cases and discussion groups when adjusted for their grade point average. We have, therefore, increased the sensitivity of our test by decreasing the unexplained variance. We have accounted for more of the variance in clinical performance by knowing GPA and teaching strategy than we did by knowing teaching strategy alone.

The third line of the table shows the error variance (see Table 24.5❹), that is, all the variance that is left unexplained after the between-groups and covariate sources have been accounted for. When the covariate is a good linear fit, the error variance will be substantially reduced. This is evident if we compare the error sums of squares in Tables 24.5A and B for the ANOVA and ANCOVA of the same data. In fact, if we look at the error (within groups) sum of squares for the ANOVA ($SS_e = 5360.33$), we can see that it is equal to the combined sums of squares for the covariate and the error component in the ANCOVA (4977.26 + 383.07 = 5360.33). By removing the effect of GPA from the unexplained variance, we have left less variance unexplained. Therefore, the ANCOVA allows us to demonstrate a statistical difference between the groups, where the ANOVA did not.

Assumptions for Analysis of Covariance

Before running an ANCOVA, several assumptions should be satisfied to assure validity of the analysis.

Linearity of the Covariate.   The analysis of covariance model is appropriate only if there is a linear relationship between the covariate and the dependent variable. It is most effective when $r > .60$.[6] For example, it would be unreasonable to use height or weight as a covariate for clinical performance. The researcher should check correlations before starting a study, to be sure that data are being collected on a useful covariate. Relationships that are curvilinear will invalidate the analysis of covariance, although the relationship may be made linear by mathematical transformation.

Homogeneity of Slopes.   The ANCOVA requires that the slopes of the regression lines for each group be parallel. Unequal slopes indicate that the relationship between the covariate and dependent variable is different for each group. Therefore, the adjusted means will be based on different proportional relationships, and their comparison will be meaningless. A test for **homogeneity of slopes** should be done before the ANCOVA is attempted, to be sure that the procedure is valid.[6] The null hypothesis for this test states that the regression coefficients (slopes) for the two groups will not be significantly different: $H_0: \beta_1 = \beta_2$. If GPA is a "good" covariate, then it will allow adjustments based on proportional values that are the same in both strategy groups.

Independence of the Covariate.   The variable chosen as the covariate must be related to the dependent variable, but must also be independent of the treatment effect; that is, the independent variable cannot influence the value of the covariate. For example, suppose we wanted to study the effect of a general exercise program on balance, using lower extremity strength as a covariate. If we were to measure the subjects' strength after the treatment was completed, we might find that the exercise program increased the strength of the lower extremities. Therefore, the strength value would not be independent of the treatment effect and would not be a valid covariate. To avoid this situation, covariates should always be measured prior to initiation of treatment.

Reliability of the Covariate.   The validity of the ANCOVA is also founded on the assumption that the covariate is not contaminated by measurement error.[6] Any error found in the covariate is compounded when the regression coefficients and adjusted means are calculated. Therefore, justification for using the adjusted scores is based on accuracy of the covariate. Although it may be impossible to obtain totally error-free measurement, every effort should be made to ensure the greatest degree of reliability possible.

Using Multiple Covariates

The analysis of covariance can be extended to accommodate any number of covariates. There may be several characteristics that are relevant to understanding the dependent variable. For example, if we wanted to compare strength at different age ranges, we might use a combination of height, weight, limb girth, or percentage body fat as covariates. With multiple covariates, the analysis of covariance involves multiple regression procedures, where several X variables are correlated with one Y variable, and a predicted value for Y is determined, based on those covariates that are most highly correlated. Multiple regression techniques are discussed further in Chapter 29.

When several covariates are used, the precision of the analysis can be greatly enhanced, as long as the covariates are all highly correlated with the dependent variable and not correlated with each other. If, however, the covariates are correlated with each other, they provide redundant information and no additional benefit is gained by including them. In fact, using a large number of interrelated covariates can be a disadvantage, because each covariate uses up one degree of freedom in the analysis. This decreases the degrees of freedom left for the error term, which increases the F needed for significance between groups. The analysis then loses statistical power. With smaller samples, this could have a biasing effect.

It is important, therefore, to make educated choices about the use of covariates. Previous research and pilot studies may be able to document which variables are most highly correlated with the dependent variable and which are least likely to be related to each other.

Pretest-Posttest Adjustments

The ANCOVA is often used to control for initial differences between groups based on a pretest measure. When intact groups are tested or when randomization is used with small groups, the initial measurements on the dependent variable are often different enough to be of concern for further comparison. For example, suppose we were studying the effect of two exercise programs on strength. We randomly assign subjects to two groups and would like to assume that their initial strength levels are similar; however, after the pretest we find that one group is much stronger on average than the other, a difference that occurred just by chance. We can use the ANCOVA to equate both groups on their pretest scores and adjust posttest scores accordingly. The analysis between groups is then done using the adjusted posttest scores, as if both groups had started out at the same level of strength.

Researchers are often tempted to control for initial differences by using difference scores as the dependent variable in a pretest-posttest design. There are disadvantages to this approach, however, because the potential for measurement error is increased when using difference scores (see Chapter 6). In experimental studies, this situation can reduce the power of a statistical test; that is, the greater the amount of measurement error, the less likely we will find a significant difference between two difference scores, even when the treatment was really effective. Therefore, many researchers prefer the analysis of covariance for statistically controlling initial differences. This approach is not, however, a remedy for a study with poor reliability. Although some research questions may be more readily answered by the use of change scores, the researcher should consider what type of data will best serve the analysis.

Interpreting the ANCOVA

The analysis of covariance is a powerful statistical tool that has often been looked on as a cure-all for design imperfections. Although it does have the power to increase the sensitivity of a test by removing many forms of bias, it does not provide a safeguard against problems in the design of a study. The ANCOVA cannot substitute for randomization. Quasi-experimental designs that use intact groups suffer from many interpretive biases, some of which the ANCOVA is able to control better than others. Indeed, unless a covariate is totally reliable, it will introduce some biases of its own. Some researchers have used the ANCOVA to compensate for failures in their design, such as the discovery of uncontrolled variables after data collection has been started, but this is not its intent. The analysis of covariance is correctly used in situations where experimental control of relevant variables is not possible and where these factors are identified and measured at the outset.

The ANCOVA has some limitations that should be considered in this context. One major criticism is that the adjusted means are not real scores, and therefore, the generalization of data from an analysis of covariance is compromised. It is also important to realize that one covariate may be insufficient for removing extraneous effects and that the outcome of an ANCOVA could be significantly altered if different combinations of covariates were used. In addition, researchers must decide which covariates will be most meaningful, and decide early so that data are collected on the proper variables. Covariates that are quantitative variables, such as height, weight and age, provide the most precision for adjusting scores; however, dichotomous variables such as sex and disability can be used as covariates.

COMMENTARY

If Only It Were That Simple

Two issues related to generalization of regression analysis should be mentioned here. First, just as with correlation, it is important to refrain from interpreting predictive relationships as causal. Statistical associations by themselves do not provide sufficient evidence of causality. The researcher must be able to establish the methodological, logical and theoretical rationales behind such claims; that is, causal inference is a function of how the data were produced, not how they were analyzed.[7] Second, it is important to restrict generalization of predictive relationships to the population on which the data were obtained. The characteristics of subjects chosen for a regression study define this population.

Simple linear regression analysis is limited in that it accounts for the effect of only one independent variable on one dependent variable. Most behavioral phenomena cannot be explained so simply. For instance, when we examined the predictive accuracy of the regression of blood pressure on age, we established that $r^2 = .76$. This indicates that 76% of the variance in blood pressure could be predicted by knowing a woman's age; however, 24% of the variance was unaccounted for. Some other variable or variables must be identified to improve the prediction equation. Multiple regression procedures have been developed that provide an efficient mechanism for studying the combined effect of several independent variables on a dependent variable for purposes of improving predictive accuracy. We present these techniques in Chapter 29.

REFERENCES

1. Anzarut A, Chen M, Shankowsky H, Tredget EE. Quality-of-life and outcome predictors following massive burn injury. *Plast Reconstr Surg* 2005;116:791–797.
2. Szatmari P, Bryson SE, Boyle MH, Streiner DL, Duku E. Predictors of outcome among high functioning children with autism and Asperger syndrome. *J Child Psychol Psychiatry* 2003;44:520–528.
3. Wee JY, Hopman WM. Stroke impairment pedictors of discharge function, length of stay, and discharge destination in stroke rehabilitation. *Am J Phys Med Rehabil* 2005;84: 604–612.
4. Gross DP, Battie MC. Predicting timely recovery and recurrence following multidisciplinary rehabilitation in patients with compensated low back pain. *Spine* 2005;30:235–240.
5. Snedecor GW, Cochran WG. *Statistical Methods* (8th ed.). Ames, IA: Iowa State University Press, 1991.
6. Green SB, Salkind NJ, Akey TM. *Using SPSS for Windows and Macintosh: Analyzing and Understanding Data* (4th ed.). Upper Saddle River, NJ: Prentice Hall, 2004.
7. Cohen J, Cohen P. *Applied Multiple Regression/Correlation Analysis for the Behavioral Sciences.* Hillsdale, NJ: Lawrence Erlbaum Associates, 1975.

CHAPTER 25

Measures of Association for Categorical Variables: Chi-Square

Many research questions in clinical and behavioral science involve categorical variables that are measured on a nominal or ordinal scale. These questions usually deal with the analysis of proportions or frequencies within various categories. For instance, surveys often code responses that represent frequencies, such as the number of Yes–No responses to a series of items or the number of respondents who fall into certain age groups. We can then ask questions about the proportion of respondents that fall into each category. In descriptive studies we are often interested in how certain nominal variables are distributed. For example, we might want to determine the proportion of patients with right-sided or left-sided strokes who are functionally dependent or independent at discharge or the proportion of therapists who work in private practice versus institutional settings.

These types of categorical data are analyzed by determining if there is a difference between the proportions *observed* within a set of categories and the proportions that would be *expected* by chance. For example, if therapists are equally likely to work in private or institutional settings, then theoretically we would expect an equal proportion, or 50%, to fall into each category. The null hypothesis states that no difference exists between the actual proportions measured in a sample and this theoretical distribution. If the observed data depart significantly from these expected null values, we reject the null hypothesis.

The purpose of this chapter is to describe the use of several statistics that can be used to analyze frequencies or proportions. These statistics are based on **chi-square,** χ^2, which is a nonparametric statistic used to determine if a distribution of observed frequencies differs from theoretical expected frequencies. Chi-square has many applications in clinical research, in both experimental and descriptive analysis. We concentrate on two general uses of the test. A test of goodness of fit is used to determine if a set of observed frequencies differs from a given set of theoretical frequencies that define a specific distribution. A test that compares the proportion of therapists in private and institutional settings fits this model, based on a theoretical distribution of 50 : 50. Tests of independence are used to determine if two classification variables are independent of each other, that is, to examine the degree of association between them. For example, we could study the frequency of left- and right-sided stroke in terms of functional level at discharge to determine if these variables are related or independent of each other. We also discuss the use of a related procedure called the McNemar test, for examining frequencies of correlated samples. In addition, several other coefficients of association for categorical data will be described.

THE CHI-SQUARE STATISTIC

As we discuss the different applications of the χ^2 statistic, it is important to keep in mind two general assumptions: (1) *Frequencies represent individual counts,* not ranks or percentages. This means that data in each category represent the actual number of persons, objects, or events in those categories, not a summary statistic. (2) *Categories are exhaustive and mutually exclusive.* Therefore, every subject can be assigned to an appropriate category, but only one. Repeated measurement or assignment is not appropriate; that is, no one individual should be represented in more than one category. The characteristics being measured should be defined with enough specificity to avoid any overlaps in group assignment.

Chi-square is defined by*

$$\chi^2 = \sum \frac{(O - E)^2}{E} \tag{25.1}$$

where O represents the **observed frequency** and E represents the **expected frequency**. As the difference between observed and expected frequencies increases, the value of χ^2 will increase. If observed and expected frequencies are the same, χ^2 will equal zero.

We illustrate the application of this statistic using a simple example. Suppose we tossed a coin 100 times. The null hypothesis states that no bias exists in the coin, and we would expect a theoretical outcome of 50 heads and 50 tails. We observe 47 heads and 53 tails. Does this deviation from the null hypothesis occur because the coin is biased, or is it only a matter of chance? In other words, is the difference between the observed and expected frequencies sufficiently large to justify rejection of the null hypothesis?

We calculate χ^2 by substituting values in the term $(O - E)^2/E$ for each category. For heads,

$$\frac{(O - E)^2}{E} = \frac{(47 - 50)^2}{50} = \frac{(-3)^2}{50} = 0.18$$

For tails,

$$\frac{(O - E)^2}{E} = \frac{(53 - 50)^2}{50} = \frac{(3)^2}{50} = 0.18$$

The sum of these terms for all categories is the value of χ^2. Therefore,

---

*Although the definitional formula for χ^2 (Eq. 25.1) is used most often, there is a computational formula that may be useful: $\chi^2 = \sum \frac{O^2}{E} - N$.

$$\chi^2 = \sum \frac{(O - E)^2}{E} = 0.18 + 0.18 = 0.36$$

We analyze the significance of this value using critical values of χ^2 found in Appendix Table A.5. Along the top of the table we identify the desired α level, say .05. Along the side we locate the appropriate degrees of freedom. In this case, $df = 1$. We will discuss rules for determining degrees of freedom for different statistical models shortly. Chi-square tests do not distinguish between one- and two-tailed tests because no negative values are possible.

The calculated value of χ^2 must be *greater than or equal to* the critical value to be significant. In this example, the observed value is less than $_{(.05)}\chi^2_{(1)} = 3.84$. Therefore, H_0 is not rejected, and we would conclude that the coin toss was fair.

GOODNESS OF FIT

In tests for **goodness of fit**, the researcher compares observed frequency counts with a known or theoretical distribution. The classical studies of heredity performed by Mendel illustrate this concept. He observed the color and shape of several generations of peas and compared the frequencies of specific color and shape combinations with a theoretical distribution based on his predictions about the role of dominant and recessive genes. When the observed distributions matched the theoretical model, his genetic theory was supported. Similarly, the coin toss described earlier is essentially a test of goodness of fit to a probability distribution. Chi-square will test the null hypothesis that the proportion of outcomes within each category will not significantly differ from the expected distribution; that is, the observed proportions will fall within random fluctuation of the expected proportions.

There are many models for testing goodness of fit. The two most common applications involve testing observed data against a **uniform distribution** across all categories and a **known distribution** within the underlying population.

Sample size for goodness of fit tests should be large enough that no expected frequencies are less than 1.0; that is, every category in the theoretical distribution of interest should expect at least one count. When this criterion is not met, sample size should be increased or categories combined to create an appropriate distribution. Note that this criterion applies to the expected frequencies, not the observed counts.

Uniform Distributions

Consider a study designed to determine if the incidence of stroke is greater on the right or the left in people over 70 years of age. If we assume that the causative factors of stroke are not biased to one side, then theoretically we would expect to see a uniform distribution, 50% right-sided and 50% left-sided strokes, in the population. This is the null hypothesis, representing chance occurrence. Suppose we obtain data from a broad sample of 130 patients, and find that 71 were affected on the right and 59 on the left. Is this distribution significantly different from the 50% ratio we expect by chance?

We use chi-square to determine if the observed frequencies fit the uniform distribution model by comparing the observed and expected frequencies using Equation (25.1).

First we must establish the expected frequencies. For a uniform distribution we do this simply by dividing the total sample equally among the categories. Therefore, if chance is operating, we would expect 50% of our sample, or 65 people, to have right-sided strokes, and 50%, or 65 people, to have left-sided strokes. We calculate $(O - E)^2/E$ for each category, as shown in Table 25.1.

In the uniform distribution goodness of fit model, degrees of freedom equal $k - 1$, where k is the number of categories. With two categories (right and left), $df = 1$. Therefore, we compare the calculated value, $\chi^2 = 1.10$, with the critical value $_{(.05)}\chi^2_{(1)} = 3.84$, obtained from Appendix Table A.5. The calculated value is less than the critical value, and we do not reject the null hypothesis. The difference between the observed and expected frequencies can be attributed to chance, and our sample fits the expected uniform distribution. According to these hypothetical data, the incidence of right- and left-sided strokes can be considered a random event.

By definition, the expected frequencies for a uniform distribution will be evenly divided among the categories. Therefore, if we studied a sample with three or four categories, we would test the observed frequencies in each category against expected frequencies of 33.3% and 25%, respectively. For example, if we assigned 130 cases to three different categories, we would expect 43.33 cases in each category. If we had four categories, we would expect 32.5 cases per category. It may seem strange to be dealing with fractions of a count in expected frequencies, as we obviously cannot have a fraction of an individual in a category; however, these values represent only theoretical values

---

TABLE 25.1   CALCULATION OF χ^2 TO TEST GOODNESS OF FIT TO A UNIFORM DISTRIBUTION: FREQUENCY OF LEFT-SIDE AND RIGHT-SIDE STROKE ($N = 130$)

A. DATA AND COMPUTATION

Side	O	E	O − E	$(O - E)^2$	$\dfrac{(O - E)^2}{E}$
Right	71	65	6	36	.55
Left	59	65	−6	36	.55
	130	130			

$$\chi^2 = \sum \frac{(O - E)^2}{E} = 1.10$$

B. HYPOTHESIS TEST

$df = (k - 1) = 1$ $_{(0.5)}\chi^2_{(1)} = 3.84$ (Table A.5)   Do not reject H_0

C. OUTPUT

Side

	Observed N	Expected N	Residual
Right	71	65.0	6.0
Left	59	65.0	−6.0
Total	130		

Test Statistics

	Side
Chi-Square	1.108
df	1
Sig.	.293

based on an infinite number of possible scores, and cannot be interpreted as representing actual expected counts.

Known Distributions

The third goodness of fit model compares a sample distribution with a known distribution within an underlying population. This is one way to document how well a sample represents its parent population. In many cases, the variable of interest is normally distributed in the population and the goodness of fit test for normal distributions should be used. In other situations, the population shows a unique distribution that can be tested against observed frequencies.

For example, suppose an investigator hypothesizes that thromboembolism is more common in individuals with certain blood types. If this is true, then we can expect to see those blood types represented among patients with thromboembolism in higher percentages than in the overall population. Suppose we study a sample of 85 patients who have experienced thromboembolism. The null hypothesis states that the disorder is not associated with blood type and that the distribution of blood types in the sample will be similar to that in the overall population. Knowing that 39% of the population has Type A blood, 9% has Type B, 5% has Type AB, and 47% has Type O,[1] we can determine what proportion of the patients should be expected to have each blood type under the null hypothesis. For example, 39% of the sample, or $(0.39)(85) = 33.15$ patients, should have Type A blood. Hypothetical observations and expected values for all four categories are shown in Table 25.2A. By looking at the column labeled $(O - E)$, we can see that there are marked differences between expected and observed frequencies, some showing less than expected and others greater than expected values.

With a known distribution, we test χ^2 with $k - 1$ degrees of freedom. In this case, $df = 4 - 1 = 3$. The calculated value of $\chi^2 = 19.94$, as shown in Table 25.2A. This value exceeds the critical value $_{(.05)}\chi^2_{(3)} = 7.82$, and we can reject the null hypothesis. These hypothetical data do not follow the population distribution, and therefore, there is reason to believe that this disorder has some association with blood type.

INTERPRETING SIGNIFICANT EFFECTS: STANDARDIZED RESIDUALS

When the results of a chi-square test are significant, we can examine the results subjectively, to determine which categories demonstrate the greatest discrepancy between observed and expected values. For this purpose we can look at a residual for each cell, which is the difference between the observed and expected frequencies, given in the column labeled $O - E$. For the blood type study, for instance, the residual for Type A is -5.15. This means that the observed proportion of Type A blood in this sample was less than expected by chance. These raw values may be difficult to interpret, however, as they are effected by the number of observed counts within each cell; that is, cells with larger counts are likely to have larger residuals. Therefore, **standardized residuals, R,**

TABLE 25.2   CALCULATION OF χ^2 FOR GOODNESS OF FIT TO A KNOWN DISTRIBUTION OF BLOOD TYPE ($N = 85$)

A. DATA AND COMPUTATION

Blood Type	% in population	O	E	O – E	$(O - E)^2$	$\dfrac{(O - E)^2}{E}$	Std. Residual
A	39%	32	39.00	−7.00	49.00	1.26	−1.12
B	9%	23	9.00	14.00	196.00	21.78	4.67
AB	5%	10	5.00	5.00	25.00	5.00	2.24
O	47%	35	47.00	−12.00	144.00	3.06	1.75
		100	100.00			$\chi^2 = 31.10$	

B. HYPOTHESIS TEST

$df = (k - 1) = (4 - 1) = 3$ $_{(0.5)}\chi^2_{(3)} = 7.82$ (Table A.5)   Reject H_0.

C. OUTPUT

Type

	Observed N	Expected N	Residual
A	32	39.0	−7.0
B	23	9.0	14.0
AB	10	5.0	5.0
O	35	47.0	−12.0
Total	100		

Test Statistics

	Type
Chi-square	31.098
df	3
Sig.	.000

are often used to demonstrate the relative contribution of each cell to the overall value of chi-square:

$$R = \frac{O - E}{\sqrt{E}} \qquad (25.2)$$

For example, using the data for Type B blood in Table 25.3A, the standardized residual is

$$R = \frac{11.35}{\sqrt{7.65}} = 4.10$$

Standardized residuals for blood types are listed in the rightmost column in Table 25.2. These residual values can be compared to determine which categories contributed most to the value of χ^2. Residuals that are close to or greater than 2.00 are generally considered important.[2] The values for blood type demonstrate that the difference between observed and expected frequencies for patients with Type B blood shows the greatest discrepancy. The positive sign for the residual indicates that the proportion of individuals with thromboembolism who have Type B blood is greater than expected by chance. The small residuals for the other blood types suggest that they do not contribute appreciably to the value of χ^2. The negative values for Types A and O indicate that those frequencies are actually represented in smaller numbers than would be expected by chance.

TESTS OF INDEPENDENCE

The most common application of chi-square in clinical research is in tests of independence. With this approach, researchers examine the association, or lack of association, between two categorical variables. This association is based on the proportion of individuals who fall into each category. These data may be obtained from randomized experiments or from descriptive studies involving classification of subject characteristics.

Many examples of these applications can be found in clinical literature. For example, Frankel et al.[3] examined outcomes of younger and older patients with traumatic brain injuries. They used χ^2 to demonstrate an age-related difference in the proportion of patients who were discharged home versus an institutional setting. Yu et al.[4] demonstrated a higher proportion of school children with wheezing and shortness of breath in school districts with greater air pollution. Monset-Couchard et al.[5] studied differences in frequency of speech problems in twins who were born at normal or small birth weight. Proctor and co-workers[6] studied patients with work-related musculoskeletal disorders, and looked at the proportion of those who completed or did not complete a functional restoration program in relation to return to work and frequency of surgeries. Epidemiologic studies often use chi-square to evaluate the effect of different exposures among diseased and nondiseased individuals.[†]

In each of the preceding studies, the research question asks if the proportions of subjects observed in each category are independent of each other. Two variables are considered independent if the distribution of one in no way depends on the distribution of the other. For example, if the presence of speech problems is independent of birth weight, then a child with a low birth weight is no more likely to have such problems than a child who was born at a normal birth weight. The null hypothesis for a test of independence states that two categorical variables are independent of each other. Therefore, when the null hypothesis is rejected following a significant χ^2 test, it indicates that an association between the variables is present.

Contingency Tables

To test the relationship between two categorical variables, data are arranged in a two-way matrix, called a **contingency table**, with R rows and C columns. To illustrate, consider the data in Table 25.3A, taken from a study by Armstrong et al.,[7] who looked at the differential effect of a total contact cast (TCC) or removable cast walker (RCW) on healing of neuropathic diabetic foot ulcers. They studied 50 patients who were randomly assigned to use either the TCC ($n = 27$) or the RCW ($n = 23$). The dependent variable was the assessment of healing over 12 weeks, scored as "healed" or "unhealed." This is a nominal level of measurement, and is appropriately analyzed

---

[†]The *Mantel–Haenszel chi-square* statistic is a variation of the chi-square test for independence, used in case-control and cohort studies, when the association between two variables is considered confounded by a third variable. The data are stratified so that the effect of the confounder is partitioned out. The Mantel-Haenszel statistic essentially adjusts the value of chi-square to account for the differential contribution of each stratum. Formulas for Mantel-Haenszel statistics can be found in most epidemiologic tests. See Chapter 28 for a discussion of confounding in epidemiologic studies.

TABLE 25.3   CALCULATION OF χ^2 FOR A 2 × 2 CONTINGENCY TABLE SHOWING FREQUENCY OF DIABETIC WOUND HEALING WITH A TOTAL CONTACT CAST (TCC) AND A REMOVABLE CAST WALKER (RCW) ($N = 50$)

A. CONTINGENCY TABLE

		Healed Yes	Healed No	Total
Cast	TCC	19	4	23
	RCW	14	13	27
	Total	33	17	50

B. COMPUTATION

Category		O	E	$O - E$	$(O - E)^2$	$\dfrac{(O - E)^2}{E}$	Std. Residual
Healed	TCC	19	15.18	3.82	14.59	0.96	0.98
	RCW	14	17.82	−3.82	14.59	0.82	−0.90
Unhealed	TCC	4	7.82	−3.82	14.59	1.87	−1.37
	RCW	13	9.18	3.82	14.59	1.59	1.26

$$\chi^2 = 5.24$$

C. HYPOTHESIS TEST

$df = (r - 1)(c - 1) = (2 - 1)(2 - 1) = 1$ $_{(0.5)}\chi^2_{(1)} = 3.84$ (Table A.5)   Reject H_0.

D. OUTPUT

Cast * Healed Crosstabulation

Cast		Healed Yes	No	Total
Total Contact				
	Count	**19**	**4**	23
	Expected Count	**15.2**	**7.8**	23.0
	% within Cast	❶ 82.6%	17.4%	100.0%
	% within Healed	57.6%	23.5%	46.0%
	Std. Residual	1.0	−1.4	
Removable				
	Count	**14**	**13**	27
	Expected Count	**17.8**	**9.2**	27.0
	% within Cast	❶ 51.9%	48.1%	100.0%
	% within Healed	42.4%	76.5%	54.0%
	Std. Residual	−.9	1.3	
Total Count		33	17	50

Chi-Square Tests

	Value	df	Sig. (2-sided)
Pearson Chi-Square	5.236	1	❷ .022
Continuity Correction (a)	❸ 3.955	1	.047
N of Valid Cases	50		

a Computed only for a 2 × 2 table; 0 cells (.0%) have expected count less than 5. The minimum expected count is 7.82.

❶ Percentages are given for each cell across each row (within Cast) and each column (within Healed).

❷ Chi-square is significant ($p = .022$).

❸ The Continuity Correction is automatically included, but is only used when there are cells with expected frequencies less than 5. It would not be applied here.

Source: Armstrong DG, Lavery LA, Wu S, Boulton A. Evaluation of removable and irremovable cast walkers in the healing of diabetic foot wounds: A randomized controlled trial. *Diabetes Care* 2005; 28:551–554.

using χ^2. The 2 × 2 contingency table shows the observed frequencies as the first entry within each cell (labeled "count").

Expected Frequencies

The null hypothesis states that there is no association between the type of cast and healing; that is, both casts will be equally effective. We begin our analysis by calculating the expected frequencies for each cell in the table. This process is somewhat more complicated when working with a contingency table, because we cannot just evenly divide the total sample among the four cells. We must account for the observed *proportions* within each variable. First we ask, what proportion of the total sample ($N = 50$) had healed or unhealed ulcers? According to the observed data, these proportions are

Healed: 33/50 = 66%

Unhealed: 17/50 = 34%

Therefore, if the null hypothesis is true, and no association exists between healing and type of cast worn, we would expect to see these same proportions in the TCC and RCW groups. This means that within each category of cast, 66% of the patients should have healed and 34% should be unhealed. Therefore, of the 23 patients who wore the TCC, 66% or [(.66)(23) = 15.18] should have healed, and 34% [(.34)(23) = 7.82] should be unhealed. Similarly, 66% of the 27 patients who wore the RCW [(.66)(27) = 17.82] should be healed, and 34% should be unhealed [(.34)(27) = 9.18]. These are the frequencies that would be expected if type of cast and healing are not related. Table 25.3B shows the expected frequencies under the column labeled "E".

We can simplify the process of calculating the expected frequency (E) for a given cell in the table using the formula

$$E = \frac{f_R f_C}{N}$$
(25.3)

where f_R and f_C represent the frequency totals for the row and column associated with that cell, respectively. Therefore, for those who wore the TCC, expected frequencies are

Healed:
$$E = \frac{(23)(33)}{50} = 15.18$$

Unhealed:
$$E = \frac{(23)(17)}{50} = 7.82$$

And for those who wore the RCW,

Healed:
$$E = \frac{(27)(33)}{50} = 17.82$$

Unhealed:
$$E = \frac{(27)(17)}{50} = 9.18$$

Interpreting Chi-Square

Table 25.3B shows the calculation of χ^2 using these data. These calculations proceed as in previous examples, with all observed and expected frequencies listed in the table (order is unimportant). The test value, $\chi^2 = 5.24$, is compared with the critical value with $(R - 1)(C - 1)$ degrees of freedom. In this case, we have two rows and two columns, with $(2 - 1)(2 - 1) = 1$ degree of freedom. From Appendix Table A.5 we obtain the critical value $_{(.05)}\chi^2_{(1)} = 3.84$. Therefore, χ^2 is significant and the null hypothesis of independence is rejected. These variables are not independent of each other. There is a significant association between the type of cast worn and healing of foot ulcers.

We can examine the frequencies within each cell to interpret these findings. The output for this analysis allows us to see how each cell contributes to the overall chi-square. As shown in Table 25.3D, the frequency within each cell is also given as a percentage of the column (% within Healed) and the row (% within Cast). For instance, 19 patients in the TCC group were healed. This represents 82.6% of all those who wore the TCC (the row %) and 57.6% of all those who were healed (the column %). If we examine the standardized residuals for these data, shown as the last entry in each cell, we can see that the two cells representing patients who were unhealed contribute most to the significant outcome. With use of the TCC, the number of patients whose ulcers were unhealed was less than expected by chance ($R = -1.4$). For those who wore the RCW, the number of patients who were unhealed was greater than expected ($R = 1.3$). It is reasonable, then, to conclude that the TCC was more effective.

Random and Fixed Models for 2 × 2 Tables

When data are arranged in a contingency table, the marginal frequencies can be generated in one of two ways. They may be *fixed effects,* in that the totals are predetermined by the experimenter. If the study were to be repeated, the same frequencies would probably be used. The levels of cast can be classified as fixed, in that the subjects were assigned to these groups. The numbers of subjects in each category of treatment were determined by the researchers. Conversely, the number of subjects appearing in each category of healing was not predetermined. This is considered a *random effect,* indicating that the numbers in these categories would probably change with repeated sampling.

A **fixed model** contingency table is created when both variables of interest are assigned. This approach is rare in clinical studies. The more common **random model** is composed of two random variables. For example, we could analyze a class of 60 students and classify them according to sex and age. The totals in each category would be different for every class that was tested. A **mixed model** is composed of one random and one fixed variable. The cast example, in which subjects were assigned to treatment groups and measured on healing, fits this model. Treatment is fixed and healing levels are random. Case-control studies use this approach, choosing a fixed number of cases and control subjects, and then examining how many in each group are exposed to a risk factor. If the study were to be repeated, the same numbers of cases and controls could be chosen, but the exposure data would vary. The significance of analyzing a fixed, random, or mixed model will be discussed shortly when we deal with issues of sample size.

TABLE 25.4   ALTERNATE COMPUTATION OF χ^2 FOR 2 × 2 CONTINGENCY TABLE

	Healed			
	Yes	**No**	**Total**	
TCC	19 (A)	4 (B)	23	
RCW	14 (C)	13 (D)	27	
Total	33	17	50	

$$\chi^2 = \frac{N(AD - BC)^2}{(A + B)(C + D)(A + C)(B + D)}$$

$$= \frac{50[(19)(13) - (4)(14)]^2}{(23)(27)(33)(17)} = \frac{1,824,050}{348,381} = 5.24$$

Calculations for 2 × 2 Tables

The 2 × 2 contingency table is a commonly used model in the analysis of frequencies. An alternative formula for calculating χ^2 can be applied, which eliminates the need for determining expected frequencies. This formula is illustrated in Table 25.4.

Sample Size Considerations—Yates' Correction for Continuity

Assumptions related to sample size with contingency tables are based on the expected frequencies. In addition to the requirement that each cell contain an expected frequency of at least 1, no more than 20% of the cells should contain expected frequencies less than 5.[8] When this occurs, the researcher may choose to collapse the table (if it is larger than 2 × 2) to combine adjacent categories and increase expected cell frequencies.

A statistical correction, known as **Yates' correction for continuity**, is often recommended to adjust χ^2 to account for small expected frequencies. This procedure reduces the size of χ^2 by subtracting 0.5 from the absolute value of $O - E$ for each category before squaring:

$$\chi^2 = \sum \frac{(|O - E| - .5)^2}{E} \tag{25.5}$$

With 2 × 2 tables, Yates' correction for continuity is given as

$$\chi^2 = \frac{N(AD - BC - N/2)^2}{(A + B)(C + D)(A + C)(B + D)} \tag{25.6}$$

A number of statistical sources suggest that Yates' correction for continuity is too conservative and unduly increases the chance of committing a Type II error.[9,10] It has been suggested that χ^2 can provide a reasonable estimate of Type I error for 2 × 2 tables when random or mixed models are used with $N \geq 8$.[11] With expected frequencies less than 5, a related procedure called the **Fisher Exact Test** is recommended for use with 2 × 2 tables.[12] This test results in the exact probability of the occurrence of the observed frequencies, given the marginal totals. The calculation of Fisher's Exact Test is quite cumbersome and is best generated by computer analysis.

McNEMAR TEST FOR CORRELATED SAMPLES

One of the basic assumptions required for use of χ^2 is that variables are independent; that is, no one subject is represented in more than one cell. There are many research questions, however, for which this assumption will not hold. For instance, we could look at a sample's responses to a question and see how many subjects answered correctly or incorrectly before and after exposure to specific information. Or we could examine the effects of a particular treatment program by looking at the presence or absence of an outcome variable, such as pain, before and after treatment. These studies use nominal variables, but in a repeated measures design. The χ^2 test is not valid under these conditions.[13]

The **McNemar test** is a form of the χ^2 statistic used with 2×2 tables that involve correlated samples, where subjects act as their own controls or where they are matched. This test is especially useful with pretest-posttest designs when the dependent variable is measured as a dichotomy in an ordinal or nominal scale. To illustrate this approach, Evans et al.[14] studied the effect of percutaneous vertebroplasty on pain and function in patients with vertebral fractures. Table 25.5A shows representative data for the use of

---

TABLE 25.5   MCNEMAR TEST: USE OF PAIN MEDICATIONS BEFORE AND AFTER VETEBROPLASTY ($N = 53$)

A. DATA

		BEFORE		Total
		Pain Meds	None	
AFTER	**Pain Meds**	A 24	B 4	28
	None	C 20	D 5	25
	Total	44	9	53

B. COMPUTATION

$$\chi^2 = \frac{(B - C)^2}{(B + C)} = \frac{(4 - 20)^2}{(4 + 20)} = 10.67$$

C. HYPOTHESIS TEST

$df = (r - 1)(c - 1) = 1$ $_{(0.5)}X^2_{(1)} = 3.84$ (Table A.5)   Reject H_0

D. OUTPUT

After * Before Crosstabulation

		Before		Total
		Pain Meds	None	
After	Pain Meds	24	4	28
	None	20	5	25
Total		44	9	53

Chi-Square Tests

	Value	Exact Sig. (2-sided)
McNemar Test		.002
N of Valid Cases	53	

Based on data from Evans AJ, et al. Vertebral compression fractures: Pain reduction and improvement in functional mobility after percutaneous polymethylmethacrylate vertebroplasty retrospective report of 245 cases. *Radiology* 2003; 226:366–372.

pain medications before and after the procedure. In this situation, the cells are not independent, and each subject is represented twice.

The cells in the correlated design follow the standard notation for a 2 × 2 table. The number of patients who demonstrate a change in the use of pain medications following the vertebroplasty are reflected in shaded cells B and C. Patients in cell B did not use pain medications prior to the procedure, but did use them afterwards. Those in cell C did use pain medications prior to the procedure, but no longer used them afterwards. Patients in cells A and D did not change their use (or nonuse) of medications.

As B and C represent the total number of patients who showed a change in their behavior, these are the only cells of interest for this analysis. Under the null hypothesis, half of those who changed should stop using medications after the procedure and half should begin using medications. We test this hypothesis using the formula

$$\chi^2 = \frac{(B - C)^2}{B + C}$$ (25.7)

which is tested against critical values of χ^2 with one degree of freedom (Appendix Table A.5). As shown in Table 25.5B, for the preceding example, $\chi^2 = 10.67$. This value is significant (Table 25.5C). We can see that the proportion of patients who stopped using medications after the vertebroplasty is substantially higher than for those who began using medications.

COEFFICIENTS OF ASSOCIATION

Sometimes a measure of association, like a correlation coefficient, is desired, as a way of expressing the degree of relationship in a set of categorical data. Chi-square tells us only if the association is significant, not if it is strong or weak.

Phi Coefficient

The **phi coefficient**, Φ, can be used to express the degree of association between two nominal variables in a 2 × 2 table.[15] Its value can range from −1.00 to +1.00, and can be interpreted as a correlation coefficient. It is based on the χ^2 statistic as follows:

$$\phi = \sqrt{\frac{\chi^2}{N}}$$ (25.8)

For the data in Table 25.5,

$$\phi = \sqrt{\frac{5.24}{50}} = .32$$

This finding indicates a relatively weak association between type of cast worn and incidence of healing. The results of the χ^2 test on these data showed that the two variables were not independent. The contingency coefficient indicates the strength of their relationship. This statistic can also be obtained using the Pearson correlation (see Chapter 23).

Contingency Coefficient

The **contingency coefficient, C,** is a measure of association that can be used with tables larger than 2 × 2, but with the restriction that the number of rows has to equal the number of columns. This value is given by

$$C = \sqrt{\frac{\chi^2}{N + \chi^2}} \tag{25.9}$$

Once again, using the data in Table 25.5

$$C = \sqrt{\frac{5.24}{50 + 5.24}} = .31$$

As these results show, the phi coefficient and the contingency coefficient will yield similar results with 2 × 2 tables.

The contingency coefficient will range from 0 to a maximum of $\sqrt{(q - 1)/q}$ where q represents the number of rows or columns in a symmetrical table. For a 2 × 2 table the upper limit of C is $\sqrt{(2 - 1)/2} = .707$. For a 3 × 3 table, this maximum will be $\sqrt{(3 - 1)/3} = .816$. Because of these differences, contingency coefficients are not directly comparable unless they are obtained from tables of equal sizes.

Cramer's V

A third measure of association based on χ^2 is **Cramer's V** coefficient, which is an alternative to the contingency coefficient when contingency tables are asymmetrical. This coefficient is designed so that the attainable upper bound is always ±1.00. The formula is

$$V = \sqrt{\frac{\chi^2}{N(q - 1)}} \tag{25.10}$$

where N is the total number of subjects, and q is the number of rows or columns, *whichever is smaller.* For example, suppose we were conducting a survey of 50 participants in a health promotion program. We ask respondents for their age (in 4 categories) and their level of satisfaction with the program (in 3 categories), so that we create a 4 × 3 contingency table. Assume that $\chi^2 = 24.00$. Because we have 4 levels of age and 3 levels of satisfaction, $q = 3$. Therefore,

$$V = \sqrt{\frac{24.00}{50(3 - 1)}} = .49$$

which represents a moderate degree of relationship, indicating that there is some association between the participants' age and level of satisfaction with the program.

Other Measures of Association

Many computer packages generate a series of coefficients associated with contingency table analyses. These statistics are not based on chi-square.

The **lambda coefficient, λ,** is used to determine how well one can predict membership in one category based on knowledge of another category. Both sets of categories should be at the nominal level. Lambda is reported in asymmetric and symmetric versions. The *asymmetric lambda* is interpreted as the improvement in predicting Y once values of X are known; that is, one nominal variable is designated as the dependent variable (Y), and the other as the independent variable (X). For instance, in the study of diabetic ulcers described ealier, we would designate the type of cast as the independent variable and level of healing as the dependent variable. In some analyses, however, the researcher is unable to specify which variable is dependent. For example, we might want to look at the relationship between side of stroke and sex, neither of which could necessarily be seen as a dependent variable. In this case, the *symmetric* version of lambda is used. Lambda ranges from 0, when there is no improvement in prediction, to 1.0, when predictions can be made without error.

Kendall's tau-b and **tau-c** are measures of association for ordinal variables that are reported in categories. Tau-b is appropriate with square tables, such 2×2, and tau-c should be used with rectangular tables where the number of rows and columns differ.

Gamma is based on the tau statistic, but ignores ties; that is, pairs that have the same classification for X and Y are eliminated from the analysis. When tables have three or more dimensions (three or more category variables, such as sex, age group and diagnosis), partial gammas can be calculated.

COMMENTARY

Uses of Chi-Square

Clinical researchers can find many uses for the chi-square statistic for data analysis and descriptive purposes. It is often useful as a way of establishing group equivalence following random assignment. For instance, once two groups have been assigned, it may be of interest to compare the numbers of males and females in each group to see if they were assigned in equal proportions. Or it may be important to determine if certain age groups are equally represented in each experimental group. Chi-square can be used to make these determinations and confirm the validity of the randomization process.

Chi-square should not be used as an alternative to more precise tests, such as the *t*-test or analysis of variance, when data can be measured on a continuous scale. Any data can be reduced to the nominal level, but this can result in a serious loss of information and is not encouraged for continuous measures. For example, if a survey requested information on an individual's age, and the exact age is given, it may not be useful to reduce the data to age intervals.

Issues of sample size are relevant to discussions of chi-square. The statistic is sensitive to increases in sample size when there is a true difference between observed and expected frequencies. With larger samples, the magnitude of these differences will usually increase, thereby increasing the value of χ^2. When samples are very small, these differences can be hidden. It is often useful to consider collapsing categories when this does not compromise the research question, and to re-examine data using larger cell frequencies; however, this should be done only when the combinations of categories are theoretically reasonable and meaningful. It may be helpful to think about potential combinations of categories prior to data analysis. It is never appropriate to make such combinations on the basis of the observed data to achieve significant outcomes. See Appendix C for a discussion of power related to chi-square.

REFERENCES

1. Volicer BJ. *Multivariate Statistics for Nursing Research.* Orlando, FL: Frune & Stratton, 1984.
2. Haberman SJ. The analysis of residuals in cross-classified tables. *Biometrics* 1984;29: 205–220.
3. Frankel JE, Marwitz JH, Cifu DX, Kreutzer JS, Englander J, Rosenthal M. A follow-up study of older adults with traumatic brain injury: Taking into account decreasing length of stay. *Arch Phys Med Rehabil* 2006;87:57–62.
4. Yu IT, Wong TW, Liu HJ. Impact of air pollution on cardiopulmonary fitness in school children. *J Occup Environ Med* 2004;46:946–952.
5. Monset-Couchard M, de Bethmann O, Relier J. Long term outcome of small versus appropriate size for gestational age co-twins/triplets. *Arch Dis Child Fetal Neonat Ed* 2004;89:F310–314.
6. Proctor TJ, Mayer TG, Theodore B, Gatchel RJ. Failure to complete a functional restoration program for chronic musculoskeletal disorders: A prospective 1-year outcome study. *Arch Phys Med Rehabil* 2005;86:1509–1515.
7. Armstrong DG, Lavery LA, Wu S, Boulton AJM. Evaluation of removable and irremovable cast walkers in the healing of diabetic foot wounds: a randomized controlled trial. *Diabetes Care* 2005;28:551–554.
8. Cochran WG. Some methods for strengthening the common χ^2 tests. *Biometrics* 1954;10: 417–451.
9. Sahai H, Khurshid A. On analysis of epidemiological data involving a 2 × 2 contingency table: An overview of Fisher's exact test and Yates' correction for continuity. *J Biopharm Stat* 1995;5:43–70.
10. Haviland MG. Yates's correction for continuity and the analysis of 2 × 2 contingency tables. *Stat Med* 1990;9:363–367.
11. Mantel N, Hankey BJ. The odds ratio of a 2 × 2 contingency table. *Am Statistician* 1975;29:143–145.
12. Dallal GE. Contingency tables. Available at: <http://www.tufts.edu/~gdallal/ctab.htm> Accessed on March 18, 2006.
13. Ottenbacher K. The chi-square test: Its use in rehabilitation research. *Arch Phys Med Rehabil* 1995;76:678–681.
14. Evans AJ, Jensen ME, Kip KE, DeNardo AJ, Lawler GJ, Negin GA, et al. Vertebral compression fractures: Pain reduction and improvement in functional mobility after percutaneous polymethylmethacrylate vertebroplasty retrospective report of 245 cases. *Radiology* 2003;226:366–372.
15. Siegel S, Castellan NJ. *Nonparametric Statistics for the Behavioral Sciences* (2nd ed.). New York: McGraw-Hill, 1988.

CHAPTER 26

Statistical Measures of Reliability

In Chapter 5 we introduced basic concepts of reliability and described how different forms of reliability can be addressed in the planning of research protocols. The purpose of this chapter is to expand on these concepts by presenting the statistical bases for estimates of reliability, including measures of correlation, agreement, internal consistency, response stability and method comparison for alternate forms. We have waited until this point in the book to present these procedures because they require application of statistical concepts that have been covered in the preceding chapters.

RELIABILITY THEORY AND MEASUREMENT ERROR

Recall from Chapter 5 that classical reliability theory partitions an observed measurement or score, X, into two components: a *true component*, T, which represents the real value under ideal and infallible conditions, and an *error component*, E, which includes all other sources of variance that influence the outcome of measurement. This theoretical relationship is expressed in the equation

$$X = T \pm E \tag{26.1}$$

We can also examine the statistical nature of this relationship by restating it in terms of *variance* (s^2). The total variance within a set of observed scores (s_X^2) is a function of both the **true variance** between scores (s_T^2) and the variance in the errors of measurement, or **error variance** (s_E^2):

$$s_X^2 = s_T^2 + s_E^2 \tag{26.2}$$

Although it is an unknown quantity, we assume that s_T^2 is fixed, because true scores will theoretically remain constant. Therefore, in a set of perfectly reliable scores, all observed differences between individual scores should be attributable to true differences between scores; that is, there is no error variance. Conversely, if we look at a set of repeated measurements from one person, and assume that the true response has not changed, then all observed variance should be the result of error. The essence of reliability, then, is based on the amount of error that is present in a set of scores. A measurement is considered

585

more reliable if a greater proportion of the total observed variance is represented by the true score variance. Thus, reliability is defined by the ratio:

$$\frac{\text{True variance}}{\text{True variance} + \text{error variance}} \quad \text{or} \quad \frac{\text{True variance}}{\text{Total variance}} \quad \text{or}$$

$$\frac{\text{Total variance} - \text{error variance}}{\text{Total variance}}$$

In statistical terminology, this relationship can be expressed as

$$r_{XX} = \frac{s_T^2}{s_T^2 + s_E^2} = \frac{s_T^2}{s_X^2} = \frac{s_X^2 - s_E^2}{s_X^2} \tag{26.3}$$

where r_{XX} is the symbol for a **reliability coefficient.**

The coefficient of reliability can take values from 0.00 to 1.00. Zero reliability indicates that all measurement variation is attributed to error. Reliability of 1.00 means that the measurement has no error, or $s_E^2 = 0$. As the coefficient nears 1.00, we are more confident that the observed score is representative of the true score.

To illustrate this application, consider the set of hypothetical data presented in Table 26.1A. These values represent ratings for six patients on a subjective pain scale, rated from 0 to 20. The first column, labeled X, lists the observed scores and their variance, $s_X^2 = 5.60$; the second column, T, shows the true scores (although in reality these are not known) and their variance, $s_T^2 = 2.40$; the last column, labeled E, shows the error component (the difference between the observed and true scores) and the error variance, $s_E^2 = 3.20$. We can verify that the observed variance is composed of true variance and error variance: $5.60 = 2.40 + 3.20$. These values can be used to calculate the reliability coefficient as follows:

$$r_{XX} = \frac{s_T^2}{s_X^2} = \frac{2.40}{5.60} = 0.43$$

Conceptually, this means that 43% of the variation in the observed scores can be attributed to variation in the true score, and the rest, 57%, is attributable to measurement error.

Of course, this approach is completely theoretical, as we can never actually know the true score or error component within a set of data. Therefore, it is necessary to use observed scores to estimate reliability. Although the procedures for obtaining these estimates will vary, the theory underlying the reliability coefficient is universally applicable; that is, reliability is a function of the amount of error variance in a set of data.

The Effect of Variance on Reliability

As reflected in the definition of reliability, statistical variance is the basis for reliability estimates. We can demonstrate that as the true variance in a set of scores decreases, the reliability coefficient will also decrease. If we look at the differences among the pain scores in Table 26.1A, we can see that the patients did not vary greatly from one another.

TABLE 26.1   PAIN MEASURES SHOWING OBSERVED SCORES (X), TRUE SCORES (T), AND ERROR COMPONENTS (E) FOR TWO HYPOTHETICAL DISTRIBUTIONS

A. Distribution with Limited Variability

Subject	X	T	E
1	12	10	2
2	10	10	0
3	8	10	-2
4	13	11	2
5	9	11	-2
6	14	14	0
ΣX	66	66	0
$\overline{X}$	11	11	0
s^2	5.60	2.40	3.20

$$r_{XX} = \frac{s_T^2}{SS_X^2} = \frac{2.40}{5.60} = .43$$

B. Distribution with Greater Variability

Subject	X	T	E
1	4	4	0
2	4	4	0
3	15	13	2
4	9	11	-2
5	12	10	2
6	10	12	-2
ΣX	54	54	0
$\overline{X}$	9	9	0
s^2	19.20	16.00	3.20

$$r_{XX} = \frac{s_T^2}{SS_X^2} = \frac{16.00}{19.20} = .8$$

True scores were in a narrow range from 8 to 14. Consequently, the variance within the observed scores is small. We also find that the differences between the observed and true scores (errors) are minimal across the six patients. Based on these observations, we might reason that these measurements should be highly reliable; however, we obtain a reliability coefficient of only .43, much lower than might be expected.

Now let us look at a similar set of hypothetical data for the same variable, shown in Table 26.1B. Note that the error components for these scores are identical to those in the first data set. This time, however, the true scores are much more variable ($s_T^2 = 16.00$), with values ranging from 4 to 15. Therefore, the observed scores also exhibit a much higher variance ($s_X^2 = 19.20$). Using these values, we can calculate a second reliability coefficient:

$$r_{XX} = \frac{s_T^2}{s_X^2} = \frac{16.00}{19.20} = 0.83$$

These data demonstrate a much stronger degree of statistical reliability than the first data set, even though the degree of error in the scores is the same! Why does this occur? Recall that reliability is based on the *proportion of the total observed variance that is attributable to error*. Therefore, for a given amount of error variance, it follows that reliability will improve as the total variance increases; that is, as the total variance gets larger, the error component will account for a smaller proportion of it.

This concept is crucial in the interpretation of reliability coefficients and in the design of reliability studies. Suppose we were interested in establishing the reliability of a new device for measuring range of back extension. We gather a large sample of "normal" individuals, all with measurements between 20 and 25 degrees of extension. Even if we are fairly consistent over successive trials, the reliability coefficient will probably be low because the total variance is so small. A low reliability coefficient can be misleading under such conditions. The solution to this problem, of course, is to include subjects that have a wider range of scores in a reliability study. We should be studying normal individuals as well as patients with hypermobility and hypomobility in back extension. Researchers should always consider the range of scores used for estimating reliability in the interpretation of reliability coefficients.

INTRACLASS CORRELATION COEFFICIENT (ICC)

The historical approach to testing reliability involved the use of correlation coefficients. In Chapter 5 we discussed the problems with this approach, in that it does not provide a measure of agreement, but only covariance (see Figure 5.1 in Chapter 5). Correlations are also limited as reliability coefficients because they are bivariate; that is, only two ratings or raters can be correlated at one time. It is not possible to assess the simultaneous reliability of more than two raters or the relationships among different aspects of reliability, such as raters, test forms, and testing occasions. As these are often important elements in reliability testing, correlation does not provide an efficient mechanism for evaluating the full scope of reliability.

Another objection to the use of correlation as a measure of reliability is based on the statistical definition of reliability; that is, correlation cannot separate out variance components due to error or true differences in a data set. Therefore, the correlation coefficient is not a true reliability coefficient. It is actually more accurate to use the square of the correlation coefficient (the coefficient of determination) for this purpose, because r^2 reflects how much variance in one measurement is accounted for by the variance in a second measurement (see Chapter 24). This is analogous to asking how much of the total variance in a set of data is shared by two measurements (the "true" variance) and how much is not shared (the error variance). If we could correlate true scores with observed scores in a set of data, the square of the correlation coefficient would be the reliability coefficient. We can confirm this interpretation using the data from Table 26.1A. For the correlation between observed and true scores, $r = .66$. Therefore, $r^2 = .43$.

To overcome the limitations of correlation as a measure of reliability, some researchers have used more than one reliability index within a single study. For instance, in a test-retest situation or a rater reliability study, both correlation and a *t*-test can be performed to assess consistency and average agreement between the data sets. This strategy does address the interpretation of agreement, but it is not useful in that it does not provide a single index to describe reliability. The scores may be correlated but significantly different (as in Table 26.1B), or they may be poorly correlated but not significantly different. How should these results be interpreted? It is much more desirable to use one index that can answer this question.

The **intraclass correlation coefficient (ICC)** is such an index. Like other reliability coefficients, the ICC ranges from 0.00 to 1.00. It is calculated using variance estimates obtained through an analysis of variance. Therefore, it reflects both degree of correspondence and agreement among ratings.

Statistically the ICC has several advantages. First, it can be used to assess reliability among two or more ratings, giving it broad clinical applicability. Second, the ICC does not require the same number of raters for each subject, allowing for flexibility in clinical studies.[1] Third, although it is designed primarily for use with interval/ratio data, the ICC can be applied without distortion to data on the ordinal scale when intervals between such measurements are assumed to be equivalent.[2] In addition, with data that are rated as a dichotomy (the presence or absence of a trait), the ICC has been shown to be equivalent to measures of nominal agreement, simplifying computation in cases where more than two raters are involved.[1,3] Therefore, the ICC provides a useful index in a variety of analysis situations.

Generalizability

Another major advantage of the ICC is that it supports the **generalizability** model proposed by Cronbach as a comprehensive estimate of reliability.[4,5] The concept of generalizability theory, introduced in Chapter 5, is based on the idea that differences between observed scores are due to a variety of factors, not just true score variance and random error. Differences occur because of variations in the measurement system, such as the characteristics of raters or subjects, testing conditions, alternate forms of a test, administrations of a test on different occasions and so on. These factors are called **facets** of generalizability.

The essence of generalizability theory is that facets contribute to measurement error as separate components of variance, distinguishable from random error. In classical reliability theory, error variance is undifferentiated, incorporating all sources of measurement error. In generalizability theory, however, the error variance is multivariate; that is, it is further partitioned to account for the influence of specific facets on measurement error. Therefore, the **generalizability coefficient** (the ICC) is an extension of the reliability coefficient:

$$ICC = \frac{s_T^2}{s_T^2 + s_F^2 + s_E^2} \qquad (26.4)$$

where s_T^2 and s_E^2 are the variances in true scores and error components, and s_F^2 is the variance attributable to the facets of interest.[6] The specific facets included in the denominator will vary, depending on whether rater, occasions or some other facet is the variable of interest in the reliability study. For example, if we include rater as a facet, then the total observed variance would be composed of the true variance between subjects, the variance between raters, and the remaining unexplained error variance.

Equation (26.4) represents a conceptual definition of generalizability. Actual calculations require the use of variance estimates that are obtained from an analysis of variance, which, of course, does not include direct estimates of true variance (as this is unknown). Theoretically, however, we can estimate true score variance by looking at the difference between observed variance among subjects and error variance ($s_T^2 = s_X^2 + s_E^2$). These estimates can be derived from an analysis of variance.

Classification of the ICC

There are actually six different equations for calculating the ICC, differentiated by purpose of the reliability study, the design of the study, and the type of measurements taken. It is necessary to distinguish among these approaches, as under some conditions the results can be decidedly different. To facilitate explanations, we will proceed with this discussion in the context of a reliability study with rater as the facet of interest; however, we emphasize that these applications are equally valid to study other facets.

Models of the ICC: Random and Fixed Effects

Shrout and Fleiss describe three *models* of the ICC.[7] They distinguish these models according to how the raters are chosen and assigned to subjects.

Model 1. In model 1, each subject is assessed by a different set of k raters. The raters are considered randomly chosen from a larger population of raters; that is, rater is a **random effect**. However, the raters for one subject are not necessarily the same raters that take measurements on another subject. Therefore, in this design there is no way to associate a particular rater with the variables being measured.[8] The only variance that can actually be assessed is the difference among subjects. Other sources of error variance, including rater or measurement error, cannot be separated out.

Model 2. Model 2 is the most commonly applied model of the ICC for assessing inter-rater reliability. In this design, each subject is assessed by the same set of raters. The raters are randomly chosen; that is, they are expected to represent the population of raters from which they were drawn, and results can be generalized to other raters with similar characteristics. Subjects are also considered to be randomly chosen from the population of individuals who would receive the measurement. Therefore, subject and rater are both **random effects**. This randomness may be only theoretical in practice; that is, we choose subjects and raters who we believe represent the populations of interest, as we do not have access to the entire population. But the intent of the study is to demonstrate that the measurement reliability can be applied to others.

Model 3. In model 3, each subject is assessed by the same set of raters, but the raters represent the only raters of interest. In this case, there is no intention to generalize findings beyond the raters involved. In this design, rater is considered a **fixed effect** because the raters have been purposely (not randomly) selected. Subjects are still considered a random effect. Therefore, model 3 is a **mixed model**. This model is used when a researcher wants to establish that specific investigators are reliable in their data collection, but the reliability of others is not relevant. Model 3 is also the appropriate statistic to measure intrarater reliability, as the measurements of a single rater cannot be generalized to other raters.[7]

Forms of the ICC: Single and Average Ratings

Each of the ICC models can be expressed in two *forms*, depending on whether the scores are single ratings or mean ratings. Most often, reliability studies are based on comparison of scores from individual raters. There are times, however, when the mean of several raters or ratings may be used as the unit of reliability. For instance, when measurements are unstable, it may be necessary to use the mean of several measurements as the individual's score to obtain satisfactory reliability. Using mean scores has the effect of increasing reliability estimates, as means are considered better estimates of true scores, theoretically reducing error variance.

The six types of ICC are classified using two numbers in parentheses. The first number designates the *model* (1, 2, or 3), and the second number signifies the *form*, using either a single measurement (1) or the mean of several measurements (k)* as the unit of analysis. For example, when using single measurements in a generalizability study, we would specify use of ICC(2,1). The type of ICC used should always be indicated.

Analysis of Variance

The ICC is based on measures of variance obtained from an ANOVA. For an interrater reliability study, rater is the independent variable; for an intrarater study, trial is the independent variable. Table 26.2 shows the arrangement of hypothetical data with rater as columns, and subjects as rows. For an intrarater study, the columns would represent trials.

Model 1: One-Way ANOVA

For model 1, a one-way analysis of variance is run, with "subjects" as the independent variable. This ANOVA partitions the total variance into two parts—the variation between-subjects and error, as shown in Table 26.3A. The between-subjects effect tells us if the subjects' scores are different from each other, which we expect. The error component represents the variation within a subject across raters. Some of this error will be due to true scores changing from trial to trial, some from rater error, and some will be

TABLE 26.2 DATA ENTERED TO TEST RELIABILITY FOR FOUR RATERS ACROSS SIX SUBJECTS

	Subject	Rater1	Rater2	Rater3	Rater4
1	1	7	8	3	5
2	2	2	4	4	1
3	3	1	2	6	1
4	4	5	5	7	2
5	5	8	9	5	6
6	6	9	10	6	7

*The designation of k equals the number of scores used to obtain the mean.

TABLE 26.3   COMPUTATION AND SPSS OUTPUT FOR ICC MODEL 1 BASED ON A ONE-WAY ANALYSIS OF VARIANCE ($k = 4$ RATERS ACROSS $N = 6$ SUBJECTS)

A. COMPUTATION

ANOVA ❶

		Sum of Squares	df	❷ Mean Square		F	Sig.
Between People		99.375	5	BMS	**19.875**	❸	
Within People	Between Items	21.792	3		7.264	2.203	❹ .130
	Residual	49.458	15		3.297		
	Total	71.250	18	WMS	**3.958**		
Total		170.625	23		7.418		

$$ICC (1, 1) = \frac{BMS - WMS}{BMS + (k - 1)WMS} = \frac{19.88 - 3.96}{19.88 + (4 - 1)3.96} = .50$$

$$ICC (1, k) = \frac{BMS - WMS}{BMS} = \frac{19.88 - 3.96}{19.88} = .80$$

The values for BMS and WMS are taken from the ANOVA as shown above; k is the number of raters (or ratings), which will be the data in columns (see Table 26.2).

B. OUTPUT

Intraclass Correlation Coefficient

			95% Confidence Interval		❺ F Test with True Value 0			
		Intraclass Correlation	Lower Bound	Upper Bound	Value	df1	df2	Sig.
Single Measures	1,1	.501	.108	.886	5.021	5	18	.005
Average Measures	1,k	.801	.326	.969	5.021	5	18	.005

One-way random effects model where people effects are random.

❶ The ANOVA is automatically run as a repeated measures analysis of variance; only the between-subjects and total within-people variance components are used for model 1.

❷ BMS = Between-subjects Mean Square (called "between-people" here).
   WMS = Within-groups Mean Square (called total "within people" here).

❸ The F-test for the between-subjects effect is not printed as part of the ANOVA. It is relevant to the ICC, however, as reliability testing depends on variance among subjects. This value can be calculated as BMS/WMS. The value of F will be reported as part of the ICC output (see ❺).

❹ This F-value is ignored.

❺ This is the F-test for the between-subjects effect, which was not reported in the original ANOVA table. This effect is significant ($p = .005$), which tells us that the subjects are different from each other. This is a necessary condition for reliability testing. The validity of the ICC will be suspect if this F-test is not significant. The value of F is equal to BMS/WMS.

unexplained. This ANOVA does not differentiate among these sources of error. Calculations for this model are shown in Table 26.3B using data from Table 26.2.

Models 2 and 3: Repeated Measures ANOVA

For model 2, the ANOVA is performed as a two-way random effects model, in which both subjects and raters are considered to be randomly chosen from a larger population.[†] Therefore, the results of the study can be generalized to other raters and other subjects. For model 3, a two-way mixed model is run, with rater as a fixed effect (not randomly chosen) and subjects as a random effect. The numerical results of the analysis will actually be the same for both random and mixed types of ANOVA. The only difference will lie in the interpretation of the data. The results of a repeated measures analysis of variance are shown in Table 26.4.

The repeated measures ANOVA partitions the variance into effects due to differences between subjects, differences between raters and error variance. The *F*-ratio associated with the rater effect reflects the difference among raters, or the extent of agreement or disagreement among them. This effect is significant when the variance due to raters is large, indicating that the raters' scores are different from each other and not reliable. In this example, the rater effect is not significant ($p = .130$). Table 26.4 shows the calculation of both forms for models 2 and 3, using data from Table 26.2.

Output for the ICC

SPSS,[‡] a commonly used software package, will generate the various forms of the ICC as part of its Reliability Analysis (under SCALE).[9,10] SAS,[§] another commonly used program, does not provide direct calculations, but a programming macro has been developed.[11] Online calculators can also be found to provide ICC values based on raw data.[12,13] Calculations by hand are straightforward once the analysis of variance is performed.

Table 26.3B shows the SPSS output[**] for model 1, and Table 26.5 shows the output for models 2 and 3. Each model is generated in two forms, for single measures and average measures. Confidence intervals are also provided. The researcher must decide which value to use, based on the design of the study.

[†]Recall that in a repeated measures ANOVA, "subjects" is considered one of the variables, so that even with only one independent variable (in this case rater), the analysis is designated as "two-way."

[‡]Statistical Package for the Social Sciences, SPSS Inc., 233 S. Wacker Drive, Chicago, Illinois 60606.

[§]SAS Institute Inc., 100 SAS Campus Drive, Cary, NC 27513.

[**]To generate ICC values in SPSS, go to SCALE > RELIABILITY ANALYSIS. Include all levels of the independent variable (raters or ratings) in the "Items" box. Click on "Statistics," and choose "Intraclass Correlation Coefficient." Choose a model from the dropdown menu (One-Way Analysis of Variance for Model 1, Two-Way Random for Model 2, or Two-Way Mixed for Model 3). Choose a Type from the dropdown menu, Absolute Agreement for Model 2 or Consistency for Model 3. An analysis of variance can be generated by checking "F test" under ANOVA. These instructions are based on versions 10.0 to 14.2 of SPSS.

TABLE 26.4   COMPUTATION OF ICC FOR MODELS 2 AND 3 BASED ON REPEATED MEASURES ANALYSIS OF VARIANCE (k = 4 RATERS ACROSS N = 6 SUBJECTS)

ANOVA ❶

		Sum of Squares	df	❷ Mean Square		F	Sig.
Between People		99.375	5	BMS	19.875	❸	
Within People	Between Items	21.792	3	RMS	7.264	2.203	❹ .130
	Residual	49.458	15	EMS	3.297		
	Total	71.250	18		3.958		
Total		170.625	23		7.418		

$$ICC\,(2, 1) = \frac{BMS - EMS}{BMS + (k - 1) + \dfrac{k(RMS - EMS)}{n}} = \frac{19.88 - 3.30}{19.88 + (4 - 1)3.30 + \dfrac{4(7.26 - 3.30)}{6}} = .51$$

$$ICC\,(2, k) = \frac{BMS - EMS}{BMS + \dfrac{(RMS - EMS)}{n}} = \frac{19.88 - 3.30}{19.88 + \dfrac{(7.26 - 3.30)}{6}} = .81$$

$$ICC\,(3, 1) = \frac{BMS - EMS}{BMS + (k - 1)EMS} = \frac{19.88 - 3.30}{19.88 + (4 - 1)3.30} = .56$$

$$ICC(3, k) = \frac{BMS - EMS}{BMS} = \frac{19.88 - 3.30}{19.88} = .83$$

The values for BMS, RMS and EMS are taken from the ANOVA as shown above; k is the number of raters (or ratings), which will be the data in columns; n is the number of subjects or rows (see Table 26.2).

❶ Model 2 uses a two-way random effects model; model 3 uses a two-way mixed model. Results of both types of ANOVA will be the same numerically.

❷ **BMS** = Between-subjects Mean Square (called "between people" here).
RMS = Between Raters Mean Square (called "between items" here).
EMS = Error Mean Square (called "residual" here).

❸ The F-test for the between-subjects effect is not printed as part of the ANOVA. It is relevant to the ICC, however, as reliability testing depends on variance among subjects. This value can be calculated as BMS/EMS. The value of F will be reported as part of the ICC output (see Table 26.5).

❹ There is no significant difference between raters (p = .130) (a good thing when you are looking for reliability!).

Interpretation of the ICC

Magnitude of the ICC

Like other forms of reliability, there are no standard values for acceptable reliability using the ICC. The ICC ranges between 0.00 and 1.00, with values closer to 1.00 representing stronger reliability. But because reliability is a characteristic of measurement obtained to varying degrees (although rarely to perfection), the researcher must determine "how much" reliability is needed to justify the use of a particular tool. The nature of the measured variable will be a factor, in terms of its stability and the precision required to make sound clinical judgments about it. As a general guideline, we suggest

TABLE 26.5   OUTPUT FOR ICC USING SPSS (SCALE > RELIABILITY ANALYSIS) (DATA FROM TABLE 26.4)

A. MODEL 2 (Two-Way Random Effects Model)—Absolute Agreement ❷

Intraclass Correlation Coefficient

	Intraclass Correlation	95% Confidence Interval		❶ F-Test with True Value 0			
		Lower Bound	Upper Bound	Value	df₁	df₂	Sig.
Single Measures	2,1 .511	.136	.886	6.028	5	15	.003
Average Measures	2,k .807	.377	.969	6.028	5	15	.003

Two-way random effects model where both people effects and measures effects are random.

B. MODEL 3 (Two-Way Mixed Model)—Consistency ❸

Intraclass Correlation Coefficient

	Intraclass Correlation	95% Confidence Interval		F-Test with True Value 0 ❶			
		Lower Bound	Upper Bound	Value	df₁	df₂	Sig.
Single Measures	3,1 .557	.146	.904	6.028	5.0	15	.003
Average Measures	3,k .834	.407	.974	6.028	5.0	15	.003

Two-way mixed effects model where people effects are random and measures effects are fixed.

❶ This is the *F*-test for the between-subjects effect, which was not reported in the original ANOVA table. This effect is significant ($p = .003$), which tells us that the subjects are different from each other. This is a necessary condition for reliability testing. The validity of the ICC will be suspect if this *F*-test is not significant. The value of *F* is equal to BMS/EMS (see Table 26.4).

❷ SPSS uses the term "Absolute Agreement" as the definition for model 2.

❸ SPSS uses the term "Consistency" as the definition for model 3.

that values above .75 are indicative of good reliability, and those below .75 poor to moderate reliability. For many clinical measurements, reliability should exceed .90 to ensure reasonable validity. **These are only guidelines, however, and should not be used as absolute standards. Researchers and clinicians must defend their judgments within the context of the specific scores being assessed and the degree of acceptable precision in the measurement.**

Rater Error

When the ICC is high, it is easy to say that reliability is good, and to express confidence in the obtained measurements. When reliability is less than satisfactory, however, the researcher is obliged to sort through alternative explanations to determine the contributing sources of error. There are two major reasons for finding low ICC values.

The first explanation is fairly obvious: The raters (or ratings) do not agree. This is not a straightforward interpretation, however, when more than two raters are analyzed.

Because the ICC is an average based on variance across all raters, nonagreement may involve all raters, some raters, or only one rater. The ICC can be considered an *average correlation* across raters and, therefore, does not represent the reliability of any individual rater. For instance, a critical look back at the data in Table 26.2 reveals that rater 3 seems to be the most out of line with the other raters. In fact, if we obtain the product-moment correlations for all possible pairs of ratings, we find that raters 1, 2 and 4 demonstrate correlations between .96 and .98, whereas the correlations of rater 3 with the other three raters are all negative and small, between −.06 and −.19 (Figure 26.1). The ICC is brought down by the "unreliable" responses of rater 3.

It is often useful, therefore, to examine the data, to determine if there is an interaction between raters and subjects; that is, are the scores dependent on what "level" of rater is doing the measuring? This type of interaction is reflected in the error variance of the repeated measures ANOVA.

When raters are reliable, there should be no interaction between raters and subjects; that is, the error variance should be small. It may be helpful to graph the results, as shown in Figure 26.1. The ratings obtained by raters 1, 2 and 4 are close and fairly parallel. The scores obtained by rater 3 are clearly incongruent. By examining both the

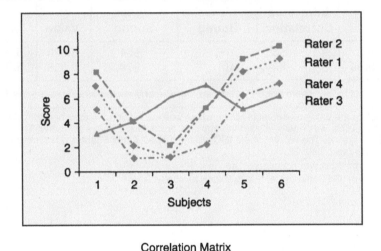

Correlation Matrix

Rater

	1	2	3	4
1	—	0.98	−0.06	0.96
2		—	−0.19	0.97
3			—	−0.14

FIGURE 26.1 Interaction among four raters. Rater 3 demonstrates inconsistent responses that are responsible for the interaction effect. All other raters show parallel responses, as suggested by the corresponding correlation coefficients.

intercorrelations and graphic evidence, we can determine that there is an interaction between rater and subject. It would be important, then, to review the circumstances of the third rater's tests, to determine why that person's ratings were not consistent with the others.

Variance

A second reason for a low ICC is one that has been discussed before in relation to the reliability coefficient; that is, the variability among subjects' scores must be large to demonstrate reliability. A lack of variability can occur when samples are homogeneous, when raters are all very lenient or strict in their scoring, or when the rating system falls within a restricted range. This effect can be checked by looking for significance of the between-subjects variance in the analysis of variance (Table 26.5❶). If subjects' scores are homogeneous, this source of variance will not be significant. It has been shown that when the between-subjects variance is not significant, the actual limits of the ICC do not match the theoretical limits of 0.00 and 1.00.[14] In fact, it is possible for ratios to range from negative to positive infinity. When a negative ICC is obtained, the value cannot be considered valid. Therefore, it is imperative that researchers be aware of the extent to which scores will naturally vary, and try to obtain heterogeneous samples whenever possible.

Choosing One Model

Although we have presented multiple values of the ICC for our example, it should be clear that only one type will be appropriate for any one study. The selection of one version should be made before data are collected, based on appropriate design considerations. In most instances, model 2 or 3 will be the appropriate choice. In some research situations, the investigator is interested in establishing the intrarater or interrater reliability of a group of clinicians for one specific data collection experience, fitting model 3. In that situation, it is of no interest if anyone else can perform the measurements with equal reliability. If, however, it is important to demonstrate that a particular measuring tool can be used with confidence by all equally trained clinicians, then model 2 should be used. This approach is appropriate for clinical studies and methodological research, to document that a measuring tool has broad application.

Model 1 is applicable in only limited circumstances. For example, Maher et al[15] performed a study to determine the interrater reliability of 25 raters who assessed the quality of published randomized controlled trials (RCTs) using the PEDro scale (see Chapter 16). The study involved a total of 120 articles, but each of the 25 raters rated from 1 to 56 RCTs. This fits the design for model 1, where subjects (in these example studies) are not all assessed by the same raters. When all raters assess all subjects, model 1 is not appropriate. Some authors have expressed a preference for using model 1 because it provides a more conservative estimate of reliability than the other models;[16] however, the conservative or liberal nature of a statistic is not an adequate rationale for its use if the model is unsuitable for the design.[7,17]

Generally, for the same set of data, model 1 will yield smaller values than model 2, and model 2 will yield smaller values than model 3. Likewise, within each model, the

ICC based on single ratings will yield a lower correlation than one based on mean ratings (see Tables 26.3 and 26.5). Because of these potential differences, the type of ICC used in a particular study should always be reported.[17]

AGREEMENT

When the unit of measurement is on a categorical scale, reliability is appropriately assessed as a measure of agreement. The simplest index of agreement is **percent agreement**. This is a measure of how often raters agree on scores given to individual subjects (or how often test-retest scores agree). The *coefficient of agreement* represents the total proportion of observations (P_O) on which there is agreement, or

$$P_O = \frac{\text{number of exact agreements}}{\text{number of possible agreements}} = \frac{\Sigma f_O}{N} \tag{26.5}$$

where Σf_O is the sum of the *frequencies of observed agreements*, and N is the number of pairs of scores that were obtained.

For example, suppose two clinicians wanted to establish their interrater reliability for evaluating level of function for self-care on a 3-point scale. They evaluate 100 patients to determine if they are independent (IND), need some assistance (ASST) or are dependent (DEP). We can summarize these data to show agreements by arranging them in an *agreement matrix*, or frequency table, as shown in Table 26.6A. The quantities along the diagonal represent the number of times both raters agreed on their ratings (f_O). (Ignore values in parentheses for now.) All values off the diagonal represent disagreements. For instance, both raters agreed on ratings of IND for 25 subjects, they agreed on ratings of ASST for 24 subjects, and they agreed on ratings of DEP for 17 subjects. They did not agree on 34 subjects. Of 100 possible agreements, 66 were achieved. Therefore, $P_O = 66/100 = .66$. The two clinicians agreed on their ratings 66% of the time. This value is fair, relative to potential perfect agreement of 100%.

There is a limitation to this interpretation, however. To determine the true reliability of categorical assignment, we must consider the possibility that some portion of the results could have occurred by chance; that is, if two raters were to assign subjects to categories completely at random, some degree of agreement would still be expected. Because of this tendency, percent agreement will often be an overestimate of true reliability. Therefore, a measure is needed that will discount the proportion of agreement that is potentially due to chance alone.

Chance Agreement: The Kappa Statistic

The **kappa** statistic, κ, is a *chance-corrected* measure of agreement. In addition to looking at the proportion of observed agreements (P_O), kappa also considers the proportion of agreements expected by chance (P_C):

$$P_C = \frac{\text{number of expected agreements}}{\text{number of possible agreements}} = \frac{\Sigma f_C}{N} \tag{26.6}$$

where Σf_C is the sum of the frequencies of agreement expected by chance.

TABLE 26.6   COMPUTATION OF PERCENT AGREEMENT AND KAPPA: AGREEMENT MATRIX FOR RATINGS OF FUNCTIONAL ASSESSMENT FOR TWO RATERS

A. DATA

		Rater 1			
		IND	**ASST**	**DEP**	**Total**
	IND	25 (15.54)	5 (11.10)	7 (10.36)	37
Rater 2 **ASST**		6 (14.28)	24 (10.20)	4 (9.52)	34
	DEP	11 (12.18)	1 (8.70)	17 (8.12)	29
	Total	42	30	28	100

B. COMPUTATIONS

$$\Sigma f_O = 25 + 24 + 17 = 66 \qquad\qquad P_O = \frac{\Sigma f_O}{N} = \frac{66}{100} = .66$$

$$\Sigma f_C = 15.54 + 10.20 + 8.12 = 33.86 \qquad\qquad P_C = \frac{\Sigma f_C}{N} = \frac{33.86}{100} = .34$$

$$\kappa = \frac{P_O - P_C}{1 - P_C} = \frac{.66 - .34}{1 - .34} = .49$$

$$\kappa = \frac{\Sigma f_O - \Sigma f_C}{N - \Sigma f_C} = \frac{66 - 33.86}{100 - 33.86} = .49$$

Chance frequencies in parentheses.

We can illustrate this application using the frequency data for functional assessment shown in Table 26.6. The number of expected chance agreements for each cell along the diagonal is calculated by multiplying the corresponding row and column margin totals, and dividing by the total number of possible agreements, or N.[††] These values are shown in parentheses. For example, for agreements on IND, the row total is 37, and the column total is 42. With $N = 100$, we determine that chance agreements on IND can be expected $(37 \times 42)/100 = 15.54$ times. Similarly, we expect both raters to come up with ratings of ASST $(34 \times 30)/100 = 10.20$ times by chance. The expected frequency for DEP is $(29 \times 28)/100 = 8.12$ times. Therefore, the total number of expected chance frequencies, Σf_C, is 33.86. The proportion of agreement expected by

---

[††]This procedure is identical to calculation of expected frequencies for the χ^2 test. See Chapter 25 for a fuller discussion of this procedure.

chance for the entire sample is $33.86/100 = 0.34$. This tells us that even if these two raters had no common grading criteria, we could expect agreement between them 34% of the time.

Thus, the proportion of observations that can be attributed to reliable measurement is defined by $P_O - P_C$, the proportion of observed agreements less the contribution of chance. The maximum possible nonchance agreements would be $1 - P_C$, or 100% less the contribution of chance. Kappa represents percent agreement based on these correction factors,

$$\kappa = \frac{P_O - P_C}{1 - P_C} \tag{26.7}$$

which is a ratio of the proportion of observed nonchance agreements to the proportion of possible nonchance agreements.

For the functional assessment data, we know the proportion of observed agreement, $P_O = 66\%$. When we calculate chance observations we note that $P_C = 34\%$. Therefore, to account for the fact that 34% of the agreement could have occurred by chance, we correct our original estimate using the formula for kappa:

$$\kappa = \frac{.66 - .34}{1 - .34} = .49$$

This indicates a lower level of agreement than the 66% obtained using percent agreement. With the effects of chance eliminated, agreement is rated at 49%. This corrected percentage is a more meaningful interpretation of reliability estimates for categorical assignments.

As shown in Table 26.6B, kappa can also be expressed in terms of frequencies to facilitate computation:

$$\kappa = \frac{\sum f_O - \sum f_C}{N - \sum f_C} \tag{26.8}$$

For all practical purposes, the lower and upper limits of kappa are 0.00 and +1.00.[18] Kappa will be zero if $P_O = P_C$, where agreement equals chance, and positive if $P_O > P_C$, where agreement is better than chance. With perfect agreement, all cells off the diagonal will equal zero; therefore, $P_O = 1.00$ and $\kappa = 1.00$. Kappa can be negative if agreement is worse than chance ($P_O < P_C$), although this is not a likely outcome in clinical reliability studies.

Weighted Kappa

For some applications, kappa is limited in that it does not differentiate among disagreements. Because it is calculated using only the frequencies along the agreement diagonal, kappa assumes that all disagreements (off the diagonal) are of equal seriousness. There may be instances, however, when a researcher wants to assign greater weight to some disagreements than others, to account for differential risks. For example, Jarvik et al[19] looked at the reliability of classifying disk herniations in patients with lumbar disk disease. They hypothesized that some misclassifications would be more serious than others, if misjudgments were made for those with protruded or extruded disks. In another clinical study, Cooperman et al[20] examined the reliability of a test for ligamentous stability at the knee, graded 0, +1, +2 or +3, with higher grades indicating less stability. They considered a disagreement between ratings of 0 and +3 to be more serious than a disagreement between 0 and +1 for diagnostic purposes and subsequent treatment decisions. When disagreements can be differentiated in this way, a modified version of the kappa statistic, called **weighted kappa,** κ_W, can be used to estimate reliability.[21]

Weighted kappa allows the researcher to specify differential weights for disagreement cells in the agreement matrix. Kappa is actually a special case of weighted kappa, where all cells along the agreement diagonal are given weights of 1.0 and all disagreements are weighted 0. By assigning different weights to the off-diagonal cells, weighted kappa essentially gives more credit for some disagreements than others.

We can illustrate this procedure once again using the functional assessment data. These data showed 66% observed agreement. In terms of clinical implications, however, we might suggest that disagreements among these grades are not all of the same importance and that weighting them would provide a more practical estimate of reliability.

Assigning Weights

Cohen[21] suggests that the assignment of weights is essentially a judgmental process. Therefore, there is no one set of weights that can be applied universally, and the value of κ_W will be sensitive to the choice of weights.[22] Weights should conform to a hypothesis that defines the relative seriousness of the disagreements.

Incremental Weights.   One approach is to look at a scale as an ordinal continuum with equal intervals, that is, an *incremental scale*.[3] For example, using the functional evaluation scale described in Table 26.6, we might hypothesize that a disagreement between IND and DEP is twice as serious as a disagreement between ASST and DEP, with IND = 3, ASST = 2 and DEP = 1. If this hypothesis is reasonable, then weights for incremental disagreements can be determined using the formula

$$w = (r_1 - r_2)^2 \tag{26.9}$$

where w is the assigned weight, and r_1 and r_2 are the scores assigned by rater 1 and rater 2 to that cell. Therefore, $r_1 - r_2$ represents the *deviation from agreement* for each cell in the agreement matrix. This type of weighting system is shown in Table 26.7A. For instance, a disagreement between IND (3) and ASST (2) would receive a weight of $(3 - 2)^2 = 1$. The same weight would be assigned to disagreements between ASST and DEP; however, a disagreement between IND (3) and DEP (1) would receive a weight of $(3 - 1)^2 = 4$. Weights of zero would automatically be assigned to all the agreement cells on the diagonal, indicating no disagreement.

Asymmetrical Weights.   In many situations, the evaluation of disagreements does not fit a uniform pattern. For instance, we might hypothesize that a disagreement between IND and DEP is more severe than a disagreement between ASST and DEP. We

---

TABLE 26.7   TWO SCHEMES FOR WEIGHTING DISAGREEMENTS ON FUNCTIONAL ASSESSMENT DATA

A. Incremental Weights

Cell weights $= (r_1 - r_2)^2$

			Rater 1	
		IND (3)	ASST (2)	DEP (1)
	IND (3)	0	1	4
Rater 2	ASST (2)	1	0	1
	DEP (1)	4	1	0

B. Asymmetrical Weights

			Rater 1	
		IND (3)	ASST (2)	DEP (1)
	IND (3)	0	2	4
Rater 2 (Criterion)	ASST (2)	3	0	1
	DEP (1)	6	1	0

---

might also suggest that the *direction* of the disagreement is important; that is, assigning a grade of IND to a patient who needs assistance is a more serious error than assigning DEP to an independent patient. If a patient who is dependent is graded IND, he might be unsafe, left alone without adequate supervision. This is more serious as an evaluation error than unnecessarily supervising a strong patient. Suppose we test the validity of a clinician's assessment of function by comparing her ratings (rater 1) with those of an "expert" (rater 2), who acts as the criterion or reference standard. We would want to assign the highest weight to an error where rater 1 says IND and rater 2 says DEP. The next highest weight might go to the converse DEP–IND disagreement. Errors between IND and ASST might be the next most serious, followed by ASST–IND. Errors between ASST and DEP might be perceived as relatively unimportant, as with either rating the patient will receive some supervision. This creates an *asymmetrical pattern* of weights, varying with the direction of disagreement.

For this type of subjective judgment, Cohen[21] suggests first choosing a weight to represent maximum disagreement and then setting the other weights accordingly. For example, as shown in Table 26.7B, we might choose weights of 6 for IND–DEP, 4 for DEP–IND, 3 for IND–ASST and 2 for ASST–IND disagreements. DEP–ASST errors would be considered least important, with a weight of 1. For convenience, weights of zero are still assigned to all agreements.

Symmetrical Weights.   A third pattern of weights can be established when the direction of disagreement is unimportant. For instance, we might argue that any disagreement between IND and DEP is twice as serious as a disagreement between IND and ASST, and that a disagreement between ASST and DEP is only minimally important. To designate a set of weights that reflect this hypothesis, we might choose a weight of 6 to represent any disagreement between IND and DEP, a weight of 3 to represent a disagreement between IND and ASST, and a weight of 1 to represent the less important disagreement between ASST and DEP. These *symmetrical weights (w)* are shown in the center of each cell in Table 26.8A.

Calculation of κ_W

The weights that are assigned to each cell in the agreement matrix are used in the calculation of weighted kappa. An obvious criticism of this procedure is based on the fact that the arbitrary assignment of weights can make the consequent value of κ_W arbitrary as well.[23] This points out the need for the researcher to operate on the basis of a hypothesis that defines the relationship among the rating categories. For instance, each of the

TABLE 26.8 COMPUTATION OF WEIGHTED KAPPA USING SYMMETRICAL WEIGHTS: TABLE OF AGREEMENTS AND DISAGREEMENTS ON FUNCTIONAL ASSESSMENT DATA[a]

A. DATA

| | | Rater 1 | | | |
		IND	ASST	DEP	Total
	IND	25 (15.54) $w = 0$	5 (11.10) $w = 3$	7 (10.36) $w = 6$	37
Rater 2 ASST		6 (14.28) $w = 3$	24 (10.20) $w = 0$	4 (9.52) $w = 1$	34
	DEP	11 (12.18) $w = 6$	1 (8.70) $w = 1$	17 (8.12) $w = 0$	29
	Total	42	30	28	100

B. COMPUTATIONS (cells with weights of zero have been omitted)

$\Sigma wf_O = 3(5) + 6(7) + 3(6) + 1(4) + 6(11) + 1(1) = 146$

$\Sigma wf_C = 3(11.10) + 6(10.36) + 3(14.28) + 1(9.52) + 6(12.18) + 1(8.70) = 229.60$

$$\kappa_W = 1 - \frac{\Sigma wf_O}{\Sigma wf_C} = 1 - \frac{146}{229.69} = .36$$

[a]Expected frequencies are in parentheses.

preceding weighting systems was based on a different theoretical rationale. The rationale used to define these weights then becomes an integral part of the hypothesis being tested.[2] For this reason, the weights used in calculating κ_W and the rationale for choosing them should be stated in a research report.

We will demonstrate the calculation of κ_W using the functional assessment data with symmetrical weights shown in Table 26.8A. Each cell in the table contains the observed frequency (f_O), the expected chance frequency (f_C, shown in parentheses), and the cell weight (w). The first step is to find the *weighted frequencies* of observed disagreement (wf_O) and chance disagreement (wf_C) for each cell in the matrix by multiplying the observed and chance frequencies by the cell weight. For example, for the first cell in the matrix, $wf_O = 0(25)$ and $wf_C = 0(15.54)$. Note that we are concerned with the *frequencies of disagreements*, not agreements as we were with kappa. Because the cells along the agreement diagonal all have weights of zero, they are effectively eliminated from the calculations.

Next we determine the sum of these terms to find the total weighted observed frequencies, Σwf_O, and the total weighted chance frequencies, Σwf_C. Weighted kappa is given by

$$\kappa_W = 1 - \frac{\Sigma wf_O}{\Sigma wf_C} \tag{26.10}$$

As shown in Table 26.8B, $\kappa_W = .36$. This value is somewhat lower than the value obtained for kappa ($\kappa = .41$).

Let us consider the implications of weighting this data. According to the frequency data, we find exact agreement in 66 of 100 tests. Kappa reduces this estimate to 49% by correcting for chance, but does not account for any differentiation in the seriousness of the 34 disagreements. Five of these disagreements were between ASST and DEP, which we consider minimally important. Of the 29 more serious disagreements, 18 were between IND and DEP (the most serious) and 11 were between IND and ASST. These serious disagreements account for more than one-quarter of the tests and 85% of all the disagreements. By accounting for these serious discrepancies, weighted kappa brings down the level of agreement further to 36%. This gives us a more meaningful estimate of the degree of reliability between these raters than kappa alone, and suggests that these raters demonstrate serious discrepancies too often.

Interpretation of Kappa

Landis and Koch[24] have suggested that values of kappa above 80% represent excellent agreement; above 60% substantial levels of agreement; from 40% to 60% moderate agreement; and below 40% poor to fair agreement. For this example, then, we have achieved only a moderate degree of reliability. **The interpretation of this outcome, like any other reliability coefficient, must depend on how the data will be used and the degree of precision required for making rational clinical decisions.**

Several factors must be considered in the application of kappa or weighted kappa. First, it is important to recognize that kappa represents an *average rate of agreement* for an entire set of scores. It will not indicate if most of the disagreement is accounted for by one specific category or rater. Therefore, in an effort to improve reliability, it is useful to subjectively examine the data when discussing results, to see where the major discrepancies lie.

A second issue, which we continue to stress for all reliability indices, is that of variance among subjects. In measures of agreement, variance is necessary to allow reasonable interpretation of reliability. In a group of subjects with homogeneous characteristics, the percentage of agreements will be necessarily high. Therefore, the reliability analysis is not really showing whether the measurement is capable of differentiating among subjects on that characteristic.

Because kappa is based on proportions, the use of very small samples can provide misleading results. For example, if two raters agree on two observations, the reliability estimate will be 100%. If they disagree on one of those observations, the rating drops to 50%. Such a variation does not accurately reflect reliability when compared with estimates of the same behavior tested many more times.

Kappa is also influenced by the number of categories used. As the number of categories increases, the extent of agreement will generally decrease. This is logical, as with more possibilities of assignment, there is room for greater discrepancy between raters. Therefore, if values of kappa are to be compared, the samples used should contain the same number of categories.

Probably the strongest limitation of kappa is that it is an analysis of exact agreement; that is, it treats agreement as an all-or-none phenomenon with no room for "close" agreement. Therefore, it is appropriate for use with nominal or ordinal data, which require that each subject be placed in an exclusive category. By definition, there can be no doubt as to whether raters achieved the same "score" for each subject. Kappa is less useful for dealing with continuous data on the interval or ratio scales, as there is no credit given for scores that remain close over several trials.

Kappa can be used with more than two raters,[1,25] although the overall rating is less informative than if separate kappas are computed for pairs of raters.[23] One advantage of using separate analyses is that it is then possible to use different rationales for setting weights for each comparison. A calculation has been derived for using kappa with multiple ratings per subject.[26] It is also possible to use the intraclass correlation coefficient, ICC, as an equivalent of weighted kappa when incremental weights are scaled according to squared disagreements ($w = (r_1 - r_2)^2$).[3]

INTERNAL CONSISTENCY

Measuring instruments are often designed as scales, composed of many items that in total should reflect the characteristic being measured. For instance, the quantitative portion of the Graduate Record Examination (QGRE) includes many items to test a student's mathematical ability. Functional scales are designed to include items related to different functional tasks. In both of these examples, the scales are actually only a sample of the possible items that could be included, although we want to draw a conclusion about an individual's performance based on the total score. If these scales are reliable, we would expect the subject to receive the same score even if we varied the items.

One assumption that is inherent in the use of such scales is the **homogeneity** of the items or their **internal consistency**. A good scale is one that assesses different aspects of the same attribute; that is, the items are homogeneous.[27] Therefore, the QGRE will not include items to assess verbal ability. A scale of physical function will reflect physical performance but not emotional function. Statistically, if the items on the scale are truly measuring the same attribute, they should be moderately correlated with each other and with the total score.[‡‡] These correlations are measures of internal consistency (see Chapter 5 for further discussion of item-total correlations).

Cronbach's Alpha (α)

The most commonly applied statistical index for internal consistency is **Cronbach's alpha (α)**.[28] It can be used for scales with items that are dichotomous (yes/no) or when there are more than two response choices (such as an ordinal scale). To illustrate the application of Cronbach's α, we will use hypothetical data from a sample of 14 patients in a rehabilitation hospital who have been assessed for function using six items: walking, climbing stairs, carrying 5 pounds, reaching for a phone, dressing (putting on a shirt), and getting in and out of a car. Each item is scored on an ordinal scale from 1 to 5, with 5 reflecting complete independence. The maximum total score, then, is 30.

Internal consistency is a reflection of the correlation among these six items and the correlation of each individual item with the total score. Cronbach's α for these data is .894, as shown in Table 26.9A. As with other correlation statistics, this index ranges from 0.00 to 1.00. Therefore, a value that approaches .90 is high, and the scale can be considered reliable.

Alpha can also be used to examine individual items to determine how well they fit the overall scale. In Table 26.9A, the means and standard deviations for each item and the total score are displayed. We can see that walking had the highest mean functional score and car transfer the lowest. In Table 26.9B we find the inter-item correlations for all six items. All item-pairs have correlations above .60 except for car transfer, which has consistently low correlations with all other items (.354 and lower). Perhaps this one variable should not be part of the scale, representing a different component of function than the other items.

To investigate this possibility, the advantage of α is that it can be computed repeatedly, each time eliminating one item from the analysis. In Table 26.9C, we see what happens to the total score when each item is deleted. In the first two columns, the mean and variance of the total score is higher when car transfer is deleted, whereas these values remain fairly stable for all other items. The third column in this panel shows the correlation of each item with the sum of the remaining items, or the **item-to-total correlation**. Only car transfer has a low correlation of .19, suggesting that this variable is not related to the other items. Each of the other five items has a correlation of approximately .80 or higher with the total. Finally, we find that alpha increases to .932 when car transfer is not included, indicating that the scale is more homogeneous when this item is omitted. These statistics suggest that car transfer

---

[‡‡]The concept of internal consistency should not be confused with content or construct validity. Internal consistency is a measure of reliability, not validity. Even if the items in a scale are correlated (a reliability issue), the scale may not be measuring what it is intended to measure (a validity issue). Internal consistency is an important characteristic of a valid scale, however.

TABLE 26.9 **OUTPUT FOR INTERNAL CONSISTENCY OF A FUNCTIONAL SCALE WITH 6 ITEMS USING CRONBACH'S ALPHA (N = 14)**

A. ITEM STATISTICS

Reliability Statistics

Cronbach's Alpha	N of Items
.894	6

Item Statistics

	Mean	Std. Deviation	N
Car	1.86	.770	14
Carry	2.79	1.251	14
Dressing	2.57	1.089	14
Reach	3.00	1.240	14
Stairs	2.36	1.336	14
Walk	3.43	1.089	14

B. CORRELATIONS

Inter-Item Correlation Matrix

	Car	Carry	Dressing	Reach	Stairs	Walk
Car	1.000	.125	.196	−.081	.278	.354
Carry	.125	1.000	.830	.843	.739	.637
Dressing	.196	.830	1.000	.797	.694	.750
Reach	−.081	.843	.797	1.000	.603	.740
Stairs	.278	.739	.694	.603	1.000	.785
Walk	.354	.637	.750	.740	.785	1.000

C. ITEM-TOTAL STATISTICS

Item-Total Statistics

	Scale Mean if Item Deleted	Scale Variance if Item Deleted	Corrected Item-Total Correlation	Squared Multiple Correlation	Cronbach's Alpha if Item Deleted
Car	14.14	28.593	.192	.566	.932
Carry	13.21	19.874	.836	.904	.854
Dressing	13.43	21.033	.856	.777	.854
Reach	13.00	20.615	.765	.916	.867
Stairs	13.64	19.632	.790	.817	.863
Walk	12.57	21.187	.837	.893	.856

should be removed from the scale, as it appears to reflect a different dimension of function than the other items.

Interestingly, several sources suggest that a scale with strong internal consistency should only show a moderate correlation among the items, between .70 and .90.[27,29–31] If items have too low a correlation, they are possibly measuring different traits. If the items have too high a correlation, they are probably redundant, and the content validity of the scale might be limited.

RESPONSE STABILITY

In addition to measuring the reliability of instruments and raters, clinical scientists are often interested in assessing the consistency or stability of repeated responses over time. **Response stability** is basic to establishing all other types of reliability, because if the response variable varies from measurement to measurement, it will not be possible to separate out errors due to the rater or instrument. Three statistical methods are commonly used to express response stability: standard error of measurement, coefficient of variation and method error.

Standard Error of Measurement

Like other forms of reliability, the concept of response stability is related to measurement error. If we were to administer a test under constant conditions to one individual an infinite number of times, we can assume that the responses would vary somewhat from trial to trial. These differences would be a function of random measurement error. Theoretically, if we could plot these responses, the distribution would resemble a normal curve, with the mean equal to the true score and errors falling above and below the mean. This distribution of measurement errors is a theoretical distribution that represents the population of all possible measurement errors that could occur for that variable. With a more reliable measurement, errors will be smaller and this distribution will be less variable. Therefore, the standard deviation of the measurement errors reflects the reliability of the response. This value is called the **standard error of measurement (SEM).**

We can use our knowledge of the normal curve to estimate the variability within repeated measurements in one individual. For example, suppose we record a series of 25 measurements of grip strength for one subject using a hand dynamometer. Let us assume that fatigue does not occur, so that the true value does not change. We can expect that this individual will produce varied scores from trial to trial because of slightly different efforts or repositioning his hand on the dynamometer—random errors of measurement. Suppose the mean score for all trials is 23 pounds with a standard deviation of 6. We can estimate, then, that there is approximately a 68% chance that this individual's true score falls within ±1 standard deviations (between 17 and 29 pounds) or a 95% chance that it falls within ±2 standard deviations (between 11 and 35 pounds). In a subsequent test, if this subject's response is 28 pounds, we would consider the score to be within the range of measurement error, that is no true difference.

When the estimate of measurement error is based on repeated measurements from a single individual, as in this example, its value will obviously be different for each subject. Therefore, the amount of error, or reliability, associated with a particular measurement will not be a constant estimate. Most often, however, it is not feasible to collect a large enough sample of repeated measurements on every subject. Therefore, we have to estimate the SEM for a set of scores obtained from a larger sample of subjects as follows:

$$SEM = s_X \sqrt{1 - r_{XX}}$$

(26.11)

where s_X is the standard deviation of the set of observed test scores on a group of subjects, and r_{XX} is the reliability coefficient for that measurement (typically obtained from previous research). For example, suppose we administer grip strength tests to a sample of 300 patients, each measured once. Assume the standard deviation of these scores is 12, and the reliability coefficient for this measurement, established by previous test-retest studies, is known to be .85. Therefore,

$$SEM = 12\sqrt{1 - .85} = 4.65$$

This value can now be used as an estimate for the entire group, based on a confidence interval.

$$95\% \text{ CI} = \text{Observed score} \pm 1.96 \text{ (SEM)}$$

$$= \text{Observed score} \pm 1.96 \text{ (4.65)} \qquad (26.12)$$

$$= \text{Observed score} \pm 9.11$$

Therefore, we can estimate that 95% of the time, the errors of measurement using this test will fall within this range. If the group mean is 30 pounds, then there is a 95% chance that the group's true mean score lies between 20.89 and 39.11. This will also provide a benchmark for evaluating individual patient performance over time.

The interpretation of standard error of measurement is dependent on the type of reliability coefficient that is used in its computation. If the estimate is based on test-retest reliability, then the SEM is indicative of the range of scores than can be expected on retesting. If the ICC is used as an indicator of rater reliability, the SEM reflects the extent of expected error in different raters' scores. The choice of reliability coefficient for calculating the SEM must be based on the ultimate purpose of predicting reliability.

Minimal Detectable Difference

In Chapter 5 we introduced the concept of **minimal detectable difference (MDD)**, which is used to define the amount of change in a variable that must be achieved to reflect a true difference. Statistics of response stability will provide estimates of this threshold. The SEM is used most often to determine if a patient's performance has truly changed from trial to trial. Values below this threshold will be considered measurement error. The more reliable an instrument, the more precise this smallest measure can be. The MDD will be discussed again in the next chapter, when we consider validity of measuring change.

Coefficient of Variation

We can also assess response stability across repeated trials by looking at the standard deviation of the responses (for one individual or a group). Variability within the responses should reflect the degree of measurement error. The standard deviation will obviously increase as the repeated scores become more disparate.

The limitation to this approach is that the standard deviation must be interpreted in relation to the size and units of the mean. For example, suppose a distribution of strength scores (in pounds) has a standard deviation of 40 lbs. If the mean of the distribution is 110, reliability will be viewed differently than if the mean is 55. In the first instance the scores are actually less variable relative to the mean. Therefore, on the basis of standard deviation alone, we cannot accurately assess the extent of error in the measurements.

To account for the relationship between the mean and standard deviation, the variability across distributions can be compared using the **coefficient of variation, CV**:

$$CV = \frac{s}{\overline{X}} \times 100 \qquad (26.13)$$

This ratio expresses the standard deviation[§§] as a *proportion of the mean*. Because both the mean and standard deviation are in the same units, this statistic will be unit free, allowing comparisons across different quantities or different studies. See Chapter 17 for a more complete discussion and sample calculations of the coefficient of variation.

Method Error

Response stability, or test-retest reliability, can also be expressed in terms of the percentage variation from trial to trial, by analyzing **method error, ME.** Method error is a measure of the discrepancy between two sets of repeated scores, or their difference scores. Larger difference scores reflect greater measurement error.

Method error is calculated using the standard deviation of the difference scores (s_d) between test and retest:

$$ME = \frac{s_d}{\sqrt{2}} \qquad (26.14)$$

This value reflects the amount of variation in the difference scores; however, just like any other standard deviation, it must be interpreted relative to the size of the mean differences. Therefore, it is converted to a percentage using the coefficient of variation:

$$CV_{ME} = \frac{2ME}{\overline{X}_1 + \overline{X}_2} \times 100 \qquad (26.15)$$

Calculation of ME and its associated coefficient of variation is illustrated in Table 26.9B for hypothetical range of motion measurements. The variation in measurement from test 1 to test 2 was 6%. The interpretation of this value will depend on the amount of error deemed acceptable by those who must use the information.

[§§]Because scores used for reliability testing are generally not intended as estimates of population parameters, the standard deviation can be calculated using N in the denominator, rather than $N - 1$.[32]

Method error is often used as an adjunct to test-retest correlation statistics, as it reflects the percentage of variation from trial to trial, which the correlation coefficient does not. In addition, unlike the correlation coefficient, method error is not affected by a lack of variation in raw scores. For instance, for the data in Table 26.10, $r = .58$. This is low, especially considering how close the two pairs of scores are. But we can also see that there is very little variability within these scores, which we know will tend to decrease the correlation coefficient or any reliability coefficient. Method error will not be affected by a restriction in range, because it looks only at the difference scores. Therefore, in situations like this example, where reliability coefficients may be misleading, method error provides a useful alternative.

Because method error is based on the variability within difference scores, it will not account for systematic variation between test 1 and test 2. Therefore, the researcher may

TABLE 26.10 COMPUTATION OF METHOD ERROR AND COEFFICIENT OF VARIATION FOR RELIABILITY TESTING

A. DATA

Subject	Test 1	Test 2	Difference (d)
1	20	17	−3
2	17	16	1
3	21	17	4
4	18	15	3
5	17	16	1
6	15	15	0
7	12	15	−3
8	24	25	−1
ΣX	144	136	$\Sigma d = 2$
$\overline{X}$	18	17.0	$\overline{d} = 0.25$
s	3.70	3.34	$s_d = 2.55$

B. COMPUTATIONS

$$ME = \frac{s_d}{\sqrt{2}} = \frac{2.55}{\sqrt{2}} = 1.$$

$$CV_{ME} = \frac{2ME}{\overline{X}_1 + \overline{X}_2} \times 100 = \frac{2(1.80)}{18 + 17} \times 10$$

$$s_{\overline{d}} = \frac{s_d}{\sqrt{n}} = \frac{2.55}{\sqrt{8}} = 0 \qquad t = \frac{\overline{d}}{s_{\overline{d}}} = \frac{.25}{.90} = 0$$

C. HYPOTHESIS TEST

$$H_0: \overline{d} = 0 \qquad _{(\alpha_2 = .05)}t_{(7)} = 2.365 \qquad \text{Do not reject } H_0$$

want to check for systematic bias by performing a paired t-test between the test and retest scores.[33] The t-ratio can be obtained directly by dividing the mean of the difference scores, $\bar{d}$, by the standard error of the difference scores, $s_{\bar{d}}$. This computation is illustrated in Table 26.10B. With $n - 1$ degrees of freedom, this value demonstrates no significant difference between test 1 and test 2.

ALTERNATE FORMS: LIMITS OF AGREEMENT

Reliability is an essential property when measurements are taken with alternate forms of an instrument. For example, clinical researchers have looked at outcomes of measuring joint range of motion with different types of goniometers, inclinometers, electrogoniometers and radiographs. Even though each instrument is different, they are all intended to result in an accurate recording of joint angles in degrees. We might want to compare different designs of dynamometers for measuring strength, different types of spirometers for assessing pulmonary function or different types of thermometers for measuring temperature. In each of these examples, we would expect these methods to record similar values. The analysis of reliability in this situation focuses on the agreement between alternative methods. We can consider two methods in agreement when the difference between measurements on one subject is small enough for the methods to be considered interchangeable.[34] This property is an important practical concern as we strive for effective and efficient clinical measurement,[35] as well as a concern for generalization of research findings.

Two analysis procedures have traditionally been applied for method comparisons. The correlation coefficient, r, has been used to demonstrate covariance among methods; however, we know this is a poor estimate of reliability, as it does not necessarily reflect the extent of agreement in the data. The second procedure is the paired t-test, (or repeated measures ANOVA) which is used to show that mean scores for two (or more) methods are not significantly different. This approach is also problematic, however, as two distributions may show no statistical difference, but still be composed of pairs with no agreement.

An interesting alternative for examining agreement across methods is an index called **limits of agreement**.[34,35] To understand this approach, consider the hypothetical distribution of 10 measurements of range of motion of straight leg raising shown in Table 26.11 for two instruments, a regular goniometer and an inclinometer. The difference between each method for each subject is calculated by subtracting the inclinometer score from the goniometer score (this direction is consistent but arbitrary). Therefore, positive difference scores reflect a higher reading for the goniometer. The mean of the difference scores is −0.1 degrees. On average, then, the differences between the methods is quite small, and certainly within acceptable clinical error range. We would be happy to find that the two instruments differed by less than one degree. On further examination, however, we can see that the amount of error varied across subjects, from zero to as much as 10 degrees. Therefore, we would be more complete in our estimate of reliability to determine the range of error that would be expected for any individual subject.

TABLE 26.11   LIMITS OF AGREEMENT: MEASUREMENT OF STRAIGHT LEG RAISING (IN DEGREES) USING TWO METHODS

A. DATA

Subject	Goniometer	Inclinometer	Difference[a]	Mean[b]
1	55	54	1	54.5
2	58	61	−3	59.5
3	70	80	−10	75.0
4	76	59	7	62.5
5	85	85	0	85.0
6	78	80	−2	79.0
7	72	70	2	71.0
8	80	75	5	77.5
9	63	68	−5	65.5
10	72	68	4	70.0
		Total	−1.0	699.5
		$\overline{X}$	−0.1	69.9
		s	5.09	9.52

B. 95% LIMITS OF AGREEMENT

$$\overline{X} \pm 2s = -0.1 \pm 10.18 = -10.28 \text{ to } 10.08$$

[a]Goniometer − Inclinometer

[b](Goniometer + Inclinometer)/2

A visual analysis can help to clarify this relationship. For example, the scatterplot of these scores is shown in Figure 26.2 (r = .86). If we draw a *line of identity* from the origin, representing agreement of scores, we can see that most of the scores are close, but not in perfect agreement. A further understanding of this relationship can be achieved by looking at the difference between methods plotted against the mean score for each subject, as shown in Figure 26.3. These plots are often called **Bland-Altman plots,** recognizing those who developed this strategy.[35] The spread of scores around the zero point helps us decide if the observed error is acceptable if we substitute one measurement method for the other. In Figure 26.3A, for example, the error appears unbiased, as differences are spread evenly and randomly above and below the zero point. Other possible patterns are shown in Figures 26.3B, which shows a pattern with no error, where all differences are zero. In Figure 26.3C we see a biased pattern, where the goniometer has consistently resulted in higher scores, resulting in positive difference scores. Figure 26.3D shows another biased pattern where error is influenced by the size of the measurement; that is, smaller angles are measured higher by the inclinometer (resulting in a negative difference score) and larger angles are measured higher by the goniometer (resulting in a positive difference score). With a biased pattern, the instruments could not be considered interchangeable.

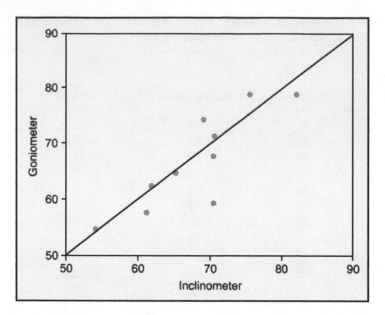

FIGURE 26.2   Example of a method comparison plot, showing the relationship between two different methods for measuring range of motion of straight leg raise. The line of identity emerges from the origin, showing how closely the two methods agree. In this example, only one score falls directly on this line.

We can examine the agreement between the two methods by looking at the spread of the difference scores. A larger variability would indicate larger errors. Statistically, this spread is reflected by the standard deviation. Assuming the errors are normally distributed,*** we would expect that approximately 95% of the difference scores would fall within two standard deviations above and below the mean of the difference scores.[34] This range is considered the **95% limits of agreement**. As shown in Table 26.11B, for the straight leg raise data the mean difference score is −0.1 degrees with a standard deviation of 5.09 degrees. Two standard deviations equal 10.18 degrees. Therefore, the difference between these two methods of measurement of straight leg raise can be expected to vary between −0.1 ± 10.18, or between −10.28 degrees and 10.08 degrees, a range of approximately 20 degrees (see Figure 26.4).

Our question, then, is would we be comfortable using either instrument, if we knew that their difference could be as much as 10 degrees higher or lower? This decision should be based on a clinical criterion and the application of the measurements. We might argue that a potential difference of 20 degrees does not suggest interchangeable methods. We are, of course, assuming that each method is reliable. These considerations have important implications for clinical analyses as well as comparison of research studies.

***Because the difference scores represent measurement error, Bland and Altman[35] suggest that they should follow a normal distribution, even if the actual measurements do not. This distribution can be checked by graphing a histogram of the difference scores.[34]

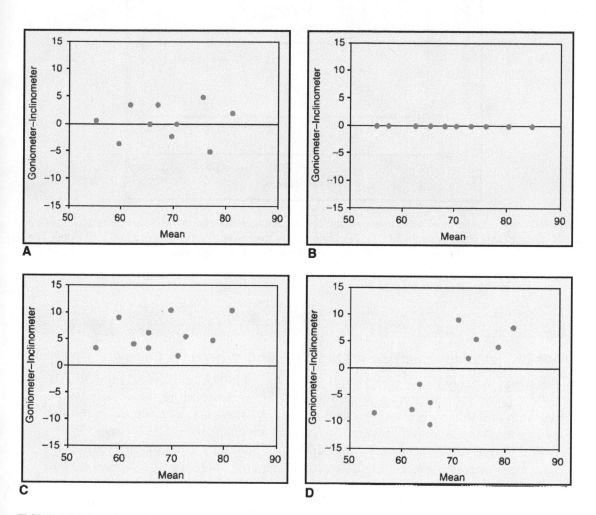

FIGURE 26.3 Plots of difference scores for straight leg raise measurements across mean scores for each subject. The center line represents zero difference. **(A)** Data from Table 26.11; **(B)** perfect agreement between two methods; **(C)** pattern with systematic bias in measurement error, in this case with the goniometer consistently producing higher scores than the inclinometer; **(D)** plot showing bias related to magnitude of the subjects' scores.

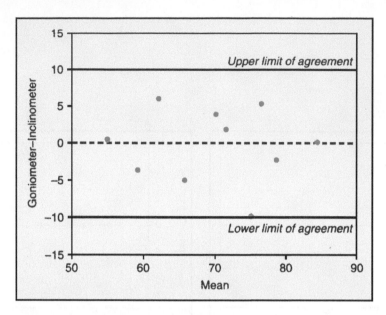

FIGURE 26.4   Difference scores between goniometer and inclinometer, plotted against mean scores for each subject (data from Table 26.11). Dashed line shows the mean difference score (−0.1 degrees). The 95% upper and lower limits of agreement represent 2 standard deviations above and below the mean difference score (−0.1 ± 10.18).

COMMENTARY

Which Reliability Coefficient Do I Use—and When Is It Enough?

Because reliability issues are so important to the validity of clinical science, the statistical bases for interpreting reliability must be understood by those who do the research and those who read research reports. What we learn from looking through professional literature is that preferred methods for analyzing reliability seem to vary with different researchers and within different disciplines. Even though statisticians have been addressing reliability issues for a long time, there is no consensus on how reliability data are handled.

Choosing a particular approach to reliability testing should be based on an understanding of the nature of the response variable, what types of interpretations are desired, and what measurement issues are of greatest concern. Consideration should be given to the scale of measurement, the amount of variability that can be expected within sample scores, and what units of measurement are used. We should be aware of the intended application of the data and the degree of precision needed to make safe and meaningful clinical decisions. These details are often overlooked, and we allow ourselves to fall into the trap of using specific standards for reliability just because they have been used by others—or stated in a textbook like this one! Guidelines are just that—not gold standards. Researchers and clinicians are obligated to justify their interpretation of acceptable reliability.

Researchers should address each of these relevant issues in their reports, so that others can interpret their work properly. Many articles are published with no such discussion, leaving the reader to guess why a particular statistic was used or standard applied. Because reliability statistics can be applied in so many ways, it is important to maintain an exchange of ideas that promotes such accountability. By having to justify our choices, we are forced to consider what a statistic can really tell us about a variable and what conclusions are warranted.

It is also important to justify a measure of reliability as a foundation for validity of a test. Reliability by itself is never enough to support the use of a particular measure. Statistics such as sensitivity, specificity and likelihood ratios must be applied to determine the clinical meaningfulness of a test (see Chapter 27). Reliability is necessary but not sufficient to assure validity; however, sometimes a test will have only moderate reliability, but may still provide strong diagnostic information because of the nature of the disorder being evaluated. All measurements will have some degree of error. Our concern with the consequences of this error will depend on how we will use the measurement in our decision making. There are several examples of measurements that have only moderate kappa or ICC values, but have strong sensitivity or likelihood ratios, suggesting that the tests are useful for identifying those who have a certain disorder.[36] Reliability is one measurement property that must be considered—an important one to be sure, but not the only one.

REFERENCES

1. Bartko JJ, Carpenter WT, Jr. On the methods and theory of reliability. *J Nerv Ment Dis* 1976;163:307–317.
2. Tinsley HEA, Weiss DJ. Interrater reliability and agreement of subjective judgments. *J Counseling Psychol* 1975;22:358–376.
3. Fleiss JL, Cohen J. The equivalence of weighted kappa on the intraclass correlation coefficient as measures of reliability. *Educ Psychol Meas* 1973;33:613–619.
4. Cronbach LJ, Gleser GC, Nanda H, Rajaratnam N. *The Dependability of Behavioral Measurements: Theory of Generalizability for Scores and Profiles.* New York: Wiley, 1972.
5. Mitchell SK. Interobserver agreement, reliability, and generalizability of data collected in observational studies. *Psychol Bull* 1979;36:376–390.
6. Berk RA. Generalizability of behavioral observations: A clarification of interobserver agreement and interobserver reliability. *Am J Ment Defic* 1979;83:460–472.
7. Shrout PE, Fleiss JL. Intraclass correlation: Uses in assessing rater reliability. *Psychol Bull* 1979;86:420–428.
8. Nichols DP. Choosing an Intraclass Correlation Coefficient. Available at: <http://www.ats.ucla.edu/STAT/spss/library/whichicc.htm> Accessed on March 7, 2006.
9. Green SB, Salkind NJ, Akey TM. *Using SPSS for Windows and Macintosh: Analyzing and Understanding Data* (4th ed.). Upper Saddle River, NJ: Prentice Hall, 2004.
10. Yaffee RA. Enhancement of reliability analysis: Application of intraclass correlations. Available at: <http://www.nyu.edu/its/statistics/Docs/intracls.html> Accessed September 23, 2006.
11. Hamer RM. Sample 537: Compute six intraclass correlation measures. Available at: <http://support.sas.com/ctx/samples/index.jsp?sid=537> Accessed March 7, 2006.

12. Intraclass correlation calculator. Stats toolbox (Concordance). Available at: <http://department.obg.cuhk.edu.hk/researchsupport/IntraClass_correlation.asp> Accessed March 7, 2006.

13. Intraclass correlation calculator. Available at: <http://sip.medizin.uni-ulm.de/informatik/projekte/Odds/icc.html> Accessed March 7, 2006.

14. Lahey MA, Downey RG, Saal FE. Intraclass correlations: There's more there than meets the eye. *Psychol Bull* 1983;93:586–595.

15. Maher CG, Sherrington C, Herbert RD, Moseley AM, Elkins M. Reliability of the PEDro scale for rating quality of randomized controlled trials. *Phys Ther* 2003;83:713–721.

16. Riddle DL, Finucan SD, Rothstein JM, Walker ML. Intrasession and intersession reliability of hand-held dynamometer measurements taken on brain-damaged patients. Author's response. *Phys Ther* 1989;69:192–194.

17. Krebs DE. Declare your ICC type. *Phys Ther* 1986;66:1431.

18. Cohen J. Coefficient of agreement for nominal scales. *Educ Psychol Meas* 1960;20:37–46.

19. Jarvik JG, Haynor DR, Koepsell TD, Bronstein A, Ashley D, Deyo RA. Interreader reliability for a new classification of lumbar disk disease. *Acad Radiol* 1996;3:537–544.

20. Cooperman JM, Riddle DL, Rothstein JM. Reliability and validity of judgments of the integrity of the anterior cruciate ligament of the knee using the Lachman's test. *Phys Ther* 1990;70:225–233.

21. Cohen J. Weighted kappa: Nominal scale agreement with provisions for scale disagreement or partial credit. *Psychol Bull* 1968;70:213–220.

22. Graham P, Jackson R. The analysis of ordinal agreement data: Beyond weighted kappa. *J Clin Epidemiol* 1993;46:1055–1062.

23. Maclure M, Willett WC. Misinterpretation and misuse of the kappa statistic. *Am J Epidemiol* 1987;126:161–169.

24. Landis JR, Koch GG. The measurement of observer agreement for categorical data. *Biometrics* 1977;33:159–174.

25. Fleiss JL. Measuring nominal scale agreement among many raters. *Psychol Bull* 1971;76: 78–82.

26. Haley SM, Osberg JS. Kappa coefficient calculation using multiple ratings per subject: A special communication. *Phys Ther* 1989;69:970–974.

27. Streiner DL, Normal GR. *Health Measurement Scales: A Practical Guide to Their Development and Use* (3rd ed.). New York: Oxford University Press, 2003.

28. Cronbach LJ. Coefficient alpha and the internal structure of tests. *Psychometrika* 1951;16: 297–334.

29. Boyle GJ. Does item homogeneity indicate internal consistency or item redundancy in psychometric scales? *Personality Individ Differences* 1991;12:291–294.

30. Hattie J. Methodology review: Assessing unidimensionality of tests and items. *Appl Psychol Meas* 1985;9:1139–1164.

31. Nunally J, Bernstein IH. *Psychometric Theory* (3rd ed.). New York: McGraw-Hill, 1994.

32. Francis K. Computer communication: Reliability. *Phys Ther* 1986;66:1140–1144.

33. Bland M. *An Introduction to Medical Statistics* (2nd ed.). New York: Oxford University Press, 1995.

34. Ottenbacher KJ, Stull GA. The analysis and interpretation of method comparison studies in rehabilitation research. *Am J Phys Med Rehabil* 1993;72:266–271.

35. Bland JM, Altman DG. Statistical methods for assessing agreement between two methods of clinical measurement. *Lancet* 1986;327:307–310.

36. Wainner RS. Reliability of the clinical examination: how close is "close enough"? *J Orthop Sports Phys Ther* 2003;33:488–490.

CHAPTER 27

Statistical Measures of Validity

Measurement validity is an essential component of evidence-based practice, to assure that our assessment tools provide us with accurate information for decision making. Although clinicians constantly face uncertainty in patient management, many decision making strategies can be applied to reduce this uncertainty.

Concepts of measurement validity were introduced in Chapter 6. In this chapter we present statistical procedures related to the accuracy of diagnostic tools, choosing cut-off scores, the application of clinical prediction rules, and methods for measuring clinically meaningful change.

VALIDITY OF DIAGNOSTIC TESTS

Many measuring instruments are specifically designed as screening or diagnostic tools. In a traditional medical framework, a diagnostic test is used to determine the presence or absence of a disease or abnormal condition. A screening test is usually done on individuals who are asymptomatic, to identify those at risk for certain disorders, and to classify patients who are likely to benefit from specific intervention strategies. Because these procedures involve allocation of resources, present potential risks to patients and are used for clinical decision making, it is important to verify their validity.

The results of a diagnostic or screening procedure may be dichotomous, categorical or continuous. The simplest tests will have only a dichotomous outcome: positive or negative, such as pregnancy or HIV status. A categorical test would involve ratings on an ordinal scale, such as $+++, ++, +, -$ to reflect degree of sensation or reflexes. A continuous scale provides the most information regarding the outcome, such as a test measuring degrees of range of motion or hearing decibel level. Ordinal and continuous scales are often converted to dichotomous outcomes using cutoff scores to indicate a "normal" or "abnormal" response.

The Reference Standard

The ideal diagnostic test, of course, would always be accurate in discriminating between those with and without the disease or condition; it would always have a positive result for someone with the condition, whether a mild or severe case, and a negative result in everyone else. But we know that such tests are not perfect. They may miss abnormalities in those with a particular disorder, or they may identify abnormalities in those without the disorder.

We determine how good a test is by comparing the test result with known diagnostic findings obtained by a **reference standard**.* The reference standard will reflect the patient's true status, either the presence or absence of the condition. The assumption is made that the individual performing the test is blind to the true condition, eliminating possible bias. In some situations, the reference standard will be a concurrent test, such as an X-ray or blood test. In other situations, it will be obtained at a future time, as with a long-term outcome or autopsy. Sometimes there is no clear standard, and one must be defined or created. For instance, studies related to falls often use the patient's report of a fall within the past 6 months or year as the standard for being a "faller" or "nonfaller."[1] Studies of delirium in hospitalized patients have used expert opinion as the reference standard to validate measures of confusion.[2] When objective definitive standards are not available, the reference must be adequately described so that others can determine its applicability.

Sensitivity and Specificity

The validity of a diagnostic test is evaluated in terms of its ability to accurately assess the presence and absence of the target condition. A diagnostic test can have four possible outcomes, summarized in the 2×2 arrangement shown in Table 27.1. Classification is assigned according to the true presence or absence of disease (Dx+ or Dx−) versus positive or negative test results. In Table 27.1 the cells labeled a and d represent **true positives** and **true negatives**, respectively, that is, individuals who are correctly classified by the test as having or not having the target condition. Cell b reflects those who are incorrectly identified as having the condition, or **false positives**, and cell c represents those who are incorrectly identified as not having the condition, or **false negatives**.

Sensitivity is the test's ability to obtain a positive test when the target condition is really present, or the true positive rate. Using the notation presented in Table 27.1,

$$\text{Sensitivity} = \frac{a}{a + c} \qquad (27.1)$$

This value is the proportion of individuals who test positive for the condition out of all those who actually have it, or the probability of obtaining a correct positive test in patients who have the target condition. The sensitivity of a test increases as the number of persons with the condition who are correctly classified increases; that is, fewer persons with the disorder are missed.

---

*We use the designation *reference standard* in place of "gold standard," as many tests do not have a true gold standard. The reference standard is defined as the basis for determining the patient's true diagnostic status. This may or may not reflect a true gold standard measure. The researcher must operationalize the reference standard.

TABLE 27.1   SUMMARY OF ANALYSIS FOR DIAGNOSTIC TEST RESULTS

		Reference Standard True Diagnosis		Total
		Dx+	**Dx–**	**Total**
Test result	**Positive**	*a* (True positive)	*b* (False positive)	*a + b*
Test result	**Negative**	*c* (False negative)	*d* (True negative)	*c + d*
	Total	*a + c*	*b + d*	*N*

Diagnostic accuracy	(a + d)/N
Sensitivity	a/(a + c)
Specificity	d/(b + d)
False positive rate (1 − specificity)	b/(b + d)
False negative rate (1 − sensitivity)	c/(a + c)
Positive predictive value (PV +)	a/(a + b)
Negative predictive value (PV −)	d/(c + d)
Prevalence	(a + c)/N
Positive likelihood ratio (LR +)	sensitivity/1 − specificity
Negative likelihood ratio (LR −)	1 − sensitivity/specificity

Specificity is the test's ability to obtain a negative test when the condition is really absent, or the true negative rate. As shown in Table 27.1,

$$\text{Specificity} = \frac{d}{b + d} \tag{27.2}$$

This value is the proportion of individuals who test negative for the condition out of all those who are truly normal, or the probability of a correct negative test in those who do not have the target condition. A highly specific instrument will rarely test positive when a person does not have the disease.

The complement of sensitivity (1 − sensitivity) is the **false negative rate,** or the probability of obtaining an incorrect negative test in patients who do have the target disorder. The complement of specificity (1 − specificity) is the **false positive rate,** sometimes called the "false alarm" rate.[3] This is the probability of an incorrect positive test in those who do not have the target condition.

Example

To illustrate the application of these measures, let's consider a study of the validity of the Functional Reach Test (FRT) to identify elders with Parkinson's disease who are at risk for falls.[4] The FRT is designed to assess anterior-posterior stability by measuring the maximum distance an individual can reach while leaning forward over a fixed base of support.[5] Based on previous research, a cutoff score of 10 in. (25.4 cm) was used to classify subjects as "at risk" or "not at risk." Screening results were compared with a known history of falls (the reference standard), as shown in Table 27.2A.

The sensitivity of the test for this population was low, at 30%. Of the 30 patients identified as having a history of falls, only 9 tested positive using the FRT. The specificity of the test, however, was 92%. Of the 13 patients who did not have a history of falls, 12 tested negative. Therefore, although almost all of those not at risk were correctly identified (true negatives), a large percentage of patients who were at risk were missed (false negatives). The graphic in Table 27.2A illustrates these proportions.

Predictive Value

In addition to sensitivity and specificity, the usefulness of a clinical screening tool can be assessed by its feasibility. A test must demonstrate that it is an efficient use of time and resources and that it yields a sufficient number of accurate responses to be clinically useful. This characteristic is assessed by the test's predictive value. A **positive predictive value (PV +)** estimates the likelihood that a person who tests positive actually has the disease. Using the notation given in Table 27.1,

$$PV+ = \frac{a}{a + b} \tag{27.3}$$

which represents the proportion of those who tested positive who were true positives. Therefore, a test with a high positive predictive value will provide a strong estimate of the actual number of patients who have the target condition. Similarly, a **negative predictive value (PV −)** indicates the probability that a person who tests negative is actually disease free. Therefore,

$$PV- = \frac{d}{c + d} \tag{27.4}$$

which is the proportion of all those who tested negative who were true negatives. A test with a high negative predictive value will provide a strong estimate of the number of people who do not have the target condition.

For the FRT study (see Table 27.2), the positive predictive (PV+) value of 90% tells us that almost all of those who tested positive actually had a history of falls. Only one patient who tested positive was not at risk. The negative predictive value (PV−) was lower, at 36%. Therefore, only one-third of patients who tested negative were actually not at risk.

Predictive value may be of greatest importance in deciding whether or not to implement a screening program. When the positive predictive value is low, only a small portion of those who test positive actually have the target condition. Therefore, considerable resources will probably be needed to evaluate these people further to separate false positives, or unnecessary treatments will be applied. Policy decisions are often based on a balance between the use of available resources and the potential harmful effects resulting from not identifying those with the target condition.[6]

**TABLE 27.2   SUMMARY OF ANALYSIS OF SCREENING TEST RESULTS
FOR FUNCTIONAL REACH TEST (FRT) IN PERSONS
WITH PARKINSON'S DISEASE[a]**

A. DATA[b]

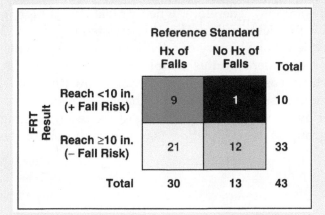

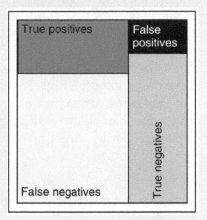

B. MEASURES OF DIAGNOSTIC ACCURACY

Diagnostic accuracy	$(a + d)/N$	$(9 + 12)/43 = 49\%$
Sensitivity	$a/(a + c)$	$9/30 = 30\%$
Specificity	$d/(b + d)$	$12/13 = 92\%$
False positive rate (1 − specificity)	$b/(b + d)$	$1/13 = 8\%$
False negative rate (1 − sensitivity)	$c/(a + c)$	$21/30 = 70\%$
Positive predictive value (PV +)	$a/(a + b)$	$9/10 = 90\%$
Negative predictive value (PV −)	$d/(c + d)$	$12/33 = 36\%$
Prevalence	$(a + c)/N$	$30/43 = 70\%$
Positive likelihood ratio (LR +)	sensitivity/1 − specificity	$.30/.08 = 3.75$
Negative likelihood ratio (LR −)	1 − sensitivity/specificity	$.70/.92 = .76$

C. CONFIDENCE INTERVALS[c]

Sensitivity = .30 (95% CI: 0.17, 0.48)

Specificity = .92 (95% CI: 0.67, 0.99)

LR+ = 3.75 (95% CI: 0.55, 27.7)

LR− = 0.76 (95% CI: 0.57, 1.005)

[a]Data from Behrmann AL, Light KE, Flynn SM, Thigpen MT. Is the Functional Reach Test useful for identifying falls risk among individuals with Parkinson's disease? *Arch Phys Med Rehabil* 2002;83:538–42.

[b]Proportions obtained using interactive calculator at <http://www.cebm.net/dxtable.asp> Accessed April 12, 2007.

[c]Obtained using the confidence interval calculator available at: <http://www.pedro.fhs.usyd.edu.au/tutorial .html#part_one> Accessed October 1, 2006.

The Effect of Prevalence

Sensitivity, specificity and predictive value are influenced by the prevalence of the target condition in the population. **Prevalence** refers to the number of cases of a condition existing in a given population at any one time. For a test with a given sensitivity and specificity, the likelihood of identifying cases with the condition is increased when prevalence is high (the condition is common). Therefore, when prevalence is high, a test will tend to have a higher positive predictive value. This is illustrated in Table 27.2 for our example of fall risk. The prevalence of a history of falls is 30 out of 43 patients, or 70%. Therefore, a large proportion of patients in this sample had a history of falls, and we could expect a high PV+, which was 90%. When prevalence is low (the condition is rare), one can expect many more false positives, just by chance. A positive predictive value can be increased either by increasing the specificity of the test (changing the criterion) or by targeting a subgroup of the population that is at high risk for the target condition.

Ruling In and Ruling Out

When we consider the diagnostic accuracy of a test, high values of sensitivity and specificity provide a certain level of confidence in interpretation. If a test has high sensitivity, it will properly identify most of those who have the disorder. If the test has high specificity, it will properly identify most of those without the condition. But how do these definitions relate to confidence in diagnostic decisions? Consider these two questions:

- If a patient has a positive test, can we be confident in ruling IN the diagnosis?
- If a patient has a negative test, can we be confident in ruling OUT the diagnosis?

Sensitivity and specificity help us answer these questions, but probably not the way you would expect. When a test has *high specificity*, a positive test rules *in* the diagnosis. When a test has *high sensitivity*, a negative test rules *out* the diagnosis. Straus and colleagues[7] offer two mnemonics to remember these relationships:

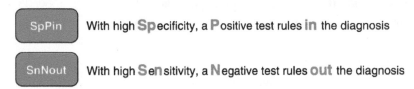

SpPin   With high **Sp**ecificity, a **P**ositive test rules **in** the diagnosis

SnNout   With high **S**e**n**sitivity, a **N**egative test rules **out** the diagnosis

Think of it this way: A highly specific test will properly identify most of the patients who do *not* have the disorder. If the test is so good at finding those who are normal, we can be pretty sure that someone with a positive test *does* have the disorder (ruling IN the diagnosis) because if he didn't have the disorder, the test would have correctly identified him as normal! Conversely, a highly sensitive test will find most of those who *do* have the disorder. Therefore, we can be pretty sure that someone with a negative test does *not* have the disorder (ruling OUT the diagnosis) because if he did have the disorder, the test would have correctly diagnosed him!

These concepts are also related to predictive value. With a more specific test, negative cases are identified more readily. Therefore, it is less likely that an individual with a positive test will actually be normal. This results in a high positive predictive value. With a more sensitive test, positive cases are identified more readily; that is, we will not miss many true cases. Therefore, it is less likely that an individual with a negative test will have the disease. This leads to a high negative predictive value.

If we use the example of the Functional Reach Test (Table 27.2), with specificity of 92% (and a PV− of 90%), we can be confident that someone with a positive test is at risk for falls. However, with sensitivity of only 30% (and a PV+ of 36%), if someone has a negative test, we cannot be sure that person is really not at risk. Because the test is not good at finding those who are at risk, having a negative test does not help us safely rule out this risk.

Pretest and Posttest Probabilities

The ultimate purpose of a diagnostic test is to help the clinician make a decision about the presence or absence of a disorder for an individual patient. The validity of a test is based on how strongly it can support a decision to rule the disorder in or out. Therefore, a test is considered a good one if it can help to increase our certainty about a patient's diagnosis.

Pretest Probabilities

When we begin to evaluate a patient by taking a history and using screening or other subjective procedures, we begin to rule in and rule out certain conditions and eventually generate a hypothesis about the likely diagnosis. This hypothesis can be translated into a measure of probability or confidence, indicating the clinician's estimate of how likely a particular disorder is present. This has been termed the **pretest probability** (or prior probability) of the disorder— or what we think might be the problem before we perform any formal testing.[8]

Finding the Pretest Probability. The process for determining a pretest probability is not an obvious one. Conceptually, it represents a "best guess" or clinical impression based on experience and clinical judgment. Clinicians may have sufficient experience with certain types of patients to estimate the probability of a diagnosis based on initial examination findings,[9,10] although such estimates are not always reliable.[11,12] Using the functional reach scenario, a clinician might have sufficient experience with patients with Parkinson's disease to generate an initial hypothesis about the patient's likelihood to fall.

Information from the literature can also be used to help with this estimate by referring to the prevalence of a disorder.[13] For instance, studies have shown that the prevalence of idiopathic scoliosis in children aged 10–16 years is 2–4%;[14] 26% of patients with orthopedic trauma have been found to experience depression;[15] 34% of children who have been enrolled in special education classes have been diagnosed with asthma;[16] the presence of postoperative delirium following hip fracture repair is estimated at 36%;[2] the prevalence of mortality 1-month following a stroke in patients with prestroke dementia is 44%.[17] These values, reported in the literature, allow the clinician to estimate the likelihood that any individual patient could have these disorders.

Suppose you are working with a patient with Parkinson's disease, and you believe she may be at risk for falling. You think it may be useful to perform a test to determine if such a risk is present. Consider the study of the Functional Reach Test once again (see Table 27.2) This study demonstrated a 70% prevalence of falls in its sample of patients with Parkinson's disease.[4] Knowing this, before you have done any further testing, your best estimate is that the pretest probability of your patient being at risk for falls is 70%.

Decision-Making Thresholds.   Being able to estimate a pretest probability is central to deciding if a condition is present and if testing or treatment is warranted. Based on the initial hypothesis and pretest probability of a condition, the clinician must decide if a diagnostic test is necessary or useful to confirm the actual diagnosis. Straus et al[7] suggest that two thresholds should be considered, as shown in Figure 27.1A. With a very low pretest probability, the diagnosis is so unlikely that testing is not useful; that is, even with a positive test, results are likely to be false positives. Therefore, treatment is not initiated and other diagnoses need to be considered.

With a very high pretest probability, the likelihood of the diagnosis is so strong that testing may be unnecessary, and treatment should just be initiated. Even with a negative test, results are likely to be false negatives. A strong pretest probability means that the results of a test are unlikely to offer any additional useful information. When the pretest probability is not definitive, however, with more intermediate values, testing is necessary to pursue the diagnosis, and treatment decisions will then be based on those results.

This approach must also take into consideration the relative severity of the disorder; the threshold for testing may vary for different conditions. For example, a patient

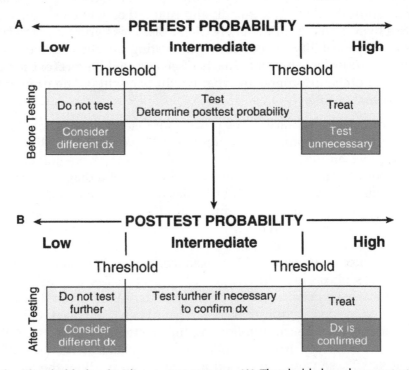

FIGURE 27.1   Thresholds for deciding to test or treat. **(A)** Thresholds based on pretest probabilities; **(B)** thresholds based on posttest probabilities. (Adapted from Straus SE, Richardson WS, Glasziou P, et al. *Evidence-Based Medicine: How to Practice and Teach EBM* (3rd ed.). Edinburgh, Churchill Livingstone, 2005, Figure 3.3, p. 85.)

may exhibit symptoms that lead a clinician to suspect the presence of a deep venous thrombosis (DVT), which is potentially life threatening. Even if the symptoms are minimal and the pretest probability is low, the clinician may feel compelled to test for the condition to safely rule it out before continuing with other interventions. At the same time, the clinician must also be able to justify that the benefits of performing the test outweigh any potential risks. A test that includes potentially harmful procedures may not be worthwhile if the condition has little consequence. Effective treatment should also be available, should the test be positive. The effort of a test is not reasonable if the results have no chance of leading to successful intervention.

Posttest Probabilities

A diagnostic test allows a clinician to revise the pretest probability estimate of the disorder.[18] Once we have the data from a test, we expect to be more confident in the diagnosis; that is, we hope to improve our certainty. The revised likelihood of the diagnosis based on the outcome of a test is the **posttest probability** (or posterior probability)—what we think the problem is (or is not) now that we know the test result. A good test will allow us to have a very high posttest probability confirming the diagnosis, or a very low posttest probability causing us to abandon it (see Figure 27.1B). When the posttest probability is not definitive, further testing may be necessary.

Likelihood Ratios

Once we have established a hypothesis that the patient may have a particular diagnosis, we want to determine if a test can make us more confident in that diagnosis. A measure called the **likelihood ratio** helps us in this effort. The likelihood ratio tells us how much more likely it is that a person has the diagnosis after the test is done; that is, it will help us determine the posttest probability. It indicates the value of the test for increasing certainty about a diagnosis,[19] or its "confirming power."[20] Likelihood ratios are being reported more often in the medical literature as an important standard for evidence-based practice. The likelihood ratio has an advantage over sensitivity, specificity and predictive values because it is independent of disease prevalence, and therefore can be applied across settings and patients.

We can determine a likelihood ratio for a positive or negative test. To understand this statistic, let's assume that a patient tests positive on the FRT. If this were a perfect test, then we would be certain that the patient is at risk for falls (true positive). But we hesitate to draw this conclusion definitively because we know that some patients who are not at risk will also test positive (false positive). Therefore, to determine if this test improves our diagnostic conclusion we must correct the true positive rate by the false positive rate. This is our **positive likelihood ratio (LR +):**

$$\text{LR+} = \frac{\text{true positive rate}}{\text{false positive rate}} = \frac{\text{sensitivity}}{1 - \text{specificity}} \tag{27.5}$$

The LR+ will tell us how many times more likely a positive test will be seen in those with the disorder than in those without the disorder. A good test will have a high positive likelihood ratio.

Now let's assume the patient has a negative test. With a perfect test we would be sure this patient was not at risk for falls. But we are still concerned about the possibility of a false negative. Therefore, to determine if a negative test improves our diagnostic conclusion, we look at the ratio of the false negative rate to the true negative rate. This is our **negative likelihood ratio (LR−)**:

$$LR- = \frac{\text{false negative rate}}{\text{true negative rate}} = \frac{1 - \text{sensitivity}}{\text{specificity}} \tag{27.6}$$

The LR− will tell us how many times more likely a negative test will be seen in those with the disorder than in those without the disorder. A good test will have a very low negative likelihood ratio.

It is important to note that likelihood ratios always refer to the likelihood of the disorder being present.[21] That's why we would like to see a high LR+, to indicate that the disorder is likely to be present with a positive test. A very low LR− means that the disorder has a small probability of being present with a negative test.

Interpreting Likelihood Ratios

The value of the likelihood ratio is somewhat intuitive, in that a larger LR+ indicates a greater likelihood of the disease, and a smaller LR− indicates a smaller likelihood of the disease. These values have been interpreted according to the following scale:[18]

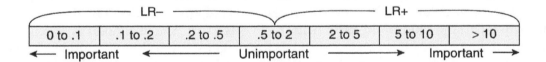

A LR+ over 5 and a LR− lower than 0.2 represent relatively important effects. Likelihood ratios between 0.2 to 0.5 and between 2 to 5 may be important, depending on the nature of the diagnosis being studied. Values close to 1.0 represent unimportant effects. A likelihood ratio of 1.0 essentially means the test is useless; that is, the true positive and false positive (or true negative and false negative) rates are the same.

Example

Let's apply this measure to the functional reach data. As shown in Table 27.2B, the LR+ = 3.75. Therefore, with a positive test, the likelihood of a patient being at risk for falls is increased by almost 4 times. This represents a potentially important value. The LR− = 0.76. This represents a small and unimportant value, close to 1.0. Therefore, based on these data, the FRT may help to improve our confidence with a positive test, but does not add important information with a negative test. Going back to the concepts of SpPin and SnNout, a large LR+ tells us that a positive test is good at ruling the disorder IN. A very low LR− tells us that the negative test is good at ruling the disorder OUT. We can confirm this by looking at the posttest probabilities.

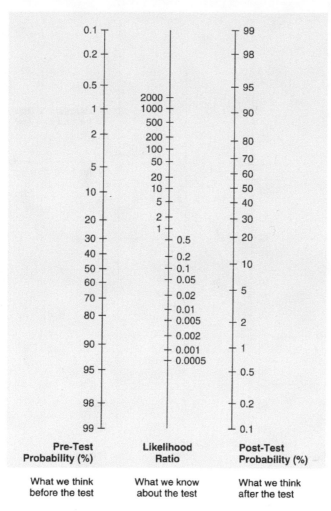

FIGURE 27.2 Nomogram to determine posttest probabilities using likelihood ratios.

Using a Nomogram to Determine Posttest Probabilities

A nomogram, shown in Figure 27.2, has been developed to determine posttest probabilities based on pretest probabilities and likelihood ratios.[22] To use the nomogram, we begin on the left by marking the pretest probability. The center line identifies the likelihood ratio. If we draw a line connecting these two points and extend it to the right margin, we find the posttest probability associated with the test.

For our example, Figure 27.3 shows a mark for 70% pretest probability based on prevalence data. Therefore, if we obtain a positive test (LR+ = 3.75), our posttest probability would approach 90%. With a positive test we have improved our confidence in this patient being at risk for falls by almost 20%. If we obtained a negative test (LR− = 0.76), our posttest probability would be approximately 60%. The patient still has a 60% chance of being at risk for falls—we have not improved our diagnostic certainty very much. Therefore, with a negative test other assessments may be necessary to accurately identify if the patient is truly not at risk.

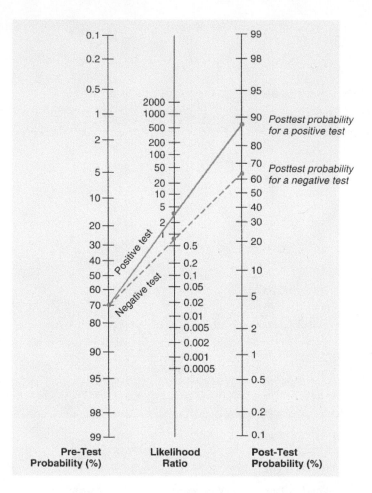

FIGURE 27.3 Use of nomogram to show posttest probability based on 70% pretest probability with LR+ = 3.75 and LR− = 0.76.

It is important to realize that the posttest probability will be dependent on the sensitivity and specificity of the diagnostic test (translated to a likelihood ratio) as well as the clinician's estimate of the pretest probability for an individual patient. For example, with a positive FRT, if we start with a pretest probability of 20%, we would get a posttest probability of 50% for a positive test. With a pretest probability of 5%, this test would increase our posttest certainty to only 15%. Where we start will influence the degree to which our certainty can be improved by the test.

Calculating Posttest Probabilities

When the nomogram is not handy, posttest probabilities can be obtained by converting the pretest probability to an odds value as follows:

1. Convert the pretest probability (prevalence) to pretest odds:

$$\text{Pretest odds} = \frac{\text{pretest probability}}{1 - \text{pretest probability}} = \frac{.70}{1 - .70} = 2.3 \tag{27.7}$$

2. Multiply the pretest odds by the likelihood ratio to get the posttest odds:

$$\text{Posttest odds} = \text{pretest odds} * \text{LR} = 2.3 * 3.75 = 8.625 \qquad (27.8)$$

3. Convert the posttest odds to the posttest probability:

$$\text{Posttest probability} = \frac{\text{posttest odds}}{\text{posttest odds} + 1} = \frac{8.625}{8.625 + 1} = .896 \text{ or } 89.6\% \quad (27.9)$$

Once again, we show that with a 70% pretest probability and a LR+ of 3.75, our posttest probability has risen to 90%. This form of calculation will usually be more precise than using the nomogram. Several Internet programs are also available for calculation of posttest probabilities.[23,24]

When Several Tests Are Needed

Applying likelihood ratios to clinical practice will necessitate a strong understanding of diagnostic principles. The threshold for making a decision about a diagnosis may not be reached until several tests have been completed. When tests are performed serially, the posttest probability for one test can be used to estimate the pretest probability for the subsequent test. This is appropriate only when the tests are independent of each other. Straus et al[7] recommend "chaining" likelihood ratios for this purpose. The posttest odds of the first test become the pretest odds for the second test. Therefore, by multiplying the new pretest odds by the likelihood ratio for the second test, we obtain the posttest odds for the second test. This can then be converted to posttest probability.

Confidence Intervals

Sensitivity, specificity and likelihood ratios can also be expressed in terms of confidence intervals (see Table 27.2C). Although these values are often not reported, they are important to understanding the true nature of these estimates.[25] Given a sample of scores, the confidence interval will indicate the range within which we can be sure the true population value will fall. Although not interpreted in terms of significance testing, confidence intervals for these measures of diagnostic accuracy will indicate the relative stability of the test's results; that is, with a wide confidence interval we would be less likely to consider the value a good estimate.[26] Calculators for confidence intervals are available on the Internet.[27,28]

Reporting Diagnostic Studies: The STARD Statement

In 2000, a consensus meeting of international researchers and journal editors resulted in a recommendation for quality reporting of diagnostic studies. This group developed the Standards for Reporting of Diagnostic Accuracy (STARD) statement, consisting of a checklist of 25 items that would allow authors to ensure they were including all relevant information in an article, including essential elements of the design and conduct of their study, the execution of tests, and their results.[29] The checklist will also allow readers to determine the potential for bias in a study, and to judge the generalizability of the results.

The STARD checklist is shown in Table 27.3. The statement has been published in several journals, and the reader is encouraged to refer to any one of these references for detailed descriptions of item criteria.[30-33] A flow diagram is also recommended to illustrate the number of participants at each stage of the study and to communicate the key elements of the design (see Figure 27.4).

TABLE 27.3 STARD CHECKLIST OF ITEMS TO IMPROVE THE REPORTING OF STUDIES ON DIAGNOSTIC ACCURACY

Section and topic	Item		on page #
TITLE/ABSTRACT/ KEYWORDS	1	Identify the article as a study on diagnostic accuracy (recommend MeSH heading 'sensitivity and specificity').	
INTRODUCTION	2	State the research questions or study aims, such as estimating diagnostic accuracy or comparing accuracy between tests or across participant groups.	
METHODS *Participants*	3	Describe the study population: the inclusion and exclusion criteria, setting and location(s) where the data were collected.	
	4	Describe participant recruitment: was recruitment based on presenting symptoms, results from previous tests, or the fact that the participants had received the index test(s) or the reference standard?	
	5	Describe participant sampling: was the study population a consecutive series of participants defined by the selection criteria in items (3) and (4)? If not specify how patients were further selected.	
	6	Describe data collection: was data collection planned before the index test and reference standards were performed (prospective study) or after (retrospective study)?	
Test methods	7	Describe the reference standard and its rationale.	
	8	Describe technical specifications of material and methods involved including how and when measurements were taken, and/or cite references for index tests and reference standard.	
	9	Describe definition of and rationale for the units, cutoffs and/or categories of the results of the index test(s) and the reference standard.	
	10	Describe the number, training and expertise of the persons executing and reading the index tests and the reference standard.	
	11	Describe whether or not the readers of the index tests and reference standard were blind (masked) to the results of the other test and describe any other clinical information available to the readers.	

TABLE 27.3 STARD CHECKLIST OF ITEMS TO IMPROVE THE REPORTING OF STUDIES ON DIAGNOSTIC ACCURACY (continued)

Section and topic	Item		on page #
Statistical methods	12	Describe methods for calculating or comparing measures of diagnostic accuracy, and the statistical methods used to quantify uncertainty (e.g. 95% confidence intervals).	
	13	Describe methods for calculating test reproducibility, if done.	
RESULTS			
Participants	14	Report when study was done, including beginning and ending dates of recruitment.	
	15	Report clinical and demographic characteristics of the study population (e.g. age, sex, spectrum of presenting symptoms, comorbidity, current treatments, recruitment centers).	
	16	Report the number of participants satisfying the criteria for inclusion that did or did not undergo the index tests and/or the reference standard; describe why participants failed to receive either test (a flow diagram is strongly recommended).	
Test results	17	Report time interval from the index tests to the reference standard and any treatment administered between.	
	18	Report distribution of severity of disease (define criteria) in those with the target condition; describe other diagnoses in participants without the target condition.	
	19	Report a cross tabulation of the results of the index tests (including indeterminate and missing results) by the results of the reference standard; for continuous results, the distribution of the test results by the results of the reference standard.	
	20	Report adverse events from performing the index tests or the reference standard.	
Estimates	21	Report estimates of diagnostic accuracy and measures of statistical uncertainty (e.g. 95% confidence intervals).	
	22	Report how indeterminate results, missing responses and outliers of the index tests were handled.	
	23	Report estimates of variability of diagnostic accuracy between subgroups of participants, readers or centers, if done.	
	24	Report measures of test reproducibility, if done.	
DISCUSSION	25	Discuss the clinical applicability of the study findings.	

Available at: <http://www.stard-statement.org/website%20stard/> Accessed April 12, 2007.

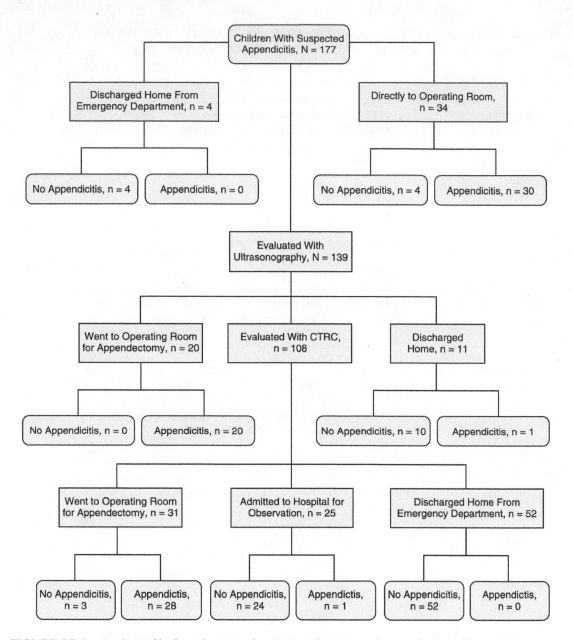

FIGURE 27.4   Study profile flow diagram of patients with suspected appendicitis evaluated in an emergency department during a 6-month study period. At each point, the accuracy of a positive or negative test is documented. (From Garcia Pena, BM et al. Ultrasonography and limited computed tomography in the diagnosis and management of appendicitis in children. *JAMA* 1999;282:1041-1046, Figure 2, p. 1044. Used with permission of the American Medical Association.)

RECEIVER OPERATING CHARACTERISTIC (ROC) CURVES

Cutoff Scores

Although continuous scales are considered preferable for screening because they are more precise, they are often converted to a dichotomous outcome for diagnostic purposes; that is, a **cutoff score** is established to demarcate a positive or negative test. For example, a specific level of blood pressure (a continuous scale) is used to determine if a patient should or should not be placed on a therapeutic regimen for hypertension. In the previous example of functional reach, a test score of less than 10 in. was considered indicative of fall risk. However, if a cutoff score of 12 in. was used, the sensitivity and specificity would be different. The problem, then, is to determine what cutoff score should be used. This decision point must be based on the relative importance of sensitivity and specificity, or the cost of incorrect outcomes versus the benefits of correct outcomes. Consider this analogy: Although there may be costs associated with unnecessary preparations in predicting a storm that does not occur (false positive), these costs would probably be considered minor relative to the danger of failing to predict a storm that does occur (false negative).

Suppose we use the Functional Reach Test to predict if an elderly individual is at risk for falling, and the individual with a low score is referred to a balance exercise program. If the individual is not truly at risk (false positive), the outcome may be considered low cost, compared to the situation where an individual who is at risk is not correctly diagnosed (false negative), not referred for treatment, and injures herself in a fall. Therefore, it might be reasonable to set the cutoff score low, to avoid false negatives, thereby increasing sensitivity. Conversely, consider a scenario where a test is used to determine the presence of a condition that requires potentially life-threatening surgery. A physician would want to avoid the procedure for a patient who does not truly have the condition. For this situation, the threshold might be set high to avoid false positives, increasing specificity. We would not want to perform this procedure unless we knew for certain that it was warranted.

Obviously, it is usually desirable for a screening test to be both sensitive and specific. Unfortunately, there is often a compromise between these two characteristics. One way to evaluate this decision point would be to look at several cutoff points, to determine the sensitivity and specificity at each point. We could then consider the relative trade-off to determine the most appropriate cutoff score. Those who use a screening tool must decide what levels of sensitivity and specificity are acceptable, based on the consequences of false negatives versus false positives. It is often necessary to combine the results of several screening tests to minimize the trade-off between specificity and sensitivity. We will discuss this approach shortly in relation to clinical prediction rules.

The ROC Curve

The balance between sensitivity and specificity can be examined using a graphic representation called a **receiver operating characteristic (ROC) curve**. This procedure actually evolved from radar and sonar detection strategies developed during World War II to improve signal-to-noise ratios. Suppose we were listening to a radio station that has a weak signal. We turn the volume up so we can hear better, but as we do so, we not only pick up the desired signal, but background noise as well. At lower volume settings, we will hear the signal more than the noise. But there will come a point, as we increase volume, that the noise will grow faster than the signal; that is, the signal has reached its full capacity, but the noise continues to increase. If we set the volume to its maximum, we may claim that the signal is strong, but the noise will be so great that the signal will be indecipherable. Therefore, the optimal setting will be where we detect the largest ratio of signal to noise.

This is essentially what we are trying to do with a diagnostic test. We want to detect the "signal" (the presence or absence of the disease—the true positive and true negative) with the least amount of interference possible (incorrect diagnoses—false positive and false negative). The ROC curve diagrams this relationship. It allows us to answer the question: How well can a test discriminate between signal and noise—can it discriminate between the presence or absence of disease?[34]

Constructing the ROC Curve

The process of constructing an ROC curve involves setting several cutoff points for a test and calculating sensitivity and specificity at each one. The curve is then created by plotting a point for each cutoff score that represents the proportion of patients correctly identified as having the condition (true positives) on the Y axis against the proportion of patients incorrectly identified as having the condition (false positives) on the X axis. The Y axis represents sensitivity, and the X axis represents one minus specificity ($1 -$ specificity).[†]

To illustrate this process, consider again the example of Functional Reach in patients with Parkinson's disease. We have created a hypothetical dataset for the sample of 43 patients who, based on their 6-month history of falls, have been identified as "at risk" (they have fallen at least once, $n = 30$) or "not at risk" (they have not fallen, $n = 13$). Table 27.4A shows the distribution of scores for the patients in each risk group, converting the continuous scores to 1-inch increments.

Table 27.4B shows the distribution of scores at 5 cutoff points. It is generally recommended that at least 5 to 6 points should be used to plot an ROC curve. We calculate the sensitivity and specificity of the test at each cutoff point. For this example, higher scores indicate better balance, and therefore, less likelihood to fall. Lower scores will result in a diagnosis of "at risk" for falls. Table 27.4B shows the number of true positive and false positive scores at each cutoff point, and the corresponding values for sensitivity and $1 -$ specificity. For example, if we use a cutoff score of 10 in., then all those with a score of 10 inches or less will be diagnosed "at risk." Those who obtained a score greater than 10 inches will be considered "not at risk." With this cutoff score, 9 individuals have been correctly identified "at risk," and 1 has been incorrectly diagnosed. This leads to a corresponding sensitivity of .30 and specificity of .92, which results in $1 -$ specificity of .08. Similarly, with a cutoff score of 12 inches, all those who obtained a score of 12 inches or less will be considered "at risk." Those with scores above 12 inches will be diagnosed "not at risk." When this cutoff score is used, 25 individuals are correctly diagnosed and 7 are incorrectly diagnosed. This leads to a corresponding sensitivity of .83 and $1 -$ specificity of .54. These values are then plotted to create the ROC curve (see Figure 27.5).

[†]If we take all those who are diagnosed negative [$(b + d)$ in Table 27.4] out of this total (100%), those who tested negative (true negatives) equal $1.00-d$ (specificity). Therefore, the remainder, or those who tested positive (false positives), would be 1.00–specificity.

TABLE 27.4   HYPOTHETICAL DATA FOR THE FUNCTIONAL REACH TEST WITH DIFFERENT CUTOFF POINTS

A. DATA

| | Known Group | |
Reach Score (Inches)	At Risk (+ Fall Hx) *n* = 30	Not at Risk (− Fall Hx) *n* = 13
>13	2	0
12.1 − 13	3	6
11.1 − 12	7	4
10.1 − 11	9	2
9.1 − 10	1	1
≤9	8	0

B. TRUE POSITIVE AND FALSE POSITIVE RATES

Cutoff Point (Positive test if ≤)	True Positives	False Positives	Sensitivity	Specificity	1 − Specificity
14	30	13	1.00	0.00	1.00
13	28	11	0.93	.15	0.85
12	25	7	0.83	.46	0.54
11	21	3	**0.70**	.77	**0.23**
10	9	1	0.30	.92	0.08
9	8	0	0.27	1.00	0.00
8	0	0	0.00	1.00	0.00

C. OUTPUT: ROC CURVE

Area Under the Curve

| Area | Std. Error | Sig. | 95% Confidence Interval | |
			Lower Bound	Upper Bound
.763	.077	.007	.613	.913

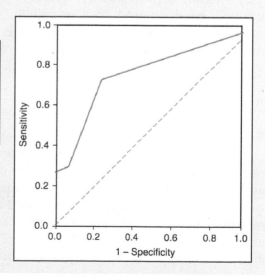

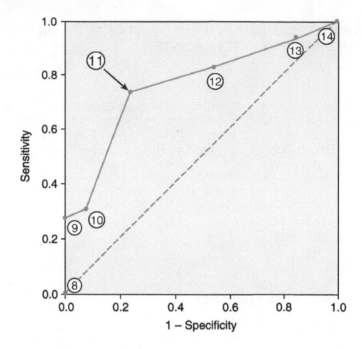

FIGURE 27.5   Receiver operating characteristics (ROC) curve for Functional Reach scores at different cutoff points (indicated by circled numbers). A cutoff score of 11, at the turn of the curve, appears to provide the best balance between true positives and false positives.

The curve is completed at the origin and the upper right hand corners, reflecting cutoff points above and below the highest and lowest scores. For example, with a cutoff score at 14, *all subjects* will be diagnosed "at risk." Therefore, all those truly "at risk" are correctly diagnosed (true positive rate is 100%), and all those "not at risk" are incorrectly diagnosed (false positive rate is 100%). Similarly, with a cutoff score of 8, *all subjects* will be diagnosed "not at risk." Therefore, all those truly "at risk" will be incorrectly diagnosed (true positive rate is zero), and all those "not at risk" will be correctly diagnosed (false positive rate is zero).

Interpreting the ROC Curve

The ROC curve is plotted on a square with values of 1.0 for sensitivity and 1 − specificity at the upper left and lower right corners, respectively. A perfect test instrument will have a true positive rate of 1.0 and a false positive rate of zero, resulting in a curve that essentially fills the square; that is, it will go from the origin to the upper left corner to the upper right hand corner. A noninformative curve occurs when the true positive and false positive rates are equal, which means that the test provides no better information than 50 : 50 chance. This curve starts at the origin and moves diagonally to the upper right hand corner (shown as the broken line in Figure 27.5).

Area under the Curve

If we wanted to compare two tests to determine which was a better diagnostic tool, we could compare ROC curves to see which curve more closely approximates the perfect curve. This provides only a visual basis of comparison, however, and a quantitative standard is more definitive. The best index for this purpose is a measure of the **area under the curve (AUC).** This value equals the probability of correctly choosing between normal and abnormal signals. This means that, given a test with an ROC curve area of .76, as in our current example, and presented with a randomly chosen pair of patients, one with the disorder and one without, the clinician would choose the correct diagnosis 76% of the time. Therefore, the area represents the ability of the test to discriminate between those at risk and those not at risk. A perfect test has an area of 1.00; using such a test would allow one to always identify the patient with disease.

Table 27.4C shows output for the area under the curve as well as a test of significance and confidence intervals. We are 95% confident that the true area under the curve will fall between 61% and 91%.

Choosing a Cutoff Point

In addition to making comparisons or describing the relative effectiveness of a test for identifying a disorder, we can also use the ROC curve to decide which cutoff point would be most useful. Most ROC curves have a steep initial section, which reflects a large increase in sensitivity with little change in the false positive rate. A relatively flat region across the top is also typical. Neither of these sections of the curve make sense for choosing a cutoff point, as they represent little change in one component of the curve. Usually, the best cutoff point will be at the point where the curve turns.[34] In Figure 27.5, a marked turn occurs at the cutoff point of 11 in., suggesting that this cutoff would provide the best balance between sensitivity and specificity for this test. At that point we would miss diagnosing risk for 9 out of the 30 individuals who have fallen, and we would incorrectly target 3 out of the 13 nonfallers. The final choice of a cutoff, however, must be based on how the clinician and patient see the impact of an incorrect identification. The ROC curve should only act as a guide for that decision.

CLINICAL PREDICTION RULES

In the previous sections we have described how sensitivity, specificity and related concepts can be used to support a diagnostic or prognostic classification based on a particular test score. In clinical practice, however, the complexity of patient conditions may require that a combination of predictors be used to support an outcome classification. Although clinical experience will often provide an intuitive sense of which findings from the history and physical examination are important for an accurate assessment, our focus on evidence-based practice demands that we strive for greater certainty in our diagnostic and prognostic assessments.[35]

Clinical prediction rules (CPR)[‡] are tools that quantify the contributions of different variables to the diagnosis, prognosis or likely response to treatment for an individual patient.[36] The objective of CPRs is to reduce uncertainty by demonstrating how specific clusters of clinical findings can be used to predict outcomes.[37]

Diagnosis

Perhaps the most obvious application of a CPR is to assist in the diagnosis of a disorder based on clinical signs. An excellent example of this application is found in the work of Stiell et al[38] who developed clinical prediction rules for the use of radiography with acute ankle injuries. They noted that many patients with ankle injuries did not have a fracture, and yet the typical response in emergency care was to order an X-ray. Estimates had shown, however, that the prevalence of fractures with ankle injuries was less than 15%. So this became an interest in efficiency and cost-savings as well as a desire for diagnostic accuracy. The prediction rules that were developed through this process have come to be known as the Ottawa Ankle Rules (based on Stiell's affiliation with Ottawa Civic Hospital), which include rules for both ankle and midfoot injuries. The indicators for ruling out a fracture are based on a lack of tenderness in specific areas of the foot or ankle, and the patient's ability to bear weight on the affected limb, even with a limp. Table 27.5 shows these guidelines, which have been validated in different countries[39] and in different populations.[40]

Systematic review of the Ottawa Ankle Rules has shown that they are 95 – 100% sensitive, with a negative likelihood ratio of 0.08.[41] If we apply this likelihood ratio to a pretest probability of 15% (based on prevalence estimates), we can see that there is less than 1.5% probability of actual fracture in those with a negative test (see Figure 27.6). Using the logic of SnNout, with a test that is highly sensitive, a negative test will effectively rule out the disorder. Therefore, a negative result using these guidelines will consistently and accurately rule out fractures after ankle or foot injury, making an X-ray unnecessary. Specificity tends to be closer to 50%, so a positive test does not necessarily mean a fracture is present, requiring an X-ray to rule out a fracture. Therefore, although there will still be some X-rays taken that do not show a fracture, the rules will effectively reduce the number of unnecessary radiographs taken.[42]

Other examples of diagnostic prediction rules include guidelines for detecting deep venous thrombosis,[43] pulmonary embolism,[44] dementia,[45] and to identify premenopausal women with low peak bone mass.[46] Guidelines have also been developed for ordering X-rays for knee injuries, called the Ottawa Knee Rules,[47,48] and cervical spine injuries, called the Canadian C-Spine Rule.[49]

Prognosis and Risk

Clinical predication rules can also be established to determine the degree to which individuals are at risk for certain outcomes. For example, Kanaya and colleagues[50] developed a CPR to identify older adults who were at risk for type 2 diabetes. They initially

---

[‡]You may also see these referred to as clinical decision rules or clinical decision guidelines.

TABLE 27.5   CRITERIA FOR THE OTTAWA ANKLE RULES

For a patient with an ankle or foot injury:

An ankle X-ray is required only if there is pain in the malleolar zone AND any one of the following:
- Bone tenderness along the distal 6 cm of the posterior edge of the fibula or tip of the lateral malleolus OR
- Bone tenderness along the distal 6 cm of the posterior edge of the tibia or tip of the medial malleolus OR
- Inability to bear weight for four steps at the time of injury and when examined.

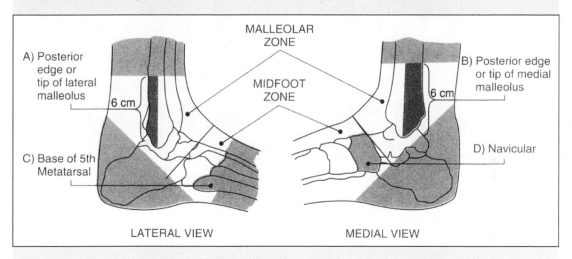

A Foot X-ray is required if there is pain in the midfoot AND

- Bone tenderness at the base of the 5th metatarsal OR at the navicular OR
- Inability to bear weight for four steps at the time of injury and when examined.

From Stiell I, Wells G, Laupacis A, Brison R, Verbeek R, Vandemheen K, Naylor D. A multicentre trial to introduce clinical decision rules for the use of radiography in acute ankle injuries. *BMJ* 1995; 311:594–597. (Figure from Google Images. <http://www.images.google.com> Accessed March 27, 2006. Reprinted with permission.)

derived the rule on a cross-sectional cohort, and then validated it using a prospective cohort of community-dwelling men and women. Of the nine variables that were initially entered into their analysis, only two demographic and two laboratory variables were significantly associated with incident diabetes. These were age ≥70 years, being female, having a fasting plasma glucose ≥95 mg/dl and triglycerides ≥150 mg/dl. They assigned points to these four risk factors and determined a total score for each participant, with scores ranging from 0 to 7 points. With a score of 4 or higher, the sensitivity of the rule was 46%, specificity 82% and LR+ = 1.9. Figure 27.7 shows the ROC curve for this analysis. Based on these results, the authors suggest that individuals who meet this threshold should receive appropriate lifestyle or pharmacologic therapies to prevent the onset of type 2 diabetes.

Other examples of prognostic clinical prediction rules include identifying risk for functional decline in older community-dwelling women,[51] identifying patients at risk

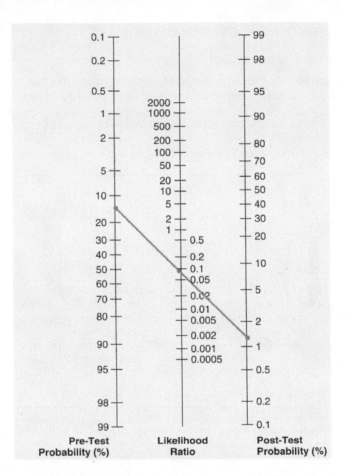

FIGURE 27.6 Nomogram showing determination of posttest probability with use of the Ottawa ankle rules. Based on 15% prevalence of ankle fractures with ankle injury, we estimate the pretest probability at 15%. With a negative likelihood ratio of .08, we obtain a posttest probability of less than 1.5%. This indicates that with a negative test, the probability of an ankle fracture is almost nil.

of complications following cardiac surgery,[52] identifying factors that lead to hospitalization with asthma,[53] and identifying workers with nonspecific back pain who are likely or not likely to return to work in good health.[54]

Response to Intervention

Clinical prediction rules have also been developed to determine the likelihood that a patient will respond positively to a specific intervention. For example, Hicks et al[55] designed a prospective cohort study to predict whether patients with nonradicular low back pain are likely to benefit from a program of stabilization exercises. They examined patients before and after an 8-week program, and assessed success based on change in the Oswestry Disability Questionnaire score. The best rule for predicting success was the presence of at least 3 of 4 variables: positive prone instability test, aberrant movements present, average straight leg raise greater than 91°, and age greater than 40 years

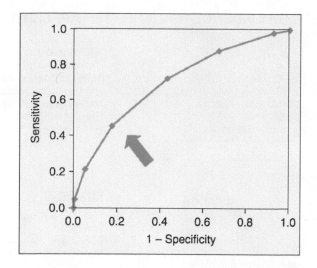

FIGURE 27.7   ROC curve for the validation of a clinical prediction rule for type 2 diabetes. The curve represents results using 0 to 7 points, based on presence of one to four risk factors. The curve turns at the point representing 4 points (arrow), with sensitivity of 46% and 1 – specificity of 17%. (Adapted from Kanaya AM, Fyr CLW, de Rekeneire N, et al. Predicting the development of diabetes in older adults. *Diabetes Care* 2005; 28:404–408. Based on data from Table 3, p. 406.)

old. This combination had a sensitivity of 56%, specificity of 86% and a LR+ of 4.0. A separate model was developed to predict failure of treatment.

Other examples of CPRs for intervention response include identifying patients who will benefit from cervical manipulation for neck pain,[56] from spinal manipulation for low back pain,[57] from the use of compression bandages for treatment of venous leg ulcers,[58] from patellar taping for anterior knee pain,[59] and those who are likely or not likely to benefit from nonarthroplasty knee surgery.[60]

Validating Clinical Prediction Rules

The development of a clinical prediction rule is a three-step process.[35] First, the factors that potentially contribute to prediction of the outcome are identified in a cohort of patients. This allows for the *derivation* of the rule, establishing which variables are most predictive. The study by Hicks et al[55] on the effectiveness of stabilization exercises is an example of this first step. Further study needs to be done to apply these results to other samples.

The second step requires *validation* of the rule in several cohorts in different settings. The study by Kanaya et al[50] looking at variables related to onset of diabetes illustrates this step. They validated the prediction rule in a sample of over 2,000 white and African-American men and women in two major cities over 5 years.

Finally, an **impact analysis** will demonstrate if the rule has changed clinician behavior and resulted in beneficial outcomes. The Ottawa Ankle Rules, for example, have been studied in many countries and settings,[61] and have been reported to significantly decrease the number of unnecessary ankle radiographs.[62] Even with the widespread acceptance of this CPR, however, researchers and clinicians continue to test its

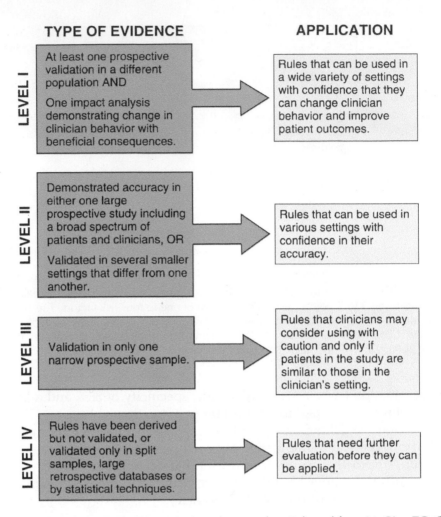

FIGURE 27.8   Levels of evidence for clinical prediction rules. (Adapted from McGinn TG, Guyatt GH, Wyer PC, et al. Users' guides to the medical literature: XXII: How to use articles about clinical decision rules. *JAMA* 2000; 284:79–84.)

validity, with various degrees of success.[63–65] An excellent review of this process is available.[66]

A hierarchy of evidence has been proposed to judge the applicability of a clinical decision rule, based on its having gone through the full process of validation (Figure 27.8).[35] Widespread use of a CPR is not recommended until it has been validated in at least one prospective study in a variety of settings and an impact analysis has demonstrated its clinical utility.

MEASURING CHANGE

So much of our clinical decision making rests on the intent to promote change or progress in a patient's or client's condition or behavior. We need to document change in a way that will be meaningful to the patient, the clinician and third-party payers. We use words like "better," "improved," "worse" or "declined" to indicate when someone's condition has changed, but these descriptors are clearly not sufficient to make reliable and valid judgments.

In Chapter 6 we introduced the concept of **responsiveness**, which is the ability of an instrument to measure true clinical change.[67] Generally, we can think of responsiveness as a ratio of signal (true change) to noise (variability or error). At this time we will consider various statistical approaches for measuring change, and the implications of these statistics for interpreting clinical data.

As we search for useful ways to evaluate change, the good news is that there is extensive literature on the concept. The bad news is that there is little agreement on the best way to express or measure change in statistical terms. We will present several alternative methods for evaluating responsiveness, but we are unable to address the full scope of this topic. The reader is urged to refer to the literature for informative debate and discussion.

A Continuum of Change

When we think about measuring a difference in response from one time to another, we can conceptualize the amount of change along a continuum, as shown in Figure 27.9. We start with the **minimum potentially detectable difference,** which will depend on the precision of the measurement tool being used. If we are using a goniometer, can we detect changes in range of motion (ROM) of less than one degree or a half degree? If we are using a survey tool, such as the Functional Independence Measure (FIM), we are restricted to differences of at least one point; that is, no fractions of a point can be counted.

Minimal Detectable Difference

Beyond the precision of the instrument, however, we are concerned with its reliability. When we address the issue of change, we must be confident that observed differences from before to after treatment reflect true change, and not simply random measurement error. The standard error of measurement (SEM), described in Chapter 26, is the most

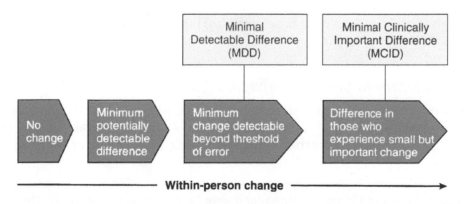

FIGURE 27.9 Reference for within-person change along a continuum.

common statistic used to determine the **minimal detectable difference (MDD)**.[§] This is the smallest amount of change that can be considered above the threshold of error expected in the measurement. Theoretically, this value can be interpreted as a property of a measurement, remaining constant across samples,[68] although it can vary depending on the reliability estimate used in its calculation. Stratford et al[69] have also shown that the SEM will vary when calculated across different ranges of initial and follow-up scores, with a smaller SEM resulting at both extremes of a scale.

The MDD is calculated using the following formula:[70]

$$MDD_{\%} = z * SEM * \sqrt{2} \qquad\qquad (27.10)$$

This estimate is most often based on the 90% ($z = 1.65$) or 95% ($z = 1.96$) confidence interval. MDD_{95} means that 95% of stable patients demonstrate a random variation of less than this amount when tested on multiple occasions.[71]

For example, Kennedy et al[72] studied patients with osteoarthritis to determine measurement stability in outcomes following total hip and knee arthroplasty. For the 6-minute walk test (6MWT), they calculated a SEM of 26.29 meters. They obtained MDD_{90}:

$$MDD_{90} = 1.65 * 26.29 * \sqrt{2} = 61.24 \text{ m}$$

This says we can expect 90% of stable patients (those who have not changed) in this population to demonstrate random variation of less than 61 meters in repeated trials of the 6MWT. Therefore, if we take measurements of the 6MWT before and after intervention, a change of 61 meters or greater would be considered true change.

Norman et al[73] have offered the interpretation that minimal differences are consistently close to 0.5 standard deviation for discriminating the threshold of change using quality of life instruments. They support their findings with psychophysiological evidence that people have a limit to their ability to discriminate tasks (such as saltiness of taste, loudness of sounds),[74] and that this limit is almost always close to 0.5 standard deviation. Therefore, they suggest that this criterion is potentially appropriate to identify the minimal detectable difference.

The MDD can be considered a conservative estimate of a patient's progress, identifying the smallest amount of change that could be interpreted as *any* improvement or decline. Therefore, using the MDD as a criterion for improvement may be thought of as having high specificity (avoiding false positives) but low sensitivity (finding many false negatives).[75]

Minimal Clinically Important Difference (MCID)

The MDD may be considered a starting point to define change, but it is typically too small to represent a meaningful difference in the patient's response. Along the continuum of change, we are concerned with identifying how much of a change will be

---

[§]This measure is also called the minimal detectable change (MDC), the smallest detectable change (SDC) or smallest real change (SRC); it has also been called the reliable change index.

important. For example, if we measure ROM of knee flexion following knee arthro-plasty, is a 5° change important? Does it indicate a meaningful difference in the patient's condition? While this may be an obvious example, consider a change of 5 mm in a visual analog scale for pain. Or a change of 5 points on the SF-36 measure of quality of life. Or a change of 5 mm in the measurement of a leg length discrepancy. Do these represent meaningful change? Would our threshold for important change vary across different groups of patients, conditions, levels of severity or cultural groups?[76]

The most common threshold for meaningful change has been called the **minimal clinically important difference (MCID)** (see Figure 27.9).** This has been defined as the smallest change in an outcome measure that is perceived as beneficial by the patient, and that would lead to a change in the patient's medical management, assuming an absence of excessive side effects and costs.[77] The criterion for just how much change is considered important is the crux of the dilemma in this process.

So how is the definition of "meaningful change" to be decided? This definition inherently reflects an element of judgment, and several perspectives must be considered.[76] For the patient, it may mean change that results in noticeable improvement in function or a reduction in symptoms. We may find, however, that patients place different values on degrees of improvement. To what extent does quality of life impact this perception? What amount of change in a score will correspond to trivial, small but important, moderate or large improvement or deterioration?[78] From the perspective of the clinician, it may mean enough change to warrant a revision in treatment or the patient's prognosis. At the institutional level, change may be viewed as important when it is sufficient to influence health care policy.[79]

Two approaches have been used to define important change. Distribution-based methods are related to a distribution of scores, with a focus on the differences in group means as well as the variance within the distribution. Anchor-based methods use an external criterion to define clinical importance.

Distribution-Based Approach

Researchers are often interested in assessing the degree of change in a group of patients, to determine the effectiveness of an intervention and to generalize results to others. For this purpose, meaningful change is determined using a **distribution-based** approach. Several indices have been used for this purpose (see Table 27.6).

Measures of Statistical Significance

One approach to evaluating an instrument's responsiveness has been to analyze change scores using a pretest-posttest design. Repeated measures *t*-tests or analyses of variance (ANOVA) are used to establish significant differences from time 1 to time 2.[84] Measurements may be taken once before and after intervention, or there may be multiple measures as individuals are followed over time.[85] This approach may involve only one group of subjects, or it may incorporate two or more groups. The assumption is made that change will occur due to treatment. Therefore, the instrument should be able to

---

**This measure is also called the minimal clinically important change (MCIC) and the minimally important change (MIC).

TABLE 27.6 DISTRIBUTION-BASED METHODS TO DETERMINE IMPORTANT DIFFERENCE

Statistic	Formula	Application and Considerations
Effect size[80,81]	$$ES = \dfrac{\overline{X}_{post} - \overline{X}_{pre}}{s_{pre}}$$	• Provides information on magnitude of change in standardized units relative to baseline standard deviation. • Difference between pretest and posttest means, divided by standard deviation of pretest scores. • Not affected by sample size, but may vary among samples with different baseline variability.
Standardized response mean[82]	$$SRM = \dfrac{\overline{X}_{post} - \overline{X}_{pre}}{s_{change}}$$	• Provides information on magnitude of change in standardized units relative to variability of change. • Will vary as a function of effectiveness of treatment.[76]
Guyatt's responsiveness index [67,83]	$$GRI = \dfrac{MCID}{\sqrt{2*MS_E}}$$	• Provides a measure of change relative to variability in scores among patients who are clinically stable. • The denominator includes the mean square error from an ANOVA, which may be obtained for test-retest reliability scores, or repeated observations in clinically stable patients.
Standard error of measurement [68]	$$SEM = s_x\sqrt{1 - r_{xx}}$$	• Assumes measurement error is relatively constant across the range of possible scores. • Based on standard deviation of change scores and test-retest reliability coefficient. • Considered by some to represent minimal detectable difference.[96]

demonstrate such change from before to after treatment, or between groups that were treated and those that were not. A statistically significant difference, then, would demonstrate that the instrument was responsive to change. A confidence interval can provide an estimate of the range of change that can be expected.

The interpretation of meaningful change can be quite different, however, if one is focused on what that change means to an individual, versus decisions based on group differences.[86] We must distinguish between the clinical significance of a particular change score for an individual patient and the statistical significance of a mean change of the same magnitude for a group of patients.[87] Guyatt et al[88] offer the example of a mean change in blood pressure of 2 mm Hg in a clinical trial, which may translate into a reduction in the number of strokes in a population. But this amount of change in an individual would probably be considered trivial, within the range of error of measurement.

Effect Size

Looking at **effect size** is generally considered more appropriate to determine if meaningful change has occurred, because it does take group variability into account. Effect size is a standardized measure of change from baseline to final measurement. Three forms of effect size have been used.

Effect Size Index (ES). The **effect size index** is a ratio of the mean change score divided by the standard deviation of the baseline scores (see Table 27.6). Therefore, a measure that has high variability in initial scores will have a smaller effect size. Cohen[81] has suggested that an effect size of .20 or less represents a small change; .50 represents moderate change; and .80 represents a large change. These values are interpreted relative to baseline variability. For instance, a moderate effect size reflects a change of at least one-half the baseline standard deviation.

Standardized Response Mean (SRM). The **standardized response mean** is another form of effect size index,[82] sometimes referred to as the efficiency index.[89] The SRM is a ratio of change from pretest to posttest divided by the standard deviation of the change scores (see Table 27.6). Therefore, a distribution that has high variability in the degree of change will have a small SRM. Cohen's criteria for small, moderate and large effect sizes are used for this index as well.

Guyatt's Responsiveness Index (GRI). A third form of effect size was proposed by Guyatt et al,[90] called the **responsiveness index.** The GRI uses an anchor-based MCID for a particular measure, or the smallest difference between baseline and posttest that would represent a meaningful benefit in a group of patients. We will discuss various methods to determine an anchor-based MCID shortly. When the MCID is not known, the difference between baseline and posttest can be used.[67] The denominator for this index is obtained from an ANOVA of repeated observations in a group of subjects who are clinically stable, which is a measure of test-retest reliability (see Table 27.6). Therefore, the denominator reflects the intrinsic variability of the instrument.[67] A disadvantage of this index is that data on stable subjects may not always be available. Once again, the values of .20, .50 and .80 are used to represent small, moderate and large effects.[91]

To illustrate the application of these measures, Quintana et al[71] studied the responsiveness of the Western Ontario and McMaster Universities Osteoarthritis Index (WOMAC) in a group of patients following total hip replacement. They calculated ES, SRM and GRI at 6 months and 2 years, as shown in Table 27.7. Of interest are the consistently higher values derived from the ES index and lower values derived from the GRI. Recall that the denominators for each of these measures will result in a

TABLE 27.7   EFFECT SIZE MEASURES OF RESPONSIVENESS FOR THE WOMAC IN PATIENTS FOLLOWING TOTAL HIP REPLACEMENT

Subscale	At 6 months			At 2 years		
	ES	SRM	GRI	ES	SRM	GRI
Pain	2.10	1.86	1.10	2.24	1.98	2.18
Function	2.34	1.80	1.45	2.58	1.97	1.79
Stiffness	1.61	1.39	0.81	1.81	1.53	1.12

Data from Quintana JM, Escobar A, Bilbao A, et al. Responsiveness and clinically important differences for the WOMAC and SF-36 after hip joint replacement. *Osteoarthritis Cartilage* 2005; 13:1076–1083, from Table III, p. 1080.

different estimate. All values are considered quite large, however, indicating that the WOMAC is a responsive instrument that is capable of reflecting important change over time.

Receiver Operating Characteristic Curves

Another way to look at responsiveness is to consider it a way of discriminating between those who have changed and those who have not. Therefore, we can look at change as a "diagnosis," or the determination of whether a clinically important change has occurred against an external standard.[92] In this context, responsiveness is described in terms of sensitivity and specificity. Sensitivity reflects the probability that someone who has truly changed will be identified has having changed. Specificity is the probability that someone who has not changed will be correctly identified. These values are then used to plot an ROC curve, as described earlier in this chapter.

For example, Stratford et al[85] looked at four questionnaires for assessing pain and function in patients with low back pain. They set different cutoff scores to represent change for each test and constructed four ROC curves. They then compared the area under the curves to determine which would be preferred for detecting change over time in this population (see Figure 27.10).

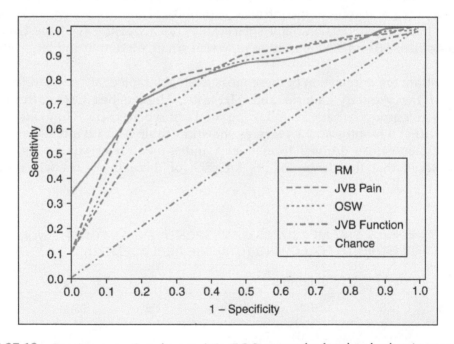

FIGURE 27.10 Receiver operating characteristic (ROC) curves for four low back pain questionnaires: Roland-Morris (RM), Jan van Breeman (JVB) pain scale and function scale, and the Oswestry (OSW). Areas under the curve were as follows: RM = 0.79; JVB pain = 0.79; JVB function = 0.66; and OSW = 0.78. A significant difference was found between the area for the JVB function questionnaire and the other three questionnaires. (From Stratford PW, Binkley J, Solomon P, et al. Assessing change over time in patients with low back pain. *Phys Ther* 1994;74:528–533, Figure p. 531. Reprinted with permission of the American Physical Therapy Association.)

Anchor-Based Approaches

In an **anchor-based** approach the magnitude of a change score is interpreted according to some clinical criterion or "anchor" that is assumed to have inherent meaning. A common anchor is the patient's ordinal rating of improvement or decline—"I feel a little better," "a lot better," "a little worse," or "a lot worse." A clinician may apply an anchor that relates to a minimal change in function or passing a threshold of impairment that points to a change in treatment or goals. The disadvantage of anchor-based methods is that they do not take into account the variability or potential measurement error in an instrument. Therefore, it is important to establish the reliability of an instrument when using it to estimate important change. Recall bias may also affect a patient's accurate estimate of improvement or decline.

Global Rating of Change

The construct of important difference has most often been evaluated using an ordinal scale, based on the patient's or clinician's subjective rating of change. Scales generally range from "a great deal worse" to "a great deal better," with as few as 5 points[71] and as many as 15 points,[77,85,93] with zero indicating no change (see Table 27.8).

For example, Beninato et al[94] used this approach to assess clinical change in function following stroke for patients who were discharged from a rehabilitation hospital. They used physician ratings on a 15-point scale to determine the MCID for the Functional Independence Measure (FIM). Based on a cutoff score of 3 (somewhat better) to distinguish those who had achieved a MCID from those who did not, they identified a

TABLE 27.8   GLOBAL RATING SCALE TO ASSESS MAGNITUDE OF CHANGE[a]

Rating	Description of Change
7	A very great deal better
6	A great deal better
5	Quite a bit better
4	Moderately better
3	Somewhat better
2	A little bit better
1	Tiny bit better, almost the same
0	No change
−1	Tiny bit worse, almost the same
−2	A little bit worse
−3	Somewhat worse
−4	Moderately worse
−5	Quite a bit worse
−6	A great deal worse
−7	A very great deal worse

[a]Adapted from Stratford PW, et al. Assessing change over time in patients with low back pain. *Phys Ther* 1994; 74:528–533.

change of 22 points in the total FIM score as a meaningful difference in function from admission to discharge. Using a cutoff of 5 (a good deal better) the MCID was 27 points, which they defined as a "moderate important clinical change."

Wolfe et al[95] have suggested that while MCID is an important minimum, a "really important difference" represents a clinically important goal. They used several outcome measures with patients with rheumatoid arthritis to reflect change at this level based on satisfaction with health, independence and disability level.

When assessing change, anchor-based methods are generally preferred over distribution-based methods because they reflect a definition of what is considered important.[96] A combined strategy, however, using both approaches, may provide a stronger foundation for understanding meaningful change.[97-99]

MDD and MCID Proportion

Group values must be interpreted with reference to their sample size and variability. We know that statistical significance is greatly influenced by the number of subjects in a sample. Therefore, with a large sample, small differences may turn out to be significant even when they are meaningless. We also recognize that a mean is a measure of central tendency, and that individuals in the sample do not all experience that amount of change—some will have achieved more and some less. Therefore, any conclusions about an individual patient's response based on a mean may be seriously flawed.

Consider, for example, a randomized trial of 1,000 patients who receive physical therapy to increase knee ROM following knee arthroplasty. Assume results show a significant mean difference of 5° ROM for patients with knee arthroplasty. While statistically significant because of high power, this is probably an unimportant difference. On the other hand, consider the same situation with a smaller sample, in which a mean difference of 5° ROM is not significant. In this case, the researcher would probably conclude that therapy is not effective. This conclusion, however, ignores the possibility that treatment could have had a heterogeneous effect,[100] and some patients may have had much larger changes in ROM. Let's assume that a minimum of 15° is considered important. We would need to look at the data to determine how many subjects actually had this much of an increase or higher, to determine if the treatment really was effective (see discussion of *Number Needed to Treat* in Chapter 28). Therefore, without looking at variability within the sample, we may be missing important information.

When studying a dichotomous variable, decisions about improvement or decline are straightforward—the patient has either gotten better or not. When dealing with a continuous measure, however, it is necessary to determine how much change is meaningful. Therefore, the proportion of individuals in a group that achieve minimal change can be considered another important benchmark to evaluate an intervention's effectiveness. **MDD** or **MCID proportion** is the percentage of patients who exceed the minimal standard of change, based either on the detectable change or the clinically meaningful change. These values can be especially useful for examining group data for program evaluation and quality assurance.[97]

In their study of responsiveness for the WOMAC, described earlier, Quintana et al[71] determined that the MDD proportion was greater than 80% for pain and function subscales, and the MDIC proportion was between 70% and 80% after 2 years following hip joint replacement. These values demonstrate that most patients in this population do consider themselves "better." In another example, in a study of the effectiveness of a fitness intervention for children with disabilities, Fragala-Pinkham et al[101] found that 59% of those with developmental disabilities exceeded the MDD, as compared to only 29% of those with neuromuscular disabilities. They suggest that these data are more informative for evaluating the effects of treatment than overall mean changes.

COMMENTARY

How Much Is Better? Finding Meaning in the Numbers

Understanding the statistical bases for measurement validity is essential as we strive to make informed evidence-based decisions. Some validity estimates are readily recognized as appropriate methods for assessing validity, such as those used to measure diagnostic accuracy. Others, such as methods for evaluating change, are still evolving, and will develop further as time goes on. The variety of indices used to assess change can be daunting, but more importantly, there is often confusion in terminology. Many authors have used "minimal detectable difference" and "minimal clinically important difference" as synonymous terms, although they have been clearly defined and distinguished. These two important benchmarks should remain distinct if we are to truly understand our measurements.

Clinical judgments regarding validity of measurements must be based on some criterion that is relevant for a particular patient. Any given study will present data from a sample that has specific properties and that has been studied in a specific context over a given time period. Clinicians must appraise that information to determine if it is appropriately applied to their patients. Published values allow us to predict our own patients' responses and give us a foundation for decision making. It is essential, however, that we remain cognizant of the limits of statistics as we apply them to our own situations.

As our understanding of validity grows, we will continue to struggle with the definitions of clinical significance. The evidence-based practitioner will benefit from more complete reporting of likelihood ratios, effect sizes and minimal change values in clinical studies. Whenever possible, confidence intervals should be used to reflect population values. Estimates are needed for different settings, age groups, disease durations and baseline conditions. Clinicians, patients and health policy analysts all want to appreciate just how much better is "better."

REFERENCES

1. Chiu AY, Au-Yeung SS, Lo SK. A comparison of four functional tests in discriminating fallers from non-fallers in older people. *Disabil Rehabil* 2003;25:45–50.
2. Sharma PT, Sieber FE, Zakriya KJ, Pauldine RW, Gerold KB, Hang J, et al. Recovery room delirium predicts postoperative delirium after hip-fracture repair. *Anesth Analg* 2005;101:1215–1220.
3. Lurie JD, Sox HC. Principles of medical decision making. *Spine* 1999;24:493–498.

4. Behrman AL, Light KE, Flynn SM, Thigpen MT. Is the functional reach test useful for identifying falls risk among individuals with Parkinson's disease? *Arch Phys Med Rehabil* 2002;83:538–542.

5. Duncan PW, Weiner DK, Chandler J, Studenski S. Functional reach: A new clinical measure of balance. *J Gerontol* 1990;45:M192–197.

6. Ibrahim MA. *Epidemiology and Health Policy.* Rockville, MD: Aspen, 1985.

7. Straus SE, Richardson WS, Glasziou P, Haynes RB. *Evidence-Based Medicine: How to Practice and Teach EBM* (3rd ed.). Edinburgh: Churchill Livingstone, 2005.

8. Davidson M. The interpretation of diagnostic test: A primer for physiotherapists. *Aust J Physiother* 2002;48:227–232.

9. Runyon MS, Webb WB, Jones AE, Kline JA. Comparison of the unstructured clinician estimate of pretest probability for pulmonary embolism to the Canadian score and the Charlotte rule: A prospective observational study. *Acad Emerg Med* 2005;12: 587–593.

10. Elstein AS, Schwarz A. Clinical problem solving and diagnostic decision making: Selective review of the cognitive literature. *BMJ* 2002;324:729–732.

11. Cahan A, Gilon D, Manor O, Paltiel O. Clinical experience did not reduce the variance in physicians' estimates of pretest probability in a cross-sectional survey. *J Clin Epidemiol* 2005;58:1211–1216.

12. Phelps MA, Levitt MA. Pretest probability estimates: A pitfall to the clinical utility of evidence-based medicine? *Acad Emerg Med* 2004;11:692–694.

13. Richardson WS, Polashenski WA, Robbins BW. Could our pretest probabilities become evidence based? A prospective survey of hospital practice. *J Gen Intern Med* 2003;18: 203–208.

14. Reamy BV, Slakey JB. Adolescent idiopathic scoloisis: Review and current concepts. *Am Family Physician* 2001;64:111–116.

15. Crichlow RJ, Andres PL, Morrison SM, Haley SM, Vrahas MS. Depression in orthopaedic trauma patients: Prevalence and severity. *J Bone Joint Surg Am* 2006;88: 1927–1933.

16. Stingone JA, Claudio L. Asthma and enrollment in special education among urban schoolchildren. *Am J Public Health* 2006;96:1593–1598.

17. Appelros P, Viitanen M. What causes increased stroke mortality in patients with pre-stroke dementia? *Cerebrovasc Dis* 2005;19:323–327.

18. Geyman JP, Deyo RA, Ramsey SD. *Evidence-Based Clinical Practice: Concepts and Approaches.* Boston: Butterworth Heinemann, 2000.

19. Altman DG, Bland JM. Diagnostic tests 2: Predictive values. *BMJ* 1994;309:102.

20. Van den Ende J, Moreira J, Basinga P, Bisoffi Z. The trouble with likelihood ratios. *Lancet* 2005;366:548.

21. Attia J. Moving beyond sensitivity and specificity: Using likelihood ratios to help interpret diagnostic tests. *Aust Prescr* 2003;26(3):111–113.

22. Center for Evidence-Based Medicine. Likelihood ratios. Available at: <http://www.cebm.net/likelihood_ratios.asp> Accessed on December 28, 2005.

23. Simon S. Children's Mercy Hospital and Clinics. Likelihood ratio slide rule. Available at: <http://www.childrens-mercy.org/stats/sliderule.asp> Accessed on August 15, 2006.

24. Center for Evidence-Based Medicine. Nomogram. Available at: <http://www.cebm.net/nomogram.asp> Accessed August 15, 2006.

25. Harper R, Reeves B. Reporting of precision of estimates for diagnostic accuracy: A review. *BMJ* 1999;318:1322–1323.

26. Poole C. Low *p*-values or narrow confidence intervals: Which are more durable? *Epidemiology* 2001;12:291–294.

27. VassasrStats. Clinical Calculator 1. Available at <http://faculty.vassar.edu/lowry/clin1.html> Accessed September 28, 2006.

28. CEBM Stats Calculator. Available at: <http://www.cebm.utoronto.ca/practise/ca/statscal/> Accessed September 21, 2007.

29. The STARD statement and standards for reporting of diagnostic accuracy studies. Available at: <http://www.stard-statement.org/website%20stard/> Accessed April 14, 2007.

30. Bossuyt PM, Reitsma JB, Bruns DE, Gatsonis CA, Glasziou PP, Irwig LM, et al. Towards complete and accurate reporting of studies of diagnostic accuracy: The STARD initiative. *Clin Radiol* 2003;58(8):575–580.

31. Bossuyt PM, Reitsma JB, Bruns DE, Gatsonis CA, Glasziou PP, Irwig LM, et al. Toward complete and accurate reporting of studies of diagnostic accuracy. The STARD initiative. *Am J Clin Pathol* 2003;119(1):18–22.

32. Bossuyt PM, Reitsma JB, Bruns DE, Gatsonis CA, Glasziou PP, Irwig LM, et al. Towards complete and accurate reporting of studies of diagnostic accuracy: The STARD Initiative. *Ann Intern Med* 2003;138(1):40–44.

33. Bossuyt PM, Reitsma JB, Bruns DE, Gatsonis CA, Glasziou PP, Irwig LM, et al. Towards complete and accurate reporting of studies of diagnostic accuracy: The STARD initiative. *BMJ* 2003;326(7379):41–44.

34. Centor RM. Signal detectability: The use of ROC curves and their analyses. *Med Decis Making* 1991;11:102–106.

35. McGinn TG, Guyatt GH, Wyer PC, Naylor CD, Stiell IG, Richardson WS. Users' guides to the medical literature: XXII: How to use articles about clinical decision rules. Evidence-Based Medicine Working Group. *JAMA* 2000;284:79–84.

36. Laupacis A, Sekar N, Stiell IG. Clinical prediction rules. A review and suggested modifications of methodological standards. *JAMA* 1997;277:488–494.

37. Wasson JH, Sox HC, Neff RK, Goldman L. Clinical prediction rules. Applications and methodological standards. *N Engl J Med* 1985;313:793–799.

38. Stiell IG, McKnight RD, Greenberg GH, McDowell I, et al. Implementation of the Ottowa ankle rules. *JAMA* 1994;271:827–832.

39. Emparanza JI, Aginaga JR. Validation of the Ottawa Knee Rules. *Ann Emerg Med* 2001;38:364–368.

40. Bulloch B, Neto G, Plint A, Lim R, Lidman P, Reed M, et al. Validation of the Ottawa Knee Rule in children: A multicenter study. *Ann Emerg Med* 2003;42:48–55.

41. Bachmann LM, Kolb E, Koller MT, Steurer J, ter Riet G. Accuracy of Ottawa ankle rules to exclude fractures of the ankle and mid-foot: Systematic review. *BMJ* 2003;326:417–423.

42. Gwilym SE, Aslam N, Ribbans WJ, Holloway V. The impact of implementing the Ottawa ankle rules on ankle radiography requests in A&E. *Int J Clin Pract* 2003;57:625–627.

43. Goodacre S, Sutton AJ, Sampson FC. Meta-analysis: The value of clinical assessment in the diagnosis of deep venous thrombosis. *Ann Intern Med* 2005;143:129–139.

44. Righini M, Bounameaux H. External validation and comparison of recently described prediction rules for suspected pulmonary embolism. *Curr Opin Pulm Med* 2004;10:345–349.

45. Gifford DR, Holloway RG, Vickrey BG. Systematic review of clinical prediction rules for neuroimaging in the evaluation of dementia. *Arch Intern Med* 2000;160:2855–2862.

46. Hawker GA, Jamal SA, Ridout R, Chase C. A clinical prediction rule to identify premenopausal women with low bone mass. *Osteoporos Int* 2002;13:400–406.

47. Stiell IG, Greenberg GH, Wells GA, McDowell I, Cwinn AA, Smith NA, et al. Prospective validation of a decision rule for the use of radiography in acute knee injuries. *JAMA* 1996;275:611–615.

48. Stiell IG, Wells GA, Hoag RH, Sivilotti ML, Cacciotti TF, Verbeek PR, et al. Implementation of the Ottawa Knee Rule for the use of radiography in acute knee injuries. *JAMA* 1997;278:2075–2079.

49. Stiell IG, Wells GA, Vandemheen KL. The Canadian C-spine rule for radiography in alert and stable trauma patients. *JAMA* 2001;286:1841–1848.

50. Kanaya AM, Fyr CL, de Rekeneire N, Shorr RI, Schwartz AV, Goodpaster BH, et al. Predicting the development of diabetes in older adults: The derivation and validation of a prediction rule. *Diabetes Care* 2005;28:404–408.

51. Sarkisian CA, Liu H, Gutierrez PR, Seeley DG, Cummings SR, Mangione CM. Modifiable risk factors predict functional decline among older women: A prospectively validated clinical prediction tool. The Study of Osteoporotic Fractures Research Group. *J Am Geriatr Soc* 2000;48:170–178.

52. Fortescue EB, Kahn K, Bates DW. Prediction rules for complications in coronary bypass surgery: A comparison and methodological critique. *Med Care* 2000;38:820–835.

53. Schatz M, Cook EF, Joshua A, Petitti D. Risk factors for asthma hospitalizations in a managed care organization: Development of a clinical prediction rule. *Am J Manag Care* 2003;9:538–547.

54. Dionne CE, Bourbonnais R, Fremont P, Rossignol M, Stock SR, Larocque I. A clinical return-to-work rule for patients with back pain. *CMAJ* 2005;172:1559–1567.

55. Hicks GE, Fritz JM, Delitto A, McGill SM. Preliminary development of a clinical prediction rule for determining which patients with low back pain will respond to a stabilization exercise program. *Arch Phys Med Rehabil* 2005;86:1753–1762.

56. Tseng YL, Wang WT, Chen WY, Hou TJ, Chen TC, Lau FK. Predictors for the immediate responders to cervical manipulation in patients with neck pain. *Man Ther* 2005;11:306–315.

57. Fritz JM, Childs JD, Flynn TW. Pragmatic application of a clinical prediction rule in primary care to identify patients with low back pain with a good prognosis following a brief spinal manipulation intervention. *BMC Fam Pract* 2005;6:29.

58. Margolis DJ, Berlin JA, Strom BL. Which venous leg ulcers will heal with limb compression bandages? *Am J Med* 2000;109:15–19.

59. Lesher JD, Sutlive TG, Miller GA, Chine NJ, Garber MB, Wainner RS. Development of a clinical prediction rule for classifying patients with patellofemoral pain syndrome who respond to patellar taping. *J Orthop Sports Phys Ther* 2006;36(11):854–866.

60. Solomon DH, Avorn J, Warsi A, Brown CH, Martin S, Martin TL, et al. Which patients with knee problems are likely to benefit from nonarthroplasty surgery? Development of a clinical prediction rule. *Arch Intern Med* 2004;164:509–513.

61. Graham ID, Stiell IG, Laupacis A, McAuley L, Howell M, Clancy M, et al. Awareness and use of the Ottawa ankle and knee rules in 5 countries: Can publication alone be enough to change practice? *Ann Emerg Med* 2001;37:259–266.

62. Nugent PJ. Ottawa Ankle Rules accurately asses injuries and reduce reliance on radiographs. *J Fam Pract* 2004;53:785–788.

63. Brehaut JC, Stiell IG, Visentin L, Graham ID. Clinical decision rules "in the real world": How a widely disseminated rule is used in everyday practice. *Acad Emerg Med* 2005;12:948–956.

64. Derksen RJ, Bakker FC, Geervliet PC, de Lange-de Klerk ES, Heilbron EA, Veenings B, et al. Diagnostic accuracy and reproducibility in the interpretation of Ottawa ankle and foot rules by specialized emergency nurses. *Am J Emerg Med* 2005;23:725–729.

65. Cameron C, Naylor CD. No impact from active dissemination of the Ottawa Ankle Rules: Further evidence of the need for local implementation of practice guidelines. *CMAJ* 1999;160:1165–1168.

66. Childs JD, Cleland JA. Development and application of clinical prediction rules to improve decision making in physical therapist practice. *Phys Ther* 2006;86:122–131.
67. Wright JG, Young NL. A comparison of different indices of responsiveness. *J Clin Epidemiol* 1997;50:239–246.
68. Wyrwich KW, Tierney WM, Wolinsky FD. Further evidence supporting an SEM-based criterion for identifying meaningful intra-individual changes in health-related quality of life. *J Clin Epidemiol* 1999;52:861–873.
69. Stratford PW, Binkley J, Solomon P, Finch E, Gill C, Moreland J. Defining the minimum level of detectable change for the Roland-Morris questionnaire. *Phys Ther* 1996;76:359–365; discussion 366–368.
70. Beaton DE, Bombardier C, Katz JN, Wright JG, Wells G, Boers M, et al. Looking for important change/differences in studies of responsiveness. OMERACT MCID Working Group. Outcome Measures in Rheumatology. Minimal Clinically Important Difference. *J Rheumatol* 2001;28:400–405.
71. Quintana JM, Escobar A, Bilbao A, Arostegui I, Lafuente I, Vidaurreta I. Responsiveness and clinically important differences for the WOMAC and SF-36 after hip joint replacement. *Osteoarthritis Cartilage* 2005;13:1076–1083.
72. Kennedy DM, Stratford PW, Wessel J, Gollish JD, Penney D. Assessing stability and change of four performance measures: A longitudinal study evaluating outcome following total hip and knee arthroplasty. *BMC Musculoskelet Disord* 2005;6:3.
73. Norman GR, Sloan JA, Wyrwich KW. Interpretation of changes in health-related quality of life: The remarkable universality of half a standard deviation. *Med Care* 2003;41:582–592.
74. Miller GA. The magic number seven plus or minus two: Some limits on our capacity for processing information. *Psychol Rev* 1956;63:81–97.
75. van der Heijde D, Lassere M, Edmonds J, Kirwan J, Strand V, Boers M. Minimal clinically important difference in plain films in RA: Group discussions, conclusions, and recommendations. OMERACT Imaging Task Force. *J Rheumatol* 2001;28:914–917.
76. Crosby RD, Kolotkin RL, Williams GR. Defining clinically meaningful change in health-related quality of life. *J Clin Epidemiol* 2003;56:395–407.
77. Jaeschke R, Singer J, Guyatt GH. Measurement of health status. Ascertaining the minimal clinically important difference. *Control Clin Trials* 1989;10:407–415.
78. Guyatt GH, Feeny DH, Patrick DL. Measuring health-related quality of life. *Ann Int Med* 1993;118:622–629.
79. Osoba D, Rodrigues G, Myles J, Zee B, Pater J. Interpreting the significance of changes in health-related quality-of-life scores. *J Clin Oncol* 1998;16:139–144.
80. Kazis LE, Anderson JJ, Meenan RF. Effect sizes for interpreting changes in health status. *Med Care* 1989;27(3):S178–S189.
81. Cohen J. *Statistical Power Analysis for the Behavioral Sciences.* (2nd ed.). Hillsdale, NJ: Lawrence Erlbaum, 1988.
82. Liang MH, Fossel AH, Larson MG. Comparisons of five health status instruments for orthopedic evaluation. *Med Care* 1990;28:632–642.
83. Guyatt GH, Bombardier C, Tugwell PX. Measuring disease-specific quality of life in clinical trials. *CMAJ* 1986;134:889–895.
84. Stratford PW, Binkley JM, Riddle DL. Health status measures: Strategies and analytic methods for assessing change scores. *Phys Ther* 1996;76:1109–1123.
85. Stratford PW, Binkley J, Solomon P, Gill C, Finch E. Assessing change over time in patients with low back pain. *Phys Ther* 1994;74:528–533.
86. Testa MA. Interpretation of quality-of-life outcomes: Issues that affect magnitude and meaning. *Med Care* 2000;38(9 Suppl):II166–174.

87. Lydick E, Epstein RS. Interpretation of quality of life changes. *Qual Life Res* 1993;2: 221–226.

88. Guyatt GH, Osoba D, Wu AW, Wyrwich KW, Norman GR. Methods to explain the clinical significance of health status measures. *Mayo Clin Proc* 2002;77:371–383.

89. Anderson JJ, Chernoff MC. Sensitivity to change of rheumatoid arthritis clinical trial outcome measures. *J Rheumatol* 1993;20:535–537.

90. Guyatt G, Walter S, Normal GR. Measuring change over time: Assessing the usefulness of evaluative instruments. *J Chron Dis* 1987;40:171–178.

91. Norman GR, Stratford P, Regehr G. Methodological problems in the retrospective computation of responsiveness to change: The lesson of Cronbach. *J Clin Epidemiol* 1997;50: 869–879.

92. Deyo RA, Centor RM. Assessing the responsiveness of functional scales to clinical change: An analogy to diagnostic test performance. *J Chronic Dis* 1986;39:897–906.

93. Stratford PW, Binkley JM, Riddle DL, Guyatt GH. Sensitivity to change of the Roland-Morris Back Pain Questionnaire: Part 1. *Phys Ther* 1998;78:1186–1196.

94. Beninato M, Gill-Body KM, Salles S, Stark PC, Black-Schaffer RM, Stein J. Determination of the minimal clinically important difference in the FIM instrument in patients with stroke. *Arch Phys Med Rehabil* 2006;87:32–39.

95. Wolfe F, Michaud K, Strand V. Expanding the definition of clinical differences: From minimally clinically important differences to really important differences. Analyses in 8931 patients with rheumatoid arthritis. *J Rheumatol* 2005;32:583–589.

96. de Vet HC, Terwee CB, Ostelo RW, Beckerman H, Knol DL, Bouter LM. Minimal changes in health status questionnaires: Distinction between minimally detectable change and minimally important change. *Health Qual Life Outcomes* 2006;4:54.

97. Haley SM, Fragala-Pinkham MA. Interpreting change scores of tests and measures used in physical therapy. *Phys Ther* 2006;86:735–743.

98. Eton DT, Cella D, Yost KJ, Yount SE, Peterman AH, Neuberg DS, et al. A combination of distribution- and anchor-based approaches determined minimally important differences (MIDs) for four endpoints in a breast cancer scale. *J Clin Epidemiol* 2004;57: 898–910.

99. Cella D, Eton DT, Lai JS, Peterman AH, Merkel DE. Combining anchor and distribution-based methods to derive minimal clinically important differences on the Functional Assessment of Cancer Therapy (FACT) anemia and fatigue scales. *J Pain Symptom Manage* 2002;24:547–561.

100. Guyatt GH, Juniper EF, Walter SD, Griffith LE, Goldstein RS. Interpreting treatment effects in randomised trials. *BMJ* 1998;316:690–693.

101. Fragala-Pinkham MA, Haley SM, Goodgold S. Evaluation of a community-based group fitness program for children with disabilities. *Pediatr Phys Ther* 2006;18:159–167.

CHAPTER 28
Epidemiology: Measuring Risk

Throughout this text, we have addressed the importance of understanding basic elements of research design and statistics for clinical decision making, especially within the context of evidence-based practice. In this chapter we will present an important perspective in health care research based on principles of epidemiology. The information from epidemiological research can have direct influence on practitioners' day-to-day choices related to diagnosis, prognosis or intervention. The purpose of this chapter is to present statistical methods for measures of disease frequency, estimates of health risks for cohort and case-control studies, and the evaluation of treatment effects in randomized trials.

THE SCOPE OF EPIDEMIOLOGY

Classically, the field of **epidemiology** is concerned with the study of the distribution and determinants of disease, injury, or dysfunction in human populations. Epidemiology literally began as the study of "epidemics," concerned primarily with mortality and morbidity from acute infectious diseases. Many of the health standards we take for granted today, such as clean water supplies, treatment of sewage and food refrigeration, can be credited to discoveries made through epidemiological investigations.

Epidemiologists try to identify those who have a specific disorder, when and where the disorder developed and what exposures are associated with its presence. Epidemiological questions often arise out of clinical experience, laboratory findings or public health concerns about the relationship between societal practices and disease outcomes. Through the analysis of health status indicators and population characteristics, epidemiologists try to identify and explain the causal factors in disease patterns.

As medical cures and treatments have been developed to control many of these problems, and as patterns of disease have changed, the scope of epidemiology has broadened. Today epidemiology includes the study of chronic disease, disability and health status. Because we are often concerned with functional problems as well as disease states, we will use the terms *disease, disorder* and *disability* interchangeably to represent health outcomes, including illness, injury and physical, psychological or social dysfunction. This approach fits with the World Health Organization's definition of health, which encompasses social, psychological and physical well-being.[1]

Epidemiology is distinguished as a research approach because of its unique concern with the identification of risk factors for disability and disease. Epidemiologic studies are generally distinguished as observational or experimental (or quasi-experimental). In observational studies there is no artificial manipulation of any of the study factors (see Chapter 13). Observational studies are categorized as *descriptive* or *analytic.* **Descriptive studies** are concerned with the distribution and patterns of disease or disability in a population. These are carried out when there is little knowledge about the state of health or frequency of disease. **Analytic studies** test hypotheses to determine if specific exposures are related to health status or disease occurrence. Case-control and cohort studies are observational analytic approaches (see Chapter 13). Randomized controlled trials (RCT) are experimental analytic studies that are designed to test the effect of interventions on health outcomes (see Chapter 10).

DESCRIPTIVE EPIDEMIOLOGY: MEASURES OF DISEASE FREQUENCY

Descriptive epidemiologic studies are done when little is known about the occurrence or determinant of health conditions. They will often provide information that can be used to set priorities for health care planning, and will generate hypotheses that can be studied using analytic methods. Descriptive studies may be presented as case reports, correlational studies, or cross-sectional surveys (see Chapter 14).

Person, Place and Time

The purpose of descriptive epidemiologic studies is to describe patterns of health, disease and disability in terms of person, place and time.

Who **experiences this disorder?**   Relevant characteristics might include age, gender, religion, race, cultural background, education, socioeconomic status, occupation and so on. This is the *demography* of the disorder. Epidemiologists try to determine if individuals with certain characteristics are more at risk for a particular disorder than others. For example, researchers have studied the increasing prevalence of type 2 diabetes in adolescents,[2] and the incidence of incontinence in women over age 45.[3]

Where **is the frequency of disorder highest or lowest?**   Epidemiologists may be concerned with identifying restricted areas within a city or large geographic areas in which disease or exposures are commonly found. They may look at environmental factors such as weather, local industry, water source and lifestyle as potential causative factors. For instance, the early studies in AIDS documented high incidence in San Francisco and New York.[4] Legionnaire's disease[5] and severe acute respiratory syndrome (SARS)[6] are other examples of diseases that had specific geographic origins (see Box 28.1).

When **does the disorder occur most or least frequently?**   The epidemiologist will compare the present frequency of a disorder with that of different time periods. When the frequency of occurrence varies significantly at one point in time, some specific time-related causative factor is sought. Seasonal variations may become obvious, or trends may be related to other historical factors. For example, researchers have found a higher incidence of hip fractures in elderly individuals during winter months,[12] and an increased rate of hospitalization due to adult asthma symptoms in spring months.[13]

Disease Frequency

The statistical measures used to describe epidemiologic outcomes focus on quantification of disease occurrence. The simplest measure of disease frequency would be a count of the number of affected individuals; however, meaningful interpretation and comparisons of such a measure would also require knowing how many people there were in the total population who could have gotten the disease and the length of time over which the occurrence of the disease was monitored. Therefore, measures of disease frequency will always include reference to population size and time period of observation. For example, we might document 35 cases of a disease within 1 year in a population of 3,200 people, or 35/3,200/year. Typically, population size is expressed in terms of thousands, such as 1,000 (10^3), 10,000 (10^4), and 100,000 (10^5). For instance, the preceding values would be expressed as 10.94 cases per 1,000 per year. To make estimates more useful, such rates are usually calculated in whole numbers, such as 1,094/100,000/year.

The number of cases of a disease that exist in a population reflects the risk of disease for that group. It describes the relative importance of the disease and can provide a basis for comparison with other groups who may have different exposure histories. The two most common measures of disease frequency are prevalence and incidence.

Prevalence

Prevalence is a proportion reflecting the number of *existing* cases of a disorder relative to the total population at a given point in time. It provides an estimate of the probability that an individual will have a particular disorder at that time. Prevalence (P) is calculated as

$$P = \frac{\text{number of existing cases of a disease at a given point in time}}{\text{total population at risk}} \qquad (28.1)$$

For example, we know that obesity has become a national concern. The National Health Interview Survey in 2000 found that the number of adults with self-reported obesity was 7,058 out of a sample of 32,375.[14] The prevalence of obesity in this population is expressed as

$$P = \frac{7,058}{32,375} = 21.8\%$$

Therefore, there is a 22% probability that any randomly selected individual from this population would be obese. Because this value reflects the cross-sectional status of the population at a single point in time, it is also called *point prevalence*.

Prevalence can also be established for a specified period in time. For example, data obtained from a random sample of 973 newspaper employees found that the number of individuals categorized as having upper limb musculoskeletal complaints after 1 year was 395.[15] The estimate of the prevalence of upper limb musculoskeletal complaints in this population during a 1-year period is, therefore, 41%. This measure, combining

BOX 28.1 The London Cholera Epidemic of 1854

The pioneering work of John Snow, a London physician in the mid-18th century, serves as the classic example of descriptive epidemiology. The era saw a cholera pandemic that caused many deaths in Europe, rivaling the plague. Following an epidemic in London in the late 1840s, Snow argued that an infectious microbe was the causal factor, not an airborne gas as most believed. Because vomiting and diarrhea were the primary symptoms of the disease, he reasoned that cholera was a pathology of the gastrointestinal tract, suggesting that something had to be ingested.[7] His hypothesis was not well accepted, however, and it was actually not until 1883 that the cholera organism was finally accepted as the causative agent.[8]

Snow noted that between 1849 and 1853, the incidence of cholera had lessened, and that during this interval an important change had taken place in the water supply of several districts in south London, which was serviced by two companies. The *Lambeth Company* had noted that water from the Thames River had become polluted, and in 1852 moved their waterworks upriver where the water was cleaner, thereby "obtaining a supply of water quite free from the sewage of London."[9] These districts were also supplied by the *Southwark and Vauxhall Company*, which continued to draw its water from the London section of the river which was just downstream from a sewer outlet.

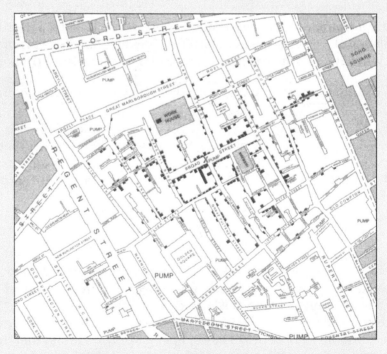

A portion of Snow's early map of Soho, 1854. The green areas show the workhouse and brewery where few or no deaths occurred. The Broad Street pump is indicated by an X.

In the summer of 1854 cholera reappeared in London. Snow recognized the potential for a "Grand Experiment" that involved thousands of people "of both sexes, of every age and occupation, and of every rank and station . . . " who were naturally divided into two groups, based on the origin of their water supply.[9] Through meticulous investigation over 7 weeks, Snow's data showed that mortality was much higher for homes supplied by the contaminated *Southwark and Vauxhall Company.*

Snow's most important investigation, however, occurred later in the summer in the Soho section of London, where a devastating outbreak of cholera killed almost 600 people within a few days at the end of August, 1854. Through door-to-door interviews, he noted that many of the deaths occurred in homes near the intersection of Broad Street and Cambridge Street, which was the location of the Broad Street water pump—supplied by *Southwark and Vauxhall.* He also found that in a workhouse on an adjacent street, surrounded by houses in which deaths had occurred, only 5 cholera deaths were seen among 535 inmates. It turned out that the workhouse had its own well. Snow visited a brewery on Broad Street and found that no deaths had occurred. The owner said the men never drank water—only beer! Snow also found that individuals who had visited the Broad Street area, and others who had purposely obtained water from that pump, had died.

In his detailed map, Snow indicated each death by a bar at each address, clearly demonstrating how the deaths clustered around the Broad Street pump. On September 7, 1854, Snow convinced the Board of Guardians of his hypothesis, and on the next day the pump handle was removed. The epidemic ended almost immediately (although it must also be noted that by then most of the residents had left the area). An investigation of the pump revealed that its well was about 28 feet deep, and that a sewer flowed within yards of the well at 22 feet down.[10]

What is most noteworthy about this history is the manner in which John Snow mounted his investigations. Brody et al[7] point out the significance of the fact that Snow did not use his map to generate his hypothesis. Rather, he developed his hypothesis from his observations and then gathered data and anecdotal information that provided cumulative evidence to support his theory that the contaminated water was the problem. The map only illustrated his data. What is all the more remarkable is that Snow formed his conclusions nearly 30 years before Louis Pasteur's work with germ theory. He called the agents that caused diseases like cholera "special animal poisons," and understood that even if scientists were unable to identify the "thing" that caused cholera, they could still have enough information to prevent further spreading of the disease.[11] These lessons were the foundation for contemporary geographic investigations into disease patterns.

Map from <http://www.hhmi.org/biointeractive/museum/exhibit99/1_snow.html> Accessed September 28, 2006.

existing with new cases of musculoskeletal complaints during the period of one year, is referred to as *period prevalence*.

Prevalence is most useful as an indicator for planning health services, because it reflects the impact of a disease on the population. Therefore, a measure of prevalence can be used to project requirements such as health care personnel, specialized medical equipment and number of hospital beds. Prevalence should not, however, be used as a basis for examining etiology of a disease because it is influenced by the length of survival of those with the disorder; that is, prevalence is a function of both the number of individuals who develop the disease and the duration or severity of the illness. Because this estimate looks at the total number of individuals who have the disease at a given time, that number will be large if the disease tends to be of long duration.

Incidence

The measure of *incidence* quantifies the number of *new* cases of a disorder or disease in the population during a specified time period and, therefore, represents an estimate of the risk of developing the disease during that time. Incidence discounts the effect of duration of illness that is present in prevalence measures. By examining incidence rates for subgroups of the population, such as age groups, ethnic groups and geographic locations, the researcher can identify those groups that demonstrate higher disease rates and target them to investigate specific exposures. Incidence can be expressed as cumulative incidence or incidence rate.

Cumulative incidence (CI) quantifies the number of individuals who become diseased during a specified time period:

$$CI = \frac{\text{number of new cases during given time period}}{\text{total population at risk}} \tag{28.2}$$

For example, in a study of low back pain 196 men who had recently taken up golf were followed over a 1-year period.[16] During that time, 16 new cases of back pain were identified. The 1-year cumulative incidence of first-time back pain for this cohort was 8% (16/196). The specification of the time period of observation is essential to the interpretation of this value. The number of cases would be perceived differently if subjects were followed for 1 or 10 years. Other issues that require consideration in interpreting a measure of cumulative incidence include the possibility that the number of individuals at risk in the cohort will vary over time, and the possibility that the condition under study is caused by other, competing risks.

Person-time. Measuring the total population at risk for cumulative incidence assumes that all subjects were followed for the entire observation period; however, some individuals in the population may enter the study at different times, some may drop out, and others who acquire the disease are no longer at risk. Therefore, the length of the follow-up period is not uniform for all participants. To account for these differences, *incidence rate* (IR) can be calculated:

$$IR = \frac{\text{number of new cases during given time period}}{\text{total person-time}} \tag{28.3}$$

As in cumulative incidence, the numerator for this estimate represents the number of new cases of the disorder; however, the denominator is the sum of the time periods of observation for all individuals in the population at risk during the study time frame, or **person-time.** For example, in the Nurses' Health Study, 121,700 female nurses were enrolled in 1976. During the period of 1976 to 1992, investigators identified 3,603 new cases of breast cancer.[17] Of the women originally enrolled, some left the study as a result of death or loss to follow-up at various times during the period, and some developed breast cancer after different amounts of time, contributing different amounts of time to the denominator. In other words, a woman who died in 1977 in an automobile crash would have contributed 1 person-year to the denominator, whereas two women who developed breast cancer in 1990 would have contributed a total of 28 person-years to the denominator.

Researchers totaled the amount of time each subject was *known to be at risk* between 1976 and 1992, and obtained the total *person-years* observed, in this case there were 1,794,565 person-years of observation. The incidence rate was, therefore,

$$IR = \frac{3,606}{1,794,565} = .002$$

or 2 cases per 1,000 person-years (2×10^{-3} years). Incidence rate is often a more efficient measure than cumulative incidence, as it allows for inclusion of all subjects, regardless of the amount of time they were able to participate. Cumulative incidence would only account for those subjects who were available for the entire study period.

The Relationship between Prevalence and Incidence

The relationship between prevalence and incidence is a function of the average duration of the outcome of interest. If the incidence of the disorder is low (few new cases occur) but the duration of the disorder is long, then the prevalence, or proportion of the population that has the disease at a given point in time, may be large. If, however, incidence is high (many new cases of the disease occur) but the disorder is manifest for a short duration (either by quick recovery or death), the prevalence may be low. For example, a chronic disease such as arthritis may have a low incidence but high prevalence. A short-duration curable condition like a common cold may have a high incidence but low prevalence, because lots of people get colds but few actually have colds at any one point in time.

Vital Statistics

Epidemiologists often use incidence measures to describe the health status of populations in terms of birth and death rates that inform us about the consequences of disease. The **birth rate** is obtained by dividing the number of live births during the year by the total population at midyear. The **mortality rate** quantifies the incidence of death in a population by dividing the number of deaths during a specific time period by the total population at the midpoint of the time period. These data are generally available through records of state vital statistics reports, census data and birth and death certificates.

The mortality rate can reflect *total mortality* for the population from all causes of death in the *crude mortality rate,* in which the total number of deaths during the year is divided by the average midyear population. This value is usually expressed as the number of deaths per 100,000 population; however, when different categories within the population differentially contribute to this rate, it may be more meaningful to look at category-specific rates. A **cause-specific rate** looks only at the number of deaths from a particular disease or condition within a year divided by the average midyear population. For instance, rates may reflect mortality specifically resulting from diseases such as cancer and heart disease or from motor vehicle accidents. The **case-fatality rate** is the number of deaths from a disease relative to the number of individuals who had the disease during a given time period.

Other commonly used categories are age, sex and race. **Age-specific rates** are probably most common because of the differential effect of many diseases across the life span. For example, if one looks at the death rate for cancer across age groups, we would find that mortality was higher for older age categories. Therefore, it may be more meaningful to present age-specific mortality rates for each decade of life, rather than a crude mortality rate; however, this results in a long list of rates that may not be useful for certain comparisons. An overall rate would be more practical, but it would have to account for the variation in rates across age categories. For instance, if we compare the crude cancer mortality rate for today versus the crude rate from 50 years ago, we would have to account for the fact that a larger proportion of the total population now falls in the older age range. Therefore, epidemiologists will often report *age-adjusted mortality rates* that reflect different weightings for the uneven categories. Methods for calculating adjusted rates are described in most epidemiology texts.

ANALYTIC EPIDEMIOLOGY: MEASURES OF ASSOCIATION AND RISK

Analytic epidemiology is concerned with testing hypotheses. Measures of association are typically derived for case-control and cohort studies (see Chapter 13), to assess the relationship between specific **exposures** and disease. These tests will establish if an association exists and the strength of that association. If an association does exist, we say that the specific exposure represents a **risk factor** for the disease.

The focus on exposures takes a broad view that reflects contemporary concerns including lifestyle practices such as smoking, substance abuse, drinking alcohol or coffee and eating foods high in cholesterol or salt; occupational hazards, such as repetitive tasks or heavy lifting; environmental influences, such as second-hand smoke, toxic waste and sunlight; and specific interventions, such as exercise, medications or treatment modalities. These exposures increase or decrease the likelihood of developing certain disorders or influence the ultimate outcome of a disorder. For example, smoking and sunlight are considered risk factors that increase the chance of developing cancer.[18,19] Stroke patients with comprehension deficits have an increased risk of poor therapeutic outcomes.[20] Exercise and higher fitness level in men with diabetes are associated with reduced risk of mortality from cardiovascular disease.[21]

This is a fundamental process in the determination of prognosis, as we attempt to predict outcomes based on patient characteristics. As with all measures of association, risk does not necessarily mean that the exposure causes the outcome.

Relative versus Absolute Effects

Analyses of association are based on a measure of effect that looks at the frequency of disease among those who were and were not exposed to the risk factor. A *relative effect* is a ratio that describes the risks associated with the exposed group as compared with the unexposed. An *absolute effect* is the actual difference between the rate of disease in the exposed and unexposed groups, or the difference in the risk of developing the disease between these two groups. To illustrate the concepts of relative and absolute effect, suppose we purchased two books, one costing $3 and the other $6. The absolute difference is $3, whereas the relative difference is that the second book is twice as expensive as the first. Therefore, the relative effect is based on the absolute effect, but takes into account the baseline value. Analogously, we can use measures of incidence of disease in exposed and unexposed groups to determine both relative and absolute effects of particular exposures.

Relative Risk

The most common measure of relative effect is **relative risk (RR)**, which indicates the likelihood that someone who has been exposed to a risk factor will develop the disease, as compared with one who has not been exposed. Relative risk is defined as the ratio of incidence of disease among the exposed subjects to the incidence of disease among the unexposed. Measures of relative risk are appropriate for use with cohort studies.

To determine risk, data are typically organized in a 2 × 2 table, called a **contingency table,** as shown in Figure 28.1. The vertical columns in the table represent the classification of disease status (the outcome), and the horizontal rows represent exposure status. To facilitate consistency in presentation and calculation, the cells in the table are designated *a, b, c,* and *d,* as shown in the figure. Therefore, cell *a* represents those who have the disease and were exposed, cell *b* represents those who do not have the disease and were exposed, and so on. The marginal totals for each row and column represent the total numbers of individuals who were exposed ($a + b$) and were not exposed ($c + d$), and the total numbers who have the disease ($a + c$) and do not have the disease ($b + d$). The sum of all four cells is the total sample size (N).

FIGURE 28.1   General format for a 2 × 2 contingency table, showing frequencies for disease and exposure.

For a cohort study, we can obtain cumulative incidence estimates for the exposed (CI_E) and unexposed (CI_0) groups. The cumulative incidence for the exposed group is the number of cases of the disease among the total exposed sample, or $a/(a + b)$. The cumulative incidence for the unexposed group is the number of cases of the disease among the total unexposed sample, or $c/(c + d)$.* Therefore,

$$RR = \frac{CI_E}{CI_0} = \frac{a/(a + b)}{d/(c + d)} \tag{28.4}$$

If the incidence rates of the outcome are the same for the exposed and unexposed groups, the relative risk is 1.0, indicating that the exposure presents no excess risk for the outcome. Therefore, a relative risk greater than 1.0 indicates an increased risk, and a relative risk less than 1.0 means that the exposure decreases the risk of developing the disorder.

Example

To illustrate this application, consider the data shown in Table 28.1A for a cohort study of the risk of hip fracture associated with leisure time physical activity.[22] Data were taken from longitudinal studies over six birth cohorts. For this example, we will look at a subsample of 130 women. The research question is: Does physical activity reduce the risk of hip fracture in elderly women?

Our first step is to determine what proportion of patients who exercised sustained a hip fracture. This is the incidence of hip fracture among exercisers, 48 out of 98, or 49%. Then we determine what proportion of sedentary patients sustained a hip fracture. This is the incidence of hip fracture for those who did not exercise, 20 out of 32, or 63%. Relative risk is the ratio of these two proportions:

$$RR = \frac{a(a + c)}{d(c + d)} = \frac{48/98}{20/32} = \frac{.49}{.63} = 0.78$$

This tells us that the risk of hip fracture was decreased among nonsedentary women; that is, those who were active at least 2 hours/week were 0.78 times as likely (less likely) to have a hip fracture as compared with those who were sedentary.

Confidence Intervals for Relative Risk

An important assumption in any research study is that we can draw reasonable inferences about population characteristics based on sample data. This assumption holds true for epidemiologic studies as well. When a risk estimate is derived from a particular set of subjects, the researcher will use that estimate to make generalizations about expected behaviors or outcomes in others who have similar exposure histories. Therefore, it is important to determine a measure of true effect using a confidence interval (see Chapter 18). For example, as shown in Table 28.1B, with an observed relative risk

---

*This calculation for relative risk is based on the assumption that all subjects in the cohort were followed for the same amount of time. When follow-up time differs, it is the person-time for exposed and nonexposed groups that should be used for marginal totals, rather than just the total number of subjects in each category.

TABLE 28.1   RELATIVE RISK: DATA FOR A COHORT STUDY SHOWING THE RELATIONSHIP BETWEEN PHYSICAL ACTIVITY AND RISK OF HIP FRACTURE IN WOMEN

A. DATA and COMPUTATION

Activity Level * Hip fx Crosstabulation

		Hip fx		
		Yes	No	Total
Activity level	≥2hr/wk	48	50	98
	Sedentary	20	12	32
	Total	68	62	130

$$RR = \frac{a/(a+b)}{d/(c+d)} = \frac{48/98}{20/32} = 0.78$$

B. OUTPUT

Risk Estimate

		95% Confidence Interval	
	Value	Lower	Upper
For cohort hip fx = Yes	.784	.560	1.097
N of Valid Cases	130		

Chi-Square Tests

	Value	df	Sig. (2-sided)
Chi-Square	1.768	1	.184
N of Valid Cases	130		

Note: Output has been edited to include only relevant data for this analysis.

Data adapted from: Hoidrup S, Sorensen T, Stroger U, et al. Leisure-time physical activity levels and changes in relation to risk of hip fracture in men and women. *Am J Epidemiol* 2001;154:60–68.

of 0.78 for the association between hip fracture and physical activity, the 95% confidence interval is 0.560 to 1.097. This interval represents a range of values within which the true population effect is expected to fall.

Confidence intervals can also be used to provide information about statistical significance by referring to the null value for relative risk, which is 1.0. We look to see if the null value is included within the 95% confidence interval. If the null value is contained within the confidence interval, and we are 95% confident that the interval contains the true population value, then we cannot rule out 1.0 as the population value. Therefore, the estimate is not considered significant. If the null value is not contained within the interval, the estimate is considered significant; that is, we are 95% sure that the null value is not the true population value. In our example, the 95% confidence interval is 0.56 to 1.097. As this interval contains the null value of 1.0, we would state that the observed association is not statistically significant at the .05 level. Therefore, we must conclude that, although the RR value shows a reduced risk for hip fracture with physical activity, this value could have occurred by chance.

Chi-square can also be used as a test of significance, to determine if the proportions differ across categories in a **crosstabulation** (see Chapter 25). In this example, the value of chi-square results in $p = .184$ (see Table 28.1B), which is not significant. This confirms the conclusion drawn from the confidence interval analysis, with a parallel interpretation. Chi-square tells us that the proportion of individuals with and without hip fracture who were in the two physical activity groups was not different from what would be expected just by chance.

Odds Ratio

A case-control study differs from a cohort study in that subjects are purposefully chosen based on the presence or absence of disease (cases or controls) and therefore, we cannot determine the rate of incidence of the disease (see Chapter 13). Relative risk is not an appropriate measure for case-control studies because we cannot calculate cumulative incidence. The relative risk can, however, be estimated using an **odds ratio (OR)**, which is calculated using the formula

$$OR = \frac{a/c}{b/d} = \frac{ad}{bc} \tag{28.5}$$

The odds ratio is interpreted in the same way as relative risk, with a null value of 1.0.

Example

Consider the data shown in Table 28.2A. These data are from a case-control study which examined the risk for developing plantar fasciitis associated with body mass index

---

TABLE 28.2   ODDS RATIO: CASE-CONTROL DATA SHOWING THE RELATIONSHIP BETWEEN BODY MASS INDEX (BMI) AND RISK OF PLANTAR FASCIITIS

A. DATA and COMPUTATION

BMI * Plantar Fasciitis Crosstabulation

		Plantar Fasciitis		
		Yes	No	Total
BMI	> 30	29	17	46
	≤ 30	21	83	104
	Total	50	100	150

$$OR = \frac{ad}{bc} = \frac{(29)(83)}{(21)(17)} = 6.74$$

B. OUTPUT

Risk Estimate

	Value	95% Confidence Interval	
		Lower	Upper
Odds Ratio for BMI	6.742	3.132	14.512
N of Valid Cases	150		

Chi-Square Tests

	Value	df	Sig. (2-sided)
Chi-Square	26.353	1	.000
N of Valid Cases	150		

Note: Output has been edited to include only relevant data for this analysis.
Source: Riddle DL, Pulisic M, Pidcoe P, Johnson RE. Risk factors for plantar fasciitis: A matched case-control study. *J Bone Joint Surg Am* 2003;85A:872–877.

(BMI).[23] The researchers assembled a sample of 50 cases and 100 controls, with a 1 : 2 match on age and gender. Among the cases, 29 individuals had a BMI over 30 (considered obese); among the controls, 17 subjects had a BMI over 30. The crude odds ratio for these data is

$$OR = \frac{ad}{bc} = \frac{(29)(83)}{(21)(17)} = 6.74$$

This means that the *odds* of developing plantar fasciitis are almost seven times greater for those who are obese than for those who are not. In other words, being obese appears to increase the risk of developing plantar fasciitis.

Confidence Intervals for the Odds Ratio

Confidence intervals can also be generated for the odds ratio to determine the significance of the ratio as an estimate of population values. As shown in Table 28.2B, the confidence interval for the relationship between plantar fasciitis and BMI is 3.13 to 14.51. This interval does not contain the null value of 1.0, and therefore, this represents a significant odds ratio.

Chi-square can also be used to determine if the proportion of individuals varies across categories. This outcome is shown in Table 28.2B, confirming the significant outcome of the confidence interval analysis.

Confounding and Effect Modification

Quite often, in the analysis of the association between a risk factor and disease, researchers seek to infer a potential causal relationship between the two. The researcher also recognizes, however, that in a study of association, cause and effect cannot be readily established (as it can in an experimental study) because other factors may contribute to the observed relationship. Alternatively, we may see no association because other factors actually obscure the relationship between exposure and outcome.

In some cases, these extraneous variables provide information important to understanding how the association varies across different subgroups, such as age or gender. In other situations, such variables create a bias in the interpretation, interfering with the true association being studied. These two complications of analysis are called confounding and effect modification.

The simplest type of analyses are based on crude data. These are data concerning the exposure status and outcome status of all subjects regardless of any other risks or characteristics. Although analyses based on crude data are often reported in the literature, most studies also require more complicated analyses to evaluate the role of other factors in the relationship of exposure and outcome. These analyses are accomplished through stratification or multivariate methods and provide adjusted measures of association. Researchers must consider the potential influence of confounding and effect modification in all analyses and account for them in the design or analysis of data as much as possible.

Confounding

Confounding variables can be thought of as nuisance variables. Confounding is introduced when extraneous variables interfere with the observed association between the exposure and outcome. A *confounder* is a variable that (1) is associated with the exposure, (2) is a risk factor for the disease independent of the exposure, and (3) is not part of the causal link between the exposure and the disease (Figure 28.2A). In other words, a confounding variable is associated with the predictor variable, but may also be a risk factor for the outcome variable, and therefore must be ruled out. Confounding occurs when the exposure can become confused or distorted by the extraneous variable.

Example. To illustrate this concept, Jackson and co-workers[24] examined the association between risk of mortality and receiving influenza vaccine in elders over 65 years. They studied 252 cases who died during an influenza season and 576 age-matched controls. The crude odds ratio for this relationship was 0.76 (95% Cl 0.47, 1.06), indicating that receiving the vaccine decreased the risk of death. The researchers were interested, however, in the potentially confounding effect of limited functional status, which (1) would be associated with not getting the vaccine, (2) would be a risk factor for mortality, and (3) is not a causal link between the vaccine and mortality. When they adjusted for the effect of functional limitations, the odds ratio was lowered to 0.59 (95% Cl 0.41, 0.83). Because older individuals who have functional limitations would be less likely to visit a clinic to get the vaccine, and mortality is also related to functional decline, the crude odds ratio was an underestimate of the protective nature of the vaccine on mortality. When function is taken into account, the actual risk of death is lower. If there were no discrepancy between the crude and unconfounded estimates, there would be no con-

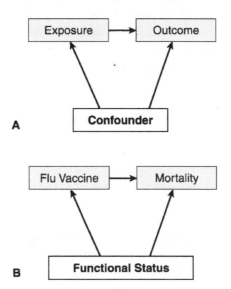

FIGURE 28.2 **A.** Relationship between exposure and outcome, both related to a confounding variable. **B.** Relationship between receiving influenza vaccine and mortality in elders, confounded by functional status.

founding. The degree of discrepancy is indicative of the extent to which function confounded the original data. By eliminating the effect of functional status, a stronger (and significant) relationship was seen between getting the vaccine and decreased mortality.

Adjusting for Confounders.   Confounding variables may or may not be present in a study, depending on the source population and how subjects are chosen. When confounding is present, the statistical outcome may not be documenting the true causal factor. A method commonly used to adjust for a potential confounder is stratification, in which the comparison between exposure and disease is done at specific levels of the potential confounder. When a study mentions that researchers "controlled" or "adjusted" for a factor in the analysis, they have tried to remove the effect of that variable as a confounder.

To evaluate the effect of confounding in an analysis, the researcher must collect information on the potentially confounding variable. If the investigator in the vaccine study did not collect data on the subjects' functional status, the analysis of the confounder would not have been possible. Therefore, the researcher must be able to predict what variables are possible confounders. It is conceivable that several confounding factors will be operating in one study. In addition to controlling for confounding in the analysis, researchers can use design strategies, such as matching or homogeneous subjects, to control for these effects (see Chapter 9). For instance, in the study of influenza vaccine, if we were to restrict subjects to only those who were functionally independent, then function would not be a confounding factor.

Age and gender are often considered potential confounders in epidemiologic studies because of their common association with disease and disability, as well as being related to the presence of many exposures. Other common confounders are socioeconomic status, education level, marital status, weight, and cognitive status.

Effect Modification

In contrast to confounding, effect modification occurs when the presence of one variable modifies the association between an exposure and outcome. Where a confounder is a nuisance that needs to be controlled to get an accurate estimate of an association, an effect modifier is a real effect that helps explain the biologic relationship between the exposure and outcome.[25] Researchers attempt to cancel the effect of a confounding variable in the design or analysis of a study. Effect modifiers are studied so they can be reported.

An effect modifier will *interact* with the exposure and disease variables in such a way as to present a constant effect. It is a natural phenomenon that exists independent of the study design and will always be a factor in interpretation of risk. Effect modifiers tend to be biologically related to the variables being studied.

Example.   Researchers have studied the association between diabetes and risk of endometrial cancer, with many conflicting results. Friberg et al[26] hypothesized that this relationship could be misunderstood because of major modifiers such as physical activity. They studied a cohort of over 36,000 women over 7 years and found a relative risk

TABLE 28.3	ASSOCIATION OF DIABETES AND ENDOMETRIAL CANCER STRATIFIED BY PHYSICAL ACTIVITY: ILLUSTRATION OF EFFECT MODIFICATION		
		Number of Cases	RR (95% CI)
Total Sample	No diabetes	203	2.37 (1.51–3.74)
	Diabetes	22	
High Physical Activity	No diabetes	103	1.06 (0.43–2.60)
	Diabetes	5	
Low Physical Activity	No diabetes	100	2.67 (1.58–4.53)
	Diabetes	17	

Source: Friberg E, Mantzoros CS, Wolk A. Diabetes and risk of endometrial cancer: A population-based prospective cohort study. *Cancer Epidemiol Biomarkers Prev* 2007;16:276–280.

of endometrial cancer of 2.37, adjusted for age, for women diagnosed with diabetes as compared to women without diabetes.

They then stratified the sample by physical activity (see Table 28.3). For diabetics with high physical activity, they found a RR for endometrial cancer of 1.06 as compared to those without diabetes who were active. Therefore, physically active diabetics were essentially at no increased risk of cancer. For diabetics with low physical activity, however, they found a RR of 2.67. The risk associated with endometrial cancer increased by more than two times for those who did not exercise. The fact that the risk estimates are different for each stratum indicates that physical activity interacts with diabetes as an effect modifier; that is, the association between diabetes and endometrial cancer is significantly modified by physical activity.

Pooled Risk Estimates

When data are stratified, separate risk estimates are calculated for each stratum; however, it is usually more useful to consider a single overall estimate that reflects the association between exposure and disease with the confounding factor taken into account. Several statistical techniques can be used to accomplish this, although the most commonly used procedures belong to a set of estimates proposed by Mantel and Haenszel.[27] The **Mantel–Haenszel pooled risk estimate** provides a weighted summary value that can be used to report the relative risk associated with a specific exposure *adjusted* for the confounding variable. When the Mantel-Haenszel estimate differs from the crude risk estimate, it is the Mantel-Haenszel estimate that should be reported. It is most appropriately used when the stratum-specific relative risks are uniform, that is, when there is no effect modification. Formulas used to calculate Mantel-Haenszel estimates of relative risk for case-control and cohort studies are given in Table 28.4. The numerators and denominators in these formulas represent the sum of the expressions for each stratum.

TABLE 28.4   MANTEL-HAENSZEL POOLED ESTIMATES FOR RELATIVE RISK FOR COHORT AND CASE-CONTROL STUDIES

Cohort Study (with count denominators)

$$RR_{MH} = \frac{\sum \frac{a(c + d)}{N}}{\sum \frac{c(a + b)}{N}}$$

Case-Control Study

$$RR_{MH} = \frac{\sum \frac{ad}{N}}{\sum \frac{bc}{N}}$$

ANALYTIC EPIDEMIOLOGY: MEASURES OF RISK BASED ON TREATMENT EFFECT

When making clinical decisions regarding the effectiveness of interventions, we generally want to know if a treatment will improve the patient's condition, or if it will prevent or decrease the risk of an adverse event. Randomized controlled trials (RCT) are the most effective approach for answering these questions, and we typically use a statistical test to compare groups on means or proportions to determine if they are different from each other after the treatment. Such a conclusion is limited, however, because it does not tell us if the difference is clinically important, nor does it help us estimate the likelihood that our own patient will respond favorably. We know that even with a well-established intervention, patients do not all respond the same way. Some will improve and others will not; some will experience an adverse outcome, and others will be fine. So how can we determine the likelihood that our particular patient will benefit from the intervention?

In addition to specific measures of change, then, we may also consider the outcome of treatment in terms of an "event," which is classified as a success or failure. The success of a treatment is usually determined as a beneficial outcome based on a specific threshold, which may be related to an impairment or functional activity. For instance, back pain is relieved or reduced by a certain percent; a child is able to utter a given number of sentences without stuttering; an obese patient loses a certain amount of weight; a patient with congestive heart failure is able to increase walking tolerance by a given distance. Success may also be indicated by whether an adverse outcome is prevented. For example, a patient may be given a drug to control hypertension to prevent stroke. If the patient subsequently suffers a stroke, he has experienced an adverse outcome. In a RCT, the success of the intervention is reflected by the difference in beneficial or adverse outcomes between treatment and control groups. The concept of relative risk (RR) can be used here in reference to treatment effect, indicating if the risk of a particular outcome for the control group is higher or lower than for the treatment group.

Example

Let's put this in the context of a rehabilitation example. A group of researchers studied the effect of exercise and manipulative therapy for reducing cervicogenic headaches.[28] They measured pain intensity and duration as well as the frequency of headaches over a 7-week treatment period. We can appreciate the effect of treatment by setting a threshold that identifies a successful outcome, based on clinically important change. In this study, in addition to the typical comparisons between group means for pain and duration, the authors set a standard of 50% or better reduction in headache frequency as a benchmark for "success" of treatment. If the reduction in recurrence of headache was less than 50%, it was considered an adverse outcome.

Table 28.5A shows the results of this study for the comparison of combined manipulative therapy and therapeutic exercise with a control. We can see that of the 49 patients who received the experimental intervention, 9 had recurring headaches. Of the 48 patients in the control group, 34 had recurring headaches.

Event Rates and Risk Reduction

We can examine differences between group responses in terms of "event rates," or the proportion of subjects in the experimental and control groups that achieved an adverse or successful outcome. We calculate two values: an **experimental event rate (EER)** for those receiving the intervention and a **control event rate (CER)** for the control group, as shown in Table 28.5B. For this study, the EER is 18% and the CER is 71%. These values indicate the risk of headaches recurring for each group. But how do they compare?

The ratio of these two values is the **relative risk (RR)** associated with the intervention:

$$RR = \frac{EER}{CER} \tag{28.6}$$

As shown in Table 28.5B, the RR associated with this intervention is .25. This means that the intervention group was only one-quarter as likely to experience a recurrence of headache as the control group.

Risk Reduction

This effect is better understood, however, as a relative value that reflects the *decrease in risk* associated with the intervention, called the **relative risk reduction (RRR)**, which is equal to:

$$RRR = \frac{CER - EER}{CER} \tag{28.7}$$

As shown in Table 28.5B, RRR = .75 for the headache study. This tells us that there is a 75% reduction in risk for recurring headaches associated with the intervention compared to the control.

As we have discussed before, the disadvantage of RRR is that a relative value does not tell us anything about the actual size of the effect. Figure 28.3 illustrates this limitation. Consider alternative results for a hypothetical comparable study (Study B), where

TABLE 28.5 **CALCULATION OF MEASURES OF TREATMENT EFFECT FOR A RANDOMIZED CONTROLLED TRIAL OF EXERCISE AND MANIPULATIVE THERAPY FOR CERVICOGENIC HEADACHES**

A. DATA

Treatment Outcome

	FAILURE < 50% reduction in headaches	**SUCCESS** ≥ 50% reduction in headaches	**Total**
Manipulation + Exercise	9 a	40 b	49 $a + b$
Control	c 34	d 14	48 $c + d$
Total	43 $a + c$	54 $b + d$	97

B. RISK MEASURES

Experimental event rate (EER)	EER = $a/a + b$	EER = 9/49 = .18
Control event rate (CER)	CER = $c/c + d$	CER = 34/48 = .71
Relative risk (RR)	RR = EER/CER	RR = .18/.71 = .25
Relative risk reduction (RRR)	RRR = (CER − EER)/CER	RRR = .53/.71 = .75
Absolute risk reduction (ARR)	ARR = CER − EER	ARR = .71 − .18 = .53
Number needed to treat (NNT)	NNT = 1/ARR	NNT = 1/.53 = 1.9

C. CONFIDENCE INTERVALS FOR ARR AND NNT

$$95\% \text{ CI} = \text{ARR} \pm 1.96 \text{ (SE)}$$

$$SE = \sqrt{\frac{\text{EER}(1 - \text{EER})}{n_{Exp}} + \frac{\text{CER}(1 - \text{CER})}{n_{control}}} = \sqrt{\frac{.18(1 - .18)}{49} + \frac{.71(1 - .71)}{48}} = .085$$

For ARR: $95\% \text{ CI} = .53 \pm 1.96 \, (.085) = .53 \pm .167 = .363, .697$

For NNT: $95\% \text{ CI (NNT)} = \dfrac{1}{.697}, \dfrac{1}{.363} = 1.43, 2.75$

Source: Jull G, Trott P, Potter H et al. A randomized controlled trial of exercise and manipulative therapy for cervicogenic headache. *Spine* 2002;27:1835–1843.

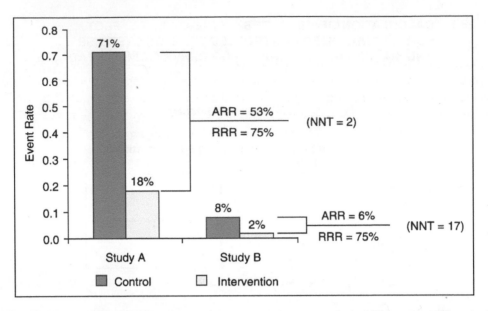

FIGURE 28.3   Results from two studies of treatment for cervicogenic headache, illustrating the important difference in absolute and relative risk measures. Bars represent the event rates for the intervention and control groups, indicating the number of patients who did NOT benefit from treatment. Both studies show a reduced risk with intervention. Although the relative risk reduction (RRR) is the same for both studies, the absolute risk reduction (ARR) and number needed to treat (NNT) are substantially different. Source (for Study A): Jull G, Trott P, Potter H, et al. A randomized controlled trial of exercise and manipulative therapy for cervicogenic headache. *Spine* 2002;27:1835–1843.

the EER was 8% and the CER was 2%. These effects are certainly not clinically meaningful, and yet their RRR would also be .75.

A more clinically useful measure is the **absolute risk reduction (ARR)**, which indicates the actual difference in risk between the groups, easily calculated by:

$$ARR = CER - EER \tag{28.8}$$

For the headache example, then, ARR = .53. There is a 53% absolute reduction in risk of recurring headaches associated with the intervention. If we look at the hypothetical study (B) in Figure 28.3, we can see that the ARR = .06, only a 6% reduction in risk. Therefore, the absolute risk reduction is a better reflection of the true difference in the studies' outcomes.

This example illustrates the importance of considering baseline risk when interpreting risk reduction.[29] The control event rate can be used as an estimate of the risk for all subjects at the start of the study, before intervention is applied. Although a RRR of 75% would be considered impressive, we can see that this value is not meaningful when the baseline risk is only 8%. This absolute risk reduction indicates that the treatment will be of minor benefit in Study B. Compare that to a baseline risk of 71% for study A, and we can see that treatment will be of greater benefit.

Number Needed to Treat

The degree of risk reduction should help us decide whether a treatment is worth pursuing, based on the likelihood that the outcome will be successful (avoiding an adverse event). The ARR, however, does not provide the clinician with a clinical value that can be used to estimate the number of patients that would need to be treated before benefit will be observed. The **number needed to treat (NNT)** was developed as a statistic that provides information about effectiveness in terms of patient numbers.[30] The NNT is defined as the number of patients that would need to be treated to prevent one adverse outcome or to achieve one beneficial outcome in a given time period. It can be calculated for any trial that reports a binary outcome.[31]

The NNT is easily calculated as the reciprocal of the ARR:

$$\text{NNT} = \frac{1}{\text{ARR}} \tag{28.9}$$

where ARR is expressed as a decimal. A large treatment effect will translate to a small number needed to treat.

If the NNT is 1.0, this means that we would need to treat 1 patient to avoid 1 adverse outcome; that is, every patient will benefit from treatment. This is, of course, the ideal, although not often the case. The closer to 1.0, the better the NNT. For the headache example, the NNT is 1.9 (shown in Table 28.4B), which is rounded up to 2.0. Therefore, we would need to treat 2 patients with manipulative therapy and exercise to prevent a recurrence of headaches in 1 patient; that is, 1 out of 2 patients will experience a successful outcome. If the absolute risk reduction is zero (no difference between CER and EER), the treatment has had no effect, and the NNT will be infinity. We would need to treat an infinite number of people to see any benefit.

Confidence Intervals for NNT

The NNT is a point estimate, and therefore, as with other estimates, it should be presented with a confidence interval for accurate interpretation.[31] The confidence limits for NNT are the reciprocals of the confidence limits for ARR, in reverse order. See Table 28.5C for formulas and sample calculations. The null value for ARR is zero, which converts to infinity for the NNT.[†] For the headache study, we are 95% confident that the true population ARR is between 36% and 70%. We are 95% confident that the NNT falls between 1.43 and 2.75.

Number Needed to Harm (NNH)

The NNT reflects the *prevention* of an adverse event, which is generally seen as a successful outcome. For example, treatment for hypertension should prevent adverse events such as stroke, heart attack or death. We can also apply this concept to evaluate serious side effects, risks or complications that occur from treatment, outside of the

---

[†]A confidence interval that contains infinity includes the possibility of no benefit.[32]

intended effects. When an intervention poses excess risk to the patient, we would want to assess the **absolute risk increase (ARI)** associated with it. The reciprocal of this value is called the **number needed to harm (NNH)**, which indicates the number of patients who would need to be treated to cause 1 adverse outcome.[‡] The larger the NNH, the less likely a patient is to experience an adverse outcome. An NNH of 100 would mean that we would need to treat 100 patients to cause one adverse event. An NNH of 1.0 would mean that every patient would experience an adverse event.

The NNH should be considered along with the NNT to evaluate the benefit and harm of an intervention.[32] For example, a systematic review of the effects of aspirin for treatment of acute pain analyzed the effectiveness of a 600 mg dose for at least 50% pain relief, with an NNT of 4.4 (95% CI 4.0, 4.9).[33] They also reported an NNH of 38 (95% CI 22,174) for the side effect of gastric irritation. According to this analysis, if 38 patients were treated, 9 would achieve a positive outcome, and 1 patient would be expected to experience gastric irritation.

Cautions in Interpretation of NNT

In terms of clinical decision making, NNT and NNH provide a useful number to help a clinician and patient decide if one or another treatment is worth pursuing, weighing their potential benefit or harm. The NNT is a particularly useful measure for expressing the relative effectiveness of different interventions. It quantifies the effort required to obtain a beneficial outcome. Several factors must be considered, however, when comparing values of NNT across different interventions or studies.

1. **The NNT must be interpreted in terms of a time period for treatment and follow-up.** The duration of the treatment may make a difference in the frequency of expected positive and negative outcomes. Generally, the NNT will be smaller for an intervention of longer duration.[34] The comparison of NNT values for different treatments is only valid when the outcome is measured within the same time period. For instance, for the headache study the report should read: The NNT was 2 over 7 weeks.

2. **The interpretation of the NNT will depend on baseline risk.** Because some patients will have a greater risk of an adverse outcome before treatment begins, the NNT must be adjusted to account for low and high baseline risks. It may not be reasonable to assume that the same relative risk applies to all patients.[32] The patient's age, gender or initial severity may alter the relative risk associated with the intervention. Therefore, when extrapolating NNT measures from the literature, the baseline risk must be taken into account. The control event rate can be used as an indicator of the baseline risk without treatment.

3. **To compare NNTs, the outcomes of interest must be the same.** For example, in the evaluation of exercise programs, an NNT of 20 for preventing falls in the elderly may be interpreted differently from an NNT of 20 for preventing hip

---

[‡]The ARI and NNH are calculated using the same equations as ARR and NNT, except that the experimental event rate should be smaller than the control event rate.

fracture. The NNT for a drug treatment to reduce hypertension will be different if the outcome is stroke, heart attack or death. In the study of cervicogenic headache, the threshold for success was set at 50%. If this threshold were changed, the resulting NNTs would not be comparable.

4. **The validity of the clinical trial must also be taken into account.** Because NNTs are used to make individual patient decisions and to support reimbursement policies, the degree to which research studies represent actual clinical expectations will influence the application of effective treatments.[35] Both internal and external validity must be considered. Replication is important to determine if results stand up to different samples.

5. **There are no standard limits for NNT (or NNH) that dictate a decision.** Like all research results, NNT should be incorporated into decision making along with the clinician's experience and judgment, the patient's preferences and the nature of the disorder that is being treated.[32] For some interventions an NNT of 2 or 3 would be considered good, whereas for others an NNT of 20 or 40 may still be considered clinically effective. Similarly, an acceptable NNH will be determined by the severity of the risks, balanced with the probable benefit. Therefore, the value of NNT and NNH should always be interpreted within the context of a specific disorder, treatment, outcome, disease severity and time period. For example, a review of treatments for hypertension to prevent stroke reported a NNT for moderate hypertensive patients of 13, and a NNT for mildly hypertensive patients of 167.[36] The recommendations for clinical management of these patients would obviously be quite different.

COMMENTARY

A New View of Outcomes

A traditional biomedical model defines health narrowly as the absence of *disease*. Based on this definition, epidemiologists collect data to determine frequency of occurrence of disease and risk factors for disease. Under this model, we open ourselves to looking at risk factors which have an effect at the biological level of the individual. Using a more complete model of health, epidemiology is able to focus on the occurrence of health-related states and risk factors related to physical, social and psychological health status as well. The *International Classification of Functioning and Disability* model, described in Chapter 1, provides an excellent framework for this approach. We can begin to look at the concept of risk in terms of impairments that lead to physical disability, and use measures of risk to help us set priorities and evaluate outcomes. This chapter has provided a broad view of epidemiology and has used the terms condition, disorder, disease and outcome interchangeably.

Most clinicians do not learn about epidemiologic approaches in basic research courses, and are not familiar with the use of measures of disease frequency, odds ratio or relative risk, number needed to treat, sensitivity and specificity or likelihood ratios. This is unfortunate, as there are many opportunities to answer important clinical questions using these techniques. As the literature continues to expand its use of these procedures, we must understand their applications to apply research findings to our clinical practice.

Questions that are appropriate for clinical epidemiologic study may deal with specific interventions or screening tests, perhaps in a randomized clinical trial format, but may also be concerned with larger decision and policy issues that have direct application to practice. They can often be effectively answered using case-control methodology or analysis of cohort data. Decisions regarding choice of intervention, who gets intervention (including prevention) and the intensity and frequency of intervention may be aided by an understanding of the relative risks associated with specific patient characteristics, activities or treatments. We may understand the physiological rationale for applying specific exercises for reducing pain or improving mobility, but do we know what factors may alter the success of our treatments, or which patients are more likely to improve? Such information can provide new insight into the rationales we use for making treatment decisions.

As health care professionals strive to embrace evidence-based decision making, the concepts covered in this chapter must become a more regular part of the rehabilitation literature. The reliance on statistical significance as a basis for diagnosis, prognosis or treatment must move to the consideration of likelihood ratios, clinical effect, risk and number needed to treat. These statistical tools will help clinicians make clinical decisions under conditions of uncertainty, and will improve the odds of those decisions being correct. In the end, the clinician will integrate information from the literature, his own knowledge, experience and judgment and the patient's preferences to arrive at a decision that uses the evidence to its best advantage.

REFERENCES

1. World Health Organization. Constitution. *WHO Chronicle* 1947;1:29.
2. Molnar D. The prevalence of the metabolic syndrome and type 2 diabetes mellitus in children and adolescents. *Int J Obes Relat Metab Disord* 2004;28 Suppl 3:S70–74.
3. Swanson JG, Kaczorowski J, Skelly J, Finkelstein M. Urinary incontinence: Common problem among women over 45. *Can Fam Physician* 2005;51:84–85.
4. Hardy AM, Allen JR, Morgan WM, Curran JW. The incidence rate of acquired immunodeficiency syndrome in selected populations. *JAMA* 1985;253:215–20.
5. Fraser DW, Tsai TR, Orenstein W, Parkin WE, Beecham HJ, Sharrar RG, et al. Legionnaires' disease: Description of an epidemic of pneumonia. *N Engl J Med* 1977;297: 1189–1197.
6. Tsang KW, Ho PL, Ooi GC, Yee WK, Wang T, Chan-Yeung M, et al. A cluster of cases of severe acute respiratory syndrome in Hong Kong. *N Engl J Med* 2003;348:1977–1985.
7. Brody H, Rip MR, Vinten-Johansen P, Paneth N, Rachman S. Map-making and myth-making in Broad Street: The London cholera epidemic, 1854. *Lancet* 2000;356:64–68.
8. Bentivoglio M, Pacini P. Flippo Pacini: A determined observer. *Brain Res Bull* 1995; 38:161–165.
9. Snow J. *On the Mode of Communication of Cholera*, 2nd ed. London: John Churchill, 1855.

10. John Snow 1813–1858. From BBC Online, 2001. Available at: <http://www.ph.ucla.edu/epi/snow/bbc_snow.htm> Accessed September 25, 2006.

11. One-hundred-fifty year old lessons of John Snow still relevant today. Available at: <http://www.newsroom.msu.edu/site/indexer/2112/content.htm> Accessed September 27, 2006.

12. Jacobsen SJ, Goldberg J, Miles TP, Brody JA, Stiers W, Rimm AA. Seasonal variation in the incidence of hip fracture among white persons aged 65 years and older in the United States, 1984–1987. *Am J Epidemiol* 1991;133:996–1004.

13. Chen CH, Xirasagar S, Lin HC. Seasonality in adult asthma admissions, air pollutant levels, and climate: A population-based study. *J Asthma* 2006;43:287–292.

14. Centers for Disease Control and Prevention. National Center for Health Statistics. Early Release of Selected Estimates from the 2000 and Early 2001 National Health Interview Surveys (9/20/01). Available at: <http://www.cdc.gov/nchs/data/nhis/combined0901.pdf> Accessed on January 8, 2005.

15. Bernard B, Sauter S, Fine L, Petersen M, Hales T. Job task and psychosocial risk factors for work-related musculoskeletal disorders among newspaper employees. *Scand J Work Environ Health* 1994;20:417–426.

16. Burdorf A, Van Der Steenhoven GA, Tromp-Klaren EG. A one-year prospective study on back pain among novice golfers. *Am J Sports Med* 1996;24:659–664.

17. Laden F, Spiegelman D, Neas LM, Colditz GA, Hankinson SE, Manson JE, et al. Geographic variation in breast cancer incidence rates in a cohort of U.S. women. *J Natl Cancer Inst* 1997;89:1373–1378.

18. Khuder SA, Dayal HH, Mutgi AB, Willey JC, Dayal G. Effect of cigarette smoking on major histological types of lung cancer in men. *Lung Cancer* 1998;22:15–21.

19. Bajdik CD, Gallagher RP, Hill GB, Fincham S. Sunlight exposure, hat use, and squamous cell skin cancer on the head and neck. *J Cutan Med Surg* 1998;3:68–73.

20. Paolucci S, Matano A, Bragoni M, et al. Rehabilitation of left brain-damaged ischemic stroke patients: The role of comprehension language deficits. A matched comparison. *Cerebrovasc Dis* 2005;20:400–406.

21. Church TS, LaMonte MJ, Barlow CE, Blair SN. Cardiorespiratory fitness and body mass index as predictors of cardiovascular disease mortality among men with diabetes. *Arch Intern Med* 2005;165:2114–2120.

22. Hoidrup S, Sorensen TI, Stroger U, Lauritzen JB, Schroll M, Gronbaek M. Leisure-time physical activity levels and changes in relation to risk of hip fracture in men and women. *Am J Epidemiol* 2001;154:60–68.

23. Riddle DL, Pulisic M, Pidcoe P, Johnson RE. Risk factors for plantar fasciitis: A matched case-control study. *J Bone Joint Surg Am* 2003;85-A:872–877.

24. Jackson LA, Nelson JC, Benson P, Neuzil KM, Reid RJ, Psaty BM et al. Functional status is a confounder of the association of influenza vaccine and risk of all cause mortality in seniors. *Int J Epidemiol* 2006;35:345–352.

25. Mortimer JA, Borenstein AR. Tools of the epidemiologist. *Alzheimer Dis Assoc Disord* 2006;20(3 Suppl 2):S35–41.

26. Friberg E, Mantzoros CS, Wolk A. Diabetes and risk of endometrial cancer: A population-based prospective cohort study. *Cancer Epidemiol Biomarkers Prev* 2007;16:276–280.

27. Mantel N, Haenszel W. Statistical aspects of the analysis of data from retrospective studies of disease. *JNCI* 1959;22:719–748.

28. Jull G, Trott P, Potter H, Zito G, Niere K, Shirley D, et al. A randomized controlled trial of exercise and manipulative therapy for cervicogenic headache. *Spine* 2002;27:1835–1843.

29. Akobeng AK. Understanding measures of treatment effect in clinical trials. *Arch Dis Child* 2005;90:54–56.

30. Weeks DL, Noteboom JT. Using the number needed to treat in clinical practice. *Arch Phys Med Rehabil* 2004;85:1729–1731.
31. Altman DG. Confidence intervals for the number needed to treat. *BMJ* 1998;317:1309–1312.
32. McQuay HJ, Moore RA. Using numerical results from systematic reviews in clinical practice. *Ann Intern Med* 1997;126:712–720.
33. Edwards JE, Oldman A, Smith L, Collins SL, Carroll D, Wiffen PJ, et al. Single dose oral aspirin for acute pain. *Cochrane Database Syst Rev* 2000:CD002067.
34. Osiri M, Suarez-Almazor ME, Wells GA, Robinson V, Tugwell P. Number needed to treat (NNT): Implication in rheumatology clinical practice. *Ann Rheum Dis* 2003;62:316–321.
35. Black HR, Crocitto MT. Number needed to treat: Solid science or a path to pernicious rationing? *Am J Hypertens* 1998;11:128S–134S; discussion 135S–137S.
36. Collins R, Peto R, MacMahon S, Hebert P, Fiebach NH, Eberlein KA, et al. Blood pressure, stroke, and coronary heart disease. Part 2, Short-term reductions in blood pressure: Overview of randomised drug trials in their epidemiological context. *Lancet* 1990;335:827–838.

CHAPTER 29
Multivariate Analysis

The technological progress of data management systems has provided clinical researchers with a sophisticated statistical framework within which to examine the multifaceted and complex relationships inherent in many clinical phenomena. **Multivariate analysis** refers to a set of statistical procedures that are distinguished by the ability to examine several response variables within a single study and to account for their potential interrelationships in the analysis of the data. These tests are distinguished from **univariate analysis** procedures, such as the *t*-test and analysis of variance, in that univariate methods accommodate only one dependent variable.

Given the types of questions being asked today and the types of data being used to examine clinical procedures, multivariate statistics have become quite important for those who do research and those who read research reports. The purpose of this chapter is to introduce the basic concepts behind several of the most commonly used multivariate methods: partial correlation, multiple regression, logistic regression, discriminant analysis, factor analysis, multivariate analysis of variance and survival analysis.

The application of multivariate procedures necessitates the use of a computer, and may require the assistance of a statistician for more advanced operations. In a short introduction such as this, it is not possible to cover the full scope of these procedures. Therefore, this discussion focuses on a conceptual understanding of multivariate tests and interpretation of the output a computer analysis will generate.

PARTIAL CORRELATION

The product-moment correlation coefficient, r, offers the researcher a simple and easily understood measure of the association between two variables, X and Y. The interpretation of r is limited, however, because it cannot account for the possible influence of other variables on that relationship. For instance, in a study of the relationship between age and length of hospital stay, we might find a correlation of .70, suggesting that older patients tend to have longer hospital stays (as shown by the shaded overlapped portion in Figure 29.1A). If, however, older patients also tend to have greater functional limitations, then the observed relationship between hospital stay and age may actually be the result of their mutual relationship with function; that is, the hospital stay may actually be explained by the patient's functional status. We can resolve this dilemma by looking at the relationship between hospital stay and age with the effect of functional status controlled, using a procedure called partial correlation.

The **partial correlation coefficient** is the correlation between two variables, X and Y, with the effect of a third variable, Z, statistically removed. For instance, in the

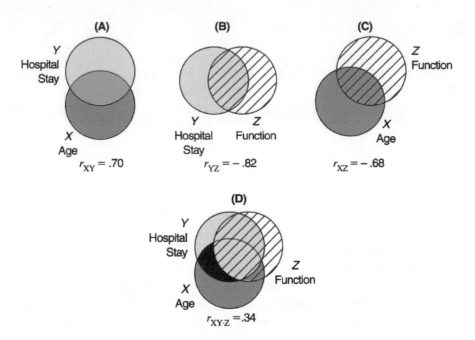

FIGURE 29.1   Representation of partial correlation between hospital stay (Y) and age (X), with the effect of function (Z) removed. In (**A**), (**B**) and (**C**), the simple correlations between each pair of variables are illustrated. In (**D**) the shaded area represents those parts of hospital stay and age that are explained by function. The black area shows the common variance in hospital stay and age that is not related to function, or their partial correlation.

preceding example, assume X is age, Y is hospital stay, and Z is functional status. We would want to know how much of the observed relationship between age and hospital stay (r_{XY}) can be attributed to the confounding influence of function, and how much is purely the relationship between age and hospital stay. The term $r_{XY \cdot Z}$ is used to represent the correlation of X and Y, with the effect of Z eliminated.

For example, suppose we are given the following correlations for a sample of 50 patients:

$$r_{XY} = .70 \text{ (hospital stay with age)}$$

$$r_{XZ} = -.82 \text{ (hospital stay with function)}$$

$$r_{YZ} = -.68 \text{ (function with age)}$$

We "remove" the effect of function from r_{XY} by first determining how much of the variance in both hospital stay and age is explained by function, as shown in Figure 29.1B and C. The overlapped, shaded portions represent the correlation between the two variables. Figure 29.1D shows how these relationships intersect. Once we remove the effect of function, the remaining overlap between hospital stay and age is reduced (the black area in Figure 29.1D). This area represents the relationship between hospital stay and age with the effect of function canceled out. This is the partial correlation.*

For the data in our example, $r_{XY \cdot Z} = .34$. When we compare this partial correlation to the original correlation of X and Y ($r_{XY} = .70$), we can see that age and hospital stay no longer demonstrate as strong a relationship. A large part of the observed association between them could be accounted for by their common relationship with functional status.

The term $r_{XY \cdot Z}$ is called a **first-order partial correlation,** because it represents a correlation with the effect of one variable eliminated. The simple correlation between X and Y is called a **zero-order correlation.** The significance of a first-order partial correlation can be determined by referring to critical values of r in Appendix Table A.4, using $n - 3$ degrees of freedom. Partial correlation can be expanded to control for more than one variable at a time. A *second-order partial correlation* is symbolized by $r_{XY \cdot Z_1 Z_2}$. This value can be checked for significance using Table A.4 with $n - 4$ degrees of freedom. This process can continue with higher order partial correlations.

Partial correlation is a useful analytic tool for eliminating competing explanations for an association, thereby providing a clearer explanation of the true nature of an observed relationship and ruling out extraneous factors.

MULTIPLE REGRESSION

Multiple regression is an extension of simple linear regression analysis, described in Chapter 24. The multiple regression equation allows the researcher to predict the value $\hat{Y}$ using a set of several independent variables. It can accommodate continuous and categorical independent variables, which may be naturally occurring or experimentally manipulated. The dependent variable, Y, must be a continuous measure. A common purpose of regression analysis is prognostic, predicting a given outcome based on identified factors. For instance, Stineman and Williams[1] developed a model to predict rehabilitation length of stay based on the patient's admitting diagnosis, referral source and admission functional status. A second purpose of regression is to better understand a clinical phenomenon by identifying those factors associated with it. To illustrate this application, Walker and Sofaer[2] studied sources of psychological distress in patients attending pain clinics. They identified that 60% of the variance associated with psychological distress was explained by a combination of fears about the future, regrets about the past, age, practical help, feeling unoccupied and personal relationship problems. This type of analysis will often present opportunities for the analysis of theoretical components of constructs.

The Regression Equation

Recall that the regression equation, $\hat{Y} = a + bX$, defines a line that can be used to make predictions, with an inherent degree of random error. This error, or **residual variance**, represents variance in Y that is not explained by the predictor variable, X. For example,

---

*The partial correlation coefficient is calculated using the formula $r_{XY \cdot Z} = \dfrac{(r_{XY} - r_{XZ} r_{YZ})}{\sqrt{[1 - r_{XZ}^2][1 - r_{YZ}^2]}}$

suppose we were interested in predicting cholesterol level using body weight as the independent variable, with $r = .48$ and $r^2 = .23$. Based on the limited strength of this relationship, we would expect that a regression equation would provide estimates of cholesterol that would be different from actual values, as body weight by itself does not adequately explain cholesterol level. Therefore, the remaining unexplained variance in cholesterol (77%) must be a function of other factors. For instance, cholesterol may also be related to variables such as blood pressure, gender, age, weight or diet. If we were to add these variables to the regression equation, the unexplained portion of variance would probably be decreased (although not necessarily completely). This expanded analysis results in a **multiple regression equation.**

In multiple regression, the regression equation accommodates multiple predictor variables:

$$\hat{Y} = a + b_1X_1 + b_2X_2 + b_3X_3 + \ldots + b_kX_k \qquad (29.1)$$

where $\hat{Y}$ is the predicted value for the dependent variable, a is a **regression constant**, and b_1, b_2, b_3 through b_k are **regression coefficients** for each independent variable. The subscript, k, denotes the number of independent variables in the equation.[†] Like simple linear regression, multiple regression is also based on the concept of least squares, so that the model minimizes deviations of $\hat{Y}$ from Y.

Once regression coefficients and a constant are obtained, we can predict values of $\hat{Y}$ by substituting values for each independent variable in the equation. For instance, suppose we wanted to evaluate the predictive relationship between serum blood cholesterol (CHOL) and potential contributing factors including age (AGE), daily dietary fat intake in grams (DIET), gender (GENDER), systolic blood pressure (SBP), and weight (WT). Table 29.1A shows the intercorrelations among these variables. The coefficients for the regression equation are shown in Table 29.1B❹, including the constant:

$$\hat{Y} = 19.116 + .012(\text{AGE}) + 3.094\,(\text{DIET}) + .218\,(\text{SBP}) + 4.158\,(\text{GENDER}) + .511\,(\text{WT})$$

Based on this equation, for a 34-year-old subject, with DIET = 20.0 g, GENDER = 1 (coded for male), SBP = 100 mmHg and WT = 150 pounds, we can predict cholesterol value as follows:

$$\text{CHOL} = 19.116 + .012(34) + 3.094(20.0) + .218(100) + 4.158(1) + .511(150) = 184.01$$

If this person's true cholesterol level was 175, the residual would be $175 - 184.01 = -9.01\ (Y - \hat{Y})$. Scatter plots can also be requested to analyze the residuals, typically plotting the predicted values on the X-axis against the residuals on the Y-axis. Visual analysis of residuals can reveal if the assumption of linearity in the data is violated (see Chapter 24, Figure 24.6).

[†]The number of independent variables included in the regression equation is effectively limited by the sample size. Power analysis can be done to estimate the number of subjects that would be needed to identify a significant effect, based on the number of independent variables in the equation. See Appendix C.

TABLE 29.1 **OUTPUT FOR MULTIPLE REGRESSION ANALYSIS: PREDICTION OF CHOLESTEROL LEVEL FROM AGE, DIET, BLOOD PRESSURE, GENDER AND WEIGHT ($N = 100$)**

A. CORRELATIONS

		Chol	Age	Diet	SBP	Gender	WT
CHOL	Pearson r	1.000	.063	.634	.109	.000	.481
	Sig (2-tailed)		❶ .266	.000	.140	.500	.000
AGE	Pearson r		1.000	.121	−.125	.125	.010
	Sig (2-tailed)			.116	.108	.108	.462
DIET	Pearson r			1.000	.099	−.039	−.207
	Sig (2-tailed)				.164	.351	.019
SBP	Pearson r				1.000	.011	−.005
	Sig (2-tailed)					.455	.482
GENDER	Pearson r					1.000	−.038
	Sig (2-tailed)						.353

B. REGRESSION OUTPUT

Model Summary

Model	R	R Square	Adjusted R Square	Std. Error of the Estimate
1	.731	❷ .534	❸ .509	42.613

ANOVA

Model	Sum of Squares	df	Mean Square	F	Sig.
1 Regression	195314.30	5	39062.86	21.512	.000
Residual	170691.00	94	1815.86		
Total	366005.30	99			

Coefficients

Model	Unstandardized Coefficients ❹ B	Std. Error	Standardized Coefficients ❺ Beta	❻ t	Sig.
1 (Constant)	19.116	41.817		.457	.649
AGE	❼ 1.150E-02	.313	.003	.037	.971
DIET	3.094	.410	.553	7.549	.000
SBP	.218	.276	.056	.788	.433
GENDER	4.158	8.612	.034	.483	.630
WT	.511	.100	.368	5.107	.000

❶ Two-tailed significance level for each correlation coefficient is shown as the second value in each cell.

❷ R^2 value for multiple regression equation.

❸ Adjusted R^2 for multiple regression equation.

❹ Regression coefficients for each variable in the equation.

❺ Standardized regression coefficients (beta weights).

❻ Test of significance of regression coefficients for each independent variable. Values for the constant are ignored.

❼ The designation E indicates an exponent. A positive exponent moves the decimal place to the right; a negative exponent moves the decimal place to the left. In this case, the decimal place will be moved two places to the left. Therefore, for AGE $B = 0.0115$.

Regression coefficients are interpreted as *weights* that identify how much each variable contributes to the explanation of Y. As part of the regression analysis, a test of significance is performed on each regression coefficient, to test the null hypothesis, $H_0: b = 0$. Depending on the statistical package this will be done using either an F-test or a t-test, as shown in Table 29.1B❻. In this example, the coefficients for AGE, GENDER and SBP are not significant ($p > .05$). Therefore, these three variables are not making a significant contribution to the prediction of cholesterol level.

Standardized Regression Coefficients

Researchers often want to establish the relative importance of specific variables within a regression equation. The regression coefficients cannot be directly compared for this purpose because they are based on different units of measurement. When it is of interest to determine which variables are more heavily weighted, we must convert the weights to standardized regression coefficients, called **beta weights**. These standardized values are interpreted as relative weights, indicating how much each variable contributes to the value of $\hat{Y}$. For example, the beta weights listed in Table 29.1B❺ show that DIET and WT are the most important variables for predicting cholesterol. The sign of the beta weight indicates the positive or negative relationship between each variable and Y, but only the absolute value is considered in determining the relative weight. Some authors present beta weights in addition to regression coefficients in a research report, to provide the reader with a full and practical interpretation of the observed relationships.

Multicolinearity

A problem occurs in the interpretation of beta weights if the independent variables in the regression equation are correlated with each other. This situation is called **multicolinearity.** The coefficients assigned to variables within the equation are based on the assumption that each variable provides independent information, contributing a unique part of the total explanation of the variance in Y. If independent variables are related to each other, the information they provide to the model is partially redundant. In that case, one variable may be seen as contributing a lot of information, and the second variable may be seen as contributing little; that is, one variable may have a larger beta weight. Each variable may be highly predictive of Y when used alone, but they are redundant when used together. This situation can be avoided by determining the intercorrelations among predictor variables prior to running a regression analysis and selecting independent variables that are not highly correlated with each other.

The interpretation of multicolinearity is based on the concept of partial correlation; that is, each regression coefficient represents the importance of a single variable after having accounted for the effect of all other variables in the equation. Therefore, the value of a regression coefficient is dependent on which other independent variables are in the equation. With different combinations of variables, it is likely that a particular regression coefficient will vary. It is important to remember, therefore, that the relationships defined by a regression equation can be interpreted only within the context of the specific variables included in that equation.

Accuracy of Prediction

The overall association between Y and the complete set of independent variables is defined by the **multiple correlation coefficient, R.** This value will range from 0.00 to 1.00; however, because R represents the cumulative association of many variables, its interpretation is obscure. Therefore, its square (R^2) is used more often as an explanation of the functional relationship between Y and a series of X values.

As an analogue of r^2, the value of R^2 represents the proportion of the total variance in Y that is explained by the set of independent variables in the equation; that is, it is the *variance attributable to the regression*. R^2 is the statistic most often reported in journal articles to indicate the accuracy of prediction of a regression analysis. Higher values of R^2 reflect stronger prediction models. The complement, $1 - R^2$, is the proportion of the variance that is left unexplained, or the variance attributable to deviations from the regression. Table 29.1B❷ shows that $R^2 = .534$ for the cholesterol analysis, indicating that this group of variables accounts for slightly more than half of the variance in cholesterol.

An *adjusted* R^2 is also generated for the regression (Table 29.1B❸). This value represents a chance-corrected value for R^2; that is, we can expect some percent of explained variance to be a function of chance. Some researchers prefer to report the adjusted value as a more accurate reflection of the strength of the regression, especially with a large number of variables in the equation.

Many regression programs will also generate a value for the **standard error of the estimate (SEE),** as shown in Table 29.1B. This value represents the degree of variability in the data around the multidimensional "regression line," reflecting the prediction accuracy of the equation (see Chapter 24 for discussion of the SEE).

Analysis of Variance of Regression

A multiple regression analysis generates an analysis of variance to test the linear fit of the equation. The ANOVA partitions the total variance in the data into the variance that is explained by the regression and that part that is left unexplained, or the residual error. The degrees of freedom associated with the regression will equal k, where k represents the number of independent variables in the equation. The probability of F associated with the regression will indicate if the equation provides an explanation of Y that is better than chance. The ANOVA in Table 29.1B demonstrates a significant model for the cholesterol data ($F = 21.512, p < .001$).

Stepwise Multiple Regression

Multiple regression can be run by "forcing" a set of variables into the equation, as we have done in the cholesterol example. With all five variables included, the equation accounted for 53% of the variance in cholesterol values, although the results demonstrated that the four independent variables did not all make significant contributions to that estimate. We might ask, then, if the level of prediction accuracy achieved in this analysis could have been achieved with fewer variables. To answer this question, we can use a procedure called **stepwise multiple regression**, which uses specific statistical criteria to retain or eliminate variables to maximize prediction accuracy with the smallest number of predictors. It is not unusual to find that only a few independent variables will explain almost as much of the variation in the dependent variable as can be explained by a larger number of variables. This approach is useful for honing in on those variables that make the most valuable contribution to a given relationship, thereby creating an economical model.

Stepwise regression is accomplished in "steps" by evaluating the contribution of each independent variable in sequential fashion.[‡] First, all proposed independent variables are correlated with the dependent variable, and the one variable with the highest correlation is entered into the equation at step 1. For our cholesterol example, Table 29.1A shows us that DIET has the highest correlation with CHOL ($r = .634$). Therefore, DIET will be entered on the first step. With this variable alone, $R^2 = .401$ (see Table 29.2❷). The regression coefficients for this first step are shown in Table 29.2❸:

$$\hat{Y} = 121.65 + 3.55(\text{DIET})$$

At this point, the remaining variables (those "excluded" from the equation) are examined for their partial correlation with Y, that is, their correlation with CHOL with the effect of DIET removed (see Table 29.2❹). The variable with the highest significant partial correlation coefficient is then added to the equation, in this case, WT (partial $r = .462, p = .000$). Therefore, WT is added in step 2 (see Table 29.2❺). With the addition of this variable, we have achieved an R^2 of .529 (see Table 29.2❻), only slightly lower than the value obtained with the full model. The adjusted R^2 is higher, however, because there are fewer variables in this model.

Another criterion for entry of a variable is its **tolerance level**. Tolerance refers to the degree of colinearity in the data. Tolerance ranges from 0.00, indicating that the variable is perfectly correlated with the variables already entered, to 1.00, which means that the other variables are not related (see Table 29.2❼). The higher the tolerance, the more new information a variable will contribute to the equation. Some computer programs will automatically generate tolerance levels for each variable. Others offer options that must be specifically requested to include tolerance values (colinearity statistics) in the printout.

The stepwise regression continues, adding a new variable at each successive step of the analysis if it meets certain *inclusion criteria*; that is, its partial correlation is highest

---

[‡]Stepwise procedures may be classified as *stepwise, forward* or *backward* inclusion. Forward inclusion means that the model starts with no variables, and adds variables one by one until the inclusion criterion is satisfied. This procedure is differentiated from stepwise regression in many statistical programs. While both proceed using a forward selection method, adding a new variable at each step, the stepwise procedure can also remove a variable at any step, if that variable no longer contributes significantly to the model, given the current variables in the equation. The procedure will specify a significance criterion to enter variables as well as to remove them. In the backward inclusion method, the model starts with all variables in the equation, and partial correlations are calculated as if each one were the last variable to be entered. Using criteria for removal, the variable with the smallest partial correlation is taken out. Steps proceed until no remaining variables are qualified for removal.

TABLE 29.2 OUTPUT FOR STEPWISE MULTIPLE REGRESSION ANALYSIS: PREDICTION OF CHOLESTEROL

Variables Entered/Removed[a]

Model	Variables Entered	Variables Removed	Method
1	DIET ❶		. Stepwise
2	DIET, WT ❺		. Stepwise

[a] Dependent variable: CHOL

Model Summary

Model	R	R Square	Adjusted R Square	Std. Error of the Estimate
1	.634	❷ .401	.395	47.285
2	.728	❻ .529	.520	42.145

ANOVA

Model	Sum of Squares	df	Mean Square	F	Sig.
1 Regression	146890.940	1	146890.940	65.698	.000
Residual	219114.370	98	2235.861		
Total	366005.30	99			
2 Regression	193715.449	2	96857.724	54.531	.000
Residual	172289.861	97	1776.184		
Total	366005.310	99			

Coefficients

Model	Unstandardized Coefficients B	Unstandardized Coefficients Std. Error	Standardized Coefficients Beta	t	Sig.
1 (Constant)	❸ 121.654	12.378		9.829	.000
DIET	3.547	.438	.634	8.105	.000
2 (Constant)	❽ 48.210	18.064		2.669	.009
DIET	3.122	.399	.558	7.831	.000
WT	.508	.099	.366	5.134	.000

Excluded Variables

Model	Beta In	t	Sig.	Partial Correlation	Collinearity Statistics ❼ Tolerance
1 AGE	−.014	−.173	.863	−.018	.985
SBP	.047	.599	.550	.061	.990
GENDER	.024	.311	.756	.032	.999
WT	.366	5.134	.000	❹ .462	.957
2 AGE	−.001	−0.11	.991	❾ −.001	.984
SBP	.057	.806	.422	.082	.990
GENDER	.036	.507	.613	.052	.998

❶ DIET is entered on the first step. ❷ The R^2 associated with DIET is .401.
❸ The regression equation with only DIET entered is $\hat{Y} = 121.854 + 3.547(DIET)$.
❹ Of the remaining variables, WT has the highest (and only significant) partial correlation with CHOL.
❺ WT are entered on the second step. ❻ The R^2 with DIET and WT added is now .529.
❼ Collinearilty statistics show that WT has the lowest tolerance, indicating it has the least redundancy with DIET of the remaining variables.
❽ In step 2 WT is added. The regression equation is now $\hat{Y} = 48.210 + 3.122(DIET) + 0.508(WT)$.
❾ After step 2, there are no additional significant partial correlations. The regression stops.

of all remaining variables, and the test of its regression coefficient is significant. This process continues until, at some point, either all variables have been entered or the addition of more variables will not significantly improve the prediction accuracy of the model. In the current example, Table 29.2❸ shows us that none of the partial correlations of the remaining three variables is significant. Therefore, no further variables were entered after step 2. As shown in Table 29.2❹, the final model for the stepwise regression is

$$\hat{Y} = 48.21 + 3.12(\text{DIET}) + .508(\text{WT})$$

Note that the coefficients in the equation have changed with the addition of WT as a variable. There are times when no variables will be entered if none of them satisfy the minimal inclusion criteria. In that case, the researcher must search for a new set of independent variables to explain the dependent variable.

Dummy Variables

One of the general assumptions for regression analysis is that variables are continuous; however, many of the variables that may be useful predictors for a regression analysis, such as gender, occupation, education and race, or behavioral characteristics such as smoker versus nonsmoker, are measured on a categorical scale. It is possible to include such qualitative variables in a regression equation, although the numbers assigned to categories cannot be treated as quantitative scores. One way to do this is to create a set of coded variables called **dummy variables**.

In statistics, **coding** is the process of assigning numerals to represent categorical or group membership. For regression analysis we use 0 and 1 to code for the absence and presence of a dichotomous variable, respectively. All dummy variables are dichotomous. For example, with a variable such as smoker–nonsmoker, we code $0 = \text{nonsmoker}$ and $1 = \text{smoker}$. For sex, we can code male $= 0$ and female $= 1$. In essence we are coding 1 for female and 0 for anyone who is not female. We can use these codes as scores in a regression equation and treat them as interval data.

For instance, we could include gender as a predictor of cholesterol level, to determine if men or women can be expected to have higher cholesterol levels. Assume the following regression equation was obtained:

$$\hat{Y} = 220 - 27.5X$$

Using the dummy code for females, $\hat{Y} = 220 - 27.5(1) = 194.5$, and for males $\hat{Y} = 220 - 27.5(0) = 220$. With only this one dummy variable, these predicted values are actually the means for cholesterol for females and males. The regression coefficient for X is the difference between the means for the groups coded 0 and 1.

When a qualitative variable has more than two categories, more than one dummy variable is required to represent it. For example, consider the variable of college class, with four levels: freshman, sophomore, junior and senior. We could code these categories with the numbers 1 through 4 on an apparent ordinal scale; however, these numerical values would not make sense in a regression equation, because the numbers have no quantitative meaning. A senior is not four times more of something than a freshman. Therefore, we must create a dichotomous dummy variable for each category, as follows:

$$X_1 = 1 \text{ if a freshman}$$
$$0 \text{ if not a freshman}$$
$$X_2 = 1 \text{ if a sophomore}$$
$$0 \text{ if not a sophomore}$$
$$X_3 = 1 \text{ if a junior}$$
$$0 \text{ if not a junior}$$

Each variable codes for the presence or absence of a specific class membership. We do not need to create a fourth variable for seniors, because anyone who has zero for all three variables will be a senior. We can show how this works by defining each class with a unique combination of values for X_1, X_2 and X_3:

	X_1	X_2	X_3
Freshman	1	0	0
Sophomore	0	1	0
Junior	0	0	1
Senior	0	0	0

The number of dummy variables needed to define a categorical variable will always be one less than the number of categories.

Suppose we wanted to predict a student's attitude toward the disabled, on a scale of 0 to 100, based on class membership. We might develop an equation such as

$$\hat{Y} = 85 - 55X_1 - 25X_2 - 15X_3$$

Therefore, the predicted values for each class would be

Freshman: $\hat{Y} = 85 - 55(1) - 25(0) - 15(0) = 30$

Sophomore: $\hat{Y} = 85 - 55(0) - 25(1) - 15(0) = 60$

Junior: $\hat{Y} = 85 - 55(0) - 25(0) - 15(1) = 70$

Senior: $\hat{Y} = 85 - 55(0) - 25(0) - 15(0) = 85$

Several dummy variables can be combined with quantitative variables in a regression equation. Because so many variables of interest are measured at the nominal level, the use of dummy variables provides an important mechanism for creating a fuller explanation of clinical phenomena. Some computer programs will automatically generate dummy codes for nominal variables. For others, the researcher must develop the coding scheme.

LOGISTIC REGRESSION

Many questions of prediction or explanation involve outcomes that are categorical. For example, we might ask why some individuals experience recurrent falls. VanSwearingen et al[3] identified mobility and functional characteristics that could predict whether a person did or did not have a history of falls. We might look for factors related to whether or not a patient returns to work following rehabilitation. Cifu et al[4] examined several measures of physical and psychological function as predictors of successful return to work one year after traumatic brain injury. These examples illustrate the application of **logistic regression**, where the dependent variable has only two values—the occurrence or nonoccurrence of a particular event, or the presence or absence of a condition, typically coded 0 and 1.[§] We cannot use multiple regression for this purpose, as a categorical dependent variable cannot meet the assumption of a normal distribution (see Chapter 24, Figure 24.5). The independent variables in logistic regression may be continuous, ordinal or categorical. Logistic regression can be run using a full set of independent variables, or it may be run using a stepwise procedure.

The Logistic Regression Model

In logistic regression, rather than predicting the value of an outcome variable, we are actually predicting the probability of an event occurring. Using the regression equation, we determine if the independent variables can predict whether an individual is likely to belong to the group coded 0 (the reference group) or the group coded 1 (the target group). Consider the following hypothetical example. Suppose we wanted to predict the discharge disposition for patients following rehabilitation, as either "return to home" (coded 0) or "long-term care" (coded 1). We would like to set appropriate goals and begin suitable discharge planning as soon as possible, and we would like to determine if characteristics upon admission will be useful predictors of discharge status. We will use the following variables, coded as present (1) or absent (0), except for age, which is continuous:

Functional status	ADL	0 = independent; 1 = limited
Age	AGE	Continuous
Marital status	MAR	0 = married; 1 = not married
Gender	GENDER	0 = male; 1 = female

We will examine data from 100 patients, 46 of whom went to long term care (LTC). The statistical question is: What is the likelihood that an individual will be discharged to LTC given this combination of factors? The results of a logistic regression for these variables are shown in Table 29.3.

[§]Logistic regression can be used when the outcome variable has more than two categories, an approach that is beyond the scope of this text.

TABLE 29.3 **OUTPUT FOR LOGISTIC REGRESSION ANALYSIS: RISK FACTORS ASSOCIATED WITH DISCHARGE DISPOSITION IN ELDERLY PATIENTS ($N = 100$)**

Classification Table[a] ❶

			Predicted		
			Discharge		**Percentage Correct**
	Observed		**Home**	**LTC**	
Step 1	**Discharge** **Home**		46	8	85.19
	LTC		9	37	80.43
	Overall Percentage				83.00

[a] The cut value is .50

Variables in the Equation

	❷ B	SE	df	❸ Sig.	❹ Exp(B)	❺ 95% CI for Exp(B) Lower	Upper
ADL	2.384	.656	1	.0003	10.848	3.000	39.192
AGE	.104	.046	1	.0236	1.110	1.014	1.215
MAR	2.935	.662	1	.0000	18.822	5.147	68.808
GENDER	−.018	.642	1	.9778	.982	.279	3.459
Constant	−11.167	3.984	1	.0051			

❶ Classification results compare predicted outcomes using the logistic regression to actual observed results (see Figure 29.2).
❷ Regression coefficients for each variable in the logistic regression.
❸ Significance levels (*p*) for each regression coefficient.
❹ Odds ratios associated with each variable, based on the exponent of the regression coefficient.
❺ Confidence intervals for the odds ratios. If the null value of 1.0 is contained within the interval, the odds ratio is not considered significant. Only GENDER is not significant.

The Logistic Function

We can think of the **logistic function** as a linear combination of these variables, similar to the linear regression equation. The likelihood of the predicted outcome is based on the odds of being discharged to LTC, or more accurately, the logarithm of the odds:

$$Z = a + b_1X_1 + b_2X_2 + b_3X_3 + b_4X_4 + b_5X_5 \qquad (29.2)$$

where Z is the natural logarithm of the odds, called a **logit**, a is a regression constant, and b is the regression coefficient. Even though we are using a different mathematical base (logarithms), this equation is conceptually the same as the multiple regression equation—but with two major differences. First, the dependent variable (the logit) is a dichotomous outcome, resulting in prediction of group membership. Second, where multiple regression uses the least squares criterion for finding the equation with the smallest residuals, logistic regression uses the concept of **maximum likelihood**, which means that the equation will present the "most likely" solution that demonstrates the best odds of achieving accurate prediction of group membership.

Coefficients for the logistic regression for our discharge status question are shown in Table 29.3❷ This logistic regression equation would, therefore, be written:

$$Z = -11.167 + 2.384(ADL) + .104(AGE) + 2.935(MAR) - .018(GENDER)$$

Predicted Probabilities

We can use the coefficients in the logistic regression equation to predict the probability that an individual belongs to the target group, as follows:

$$\text{Probability} = \frac{e^z}{1 + e^z} \quad \text{or} \quad \frac{1}{1 + e^{-z}} \tag{29.3}$$

where e is the base of the natural logarithm.** The probability associated with the outcome will be 0 if the subject is discharged home, and 1 if long-term care. We can expect, however, that the logistic regression will yield probabilities between 0 and 1. A value closer to 1.0 (above .5) will suggest a probability in favor of discharge to long-term care, and a value closer to zero (below .5) would predict that this event is not likely to occur; that is, the subject is likely to be discharged home. A probability of .5 would mean that the individual has an equal likelihood of either outcome.

When this model is applied to an individual's data, we obtain the probability of that individual being discharged to long-term care. Consider, for example, a subject who ultimately was discharged to LTC, who had the following scores: ADL = 1, AGE = 78, MAR = 1 and GENDER = 0,

$$Z = -11.167 + 2.384(1) + .104(78) + 2.935(1) - .018(0) = 2.264$$

Therefore,[††]

$$\text{Probability (discharge to LTC)} = \frac{e^{2.264}}{1 + e^{2.264}} \quad \text{or} \quad \frac{1}{1 + e^{-2.264}} = .91$$

Using this model, we would have correctly predicted that this individual would be discharged to LTC, as the probability is greater than .5.

Let's look at another example for a subject who was also discharged to LTC, with the following data: ADL = 1, AGE = 80, MAR = 0, and GENDER = 0:

$$Z = -11.167 + 2.384(1) + 2.935(0) - .018(0) + .104(80) = -0.463$$

[**]Find the key marked e^x on your scientific calculator.
[††]The value $e^{2.264} = 9.62$ and $e^{-2.264} = .104$.

Therefore,

$$\text{Probability (discharge to LTC)} = \frac{e^{-0.463}}{1 + e^{-0.463}} \text{ or } \frac{1}{1 + e^{-(-0.463)}} = .39$$

We would incorrectly predict that this individual would be discharged home because the probability is less than .5.

A histogram helps us visually understand how these predictions are interpreted. In Figure 29.2 we see such a graph of the predictions for subjects in this example, where the symbol "0" represents those who were actually discharged home, and the symbol "1" represents those who went to long-term care. The X axis shows the predicted probabilities associated with each individual's scores. In this instance, probabilities above .5 are assigned to group 1, whereas probabilities of .5 or below are assigned to the group coded 0. Therefore, on the left half of the graph we can see that nine of those who actually went to long-term care (coded 1) were predicted to go home, whereas on the right half we find that eight of those who went home (coded 0) were predicted to go to long-term care. These incorrect classifications are shaded on the graph. Classification results are also given in Table 29.3❶. A total of 83% of the sample was correctly classified using this logistic model. Over 80% of those who actually went to long-term care (1) were

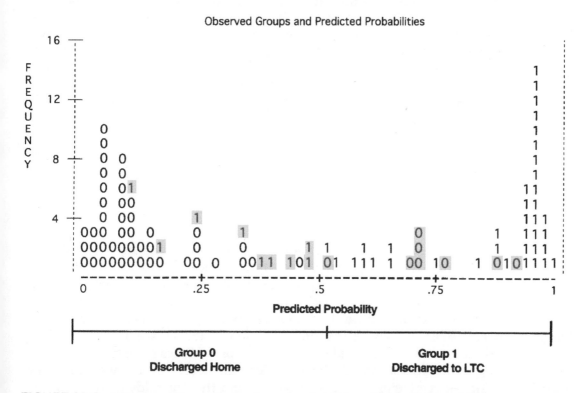

FIGURE 29.2 Histogram (*N* = 100) of estimated probabilities of being discharged home (0) versus discharged to long term care (1), derived from logistic regression. Each symbol represents one subject. Shaded symbols represent misclassifications using a cutoff score of .50. (*Histogram obtained using SPSS 8.0 logistic regression procedure.*)

correctly classified; approximately 85% of those who went home (0) were correctly assigned using the logistic regression model.

The histogram also allows us to see the effect of using this model and the consequences of misclassification. For instance, in this example we can see that most of the misclassifications occur in the region around .5. In setting discharge plans, we might want to reserve judgment for this group. We would be more confident, however, in setting up home discharge plans for those with probabilities below .25, and similarly confident in securing a bed in a skilled nursing facility for those with probabilities above .75.

The Odds Ratio

It is generally more useful to interpret regression coefficients in terms of *odds* rather than probability. Odds tell us how much more likely it is that an individual belongs to the target group than the reference group. If the odds are 1.00, then either outcome is equally likely. With odds greater than 1.00, the individual is more likely to belong to the target group; conversely, with odds less than 1.00, the individual is more likely to belong to the reference group.

The **odds ratio** is used to estimate the odds of membership in the target group, given the presence of specific independent variables (see Chapter 28 for discussion of the odds ratio). The regression coefficient in the equation is the logarithm of the odds for each independent variable. Therefore, an odds ratio can be computed for each variable by using the regression coefficient as the exponent of e (see Table 29.3❹). For a subject who is limited in ADL (ADL = 1), the odds of going to LTC are $e^{2.384} = 10.848$. This number represents the odds of going to LTC with a one-unit change in the value of X. With a dichotomous variable, this means that an individual who is limited in ADL is almost 11 times more likely to go LTC as compared to one who is independent (a change from 0 to 1 for ADL). Confidence intervals can also be determined for each odds ratio (see Table 29.3❺). A significant odds ratio will not contain the null value, 1.0, within the confidence interval. We can see that this is true for the odds ratios associated with ADL and MARital status.

Adjusted Odds Ratio

When the logistic regression equation includes several independent variables, as in our example, each odds ratio is actually corrected for the influence of the other variables. Just as independent variables in multiple regression exhibit colinearity, independent variables with logistic regression will affect each other. This is an important consideration for prediction models. For instance, if we were to look at the simple association between discharge status and ADL, we would find an odds ratio of 15.909 (see Table 29.4). This means that individuals who are limited in ADL are almost 16 times more likely to be discharged to long-term care than those who are independent. However, if we look at the results of the logistic regression in Table 29.3❹, we find that the odds ratio associated with ADL is 10.848. This discrepancy is a function of the other variables in the equation; that is, the odds ratio for ADL is *adjusted* for the influence of the other factors. Therefore, the odds ratios shown in Table 29.3❹ are considered **adjusted odds ratios.**

TABLE 29.4 **ODDS RATIO (OR) ASSOCIATED WITH DISCHARGE STATUS AND FUNCTIONAL INDEPENDENCE (ADL)**

ADL		Discharge		TOTAL
		Long-Term Care (1)	Home (0)	
Limited	(1)	35	9	44
Independent	(0)	11	45	56
	TOTAL	54	46	100

$$OR = \frac{ad}{bc} = \frac{(35)(45)}{(9)(11)} = 15.909$$

Continuous Variables

When an independent variable is continuous, the interpretation of logistic regression is more complex. Consider the effect of AGE on discharge status, with an odds ratio of 1.11. Remember that an odds ratio of 1.0 indicates that either outcome is equally likely. Because the odds ratio relates to the relative increase in odds with a one-unit increase in X, we can interpret this value as the odds associated with a 1-year difference in age, such as from 87 to 88, or any other 1-year difference. Therefore, with a 1-year difference in age, the odds of going home or to long-term care are essentially even. As the unit difference increases, however, we must multiply the regression coefficient for age (B = .104, Table 29.3❷) to obtain the odds ratio. With a 2-year difference in age, then, we determine the odds ratio by $e^{(2\times.104)} = 1.23$. Not much of a change. To determine the odds related to a 10-year difference in age, we find $e^{(10\times.104)} = 2.83$. Now the odds of going to long-term care are almost three times greater for someone who is 80 as compared to someone who is 70, or for someone who is 75 compared to someone who is 65. Many researchers choose to categorize continuous variables to simplify this interpretation.

Presentation of Results

The presentation of results from a logistic regression will depend on the research question. In many research situations, the investigator is actually interested in one particular variable, but wants to control for potential confounders. Using our discharge study, we might be specifically interested in the effect of function on discharge status, but we would want to account for the influence of demographic factors. In that case we might report that the odds ratio for ADL was 10.848, adjusted for age, marital status and gender.

Alternatively, we could approach this analysis using a broader question, asking which of these four factors is related to discharge status. For this approach, we would summarize results, suggesting that ADL and MARital status are most influential in predicting discharge status, adjusted for age and gender. In addition to the increased likelihood of going to LTC if the patient is functionally limited, those who are not married are almost 19 times more likely to be sent to LTC than those who are married.

Another consideration in presenting results is the significance associated with each independent variable. In the current example, only ADL and MARital status have significant regression coefficients (Table 29.3❸). Some authors will present coefficients and odds ratios for all independent variables, regardless of their significance. Others will provide odds ratios only for significant variables.

DISCRIMINANT ANALYSIS

Discriminant analysis is another analogue of multiple regression, also used when the dependent variable is categorical. It is a technique for distinguishing between two or more groups based on a set of characteristics that are predictors of group membership. Based on the equation generated by the discriminant analysis, subjects are classified according to their scores, and the model is then examined to see if the classifications were correct. Discriminant analysis has an important distinction from logistic regression, in that the independent variables are assumed to be normally distributed, and variances are assumed to be equal across groups. Dichotomous independent variables can be used, but with a mixture of continuous and dichotomous variables, discriminant analysis may be less than optimal.

The ability to classify individuals into distinct groups can be useful in many areas of clinical and behavioral science, for purposes of prevention, evaluation, screening, and diagnosis. For example, Ermer and Dunn[5] studied three groups of children: with autism, attention deficit disorder and without disabilities. The researchers conducted a discriminant analysis to determine if these groups could be differentiated on the basis of their scores on nine factors of a Sensory Profile. Nearly 90 percent of the cases were correctly classified using the resulting model, supporting its validity.

The discriminant analysis develops a statistical model, called a **discriminant function,** that will allow us to describe the existing groups and to assign new individuals to a group when it is not known to which group they belong. Discriminant analysis can be performed using a fixed set of variables or in a stepwise manner to reduce the discriminant function to a minimum of relevant variables.

To demonstrate this process, consider a hypothetical example in which we are interested in distinguishing between athletes who are likely to sustain an injury over the course of a season (designated group 1) versus those who will remain uninjured (designated group 0). Using a group of athletes from one school, we will consider overall strength, flexibility, balance and time in play as risk factors. To illustrate these relationships, consider only the first two variables for a moment. In Figure 29.3 we have plotted scores representing strength (Y) and flexibility (X) for injured and noninjured groups. In Figure 29.3A, the variables clearly discriminate between the groups, with those who were not injured demonstrating greater strength and flexibility; however, even with this degree of separation, we can see that discrimination will not be totally accurate because there is some overlap between the groups. Figure 29.3B represents a different situation, where there is much less differentiation between the groups, and it is likely that the independent variables would not be successful in distinguishing between them. When we incorporate many more variables into the analysis, we cannot visualize discrimination in a two-dimensional plot, but we can extend this illustration conceptually to visualize the discrimination between groups in multiple planes.

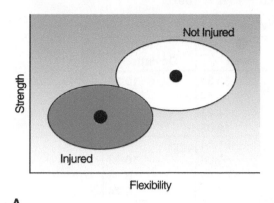
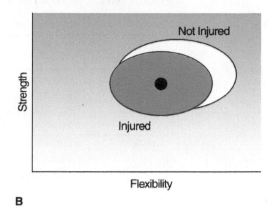

A   **B**

FIGURE 29.3   Basis for discriminant analysis. In **A**, groups are different in levels of strength and flexibility. In **B**, the variables do not discriminate between the groups.

The Discriminant Function

Any number of predictor variables can be used to develop the **discriminant function**, which is analogous to the multiple regression prediction equation. The equation takes the form:

$$D = a + d_1X_1 + d_2X_2 + d_3X_3 + \ldots + d_kX_k \tag{29.4}$$

where D is the *discriminant score*, a is a constant, d is the *discriminant function coefficient*, and k is the number of predictor variables in the equation. The discriminant score for each subject is calculated by substituting scores for each predictor variable into the equation (see Table 29.5❺). The purpose of the discriminant function is to determine the linear combination of variables that makes the groups as statistically distinct as possible; that is, it provides maximum discrimination between the groups. Discriminant function coefficients are often expressed as *standardized coefficients*, without a constant in the equation, similar to a beta weight in linear regression.

When more than two criterion groups are used, discriminant analysis becomes more complex, necessitating the development of more than one discriminant function. With k groups, we will require $k - 1$ discriminant functions. For example, in the study by Ermer and Dunn,[5] where three groups were used, two discriminant functions were generated, one distinguishing normal children from the two disabled groups, and the second distinguishing the two disabled groups from each other.

The ability of the discriminant function to distinguish between groups can be assessed in several ways. The statistics associated with the equation are shown in Table 29.5. An **eigenvalue** (see Table 29.5❷) is a measure of variance, indicating how well the discriminant function discriminates between the groups; the higher the eigenvalue, the greater the discrimination.[‡‡] This value is difficult to interpret, however, as it has no

---

[‡‡]An eigenvalue is analogous to an F ratio, the ratio of the between-groups sum of squares to the within-groups sum of squares that would be generated in an analysis of variance, with group as the independent variable and the discriminant function as the dependent variable (the discriminant function is interpreted as a weighted sum of the values on the predictor variables).

TABLE 29.5 SELECTED OUTPUT FOR DISCRIMINANT ANALYSIS: RISK FACTORS ASSOCIATED WITH ATHLETIC INJURY ($N = 109$)

Group Statistics

Injury Group		❶ Mean	Std. Deviation
No injury	BALANCE	33.37	10.25
	FLEXIBILITY	65.44	13.70
	STRENGTH	14.23	5.48
	TIMEINPLAY	19.03	8.26
Injury	BALANCE	21.64	4.78
	FLEXIBILITY	40.38	16.32
	STRENGTH	22.94	8.56
	TIMEINPLAY	26.78	6.74

Eigenvalues

Function	❷ Eigenvalue	% of Variance	❸ Canonical Correlation
1	1.898	100.00	.809

Wilks' Lambda

Test of Function	Wilks' Lambda	Chi-square	df	❹ Sig.
1	.345	111.711	4	.000

Unstandardized Canonical Discriminant Function Coefficient

❺	Function 1
BALANCE	.055
FLEXIBILITY	.040
STRENGTH	−.081
TIMEINPLAY	−.052
Constant	−1.016

Standardized Canonical Discriminant Function Coefficient

❻	Function 1
BALANCE	.448
FLEXIBILITY	.592
STRENGTH	−.572
TIMEINPLAY	−.395
Constant	

Classification Results[a] ❼

	Injury Group	Predicted Group Membership No Injury	Predicted Group Membership Injury	Total
Count	No injury	56	3	59
	Injury	7	43	50
%	No injury	94.9	5.1	
	Injury	14.0	86.0	

[a]90.8% of original group patients correctly classified.

❶ Group means for each variable.

❷ The eigenvalue is a reflection of the proportion of variance that is accounted for by the discriminant function.

❸ The canonical correlation is the correlation between the two sides of the equation, that is, between group membership and the discriminant function (the weighted sum of the independent variables).

❹ Chi-square tests the significance of the canonical correlation. In this case, $p = .000$, which is significant. If p is greater than .05, it would suggest that the discriminant function does not significantly account for differences between groups.

❺ The unstandardized coefficients are used to create the discriminant function, including a constant:

$$D = -1.016 + .055(BALANCE) + .04(FLEXIBILITY) - .081(STRENGTH) - .052(TIME)$$

❻ The standardized coefficients are similar to beta weights in a multiple regression analysis, with no constant:

$$D = .448(BALANCE) + .592(FLEXIBILITY) - .572(STRENGTH) - .395(TIME)$$

where each variable is expressed as a standardized z-score.

❼ Classification results of the discriminant analysis.

upper limit. Therefore, it is usually preferable to use a measure of correlation that ranges from 0 to 1, similar to the interpretation of R^2. The **canonical correlation** expresses this relationship, conceptually serving as a correlation of group membership with the discriminant function (see Table 29.5❸). The square of the canonical correlation reflects the extent to which the variance in scores in the discriminant function account for differences among the groups. In this example, with a canonical correlation of .809, approximately 66% of the variability in scores is accounted for by the differences between injured and noninjured athletes. A chi-square test is used to determine the significance of this relationship (see Table 29.5❹).

Classification

Probably the most useful test of the discriminant function is the degree to which it accurately predicts group membership. Obviously, when we calculate D it will not be exactly equal to 1 or 0. Therefore, a cutoff score must be defined, below which subjects are assigned to group 0 and above which they are assigned to group 1. The discriminant analysis will establish the coefficients and cutoff score that will maximize accuracy of classification. Unless the predictor variables are completely different from each other, with no overlapping variance (correlation), we can anticipate that this classification will not be 100% correct. A summary of classification results is included as the final step in the discriminant analysis. Because we know the true group assignment for each subject, we can determine if the discriminant function has correctly classified each individual. For example, Table 29.5❼ shows the results of the discriminant analysis for classifying athletes who were and were not injured. This summary shows that of those who actually had no injury, 94.9% were correctly classified, and of those who were injured, 86.0% were correctly classified. In the entire sample of 109 subjects, 90.8% were placed in the correct group by the discriminant function. This would be considered excellent discrimination. Therefore, based on these hypothetical data, measures of strength, flexibility, balance and time in play will be useful predictors of an athlete's risk of injury.

In essence, analysis of variance and the *t*-test for independent samples are special forms of discriminant analysis. Questions that are analyzed using these tests would often be equally well suited to discriminant analysis, and results would be identical; that is, where groups are significantly different using an analysis of variance, the discriminant analysis would show that the predictor variables are capable of discriminating among the groups. For instance, using the current example, we could have done five separate *t*-tests to determine if the injured and noninjured athletes were different from each other for each of the five identified risk factors. The discriminant analysis approach is more useful, however, when several measured variables are studied, accounting for their interdependence in the analysis, and controlling for potential Type I errors with multiple univariate analyses.

FACTOR ANALYSIS

The technique of **factor analysis** is quite different from any of the statistical procedures we have examined thus far. Rather than using data for comparison or prediction, factor analysis takes an exploratory approach to data analysis. Its purpose is to examine the structure within a large number of variables, in an attempt to explain the nature of their interrelationships. This procedure is more controversial than other analytic methods because it leaves room for subjectivity and judgment; however, factor analysis makes an important contribution to multivariate methods because it can provide insights into the nature of abstract constructs and allows us to superimpose order on complex phenomena.

The concept of factor analysis is illustrated in Figure 29.4. The larger set of variables at the top is composed of several overlapping circles with various degrees of "gray" or "green." We can assume that there is some relationship among circles that have similar shades. Through factor analysis, these variables are reorganized into two relatively independent circles, each one representing a set of related variables. Each set of green and gray variables represents a unique *factor*. A factor consists of a cluster of variables that are highly correlated among themselves, but poorly correlated with items on other factors. Therefore, we assume that circles with blue shades are related to other circles with green, but not to circles with gray, and vice versa.

Developing Factors

In real terms, we use factor analysis to examine a large set of variables that represents elements of an abstract construct, and to reduce it to a smaller, more manageable set of underlying concepts. For example, we could examine a large set of behaviors within an

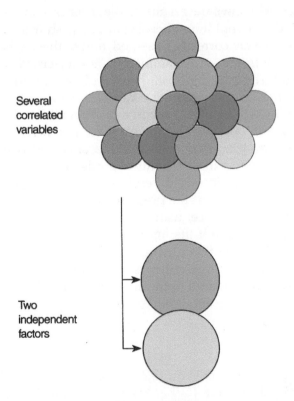

Several
correlated
variables

Two
independent
factors

FIGURE 29.4   Conceptual representation of factor analysis.

individual and categorize them as representing different conceptual elements of the person's psychological state. Loss of appetite, lack of motivation and withdrawal might reflect underlying "depression." Sleeplessness, inability to concentrate, and nail biting might be indicative of "anxiety." Depression and anxiety would each be composed of a set of related elements, with each set of elements unrelated to the other set. The inter-correlation of variables within a factor suggests that those variables, taken together, represent a singular concept that can be distinguished from other factors. Therefore, depression can be distinguished from anxiety.

We might also be interested in the relative strength of the association between each of the variables within a factor and the concept that the factor represents. For instance, what is the relationship between sleeplessness and the concept of anxiety? In addition to grouping variables into factors, factor analysis also weights each variable within a factor. These coefficients, called **factor loadings**, are measures of the correlation between the individual variable and the overall factor.

The determination of what variables make up a factor is not determined a priori. The factor analysis approaches a set of data by looking at the intercorrelations among all the variables and arranging them into sets of statistically related variables. Through a complex series of manipulations that can only be envisioned by a computer, the analysis derives the factors and shows which variables fit best into each factor.

Example

To demonstrate this application using a practical example, suppose we are interested in studying behaviors that are related to chronic pain in a sample of 150 patients with low back pain. For this hypothetical example, we will examine seven variables (although many more would probably be of interest in such a study). These variables have all been measured on a 5-point Likert scale, based on the frequency with which each behavior is observed, from 1 = "never observed" to 5 = "almost always observed." The seven variables are (1) COMPLAINs about pain; (2) CHANGES position frequently while sitting; (3) GROANS, moans, or sighs; (4) RUBS painful body parts; (5) ISOLATEs herself or himself; (6) MOVES rigidly and stiffly; and (7) drags feet when WALKING. We will interpret a computer printout for a factor analysis on these seven variables.

Extraction of Factors

The first step in a factor analysis is the creation of a correlation matrix for all the test items. On the basis of these correlations, the factor analysis attempts to identify the **principal components**[§§] of the data; that is, the analysis proceeds to identify sets of variables that are linearly correlated with each other. Conceptually, this method looks at the data in a multidimensional space and configures the variables in all possible combinations to determine groupings that "go together" statistically; that is, they demonstrate

---

[§§]There are actually several different approaches to factor analysis, of which *principal components analysis* (PCA) is one. As this is the more common approach reported in the literature, we have chosen to present it here. Those interested in other approaches should consult manuals for different statistical packages, as well as references listed at the end of this chapter.

strong correlations. These clustered variables represent "components" of the total data set and are derived through a process called *extraction*. The process is as mathematically complex as it sounds.

Principal components analysis "extracts" a factor from the overall data matrix by determining what combination of variables shows the strongest linear relationship and accounts for a large portion of the total variance in the data. The first factor that is "extracted" will account for as much of the variance in the data as possible. The second factor represents the extraction of the next highest possible amount of variance from the remaining variance. Each successive factor that is identified "uses up" another component of the total variance, until all the variance within the test items has been accounted for. These factors are abstract statistical entities only. This process does not indicate which variables are related to which factors.

As shown in the printout in Table 29.6❶, this analysis has extracted seven factors. The number of factors derived from a set of variables will always equal the number of variables, as it does here. These factors are statistical representations of variance and cannot be interpreted as any real concept yet. The computer is simply looking at patterns within the data and manipulating numbers. It will not be until the end of the analysis that these "factors" will make sense.

Even though seven factors have been identified, several of these factors account for small amounts of variance, and do not really contribute to an understanding of the structure of the data. We can usually characterize the data most efficiently using only the first few components. Therefore, we need to establish a cutoff point to limit the number of factors for further analysis. The statistic used to set this cutoff is called an **eigenvalue** (Table 29.6❷). Eigenvalues tell us how much of the total variance is explained by a factor. Factor 1 will always account for more variance than the other factors (in this example 27.1%). The most common approach restricts retaining factors to those with an eigenvalue of at least 1.00. Using this criterion, then, we limit further analysis to the first four factors, which taken together account for 72.5% of the variance in the data (see Table 29.6❸). Alternatively, the researcher may specify the number of factors to be used.

The result of a principal components analysis is a factor matrix (see Table 29.6❹), which contains the factor loadings for each variable on each factor. Loadings are interpreted like correlation coefficients, and range from 0.00 to ±1.00. Ideally we want each variable to have a loading close to 1.00 on one factor and loadings close to 0.00 on all other factors.*** Factor loadings greater than .30 or .40 are generally considered indicative of some degree of relationship. We consider only the absolute value of the loading in this interpretation. The sign indicates if the variable is positively or negatively correlated with the factor.

Unfortunately, this factor matrix is usually difficult to interpret because it does not provide the most unique structure possible; that is, several variables may be "loaded" on more than one factor. For instance, if we look across the row for COMPLAIN, we can

---

***The ideal outcome of a factor analysis would be the generation of factors that are composed of variables with high loadings on only that one factor. These would be considered "pure" factors. This does not always happen, however. When one variable loads heavily on two factors, those factors do not represent unique concepts, and there is some correlation between them. The researcher must then reconsider the nature of the variables included in the analysis and how they relate to the construct that is being studied.

TABLE 29.6   SELECTED OUTPUT FOR FACTOR ANALYSIS: SEVEN MEASURES RELATED TO CHRONIC PAIN BEHAVIOR ($N = 100$)

Total Variance Explained

❶ Component	Initial Eigenvalues		
	❷ Total	**% of Variance**	**Cumulative %**
1	1.89	27.1	27.1
2	1.12	15.9	43.0
3	1.06	15.1	58.1
4	❸ 1.01	14.4	72.5
5	0.84	11.9	84.4
6	0.78	11.1	95.5
7	0.30	4.5	100.0

Extraction Method: Principal Component Analysis

Factor Matrix ❹

	Factor			
	1	**2**	**3**	**4**
COMPLAIN	0.55	−0.28	0.27	−0.42
CHANGES	0.19	−0.74	0.05	−0.32
GROANS	0.31	−0.60	0.29	−0.17
RUBS	0.27	0.36	0.73	−0.01
ISOLATE	.028	0.01	0.34	0.80
MOVES	0.87	0.04	−0.25	−0.06
WALKING	0.75	0.08	−0.43	0.24

Rotated Factor Matrix ❺

	Factor			
	1	**2**	**3**	**4**
COMPLAIN	0.24	0.72	0.19	−0.11
CHANGES	0.19	−0.24	0.74	−0.24
GROANS	0.01	0.73	−0.17	0.08
RUBS	−0.12	0.25	0.71	0.38
ISOLATE	0.14	−0.04	0.00	0.90
MOVES	0.86	0.27	0.14	−0.00
WALKING	0.89	−0.02	−0.05	0.14

Rotation Method: Varimax Rotation

❶ Seven components are identified in the data, corresponding to the number of variables entered.

❷ The eigenvalues reflect the amount of variance accounted for by each component.

❸ Using the 1.0 cutoff for the eigenvalue, we will stop at four factors, accounting for a cumulative 72.5% of the variance in the data.

❹ Unrotated factors

❺ Rotated factors matrix shows largest loading for each variable (in gray).

see that factor loadings are moderately strong for both Factors 1 and 4. Therefore, the next step is to develop a unique statistical solution so that each variable relates highly to only one factor. This process is called *factor rotation.*

Factor Rotation

Factor rotation is also a complex, multidimensional concept. Envision multiple axes in space, all intersecting at a central point, each one representing one factor. In this example, we would imagine four planes, or axes, one for each of the four factors we have identified. Each of the seven variables sits somewhere in this four-dimensional space, with factor loadings that identify its location relative to each of the four axes. The factor loadings can be considered multidimensional coordinates. In the ideal solution to this analysis, each of the variables would be located directly on one of the axes, which would indicate that the variable was "loaded" on that factor. We would then be able to identify which variables "belonged" to each factor.

We can illustrate this concept more simply using a two-dimensional example. Assume we have identified only two factors, Factor 1 and Factor 2. We could plot each of the seven variables against these two axes, as shown in Figure 29.5A.[ttt] The vertical axis represents Factor 1 and the horizontal axis represents Factor 2. As we can see, none of the variables sits directly on either of the axes. Some variables are located close to the origin, indicating that they are not related to either factor (their factor loading is small). The other variables sit in space somewhere between the two

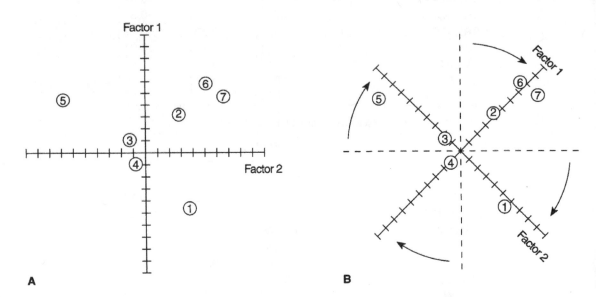

FIGURE 29.5   Orthogonal rotation of factor axes.

[ttt]For this illustration, the factor loadings are hypothetical. We cannot use the factor loadings given in Table 29.5, as these represent coordinates in a four-dimensional space.

factors. This plot does not present a clear "structure" in the data in terms of specific factor assignments.

If, however, we could rearrange the orientation of axes and variables, we might be able to create a structure that will help us interpret these relationships. We do this by *rotating* the two axes in such a way as to maximize the orientation of variables near one of the axes. There are actually several ways that factor axes can be statistically rotated to arrive at this solution. In this example, we have used the most common approach, called **varimax rotation**, which tries to minimize the complexity of the loadings within each factor.[‡‡‡]

This rotation is shown in Figure 29.5B. The rotation improves the spatial structure of the variables so that distinct factors are now visible; that is, several of the variables lie directly on or close to one of the axes. We find that variables 2, 6 and 7 now have the closest orientation to Factor 1, and variables 1 and 5 have the closest orientation to Factor 2. Variables 3 and 4, still clustered around the origin, show little or no relationship to either factor. This type of two-dimensional plot can be requested as part of a computer analysis for combinations of factors.

This form of rotation is called **orthogonal rotation** because the axes stay perpendicular to each other as they are rotated. This means that the two factors are independent of each other (orthogonal means independent); that is, they maintain maximal separation. **Oblique rotation**, used less often, allows the axes to change their orientation to each other. Therefore, some variables could be close to both factors, and the factors would be correlated. This might lead to a more realistic solution in some cases; however, the orthogonal solution will typically be easier to interpret, and in many cases will provide a comparable solution to oblique rotation.

In the actual factor analysis, this rotation process is carried out for all four planes simultaneously. Clearly, it would be impossible to conceive of this type of analysis without a computer. We must visualize a spatial solution that provides the one best linear combination for all variables.

This process results in the creation of a *rotated factor matrix* shown in Table 29.6❺. This matrix provides new factor loadings that represent the spatial coordinates of each variable in the reoriented multiaxial rotated solution. This new configuration should provide a cleaner statistical picture. We interpret this information by looking across each row of the matrix to determine which factor has the highest loading for that variable. We have highlighted the one loading for each variable that shows the strongest relationship to one of the factors. MOVES and WALKING load highest on Factor 1; COMPLAIN and GROAN load highest on Factor 2; CHANGES and RUBS load highest on Factor 3; and ISOLATE is loaded highest on Factor 4.

[‡‡‡]Other forms of rotation that are used less often are *quartimax rotation*, which is based on simplifying row loadings, and *equimax rotation*, which simplifies loadings on rows and columns. Each of these methods will result in a slightly different positioning of the axes. Varimax rotation is used most often because it generally presents the clearest factor structure. For some analyses it may be necessary to try different solutions to develop the one that best differentiates factors. Fortunately, these processes are easily requested in a computer analysis. It is important to recognize that different mathematical solutions can be generated, depending on the rotation approach used.

Naming Factors

The final solution to a factor analysis is the naming of factors according to a common theme or theoretical construct that characterizes the important variables in the factor. This is a subjective and sometimes difficult task, especially in situations where the variables within a factor do not have obvious ties. The computer runs the analysis without any preconceived judgments on its part as to what "should" go together or what combinations "make sense." The researcher must look for commonalties and theoretical relationships that will explain the statistical outcome. When the factor labels are not so obvious, it may be necessary to re-examine the very nature of the construct being studied.

Table 29.7 shows how we have assigned the seven variables to four factors, using the strongest factor loadings for each variable as the criterion. Factor 1 could be called "mobility." Factor 2 could be labeled "verbal complaints." Factor 3 is concerned with "nonverbal complaints," and Factor 4 is associated with "nonsocial behavior." We are able to specify the percentage of the total variance in the data that each factor explains, using the information given in Table 29.6. Together, these four factors account for 72.5% of the total variance. Table 29.7 illustrates the type of information that would be included in a published report of factor analysis.

What we have, then, is a set of variables that contribute to a construct we are calling "chronic pain behavior." The variables demonstrate different components of this construct. We can begin to understand the structure of pain behavior by focusing on four elements that we have called mobility, verbal complaints, nonverbal complaints, and nonsocial behavior. As we move forward in this research, we can explore how each of these elements contributes to a patient's reactions to treatment, interactions with family, participation in social activities, and so on. The factor analysis has provided a framework from which we can better understand these types of theoretical relationships.

TABLE 29.7   FACTOR LOADINGS ON FOUR FACTORS RELATED TO CHRONIC PAIN BEHAVIOR

Factor 1: Mobility		Factor 2: Verbal Complaints	
Variable	**Loading**	**Variable**	**Loading**
MOVES	0.86	COMPLAIN	0.72
WALKING	0.89	GROANS	0.73
% Variance: 27.1%		% Variance: 15.9%	

Factor 3: Nonverbal Complaints		Factor 4: Nonsocial Behavior	
Variable	**Loading**	**Variable**	**Loading**
CHANGES	0.74	ISOLATE	0.90
RUBS	0.71		
% Variance: 15.1%		% Variance: 14.4%	

Applications of Factor Analysis

Exploratory Analysis

Factor analysis can be used to answer many types of research questions. As an exploratory approach, it can be used to sort through a large number of variables in an effort to reveal patterns of relationships that were not obvious before. This type of analysis may represent early stages of inquiry, when concepts and relationships are not yet sufficiently understood to propose relevant hypotheses. A classic example of this approach was presented by Thurstone and Thurstone[6] in their studies of intelligence. They factor analyzed 60 tests and identified six primary abilities: verbal, number, spatial, word fluency, memory, and reasoning. Through repeated testing, these have come to be accepted as some of the elements that underlie the construct of intelligence, and are used as the basis for many intelligence tests.

Reduction of Data

Factor analysis can also be used to simplify a test battery, by determining which elements of the test are evaluating the same concepts. This approach can result in reducing the number of items that are used, or it may provide the basis for creating composite summary scores for each concept. For example, Jette[7] used factor analysis to look at a set of 45 items on a functional capacity evaluation, with the intent of reducing the number of items without sacrificing the comprehensiveness of the assessment. The test items were structured into factors that identified distinct functional constructs, such as physical mobility, personal care, home chores, transfers and kitchen chores. Jette suggested that two or more items from each functional category should be assessed as part of the evaluation, substantially reducing the time needed to complete the test, while maintaining the validity of the information it produces. This method of sorting through a large number of items is preferable to the intuitive or empirical classification of functional tasks into categories.

Factor Scores

One of the most interesting uses of factor analysis is the creation of a smaller set of composite scores, to be used as evaluative data or to be used as data in a statistical analysis. Subscores are created for each factor by multiplying each variable value by a weighting, and then summing the weighted scores for all variables within the factor. This result is called a **factor score**. The advantage of using composite scores is that the total number of variables needed for further analysis is decreased. This, in turn, will improve variance estimates for analyses such as regression or discriminant analysis. For example, Warren and Davis[8] used a discriminant analysis to differentiate patients with running-related injuries. They started with 72 anatomical variables and performed a factor analysis to reduce these data to nine factors. Factor scores for each factor were then used as predictors in a discriminant analysis to predict membership in six pain groups. This simplified the analysis, which would have been quite cumbersome with 72 variables. Unfortunately, their classification was successful for only 29.1% of their cases, and they concluded that the identified factors were not good predictors of type of pain.

Construct Validity

Many behavioral and clinical constructs, such as intelligence or motor development, cannot be measured directly. Therefore, they must be defined by relevant measurable variables that together form a conceptual package, indicative of the construct. Most tests of this sort contain many items that supposedly evaluate different components of the construct. These components can be considered factors, each one addressing a separate concept within the total construct. The construct validity of these tests must be established to document that they are indeed measuring the abstract behavior they supposedly define. This approach is basically one of theory testing; that is, the results of testing should conform to the theoretical premise for the construct. For example, suppose we developed a new intelligence test for use with learning-disabled children. If we accept the theoretical premise of intelligence defined by Thurstone and Thurstone,[6] then we could hypothesize, a priori, which variables or test items should go together to reflect each of the six primary abilities. After the test is administered to a large sample, the scores can be factor analyzed, and we should see factors emerge that fit with this theory. If the factors do not match the hypothesized variable groupings, the test items are probably not measuring what they were intended to measure. This approach to construct validity testing is an important one that should be replicated on several samples before any conclusions are drawn about the appropriate or inappropriate inclusion of test items.

Hypothesis Testing

Factor analysis can also be used to support research hypotheses, when the focus of treatment or intervention is a set of behaviors that define a construct. For instance, educators could evaluate the effects of changes in professional curricula, such as moving from a fact-based to a problem solving approach, by examining differences in factor structure before and after program changes. One would expect to find different loadings and combinations of variables following this type of change.[9] Because of the complex and interactive nature of curriculum characteristics, it would be difficult to evaluate change using only individual variables that represent small pieces of overall performance.

Limitations of Factor Analysis

Although factor analysis has a unique statistical role in multivariate analysis, its subjectivity is often the basis for serious criticism. Researchers must be cautious about how "factors" are interpreted, as they are not real measurement entities, but only hypothetical statistical concepts. Giving a factor a name does not make it real. Similar analyses on different samples may organize data differently, as will other approaches to a single analysis, such as different methods of extraction or rotation. These differences can alter a factor's essential meaning. Indeed, factor analysis may generate factors that are totally uninterpretable within the framework of the research question. Because of the subjective and judgmental nature of some decisions, we recommend consulting an experienced statistician to document the rationale for using particular methods under specific research conditions.

CLUSTER ANALYSIS

Researchers are often interested in the underlying structures in a set of data. We can look at such structures in two ways. Factor analysis is one approach to determine how clusters of correlated variables contribute to that structure. In an analogous process, **cluster analysis** looks for groupings of people that demonstrate similar characteristics. Rather than generating factors of variables, this analysis generates homogenous clusters of subjects.

To illustrate this approach, Michel et al[10] studied the prognosis of functional recovery in patients who had experienced a hip fracture. They looked at prefracture characteristics as well as function and mobility measures 1 year postsurgery. Their analysis generated 4 clusters of patients with similar profiles in terms of 13 predictor variables and 7 outcome variables.

Figure 29.6 shows the hierarchical structure, or cluster tree, that was generated for this study. The researchers started with 207 patients. Cluster analysis moves in a hierarchical fashion, reorganizing the data in steps to determine how the patients' characteristics relate to each other. In the first iteration, two groups were created, with 79 and 128 subjects. These groupings were further reduced in successive steps. The authors noted that the first cluster ($n = 79$) was clearly homogeneous, as it stayed intact until the seventh step. The second cluster ($n = 128$) was sufficiently heterogenous to form two more smaller groupings of 89 and 39 subjects in the third step. The smaller of these two clusters stayed intact through the next step, whereas the larger cluster was further classified into groupings of 27 and 62 subjects. These two clusters stayed intact through one more step, indicating a reasonable level of homogeneity in these subjects.

This pattern led the researchers to determine that the classification using four clusters was the best organization to describe this sample. Beyond four clusters, the groupings became too small to allow meaningful descriptions. Just as with factor analysis, this statistical technique has room for judgment in exploring the data.

Table 29.8A shows a small portion of the data that were generated to describe these clusters. We can see, for instance, that Cluster 1 was younger, had better mobility, and the shortest hospital stay; Cluster 2 had a longer hospital stay and low mobility; Cluster 3 had a larger number of patients in a nursing home, but no one who was disoriented; and patients in Cluster 4 were most likely to live in a nursing home, be disoriented, and have poor mobility.

The researcher is responsible for classifying the clusters by describing the characteristics that distinguish them. For this example, the researchers looked specifically at measures of ambulation and function prior to fracture and 1 year following surgery, to show how the members of each cluster varied. In Table 29.8B we can see that the patients in Cluster 1 were high functioning before and after their hip fracture. Those in Cluster 2 were functional prior to the fracture, but showed limitations 1 year later. Those in Cluster 3 were already limited prior to their fracture, and declined even further in ambulation

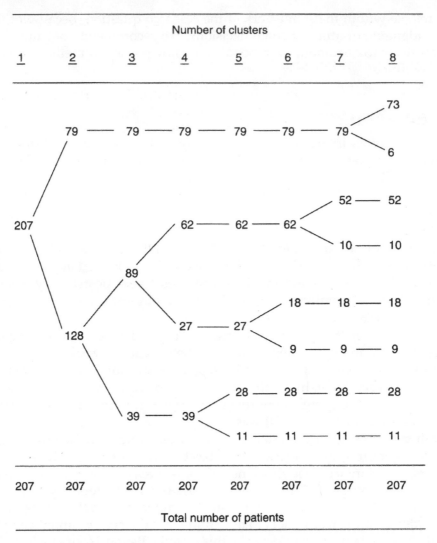

FIGURE 29.6   Number and size of clusters at successive steps in a study of functional recovery following hip fracture. (From Michel JP, Hoffmeyer P, Klopfenstein C, et al. Prognosis of functional recovery 1 year after hip fracture: Typical patient profiles through cluster analysis. *J Gerontol* 2000;55:M508–515, Figure 1, p. 511. Used with permission of the Gerontological Society of America.)

1 year later. And those in Cluster 4 started with some limitations and declined in both function and ambulation 1 year later. By understanding how these profiles emerge, clinicians can develop specific management strategies that are appropriate to their patients.

MULTIVARIATE ANALYSIS OF VARIANCE

Many clinical research designs incorporate tests for more than one dependent variable. For example, if we were interested in the physiological effects of exercise, we might measure heart rate, blood pressure, respiration, oxygen consumption, and other related variables on each subject at the same time. Or if we wanted to document muscle activ-

TABLE 29.8 **PROFILE OF FOUR CLUSTERS OF PATIENTS FOLLOWING HIP FRACTURE (*N* = 207)**

A. CLUSTER CHARACTERISTICS

	CLUSTER 1 *n* = 79 (38%)	CLUSTER 2 *n* = 62 (30%)	CLUSTER 3 *n* = 27 (13%)	CLUSTER 4 *n* = 39 (19%)
Mean age (y)	78.2	83.8	84.0	85.9
Living in nursing home (%)	5.1	4.8	37.0	64.1
Disoriented (%)	6.3	16.1	0.0	38.5
Self-reported mobility (%)	93.7	24.2	37.0	7.7
Mean number of hospital days/yr	45.8	96.1	60.3	78.2

B. CLASSIFICATION OF CLUSTERS[a]

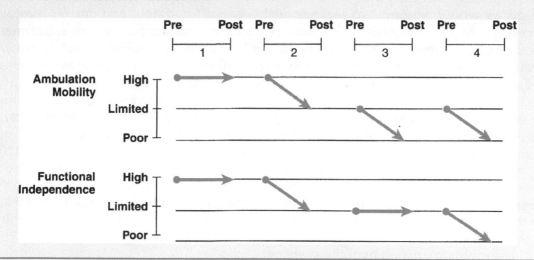

Adapted from Michel JP, Hoffmeyer P, Klopfenstein C, et al. Prognosis of functional recovery 1 year after hip fracture: Typical patient profiles through cluster analysis. *J Gerontol* 2000; 55A: M508-M515

[a]Pre = prior to fracture; Post = 1 year post surgery

ity during a particular exercise, we might record electromyographic data from several muscles in the upper and lower extremities simultaneously. It makes sense to do this because it is efficient to collect data on as many relevant variables as possible at one time, and because it is useful to see how one person's responses vary on all these parameters concurrently. These types of data are usually analyzed using *t*-tests or analyses of variance, with each dependent variable being tested in a separate analysis.

This approach to data analysis presents two major problems. First, the use of multiple tests of significance within a single study can increase the probability of a Type I error. This means that the more tests we perform, the more likely we are to find significant differences, just by chance. The second problem is related to the univariate basis of the *t*-test and analysis of variance. The validity of these tests is based on the assumption that each test represents an independent event; however, if we measure heart rate, blood pressure, and respiration on one person, we cannot assume that the responses are unrelated. Most likely, changes in one variable will influence the others. Therefore, these responses are not independent events and should not be analyzed as if they were.

The purpose of a **multivariate analysis of variance (MANOVA)** is to account for the relationship among several dependent variables when comparing groups. This test can be applied to all types of experimental designs, including repeated measures, factorial designs, and analyses of covariance. In many situations, a MANOVA can be more powerful than multiple analyses of variance if the dependent variables are correlated.

Statistical Hypotheses for Multivariate Analyses

To illustrate the concept of multivariate analysis, suppose we wanted to measure systolic blood pressure (SBP) and diastolic blood pressure (DBP) to study the effects of three different medications for reducing hypertension. Hypothetical means for such a study are shown in Table 29.9. If we were to use a standard analysis of variance for this study, we would perform two separate analyses, one for systolic and one for diastolic presssure. In each analysis, we would compare means across the three treatment groups. In a multivariate model, we no longer look at a single value for each treatment group, but rather we are concerned with the overall effect on both dependent variables. We conceptualize this effect as a multidimensional value, called a **vector**. The mean vector, $\overline{V}$, for each group represents the means of all dependent variables for that group. In statistical terms, a vector can be thought of as a list of group means. In this example, there would be two values in each of the three vectors, representing systolic and diastolic blood pressure measures for each medication group. Therefore, $\overline{V}_1 = (50,120)$, $\overline{V}_2 = (60,110)$ and $\overline{V}_3 = (90,135)$. Figure 29.7 illustrates how these values would be oriented in a two-dimensional framework. The center point in each group, called the **group centroid**, represents the intersection of the means for both dependent variables, or the spatial location of the mean vector. The purpose of the MANOVA is to determine if there is a significant difference among the group centroids.

The multivariate null hypothesis states

$$H_0: \overline{V}_1 = \overline{V}_2 = \cdots = \overline{V}_k$$

where $\overline{V}$ represents the mean vector for each group. The alternative multivariate hypothesis states that at least one group has a population centroid that is different from the others. Just as with an ANOVA, follow-up tests are necessary to explain significant differences.

TABLE 29.9   MEANS FOR SYSTOLIC AND DIASTOLIC BLOOD PRESSURE FOR THREE TREATMENT GROUPS

	Treatment Group		
	1	2	3
Systolic	120	110	135
Diastolic	50	60	90

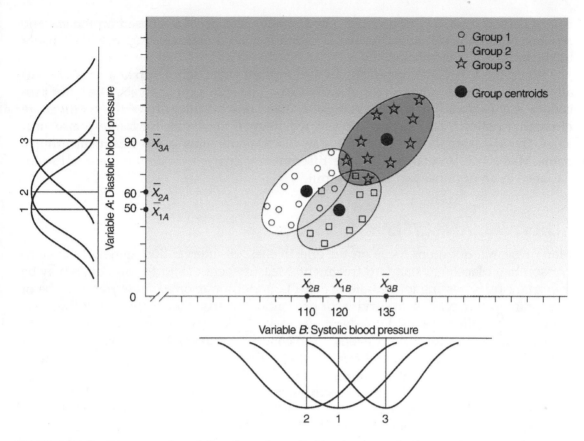

FIGURE 29.7 Representation of diastolic and systolic blood pressure for three groups in a multivariate model.

Multivariate Test Statistics

The concept behind the multivariate analysis of variance is really the same as that for the analysis of variance. The total variance in the sample is partitioned into parts that represent between-groups and error effects, although in the multivariate case, variability is measured against centroids rather than individual group means.

The statistics associated with multivariate analysis of variance are not as clear cut as using F or t in univariate models. When two groups are compared, *Hotelling's T^2* can be used, which is a multivariate extension of Student's t-test. With more than two groups, four statistical procedures are usually reported in a computer analysis: Wilk's lambda, the Hotelling-Lawley trace, the Pillai-Bartlett trace, and Roy's maximum characteristic root (MCR). Each of these tests is a variance ratio, although each has a slightly different interpretation. For the sake of consistency in generating critical values for these statistics, most programs convert these values to F-values.

Unfortunately, statisticians are not in agreement as to which one of these procedures should be used. In most cases, the tests yield similar results. The rationale for choosing one test over the others is based on a complex consideration of statistical power and how well the assumptions underlying each test are met. Rather than attempt to define these rationales, a task that goes beyond the scope of this text, we encourage researchers to consult with a statistician to make these decisions based on the specific research situation. We advise that Wilks' lambda is used most often, and will probably be the most easily interpreted.

When the MANOVA demonstrates a significant effect, follow-up analyses are usually based on univariate analyses of variance or a discriminant analysis. The latter procedure is considered preferable, because it maintains the integrity of the multivariate research question. Discriminant analysis will show if the values for the response variables, in this example SBP and DBP, can discriminate among the treatment groups. Some MANOVA programs will offer discriminant analysis or univariate analyses of variance as an optional part of the output.

SURVIVAL ANALYSIS

Many research questions focus on the effectiveness of intervention, generally in comparison to a placebo or standard treatment. Measurement of short-term effects may be important for assessing immediate benefit. Long-term outcomes, however, may be of greater interest in relation to survival or prevention because they better reflect the intervention's true effectiveness. Long-term effects are typically evaluated with reference to survival time to an identified "event." The concept of **survival analysis** is important to understanding prognosis and treatment effectiveness. It answers questions relating to time: "How long will it be before I am better?" "How long am I going to live?" "When in the future will the risk of recurrence of my disorder decrease?"

For many diseases, such as cancer or cardiovascular disease, the terminal event of interest is death. Life expectancy can also be examined in relation to functional conditions. For example, Strauss et al[11] looked at decline in function and life expectancy in older persons with cerebral palsy. They were able to demonstrate that survival rates of ambulatory older adults were only moderately worse than the general population, but were much poorer for those who had lost mobility. Survival time can also refer to other events, such as time to relapse, injury or loss of function. For instance, Ruland et al[12] used survival analysis to examine time to recurrence of stroke. Grossman and Moore[13] followed the longitudinal course of aphasia to determine how grammatical and working memory factors contribute to decline of sentence comprehension. Researchers have also looked at the prognosis of walking capacity in patients with rheumatoid arthritis who underwent multiple arthroplasty.[14] They found that within the first 5 years after the first surgery, 92% of patients were still able to walk independently. This decreased to 79% in the 10th year, and 60% in the 15th year.

Censored Observations

Estimates of survival present a special dilemma for analysis because it is not possible to follow all subjects to the event of interest. Even in long-term studies, there will be an end to data collection and some patients will not have reached the terminal event at that point. Therefore, we could not know how long these subjects will "survive." Subjects may drop out of a study, leaving their end point undocumented. There may also be a variation in the onset of disease or treatment, often resulting in patients entering a study at different times.

When individuals are followed for this type of analysis, those who have not yet reached the terminal event by the end of the study are considered **censored observations**. These censored survival times will underestimate the true (but unknown) time to the event because it will occur beyond the end of the study.[15] Therefore, special methods of analysis are needed to account for censored data.

Methods of Analysis for Survival Data

Techniques such as analysis of variance and regression are often used to follow a subject's responses over time. Because of censored observations, however, they are not appropriate for survival analysis. Taking a mean survival time for a cohort of patients will be misleading because the mean will continually change as different individuals reach the terminal event. A mean survival time can actually only be accurate when all subjects in the cohort have reached that end point.

Life Tables

The oldest method of analyzing survival was developed in the 17th century using actuarial or **life tables** (see Box 29.1). In this approach, time intervals are created to provide estimates of an individual's probable survival, a technique still used by insurance companies to establish premiums. Within each interval, several indices can be computed.

- The **number of cases at risk** is the number of individuals who enter the time interval (those who have survived) minus half the number of cases lost to follow-up within that interval.
- The **proportion failing** is the ratio of the number of cases who did not survive into the interval, divided by the number of cases at risk. The **proportion surviving** is 1 minus the proportion failing.
- The **probability density** is the probability of reaching the terminal event in the given time interval per unit of time. It is computed as the proportion surviving at the start of the interval minus the proportion surviving at the end of the interval, divided by the width of the interval.
- The **hazard rate** is the probability that an individual who has survived to the beginning of a time interval will reach the terminal event during that interval. It is the number of individuals who reach the event divided by the mean number of surviving cases at the midpoint of the interval.
- The **survival function** is a cumulative proportion of cases surviving up to the given interval. It is computed by multiplying the probabilities of survival across all previous intervals.
- The **median survival time** is the point at which the cumulative survival function is equal to 0.5, or the 50th percentile. Because of censored observations, this will not necessarily be the same as the time up to which 50% of the sample survived.

Kaplan-Meier Estimates

The most common method of determining survival time is the **Kaplan-Meier product limit method**, which does not depend on grouping data into specific time intervals.

BOX 29.1 Halley's Life Table

Edmund Halley (1656–1742) was a 17th century mathematician and astronomer, who is famous for identifying the recurrence of a comet every 79 years, now called Halley's Comet. But did you know that he was also responsible for developing the process of estimating life insurance premiums?

In 1693 Halley published the first life table that presented mortality data for the city of Breslau, Germany based on specific ages for the five years between 1687 and 1691. With a city population of 34,000, he documented 6,193 births and 5,869 deaths per year. He showed that on average 348 died yearly in the first year of life, and another 198 died between 1 and 6 years of age. His table (below) showed mortality from ages 7 through 100, with the mortality figures listed below each age (11 people died at age 7; 11 people died at age 8, and so on). He noted how deaths in teen years decreased markedly, and that after age 70 the number increased, with a gradual decline in later years until "there be none left to die."

```
  7 . 8  9 .   . 14    . 18 . 21 . 27 . 28 . . 35 .
 11 . 11 . 6 .  5½ . 2 . 3½  5 6  4½ 6½  9 .  8 . 7 . 7 .

 36 .   42 .     45        49 54 .  55 . 56    .  63
  8 . 9¼  8 . 9 . 7 . 7  . 10 11 .   9 .  9 . 10 . 12

    70 71 . 72      77      81      84 .    90   91 .
 9¼  14  9 . 11  9½    6 . 7 . 3 . 4 .   2 . 1 . 1.   1 .

 98 . 99 . 100 .
  0 . ⅕ . ⅗
```

Halley cited several uses for his table. First, it could be used to determine the number of men in the city eligible to bear arms between the ages of 18 and 56, with the assumption that those under 18 were "too weak to bear the *Fatigues of War* and the *Weight of Arms*, and [those over 56 were] too crasie [sic] and infirm from *Age*, notwithstanding particular *Instances* to the contrary" (italics from original text).

Second, the table identified different mortality rates in specific age groups. And third, the data could be used to estimate of the price of life insurance and the valuation of annuities, based on the probability that the person would survive to collect the installment. Halley's work was considered the founding of actuarial science, and resulted in a profitable insurance practice for the British government.

Source: Halley E. An estimate of the degrees of mortality of mankind, drawn from curious tables of the births and funerals at the city of Breslaw, with an attempt to ascertain the price of annuities on lives. *Philosophical Transactions of the Royal Society of London* 1693;17:596–610, 654–656.

This approach generates a step function, changing the survival estimate each time a patient dies (or reaches the terminal event). Graphic displays of survival functions computed with this technique provide a useful visual understanding of the survival function as a series of steps of decreasing magnitude. This method can account for censored observations over time. Confidence intervals can also be calculated.

The Kaplan-Meier estimate can also be used to compare groups of patients. Figure 29.8 shows survival curves over a 5-year period for a cohort of elderly men and women who participated in an aging study.[16] Subjects were differentiated on the basis of their gait abnormalities. The graph shows that subjects had a greater risk of death or institutionalization if they exhibited abnormal gait characteristics, than if they had a normal gait. The distinction between the groups became most evident after the first year of follow-up. By looking at the survival rate along the Y-axis, we can see that the median survival time for those with abnormal gait was approximately 3 years, and for those with normal gait approximately 4.5 years.

Cox Proportional Hazards Model

Survival time is often dependent on many interrelated factors that can contribute to increased or decreased probabilities of survival or failure. A regression model can be

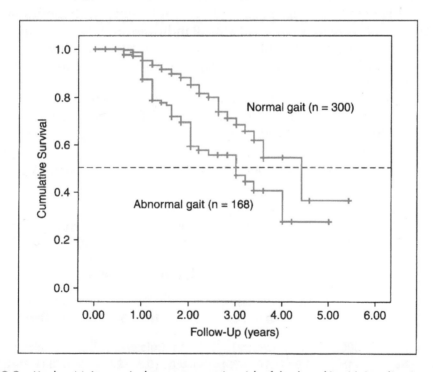

FIGURE 29.8   Kaplan-Meier survival curve comparing risk of death and institutionalization over 5 years for subjects with abnormal gaits and those with normal gaits. The small vertical tick marks represent censored observations. The median survival time is determined by looking at the 50% cumulative survival rate along the Y-axis (horizontal line). (Adapted from Verghese J et al. Epidemiology of gait disorders in community-residing older adults. *J Am Geriatr Soc* 2006; 54:255–261, Figure 1, p. 259. Used with permission of Blackwell Publishing.)

used to adjust survival estimates on the basis of several independent variables. Standard multiple regression methods cannot be used because survival times are typically not normally distributed—an important assumption in least squares regression. And of course, the presence of censored observations presents a serious problem. The most commonly used method is the **Cox proportional hazards model**, which is conceptually similar to multiple regression, but without assumptions about the shape of distributions. For this reason, this analysis is often considered a nonparametric technique.

The proportional hazards model is based on the **hazard function**, which is related to the survival curve. This function represents the risk of dying (or the terminal event) at a given point in time, assuming that one has survived up to that point. The dependent variable is the hazard (risk), and the independent variables, or covariates, are those factors thought to explain or influence the outcome. Variables may be continuous, dichotomous or ordinal.[17] Factors such as age, gender, occupation and so on, are typically used for this purpose. When treatment is used as an independent variable, the model allows for comparison of the hazard, and therefore survival time, associated with placebo compared to treatment.

Like odds ratios generated from a logistic regression, a **hazard ratio (HR)** can be generated from coefficients in the hazard function. A HR of 1.0 indicates that there is no excess risk associated with the covariates. A value greater than 1.0 indicates that a covariate is positively associated with the probability of the terminal event—thereby decreasing survival. A HR less than 1.0 indicates that the covariate is protective, decreasing the probability of the terminal event, and thereby increasing survival time. Confidence intervals can be expressed for the hazard ratio to indicate significance, with a null value of 1.0. Table 29.10 shows a portion of the data from the study of gait abnormalities. We can see that those who had moderate to severe gait abnormalities were 3.7 times more likely to die and 2.6 times more likely to become institutionalized than those with normal or mildly abnormal gaits. The confidence intervals for these hazard ratios do not contain 1.0, and therefore are significant. These values were generated from a Cox regression that included age and sex as covariates.

TABLE 29.10   **RISK OF DEATH, INSTITUTIONALIZATION OR BOTH OVER 5 YEARS BASED ON GAIT STATUS, ADJUSTED FOR AGE AND SEX**

Gait	N = 468	Hazard Ratio (95% CI)		
		Institutionalization (n = 75)	Death (n = 30)	Institutionalization or Death (n = 99)
Normal	300	1.0 (reference)	1.0 (reference)	1.0 (reference)
Mild Abnormality	118	1.99 (1.18–3.36)	0.89 (0.32–2.51)	1.76 (1.01–2.84)
Moderate-Severe	50	2.67 (1.47–4.84)	3.66 (1.62–8.29)	3.18 (1.94–5.21)

Source: Verghese J et al. Epidemiology of gait disorders in community-residing older adults. *J Am Geriatr Soc* 2006;54:255–261.

COMMENTARY

Can We Keep It Simple?

Multivariate analyses have become popular in behavioral research because of the increased availability of computer programs to implement them. Their applications are, however, not well understood by many clinical researchers, and many studies using multivariate designs are still analyzed using univariate methods.

Multivariate techniques can accommodate a wide variety of data and are able to account for the complex interactions and associations that exist in most clinical phenomena. Many research questions could be investigated more thoroughly if investigators considered multivariate models when planning their studies. We have limited this chapter to a discussion of the conceptual elements of multivariate analysis, but with enough of an introduction to terminology and application that the beginning researcher should be able to communicate effectively with a statistician and follow the computer output. This information will also facilitate understanding research reports that present the results of these analyses.

Although we have emphasized the potential for improving explanations of clinical data using multivariate methods, we must also include the caveat that clinical research need not be complicated to be meaningful. A problem is not necessarily better solved by a complex analysis, nor should such an approach be taken just because computer programs are available. The indiscriminate use of multiple measurements is not a useful substitute for a well defined study with a select number of variables. To be sure, the results of multivariate analyses are harder to interpret and involve some risk of judgmental error, such as in factor analysis. In addition, multivariate tests require the use of larger samples. Many important and concise research questions can be answered using simpler methods and designs. Many clinical variables can be studied effectively using a single criterion measure. On the other hand, simple analysis is not necessarily better just because the interpretation of results will be easier and clearer. The choice of analytic method should be based on the research question and the theoretical foundation behind it. When dealing with constructs that reflect several abstract phenomena, multivariate methods offer the most powerful means for developing and explaining theory. The purpose of this chapter was to present alternatives that provide the researcher with useful choices for planning the most effective study possible.

REFERENCES

1. Stineman MG, Williams SV. Predicting inpatient rehabilitation length of stay. *Arch Phys Med Rehabil* 1990;71:881–887.
2. Walker J, Sofaer S. Predictors of psychological distress in chronic pain patients. *J Adv Nurs* 1998;27:320–326.
3. VanSwearingen JM, Paschal KA, Bonino P, Chen T. Assessing recurrent fall risk of community-dwelling frail older veterans using specific tests of mobility and the Physical Performance Test of Function. *J Gerontol* 1998;53A:M457–M464.

4. Cifu DX, Keyser-Marcus L, Lopez E, Wehman P, Kreutzer JS, Englander J, et al. Acute predictors of successful return to work 1 year after traumatic brain injury: A multicenter analysis. *Arch Phys Med Rehabil* 1997;78:125–131.
5. Ermer J, Dunn W. The sensory profile: A discriminant analysis of children with and without disabilities. *Am J Occup Ther* 1998;52:283–290.
6. Thurstone L, Thurstone T. *Factorial Studies of Intelligence.* Chicago: University of Chicago Press, 1941.
7. Jette AM. Functional capacity evaluation: An empirical approach. *Arch Phys Med Rehabil* 1980;61:85–89.
8. Warren BL, Davis V. Determining predictor variables for running-related pain. *Phys Ther* 1988;68:647–651.
9. Bray JH, Maxwell SE. *Multivariate Analysis of Variance.* Beverly Hills, CA: Sage Publications, 1986.
10. Michel JP, Hoffmeyer P, Klopfenstein C, et al. Prognosis of functional recovery 1 year after hip fracture: Typical patient profiles through cluster analysis. *J Gerontol* 2000; 55:M508–515.
11. Strauss D, Ojdana K, Shavelle R, Rosenbloom L. Decline in function and life expectancy of older persons with cerebral palsy. *NeuroRehabilitation* 2004;19:69–78.
12. Ruland S, Richardson D, Hung E, Brorson JR, Cruz-Flores S, Felton WL, 3rd, et al. Predictors of recurrent stroke in African Americans. *Neurology* 2006;67:567–571.
13. Grossman M, Moore P. A longitudinal study of sentence comprehension difficulty in primary progressive aphasia. *J Neurol Neurosurg Psychiatry* 2005;76:644–649.
14. Shinomiya F, Mima N, Hamada Y, Fuzimura T, Matsumoto S, Okada M, et al. Long-term outcome of patients with rheumatoid arthritis treated by multiple arthoplasty. *Mod Rheumatol* 2005;15:241–248.
15. Clark TG, Bradburn MJ, Love SB, Altman DG. Survival analysis part I: Basic concepts and first analyses. *Br J Cancer* 2003;89:232–238.
16. Verghese J, LeValley A, Hall CB, Katz MJ, Ambrose AF, Lipton RB. Epidemiology of gait disorders in community-residing older adults. *J Am Geriatr Soc* 2006;54:255–261.
17. Bradburn MJ, Clark TG, Love SB, Altman DG. Survival analysis part II: Multivariate data analysis—and introduction to concepts and methods. *Brit J Cancer* 2003;89:431–436.

CHAPTER 30
Data Management

An important part of the research planning process is the development of a data management plan that specifies how data will be recorded, organized, reduced and analyzed. This plan begins with the research proposal, specifying the research question, hypotheses and design. Before any data are collected, the researcher must be able to identify what variables will be measured, using what instruments and units of measurement. Those who will collect data may need to be trained and reliability assessments done. Undoubtedly, some of these plans will change once the project has begun, but nothing should begin without a firm plan in place. This planning requires knowledge of data coding and format requirements, statistics and computers. The purpose of this chapter is to describe procedures for setting up data to be entered into a computer and analyzed with statistical programs.

CONFIDENTIALITY AND SECURITY OF DATA

The research proposal will include a plan for handling data, including maintaining confidentiality of participant information. All subjects should be assigned a unique ID number that is not related to their name, medical unit number, Social Security number or other personal identifier. Documents for data collection should include the subject ID only. A list of subject names, addresses or phone numbers and corresponding ID codes can be kept separate and secured from other files in case participants need to be contacted.

As part of informed consent, subjects should be assured that their personal information, data from medical records and data collected as part of the project will only be accessed as necessary for research. The institutional review board (IRB) that approves the project will want to know the type of data to be collected, the purposes for which the data will be used, who will have access to records, and what safeguards have been put in place for security and confidentiality (see Chapter 3). Many countries have regulations in place that define these standards. In the United States, these are part of the Privacy Rule of the Health Insurance Portability and Accountability Act (HIPAA).[1] In Canada, they are incorporated into the Tri-Council Policy Statement: Ethical Conduct for Research Involving Humans.[2]

MONITORING SUBJECT PARTICIPATION

Throughout the project, researchers should have procedures in place to keep accurate and complete records of subject involvement. Records should indicate how many subjects were recruited and why some were not eligible, how many agreed to participate, and how many eventually did participate. Attrition should be monitored, and reasons noted if possible. Changes to the research protocol must be described. Initial group assignments and deviations from these assignments should be documented. This information is relevant to the validity of the project and will be important if the researcher wants to complete an intention to treat analysis (see Chapter 9).

STATISTICAL PROGRAMS

The number of statistical packages for use on a microcomputer has grown dramatically, many at reasonable prices. The two most commonly used programs are SPSS (Statistical Package for the Social Sciences)* and SAS (Statistical Analysis System).† SPSS has traditionally been used more for the social and behavioral sciences, although its use has increased in health care research. SAS is most useful in medicine and epidemiology as a biostatistics program. These packages, once available only on main frames, have been adapted for use on personal computers. Many other programs are also on the market, and it would be useless to name them here as we are sure more will be published by the time you read this. Even though these packages are all slightly different, they adhere to certain standards that are important for data management. Most programs provide a format for data entry similar to a spreadsheet. Data may also be imported into a statistical program from a spreadsheet such as Microsoft Excel®.

DATA COLLECTION FORMS

A data recording system must be carefully developed. Typically, data are collected from each subject and recorded on a separate sheet or directly into a computer program. The subject's identification code is listed, as well other relevant information such as the date, the individual collecting the data (if there is more than one investigator), the subject's group assignment and demographic information such as age, gender and diagnosis. If possible, all data should be listed in the order they will be included in the data file, to facilitate data entry. Figure 30.1 illustrates a data collection form for a study of two diet regimens in patients with diabetes.

The researcher must make decisions about how data will be recorded for each subject. Is there a level of precision in measurements that should be used, such as measuring to the nearest millimeter or half inch? The format for recording open-ended responses or qualitative data should be specified. If data are missing, the reason should be included. The importance of a well organized data collection scheme becomes most evident when the researcher begins to enter data into a computer. If data are not clearly recorded and in a consistent format, data entry will be a difficult and potentially error-ridden process.

---

*SPSS Inc., 233 S. Wacker Drive, Chicago, IL 60606 <http://www.spss.com>
†SAS Institute Inc., 100 SAS Campus Drive, Cary, NC 27513 <http://www.sas.com>

Subject ID # __4__   Date of enrollment __9/23/04__

Group Assignment: (Diet 1)   Diet 2

Subject's Age (in years) ___58___

Gender (Male) Female

Year of Onset __1998__

BASELINE   Date 11/04/04

Blood Sugar   Trial 1 ___152___   Trial 2 __155__

Weight __198__ (lbs)

FOLLOW-UP   Date 10/18/05

Blood Sugar   Trial 1 ___120___   Trial 2 __125__

Weight __179__ (lbs)

Questions at Follow-up

How many times per week (on average) do you exercise?

    0   Less than once a week

   (1) Once a week

    2   2-3 times per week

    3   4 or more times per week

  -98 Refused to answer

  -99 Don't know

   Other _____

COMMENTS

FIGURE 30.1   Sample data collection form.

DATA CODING

An essential part of the data collection plan is the development of a scheme for recording data. Some measurements produce quantitative data, such as range of motion and blood pressure. Variables such as gender, group and race produce categorical data. Surveys and qualitative studies may produce open-ended responses that must be coded.

Types of Variables

Data can be entered as numerals or characters. Quantitative data are **numeric**, having values of single or multiple digits, sometimes including decimal points, and composed of only numbers. Numeric values can be preceded by a plus or minus sign, although plus signs are assumed and not entered. Character variables, called **alphanumeric** or **string variables,** are composed of letters or characters and may include digits. String variables may be letters or words that represent variable values, such as male/female or the names of states or cities. Money values can be coded for different monetary units, with or without decimals places. Variables can also be entered as dates, using one of many acceptable forms, such as MM-DD-YYYY. Date fields can be added or subtracted to determine length of time in days, weeks, months or years.

Codes for Categorical Variables

Data for categorical variables are entered as labels. For instance, if gender is a variable, we enter either male or female as the data value. Although we can enter the full label as the data, it is much easier to code these values. Using character codes, for instance, gender could be coded F for female and M for male. It is generally recommended, however, that codes be entered as numeric data to facilitate statistical analysis, such as coding 1 for female and 0 for male. For dichotomous variables it is conventional to use 1 and 0 as codes, usually signifying the absence of a trait as zero. As a pure label it does not matter whether we code gender as 1 and 0, as 1 and 2, or any other number; however, many statistical procedures will only manipulate categorical data with 1 and 0 as the category codes (see discussion of dummy variables in Chapter 24). When the research design includes group comparisons, each subject's group assignment must be identified by a code for the **grouping variable**. Decisions about coding categorical variables should be made before data are collected. Codes should be used on data collection forms to expedite transfer of data to the computer.

Missing Data

It is not unusual for some pieces of data to be missing from a subject's record because of errors in recording, unavailability of information, nonresponses on surveys, or problems in data collection. To identify missing values, blanks are used as the default in most computer programs. Others have specific rules for identifying missing values, such as the use of a period in place of a missing datum. It is not advisable to use zeros to represent missing values, as zeroes will be read as a number and there may be true zeroes in the data. It is often useful to assign specific codes for missing values, to identify the reason for the missing information. For instance, separate codes might be used to distinguish a refusal to answer a question, a response of "Don't know," a question that was not asked, investigator error and so on. Such distinctions can be helpful for interpretation of results, especially when there are many missing data points. Missing data should be coded using numeric values that are out of range of any actual data values. For example, the code of -99 is commonly used.

DATA ENTRY

The standard structure for data entry requires that each variable is entered in a separate column, and each row represents an individual subject. Data may be typed directly into a statistical program, or it may be entered in a spreadsheet first and later imported into the statistical program. No matter how information is entered, the wise researcher will save the data often and back up the data file regularly. We have suffered with too many colleagues who have lost hours of work to take this advice lightly!

When data originate as a spreadsheet, the first row in each column should contain the variable name, which will then be read by the statistical program. To facilitate this transfer, the variable names should conform to the restrictions of the statistical program. Other than this first row, all other rows in the spreadsheet should contain only data. No embedded formulas or charts should be included. If formulas are used in specific cells, they should be converted to the actual data values before transferring to a statistical program.

Variable Names

Variable names identify each data point in a file. Every variable in the file must have a unique name. When variable names are long, abbreviations can be used. As much as possible, variable names should be readily identifiable. Certain rules apply to variable names, depending on the statistical package being used.

Many programs require that a variable name be no more than eight characters (numbers or letters), although more recent versions of some packages allow for longer variable names. Variable names typically must begin with a letter and have no spaces. Some programs allow hyphens, underscores, dollar signs or number signs within a variable name. Generally special characters such as !, ? and / cannot be used in variable names. For example, a pretest and posttest value for pain could be coded PAIN1 for the pretest and PAIN2 for the posttest. Researchers should be familiar with the requirements for the statistical package they use.

Variable Fields

Each row of data, representing a single subject's scores, is called a **record** or **case**. Each individual score, or variable value, is identified as a **field.** A case is composed of several fields of data. Fields are described according to their width, that is, the number of digits or spaces needed for the maximum possible value. The field width is described according to the format F$w.d$, where w is the total number of spaces (or field width), and d is the number of digits within the field that follow a decimal point (the F is for Format). For example, the value 7.85 takes up four spaces (including the decimal point), for a field width of F4.2. The value 3560 also takes up four spaces with no decimal places, for a field width of F4.0. The value 136.45 takes up six spaces, described as a field width of F6.2. Many programs set a default field width that can be changed by the researcher.

Labels

Because variable names must be kept short and categories are coded, it is sometimes confusing to read a printout of an analysis with many abbreviations. To facilitate reading the output, most programs will allow the researcher to specify **labels** for variable names and for category value codes. These labels can usually extend to 40–60 characters or longer. They allow the researcher to customize the printout in a way that will be convenient for interpretation. To make this happen, however, the researcher must take the time to type in all the labels. But it is worth the effort when reams of paper are sitting in front of you and you can't remember whether males are coded 1 or 0! Labels are not required, but with large data sets they are extremely useful. Labels may be listed in the data collection form.

Code Books

Code books are used to organize data and to catalog the order of entry of all variables. Variable names are listed with their abbreviations. Codes are listed to identify their values. Figure 30.2 shows a sample page from a code book for the study examining the effectiveness of two diet regimens on fasting blood sugar in patients with diabetes. Data were collected on the subjects' age, gender, and baseline and follow-up blood sugar levels. Two trials were performed for each test. Codes were developed for gender and group assignment. Subjects were also asked how often they exercised and if they were compliant with their medications. The code book is a necessary reference for all those who are involved with the study, most especially those who will analyze the data. SPSS provides this information in the Variable View of the data file.

DATA CLEANING

Once data are entered into the computer, and before analyses are run, the data should be checked against the raw data to be sure there are no discrepancies or coding errors. This process is called **data cleaning**, and although it may be time consuming and tedious, it is essential to ensure validity of the data analysis. The data file can be printed out or displayed on a computer screen and visually checked for accuracy against the original data.

Running descriptive statistics on the data will allow the researcher to see if there are obvious discrepancies. Frequency counts should be checked for all categorical variables. The output will list all the codes for each variable and the number of times that code appears in the data. It will also indicate how many subjects are counted, and if there are missing data for that variable. This allows the researcher to determine if there are mistakes in codes, or if the variable has too few entries to be useful. For continuous variables, descriptive statistics and graphs, such as histograms or plots, should be run to analyze means, minimums and maximums, to be sure that the range of scores is appropriate. In this way, the researcher can ascertain if values out of the possible range have been entered. For instance, if the maximum blood sugar score is printed as 560, the researcher knows there is an error and can go back and correct that entry. Sometimes it

Variable	Variable Label	Values	Value Labels	Missing Values	Scale	Format
1. ID	<none>				Nominal	F8
2. AGE	<none>				Ratio	F8.2
3. GENDER	<none>	0 1	Male Female		Nominal	F8
4. DIET	<none>	0 1	Diet 1 Diet 2		Nominal	F8
5. BASE1	Baseline Trial 1				Ratio	F8.2
6. BASE2	Baseline Trial 2				Ratio	F8.2
7. WEIGHT1	Baseline Weight				Ratio	F8.2
8. FOLLOW1	Follow-up Trial 1				Ratio	F8.2
9. FOLLOW2	Follow-up Trial 2				Ratio	F8.2
10. WEIGHT2	Follow-up Weight				Ratio	F8.2
11. EX	Exercise frequency	0 1 2 3 -99 -98	Less than once a week Once a week 2-3 times a week 4 or more times a week Refused to answer Don't know	-98, -99	Ordinal	F8

FIGURE 30.2   Sample page from a code book.

is useful to sort data, reordering the subjects according to the value of a particular variable, to determine if appropriate numbers have been entered.

DATA MODIFICATION

All statistical programs include processes for **data modification** or **transformation** to create new variables or to assign new codes to existing variables. For example, we might want to compute the mean of several trials to use for data analysis. Or we might have scores for several items on a scale and want to get the sum. Perhaps a continuous variable will be converted to categories. When these types of transformations are performed, a new variable is created, and must be given a new and unique variable name.

Computing New Variables

Computing a new variable requires that some arithmetic operation be performed on the existing data. All programs use the same symbols to represent logical operations. These symbols, known as **operators,** are used to create expressions that are instructions to the computer. The following symbols are used for arithmetic operations:

+	add	$A + B$
−	subtract	$A - B$
/	divide	A/B
*	multiply	$A*B$
**	exponent	$A**2$

These expressions are considered **simple expressions** because they contain one operator. When more than one operator is used, a **compound expression** is created, for instance,

$$A**2*B/(C + 1.0)$$

is a compound expression. This expression is equal to

$$\frac{(A^2)(B)}{C + 1.0}$$

When compound expressions are used, specific rules apply to the order in which operations take place. First, all expressions within parentheses are carried out. Second, adjacent operations are carried out in the following order: (1) exponentiation, (2) division and multiplication and (3) addition and subtraction. Within each of these levels, operations proceed from left to right. Therefore, in the preceding expression, the first operation will be to complete the addition $(C + 1.0)$ within the parentheses. Next, the value of A will be squared. This value will then be multiplied by B. Lastly, this product will be divided by the sum $(C + 1.0)$. If the parentheses had been left out, the expression would be read differently. Using

$$A**2*B/C + 1.0$$

the expression would read

$$\frac{(A^2)(B)}{C} + 1.0$$

To illustrate the application of these arithmetic operators, we might want to compute a mean baseline and follow-up score to use for analysis for the data in Figure 30.3. To do this, we tell the computer we want to create two new variables called BASEMEAN and FOLLMEAN using the following expressions:

$$BASEMEAN = (BASE1 + BASE2)/2$$

$$FOLLMEAN = (FOLLOW1 + FOLLOW2)/2$$

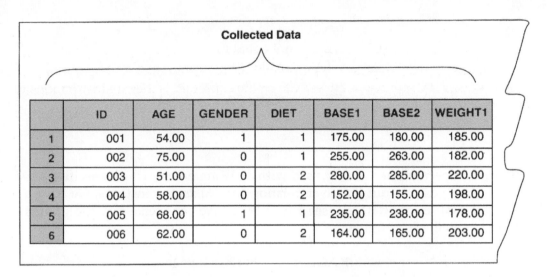

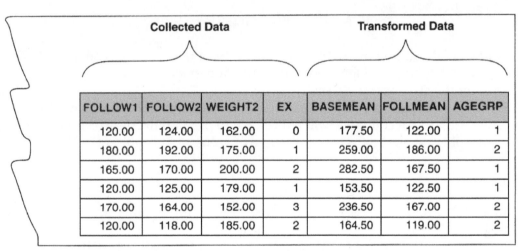

FIGURE 30.3   Data file for a pretest-posttest design, showing original data collected as part of the study and transformed data created through computing and recoding variables. Subjects are identified by ID number. All data for each subject appears on one row in the file.

Note the importance of the parentheses, so that the sum of the two items is divided by 2, and not just the value for BASE2 or FOLLOW2. When these computations are done, the values for the new variables will appear as new columns in the data file, as shown in Figure 30.3. These new variables can now be used in statistical procedures. We could, for instance, get a difference score between BASEMEAN and FOLLMEAN, and subject these values to a *t*-test. This type of data modification can also be done within spreadsheet programs.

Recoding Variables

We can also use **comparison operators** to recode variables by specifying relationships between them. Comparison operators may be specified as symbols or letter combinations:

=	EQ	equal to
∧=	NE	not equal to
>	GT	greater than
<	LT	less than
>=	GE	greater than or equal to
<=	LE	less than or equal to

Comparison operators are usually used with an IF statement, which specifies a specific operation to be carried out if a given relationship exists. For instance, we have a variable called AGE in our data set (see Figure 30.2). We can create two age groups for a comparison analysis, as follows:

$$IF\ AGE < 30,\ AGEGRP = 1$$

$$IF\ AGE >= 30,\ AGEGRP = 2$$

These statements illustrate how we specify values for a new variable called AGEGRP (shown in the last column in Figure 30.3). The actual method for setting recode values will depend on the statistical program.

When assigning values to a new variable, the researcher must be careful not to overlap any categories, or the computer will not be able to perform the desired functions. In addition, groupings should reflect the full range of values that is present in the data.

Statistical Procedures

Many statistical procedures also provide a mechanism for creating and saving new variables. For example, when running a factor analysis, factor scores are created for each subject on each factor. These values can be saved and used as variables in future analyses. When regression procedures are run, residual scores can be calculated and saved. Most programs require specific instructions for these options.

DATA ANALYSIS

Data collection is complete, all the data are entered and saved (and backed up!), and you are set to begin data analysis. If the research proposal was done well, you are ready to approach this phase of the research process in an organized way. It is a good idea to start by becoming familiar with the data by looking at descriptive statistics—frequencies for categorical variables and means for continuous variables. Histograms, line plots, stem-and-leaf plots or box plots are helpful to visually assess the shape of a distribution, and to identify gaps or outliers. For correlational data, scatterplots should be created to get a sense of the linearity and degree of relationship in the data. These initial steps are necessary to understand the scope of the data, and may suggest alternative statistical approaches. For example, transformations may be needed for nonlinear variables (see Appendix D).

The next step is the culmination of all the research efforts—to apply statistical procedures to answer the research question. This is the fun part. Some helpful hints:

To make this process efficient, prepare a list of specific hypotheses, variables and appropriate statistical procedures to guide your time at the computer. Be specific. For instance, if you intend to compare two groups, specify the *t*-test, paired or unpaired, and which variables will be used. If you run several regressions, list which are the independent and dependent variables for each one. Then you won't have to sit at the computer, faced with columns and columns of data, and wonder where to start.

Look at the output as you generate it. Examine your findings. Often, additional questions emerge and you may choose to run further tests. For instance, you may find relationships among some variables that you did not anticipate. Groups may end up having different characteristics than planned. It may be of interest to perform certain analyses on subgroups within the data. Statistical programs provide different filtering options to select subjects according to a specified criterion. You might specify that an analysis be done only on those coded 1 for gender, or only those coded for group 1.

Finally, most statistical programs include choices for creating tables or charts directly from the data. Many of these programs provide fairly sophisticated options, with a variety of fonts and colors to customize your presentation. These charts and tables can be imported into word processing or presentation programs. Many different types of charts are usually available, and it is often helpful to try out different formats to see which presents the data best.

Be sure you save your data and output so you can play with options and prepare your project for the final phase of the process—dissemination as a journal article or presentation as a platform or poster.

COMMENTARY

"Anyone can analyze data, but to really mess things up takes a computer!"

Because of the seemingly overwhelming power of computers for statistical analysis, it may seem unnecessary to become proficient in statistics. The computer seems to be able to handle the job of running statistical procedures with infinite ease, and can provide answers to statistical questions without the researcher ever having to crack a formula. The days of writing out a program and searching for the misplaced semicolon are gone. Today you need a mouse and a keyboard, and once you have entered your data and variable names you have very little else to do. Most programs will guide you through analyses by clicking on the appropriate button.

This is an oversimplification of the situation, however, for two reasons. First, the researcher must know the conceptual foundations for the statistical tests that will be used to make the appropriate choices in the first place. The computer can only carry out the instructions it is given. Programs require that the researcher sort through different options that will dictate how the procedures will be carried out. Most run at **default settings**, that is, parameters that are set at a certain level unless they are specifically changed. For instance, to run a stepwise regression procedure, variables will be included in the equation if partial correlations reach a specific level of significance.

The default setting may be .05 or .15. The analysis will run at that level unless the researcher specifies a different level in the program. In addition, there are several approaches to stepwise analysis, and these may have to be specified. Some programs will print out certain summary statistics by default, such as mean, standard deviation and range. These programs may require additional options to request different information. The researcher must know how the data should be analyzed, and what summary values are of interest, and then must be able to instruct the computer to perform the desired operations.

Second, there is an enormous amount of information generated by a computer analysis, and the interpretation of that output must be based on an understanding of the statistical procedures that were run. If data are entered incorrectly, the output will be useless. If the data are inappropriate for a particular procedure, the computer may still be able to run an analysis, but the output won't be meaningful. This situation is summed up in an important computer principle: GIGO, which means "garbage in, garbage out." The wise researcher will have sufficient knowledge of both computers and statistics to be able to make the appropriate choices and assure statistical conclusion validity for the study. When this knowledge is not sufficient, advice should be obtained from a statistical consultant.

REFERENCES

1. National Institutes of Health. HIPAA Privacy Rule: Information for researchers. Available at: <http://privacyruleandresearch.nih.gov/> Accessed August 17, 2006.
2. Canadian Institutes of Health Research, Natural Sciences and Engineering Research Council of Canada, Social Sciences and Humanities Research Council of Canada, Tri-Council Policy Statement: Ethical Conduct for Research Involving Humans. 1998 (with 2000, 2002 and 2005 amendments). Available at: <http://www.pre.ethics.gc.ca/english/policystatement/policystatement.cfm> Accessed August 17, 2006.

PART **V**

Communication

CHAPTER 31
Searching the Literature

Although most of us have had some experience obtaining references for term papers or assignments, technology has forever changed how we locate information. Our expectations have changed in terms of how quickly we want the information, the volume of data available, and virtual accessibility. These expectations have required us to become better skilled at locating and using resources.

Clinicians may go to the literature to expand their knowledge or simply to stay on top of scientific advances as part of professional development and life-long learning. They may also gather information specifically for clinical decision making as part of the framework of evidence-based practice (see Chapter 1, Figure 1.2). Using the "best research evidence" available allows the practitioner to balance that information with clinical judgment and patient values to determine the most appropriate course of action. This process, of course, assumes that the clinician is able to locate the relevant research literature.

Researchers will review the literature in the development of a research question (see Chapter 7) and the interpretation of findings. The literature review is necessary to build the rationale for a study and to help make decisions on operational definitions and methods. Researchers who conduct systematic reviews require a comprehensive approach to searching for primary sources of data on a given topic (see Chapter 16).

In other words, we all need to develop skills in searching the literature so that we can find what we want when we need it. The purpose of this chapter is to describe strategies for successful literature searches.

LIBRARY RESOURCES

There are many efficient strategies for locating research references. The library, of course, is where this process begins, whether this is an actual building or a virtual connection. Clinicians may have access to a departmental or institutional library, but medical and university libraries will usually be more complete. Most libraries today have online catalogues that allow searching by author, title or subject. Articles, books or theses that are not available at a local facility can often be obtained electronically or through interlibrary loan. Many facilities also provide access to full text downloads of articles, sometimes for a fee. Technology has greatly enhanced everyone's access to literature searches through Internet resources.

SEARCH ENGINES

Many specialized library resources are available to assist the researcher in locating references on specific topics. **Search engines** are information retrieval systems that search the Internet and electronic databases for websites, files or documents based on keywords or phrases. Meta-search engines query several other search engines and/or databases simultaneously, allowing the user access to broader resources by entering search criteria only one time.

Some search engines specialize in health and medical topics (see Table 31.1). The National Center for Biotechnology Information (NCBI), which is part of the National Library of Medicine, offers an integrated, text-based search and retrieval system called *PubMed. Scirus* focuses on scientific, scholarly, technical and medical information. *Google Scholar* searches scholarly literature in journals, theses, books, as well as material from professional societies, preprint repositories, universities and other scholarly organizations. The *OVID* search engine provides access to over 300 databases in medicine and health.

Many professional associations offer access to search engines with specific relevance to their particular field. The *Open Door* portal is available to members of the American Physical Therapy Association (APTA), providing access to full text clinical and academic journals, conference proceedings and dissertations related to rehabilitation. The American Occupational Therapy Association (AOTA) sponsors *OT Search*, available by subscription. The American Speech-Language-Hearing Association (ASHA) supports *The Dome*, a search engine for communication sciences disorders professionals, also available through subscription.

DATABASES

Databases are organized systems that allow search access for specific content or information. Bibliographic databases contain lists of citations of published and unpublished references. A computer search allows the researcher to view the full citation and abstract of a document, to determine if it is relevant. The citation can then be printed or downloaded for future reference. Citations may be displayed as the summary bibliographic reference, reference with abstract, or full text of the article.

Several databases are available for health science literature, providing listings of articles, books, theses and dissertations, and conference proceedings (see Table 31.1). Many databases can be accessed free through the Internet, while others require a subscription through an online service or CD-ROM. The list that follows is by no means exhaustive.

- The *Clinical Trials Registry* provides a regularly updated information databank about federally and privately funded clinical research. The database provides information about a trial's purpose, eligible subjects and locations. The site is geared toward non–health professionals who want to learn more about ongoing human studies research.
- The *Cumulative Index to Nursing and Allied Health Literature (CINAHL)* provides access to citations from all nursing journals as well as primary journals in more than a dozen other health disciplines, including occupational and physical

TABLE 31.1   COMMONLY USED BIBLIOGRAPHIC DATABASES

Database or Search Engine	Start of Coverage	Description	Full Text Available[a]	Subscription Required
ACP Journal Club *American College of Physicians* www.acpjc.org	1991	Structured abstracts of original articles and systematic reviews	—	✔
BMJ Clinical Evidence *British Medical Journal* www.clinicalevidence.com	1999	Updated systematic reviews on prevention and treatment	✔	✔
CINAHL *Cumulative Index to Nursing and Allied Health Literature* www.cinahl.com	1982	Abstracts and bibliographies in nursing and allied health	✔	✔
Clinical Trials Registry *National Institutes of Health* www.clinicaltrials.gov	Ongoing	Information about ongoing clinical trials	NA	—
Cochrane Central Register of Controlled Trials (CCTR) *The Cochrane Collaboration* www.cochrane.org	Ongoing	Bibliographic database of definitive clinical trials	✔	✔
Cochrane Database of Systematic Reviews *The Cochrane Collaboration* www.cochrane.org	1988	Abstracts and topic reviews	✔	✔
Database of Abstracts of Reviews of Effects (DARE) *Evidence Based Medicine Reviews* www.york.ac.uk/inst/crd	2000	Abstracts of systematic reviews of effectiveness	✔	✔
EMBASE *Excerpta Medica; Elsevier* www.embase.com	1974	Citations and abstracts on medical and drug-related subjects	Via links	✔
ERIC *Educational Resources Information Center* www.eric.ed.gov	1966	Citations and abstracts on education-related subjects	✔	—
Evidence-based Practice Centers (EPC) Reports *Agency for Healthcare Research and Quality* www.ahrq.gov/clinic/epc	NA	Reports on specific topics related to evidence-based practice	✔	—

(continued)

TABLE 31.1   COMMONLY USED BIBLIOGRAPHIC DATABASES (continued)

Database or Search Engine	Start of Coverage	Description	Full Text Available[a]	Subscription Required
Google Scholar www.googlescholar.com	Varies by database	Search engine that references several disciplines, citing theses, books, abstracts and articles	—	—
Hooked on Evidence *American Physical Therapy Association* www.hookedonevidence.com	No limit	Extractions of journal articles related to physical therapy interventions	—	APTA membership
Index to Scientific and Technical Proceedings® *Thomson Scientific* scientific.thomson.com/ products/istp/	1980	Citations and abstracts of presentations at conferences and conference proceedings	—	✔
LILACS *Latin American and Caribbean Health Sciences Information System* www3.bireme.br/abd/I/ililacs .htm	1982	Citations and abstracts of articles, books, proceedings, theses in English, Spanish and Portuguese.	—	✔
MEDLINE *National Library of Medicine* www.pubmed.gov www.pubmedcentral.gov	1966	Citations and abstracts	✔	—
National Rehabilitation Information Center (NARIC) *National Institute on Disability and Rehabilitation (NIDRR)* www.naric.com	1956	Citations and abstracts of articles, books and projects on all aspects of rehabilitation	—	—
NIOSHTIC-2 *National Institute for Occupational Safety and Health Technical Information Center (CDC)* www2.cdc.gov/nioshtic-2	1974	Database of occupational safety and health publications, grant reports, and other products supported by NIOSH	Via links	—
Open Door *American Physical Therapy Association* www.apta.org	Varies by journal	Search engine including Pro-Quest Health & Medical Complete, and Nursing and Allied Health Source	✔	APTA membership
OT Search *American Occupational Therapy Association* www.aota.org/otsearch	Varies by journal	Citations and abstracts for literature related to occupational therapy	—	✔

TABLE 31.1   COMMONLY USED BIBLIOGRAPHIC DATABASES

Database or Search Engine	Start of Coverage	Description	Full Text Available[a]	Subscription Required
OTseeker *Occupational Therapy Systematic Evaluation of Evidence University of Queensland, Australia* www.otseeker.com	No limit	Abstracts of systematic reviews and randomized clinical trials	—	—
OVID *Ovid Technologies* gateway.ovid.com	Varies by database	Citations and abstracts from a variety of databases	✔	✔
PEDro *Center for Evidence-based Physiotherapy University of Sydney* www.pedro.fhs.usyd.edu.au	1929	Abstracts of randomized clinical trials, systematic reviews and practice guidelines	Via links	—
Proquest Dissertations and Theses *Proquest CSA* www.proquest.com	1861	Citations and abstracts	✔	✔
PSYCINFO *American Psychological Association* www.apa.org/psycinfo	1800	Citations and abstracts of literature in psychology	—	✔
Public Library of Science (PLoS) www.plos.org	2004	Open access journals in medicine, biology and clinical trials	✔	—
Science Citation Index *Thomson Scientific* scientific.thomson.com/products/sci	1974	Bibliographic information on cited references	—	✔
Scirus *Elsevier* www.scirus.com	Varies by database	Searches scientific web pages; link to Networked Digital Library of Theses and Dissertations	—	—
Scopus *Elsevier* www.scopus.com	1900	Citations and abstracts of scientific, technical, medical and social science literature	✔	✔
SportDiscus *Sports Information Resource Centre, Canada* www.sirc.ca	1949	Citations and full text for sports-related references	✔	✔

(continued)

TABLE 31.1   COMMONLY USED BIBLIOGRAPHIC DATABASES (continued)

Database or Search Engine	Start of Coverage	Description	Full Text Available[a]	Subscription Required
The Dome *American Speech-Language Hearing Association* www.asha.org	Varies by publication	Search engine for speech pathology, citing articles, books, and other web resources	—	✔
Web of Knowledge® *Thomson Scientific* isiwebofknowledge.com	1900	Citations from international journals, open access resources, books, patents, proceedings, or websites	✔	✔
WorldCat *Online Computer Library Center (OCLC)* www.worldcat.org	No limit	Network of library contents and services	—	—

[a]The availability of full text depends on the journal. Some journals only make full text available to subscribers; others allow full text access after a certain amount of time has passed following initial publication; others are available to the public.

therapy, speech language pathology, cardiopulmonary technology, respiratory therapy, nutrition and social services.

- The *Educational Resources Information Center (ERIC)* hosts a database of education-related resources, sponsored by the Institute of Education Sciences of the U.S. Department of Education. A newly designed digital library allows free access, including full text availability of many journal and nonjournal materials.

- **EMBASE** is the *Excerpta Medica* biomedical database, which includes over 7,000 journals covering medicine, pharmacology and drug research, and health policy and management. EMBASE includes MEDLINE references from 1966, and additional references from 1974 on.

- The *Index to Scientific & Technical Proceedings* provides information on papers delivered at major conferences. It includes bibliographic information and abstracts from proceedings published in journals and books. This database covers topics included in the *Science Citation Index*. An *Index to Social Science and Humanities Proceedings* is also available.

- *Latin American and Caribbean Health Sciences Information System (LILACS)* is a cooperative database published since 1982 that registers health-related literature published by authors in Latin American countries. The database includes journal articles, conference proceedings, scientific-technical reports, theses, books and book chapters. LILACS indexes 670 journals published in the region, with abstracts in English, Portuguese or Spanish; only 41 of these journals are also included in MEDLINE or EMBASE. Therefore, a literature search can be substantially enhanced by including this database.[1] Subscription is required. LILACS is part of the WorldCAT network.

- *MEDLINE* is the most commonly used database in health-related sciences, indexing almost 5,000 journal titles in biomedical sciences. It is the electronic platform for the formerly published *Index Medicus.* Full references are available back to 1966, although earlier citations from 1950–1965 can be obtained through Old MEDLINE. MEDLINE is part of MEDLARS (*MEDical Literature Analysis and Retrieval System*), the computerized system of databases offered through the National Library of Medicine (NLM). This database can be accessed free through the PubMed website. PubMed also allows the search to be limited to subsets of databases that focus on AIDS, bioethics, cancer, complementary medicine, and other topics. **PubMed Central (PMC)** provides free full-text access to articles in a growing number of journals.

- *National Rehabilitation Information Center (NARIC)* houses the REHABDATA database, which contains approximately 69,000 abstracts of books, reports, articles, and audiovisual materials relating to disability and rehabilitation research, dating back to 1956. NARIC also includes the NIDRR Project Database with information on every project funded by NIDRR since 1993. Each record includes institutional and contact information, funding data, and an abstract of project goals and activities.

- *OTseeker* was developed by occupational therapists at the University of Queensland and the University of Western Sydney. It contains abstracts of systematic reviews and clinical trials related to occupational therapy, and includes ratings based on the PEDro scale. In 2006, more than 4,300 articles had been reviewed.

- *PEDro* is the Physiotherapy Evidence Database, which is an initiative of the Centre of Evidence-Based Physiotherapy out of the University of Sydney. This database includes citations and abstracts of systematic reviews, clinical trials and clinical practice guidelines related to physical therapy. All clinical trials are rated for quality using the PEDro Scale, a standardized rating scale for assessing methodologic quality (see Chapter 16).

- *ProQuest Dissertations and Theses (PQDT)* is a comprehensive collection of graduate scholarly works from universities, cataloguing more than 2 million dissertations and theses from around the world. Citations date from the first accepted U.S. dissertation in 1861, although abstracts are available only since 1980. Most are available in full text in microfilm or hard copy, and more recent titles may be obtained in electronic formats, depending on subscriptions. Proquest includes the former University Microfilms (UMI) collections through Dissertation Abstracts.

- *PsycINFO* is an abstract database sponsored by the American Pyschological Association. It covers topics in psychology, behavioral sciences and mental health, including over 2,000 journal titles, books and book chapters. Historic records are available dating back to 1802. Abstracts of dissertation titles are listed starting from 1995.

- *Public Library of Science (PLoS)* is a nonprofit organization of scientists and physicians who are committed to making medical research literature a public resource. Open-access journals are published in biology, medicine, computational biology, genetics, pathogens, and clinical trials. The inaugural journal was published in 2004.

- *SCOPUS* is available to research and academic institutions. It covers over 15,000 titles including journals, conference proceedings, books and trade publications. It includes scientific, technical, medical, and social science literature, with sources from the United States, Europe, Latin America and Asia. Scopus includes all of MEDLINE and more than 500 open access journals.

- *SportDiscus* is a database supported by the Canadian Sports Information Resource Centre (SIRC). It covers sports, exercise physiology, sports medicine, physical fitness, and biomechanics. It indexes over 2,000 journals as well as books, theses, and nonprint resources.
- *Web of Knowledge* is an integrated database that allows searching for citations, conference proceedings, websites and books in a multidiscliplinary platform. Its records cover scholarly information in the sciences, social sciences, and arts and humanities going back more than 100 years.
- *WorldCat* is a library network that allows searching collections of more than 57,000 libraries around the world. Books, theses and dissertations, as well as special collections are catalogued through this service. WorldCat is part of the Online Computer Library Center (OCLC), which provides various services to an international consortium of libraries. Most academic libraries are members of OCLC. The database identifies libraries that hold the items of interest, and will usually link directly to that library's website. The availability of the item will depend on that library's policies.

SEARCH STRATEGIES

The most important part of a literature search is deciding what terms to enter as keywords. All electronic databases will utilize some form of algorithm to generate a list of citations based on the keywords you choose. Citations will generally be brought up if the keyword is present in the title or abstract of the article. Journal articles may also have lists of keywords assigned to them by the author that are then used to index the document. Because so many words have synonyms or alternative terminology, this process can be daunting at times. It is useful to begin by brainstorming the various words that may be useful in finding articles related to your topic. Consider the pathology or diagnosis, the population, the specific treatments or measurement tools, and the outcomes of interest.

Suppose we were interested in studying physical endurance in patients who have experienced a stroke, with specific interest in the effectiveness of exercise programs. We would want to learn about the previous success of exercise programs for this population, and how endurance has been measured. Some possible keywords might include:

- Stroke
- Exercise
- Endurance
- Cerebrovascular accident (CVA)
- Therapy

Once we choose our keywords, we must consider how to combine them to generate citations that will relate to our question.

Boolean Logic

When performing a search, it is important to fine tune the choice of key words or reference terms to narrow the search. Most databases and search engines use a system called Boolean logic, named for George Boole, an English mathematician who invented it in the mid 1800s. Boolean logic utilizes three primary operators: AND, NOT and OR.*

We will illustrate the use of these operators to develop a search strategy for our question related to endurance after stroke (see Figure 31.1).

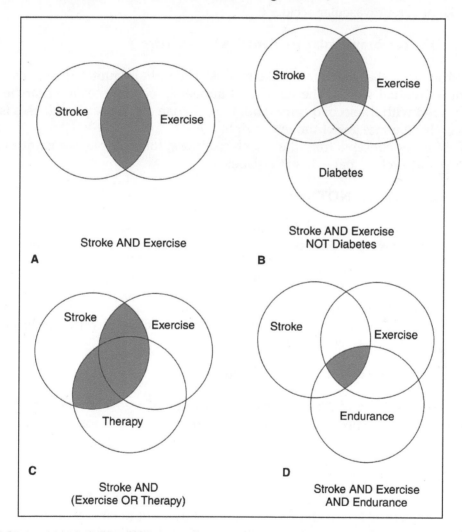

FIGURE 31.1 Samples of Boolean Logic showing the use of AND, OR, and NOT as logical operators. (**A**) AND confines the search to only references that relate to both stroke and exercise. (**B**) NOT further limits the search by excluding references related to diabetes. (**C**) OR broadens the search to include references related to either exercise or rehabilitation in addition to stroke. (**D**) AND further limits the search to include references that include all three terms.

---

*When these operators are used together, they will be read in the order of AND, NOT and OR, unless parentheses are used to indicate specific combinations that should be considered first.

AND narrows the search, requiring that all requested terms to be present. We can begin by finding references that include both of our main terms:

stroke AND exercise

This search yields 6,423 citations.[†]

OR broadens the search, usually when you want to include synonyms of the main search term. We may want to expand the search so that it includes studies that use the terms stroke or cerebrovascular accident:

(stroke OR "cerebrovascular accident") AND exercise

This has broadened the search to 6,448 citations. The term in quotes is read as a fixed string, not individual words. The terms that appear in parentheses are searched first and then paired with the second command. If more than one set of parentheses is present, the search sequence goes from left to right.

NOT excludes concepts from the search. Suppose, for example, we want to eliminate studies that exclude patients with diabetes:

stroke AND exercise NOT diabetes

This brings the search down to 6,084 citations.

We may finally want to limit our search to outcomes related to endurance:

stroke AND exercise AND endurance

The search is now limited to 439 references. Perhaps we can refine it a little more by making our terms more specific. For example, let's specify "physical endurance" to clarify the type of endurance we want to include:

stroke AND exercise AND "physical endurance"

Now our search is down to 278 citations. This is still too large a number of references, however. Let's examine how we can move through this process more effectively.

MeSH Headings

The National Library of Medicine has developed a sophisticated system of Medical Subject Headings (MeSH) that have been adopted by most databases that cite medical and health literature. Because authors will use different terminology for the same concepts, MeSH terms provide a consistent search vocabulary. MeSH consists of sets of terms in a hierarchical structure or "tree" that permits searching at various levels of specificity.[2] The tree starts with broad categories such as "Anatomy," "Disease" or

---

[†]This search was conducted using MEDLINE through PubMed on April 31, 2007.

TABLE 31.2 PARTIAL HIERARCHY OF MESH TERMS

Anatomy +[a]
Diseases +
Analytical, Diagnostic and Therapeutic Techniques and Equipment
    Anesthesia and Analgesia +
    Diagnosis +
    Equipment and Supplies +
    Surgical Procedures, Operative +
    Therapeutics
        Behavior Control +
        Electric Stimulation Therapy +
        Exercise Movement Techniques
            Breathing Exercises
            Dance Therapy
            Drainage, Postural
            Exercise
        Exercise Therapy
            Relaxation Techniques
        Hydrotherapy +
        Musculoskeletal Manipulations +
        Physical Therapy Modalities +
        Prescriptions, Non-Drug +
        Rehabilitation
            Activities of Daily Living
            Dance Therapy
            Early Ambulation
            Exercise Therapy
                Motion Therapy, Continuous Passive
            Occupational Therapy
            Rehabilitation of Hearing Impaired +
            Rehabilitation of Speech and Language Disorders +
            Rehabilitation, Vocational
        Respiratory Therapy +
Biological Sciences +
Anthropology, Education, Sociology and Social Phenomena +
Health Care +
Pharmacological Actions +

[a]The symbol + indicates that the term can be further exploded.

"Analytical, Diagnostic and Therapeutic Techniques and Equipment." More specific terms, close to 23,000 descriptors, are provided at various levels of the tree. Each heading can be further detailed in a list of subheadings. Table 31.2 shows a partial list of terms to illustrate this hierarchy.

Additional options include **exploding** the search, which means that the search will retrieve results using the selected term and all of the more specific terms in the tree.

Focusing or restricting the search means that it will be limited to documents where the subject heading is the major point of the article.

OVID provides a "Map Term to Subject" feature that shows MeSH headings for entered keywords. PubMed provides a MeSH database that will serve the same purpose. These programs provide a useful tutorial for those who are not familiar with this process.

For our current example, the term stroke is not a MeSH heading, but "cerebrovascular accident" is. There are several terms that relate to exercise, including "exercise therapy," "exercise test," "exercise movement techniques," and "exercise tolerance." The definition of "exercise therapy" is closest to our intention: "Motion of the body or its parts to relieve symptoms or to improve function, leading to PHYSICAL FITNESS, but not PHYSICAL EDUCATION AND TRAINING." MeSH terms related to endurance include "physical endurance," "sports," and "muscle fatigue." The definition for "physical endurance" is most appropriate for our purpose: The time span between the beginning of physical activity by an individual and the termination because of exhaustion.

In our search we use a slash to define our terms as MeSH headings. By combining the three terms:

cerebrovascular accident/ AND exercise therapy/ AND physical endurance/

We now obtain 9 references, substantially different from the 278 we had before!

A comprehensive search strategy for this topic is illustrated in Box 31.1, showing the scope of this process. This search was used to generate references for a systematic review.[3]

Limiting the Search

Search strategies can be refined by setting specific **limits** or **filters,** including language, dates of publication, or studies that are provided as full text. Searches can be restricted to studies of humans or animals, specific age groups or gender, or types of studies such as case studies, randomized trials, or systematic reviews. A specific author or journal can be searched. When a search yields large numbers of potential references, such limits will often provide a useful way to hone in on articles that are available and contemporary.

PubMed has developed predesigned strategies to target a search for studies on therapy (interventions), diagnosis, etiology or prognosis. These search strategies can be accessed under Clinical Queries.

Truncation and Wildcards

Most databases will recognize **truncation** and **wildcard** symbols that can be used to allow a broad interpretation of a search term, finding plurals, spelling variations and alternate forms of words. Each database specifies the symbol to be used, such as a question mark (?), an asterisk (*) or a dollar sign ($). For example, entering the term "sensitiv$" in PubMed will retrieve articles that include "sensitive" or "sensitivity." The term "wom$n" will find "woman" or "women."

BOX 31.1 Search Strategy for Studies Related to Stroke, Exercise and Endurance

Sophisticated strategies that combine MeSH headings and keywords can provide a comprehensive search. Synonyms for keywords are incorporated to target the full scope of studies related to the topic. Special abbreviations can be used to clarify where terms are found:

- exp = explode
- ab = words in abstract
- hw = word in subject heading
- pt = publication type
- ti = words in title

- tw = text words
- / = MeSH subject heading
- $ = truncation symbol
- adj4 = adjacent (within four words)
- or/ = apply OR to specified steps

The following search illustrates this process related to the effect of exercise on endurance following stroke.[3] The strategy illustrates how MeSH terms, keywords and series of search groupings can be combined to retrieve references.

1. exp Cerebrovascular accident/
2. (stroke or cva$ or cerebrovascular accident or cerebral vascular).tw
3. exp Brain injuries/
4. exp Hemiplegia/
5. (hemipleg$ or hemipar$ or brain injur$).tw
6. or/1-5
7. exp Exercise Therapy/ or exp Exercise/
8. exp Physical Fitness/
9. exp Physical Endurance/
10. treadmill.tw
11. ((aerobic or endurance or cardio$ or fitness) adj5 (train$ or program$ or protocol$ or intervention$)).tw.
12. or/7-11
13. exp Randomized Controlled Trials/
14. Clinical trial.pt
15. exp Random Allocation/
16. Random$.tw.
17. exp Cross-Over Studies/
18. Control$.tw.
19. Experimental$.tw.
20. exp Follow-Up Studies/
21. or/13-20
22. 6 and 12 and 21

Adapted from Pang MY, Eng JJ, Dawson AS, Gylfadottir S. The use of aerobic exercise training in improving aerobic capacity in individuals with stroke: A meta-analysis. *Clin Rehabil* 2006;20(2):97–111.

Broadening the Search

Related References

Several databases offer an option to search "related articles" or "similar pages," once a relevant citation has been found. By using this function, one relevant article becomes the key to a list of useful references. These references will usually be shown in order of their relevance to the original record.

Science Citation Index

Science Citation Index is a reference system that allows researchers to search based on citations (see Table 31.1), by tracking literature forward or backward, and across disciplinary boundaries. The index will identify articles, books or other sources that have cited a particular reference or author. This index is available through online subscription or DVD, usually through a library.

Other Articles' Reference Lists

The reference list at the end of published articles will provide a handy inventory of sources that were used by other authors in their review of literature. The obvious disadvantage of this approach is that you will only identify references that are older than the original article. But it is often a good place to start, and to distinguish classic references that are used repeatedly.

Sensitivity and Specificity of Literature Searches

Electronic searching can be considered a blessing or a curse by the researcher. It is certainly more efficient than the old-fashioned time-consuming hand searching through volumes of the *Index Medicus*, although at the same time it can generate substantial lists of citations that may not be relevant to the project. The incentive for developing competence in searching is the ability to avoid retrieving too many citations or long lists of irrelevant ones.

In this aspect of searching, the terms "sensitivity" and "specificity" have been applied, with meanings analogous to their use with diagnostic tests (see Chapter 27).[4] Sensitivity, also called **recall**, is the proportion of retrieved citations that are relevant, or the likelihood of finding relevant references. A sensitive search might include some irrelevant studies but is more likely to be comprehensive. Specificity, also called **precision**, is the proportion of citations that are relevant that the search is able to retrieve, or the likelihood of excluding irrelevant references. A specific search might exclude some relevant studies but is more likely to include the very relevant ones.

When a search results in too many citations, you need to improve specificity by narrowing the question, using more specific search terms, combining search terms, or setting limits. Using the "focus" option can also restrict the search. When the number of references is too small, the search needs to improve its sensitivity by broadening the question, finding better search terms, using truncation or wildcards or trying varied combinations of terms. Using the "explode" option can improve the breadth of the search. In PubMed, under Clinical Queries, choosing a "sensitive" search will explode the search to include a broad range of articles, some that may be less relevant. Choosing a "specific" search will focus the search on the most relevant articles, but will eliminate some that have less obvious relevance. A useful guide to terms that can be used to increase sensitivity or specificity has been developed for use with MEDLINE.[5]

FINDING REFERENCES FOR EVIDENCE-BASED PRACTICE

In Chapter 1 we described the process of generating a question related to a patient case (see Box 1.1) to provide an evidence base for clinical decision making. When we search the literature as part of evidence-based practice, we are not "studying" a topic, as suggested in the previous section. Instead, for this purpose we are asking a question that is spurred by a particular patient issue, and our literature search is intended to find references that will help us make a good clinical decision for management of the patient.

Using PICO

The acronym **PICO** has been used to emphasize the importance of specifying the *P*opulation (or *P*atient characteristics), *I*nterventions, *C*omparisons and *O*utcomes that are relevant to the clinical question.[6] In going through this process, it is useful to generate a thorough list of terms that can then be used as keywords in a literature search. For example, consider the following case scenario:

> A 78 year-old male patient experienced a stroke 6 months ago. He is able to ambulate with the assistance of a regular cane, but does not participate in activities because of fatigue. He has been referred to physical therapy to increase his physical endurance. The patient has discussed the benefits of exercise with his physical therapist, but is concerned about risks associated with overexertion. He asks the therapist if exercise is really effective for people like him.

The therapist wants to gather specific information that the patient will be able to use in setting his own goals for exercise. She asks the question, "Will exercise improve endurance in a patient following stroke?

We might consider the following elements important for answering this clinical question:

P	stroke, "cerebrovascular accident," CVA
I	exercise, "aerobic exercise"
C	"no exercise"
O	endurance

These terms would become useful keywords for a search. Terms in quotes are intended to be searched as a string.

Searching for Systematic Reviews

Identifying systematic reviews in a search strategy can be challenging because the phrases "systematic review" or "meta-analysis" will not always appear in the title or abstract of an article. Many search engines and databases have established specific search strategies to find these types of studies. For instance, in PubMed reviews on a given topic can be obtained by checking "systematic reviews" under Subsets on the "Limits" tab. OVID provides limits for "Reviews" or "EBM Reviews." CINAHL will allow for retrieval of systematic reviews under publication type. Systematic reviews are considered a higher level of evidence than single primary studies (see Chapter 16) because they provide a critical analysis of available literature. Clinicians will typically find systematic reviews to be a good place to start when asking a clinical question for evidence-based practice decisions.

Reviews and Abstracts for Evidence-Based Practice

Several specialized databases index reviews of published literature. **Evidence Based Medicine Reviews (EBMR)** is a collection of databases available through the Cochrane Library and OVID Technologies, containing the following resources (see Table 31.1):

- *ACP Journal Club* is a collection of structured abstracts supported by the American College of Physicians. The abstracts describe the objectives, methods, results and evidence-based conclusions of original articles and systematic reviews published in over 100 clinical journals. The abstracts are written by clinicians with specific expertise to summarize the literature and provide brief commentaries on the context, methods and clinical applications of the findings. Articles are graded for clinical relevance using star ratings from 1 (least informative) to 7 (highly relevant).
- The **Cochrane Database of Systematic Reviews** is part of The Cochrane Library. This database indexes systematic reviews of healthcare interventions. Summaries of reviews can be accessed free online, but full text requires a subscription.
- The **Cochrane Central Register of Controlled Trials (CCTR)** is an index of randomized clinical trials that have been determined to be of sufficient quality for use in systematic reviews. CCTR can be accessed through the Cochrane Library.
- The **Database of Abstracts of Reviews of Effects (DARE)** is a full text database containing critical assessments of systematic reviews from a variety of medical journals. DARE records cover topics such as diagnosis, prevention, rehabilitation, screening, and treatment.

Other review databases are also useful for research and clinical decision making (see Table 31.1):

- *BMJ Clinical Evidence* is a journal of systematic reviews related to a broad range of clinical specialties. This publication continually updates already published systematic reviews by including recently published clinical trials as well as observational studies that might not have been cited in the original paper. The reviews are intended to summarize the current state of knowledge or uncertainty about the prevention and treatment of clinical conditions, and also strives to show when good evidence is not available.

- *Evidence-based Practice Centers (EPC) Reports* are developed on topics relevant to clinical, social science/behavioral, economic, and other health care organization and delivery issues—specifically those that are common, expensive, and/or significant for the Medicare and Medicaid populations. In 1997 the Agency for Health Care Policy and Research (AHCPR), now known as the Agency for Healthcare Research and Quality (AHRQ), launched its initiative to promote evidence-based practice in everyday care through establishment of 12 Evidence-based Practice Centers (EPCs).

- **Hooked on Evidence** is available to members of the American Physical Therapy Association. This database includes extractions from clinical trials, case-control and cohort studies, case reports and single-subject design studies related to physical therapy interventions. Over 3,000 extractions were available as of 2006.

KEEPING UP WITH THE LITERATURE: EMAIL ALERTS

The volume of literature that is available in health care can be truly overwhelming, as one strives to stay up to date in an environment that is increasingly focused on evidence. Many of us subscribe to a variety of journals that concentrate on our areas of clinical interest, and just keeping up with that reading can be a daunting task. Scanning the table of contents of particular journals can be a useful habit for finding articles of interest.

A convenient strategy to maintain a current library is to subscribe to **email alert** services, which provide regular automatic updates based on a search profile that you create. These services are usually free. They deliver current citations (with abstracts) or the table of contents of selected journals directly to your email. Services such as OVID, PubMed (through My NCBI), and ProQuest offer email alerts.[7] Many journals, including *Physical Therapy, Archives of Physical Medicine and Rehabilitation, New England Journal of Medicine,* and the *Journal of Speech, Language and Hearing Research,* allow individuals to register to receive free alerts for their table of contents each month. Some journals will also send out alerts for early release of certain articles. In this day of electronic communication and information overload, it seems prudent to let technology help us sort through the many resources that are available to us!

COMMENTARY

Is the Evidence Not There—or Can't We Find It?

In the pursuit of evidence for clinical decision making, it is important for us to realize that a lack of evidence (or perhaps more accurately our inability to locate the evidence) is not the same as having evidence that an intervention or diagnostic tool is ineffective. When looking for "best evidence," the literature may be inadequate, and experience and patient preferences may be the "best" guide available.

Whatever the reason for your literature search, be it for research or clinical purposes, it can be a frustrating process if you are not knowledgeable and experienced in the use of resources available to you. Various search strategies can be employed to find an appropriate reference list for a particular topic. We cannot begin to cover all of the approaches or tips that will make this process successful and efficient. Few of us are experts in this process, and new resources are constantly becoming available. A reference librarian can be an invaluable resource to assist with a search, avoiding that terrible and futile lament, "I've spent 5 hours searching and haven't found anything!" Most search engines and databases provide tutorials and tips that can guide the researcher in using the appropriate strategies. Many libraries sponsor classes in the use of these programs as well. It is worth the effort to learn to use these programs effectively.

The number of databases that are available through online services is staggering, and new options are constantly being developed. Reference librarians and good search strategies are essential to the researcher and clinician to take advantage of these remarkable resources.

REFERENCES

1. Clark OA, Castro AA. Searching the Literatura Latino Americana e do Caribe em Ciencias da Saude (LILACS) database improves systematic reviews. *Int J Epidemiol* 2002; 31:112–114.
2. Fact Sheet: Medical Subject Headings (MeSH). Available at: <http://www.nlm.nih.gov/pubs/factsheets/mesh.html> Accessed July 10, 2006.
3. Pang MY, Eng JJ, Dawson AS, Gylfadottir S. The use of aerobic exercise training in improving aerobic capacity in individuals with stroke: A meta-analysis. *Clin Rehabil* 2006;20:97–111.
4. Searching for the best evidence in clinical journals. Available at: <http://www.cebm.net/searching.asp> Accessed April 31, 2007.
5. Health Information Research Unit. Evidence-Based Health Informatics. Search strategies for MEDLINE in Ovid syntax and the PubMed translation. Available at: <http://hiru.mcmaster.ca/hedges/> Accessed May 3, 2007.
6. Straus SE, Richardson WS, Glasziou P, Haynes RB. *Evidence-based Medicine: How to Practice and Teach EBM*, 3rd ed. Edinburgh: Churchill Livingstone, 2005.
7. HealthLinks. Email Alert Services. Available at: <http://healthlinks.washington.edu/howto/alerts.html> Accessed April 10, 2007.

CHAPTER 32
Writing a Research Proposal

The initial stages of the research process include development of the research question and delineation of methods of data collection. The success of the project depends on how well these elements have been developed and defined in advance, so that the proper resources are gathered and methods proceed with reliability and validity. The plan that describes all these preparatory elements is the **research proposal.** The proposal describes the purpose of the study, the importance of the research question, the research protocol and justifies the feasibility of the project.

The proposal can serve several purposes. First, it represents the synthesis of the researcher's critical thinking and the scientific literature to ensure that the research question is refined enough to be studied, that the assumptions and theoretical rationale on which the study is based are logical and that the method is appropriate for answering the question. Second, the well prepared proposal may constitute the body of a grant application when external funding is required. Third, it is part of an application for review by peer or administrative committees. This is the document that will be carefully scrutinized by the **Institutional Review Board (IRB)** (see Chapter 3). Fourth, the proposal enhances communication among colleagues who may be co-investigators and with consultants whose advice may be needed. Finally, the careful, detailed account of the study procedures serves as a guide throughout the data collection phase to ensure that the researchers follow the outlined rules of conduct. The research proposal, therefore, is an indispensable instrument in initiating and implementing a project.

When proposals are written as part of a grant application for funding from foundations or government agencies, the researcher must obtain the guidelines of the agency to which the proposal will be submitted. Generally, requirements and components of a proposal will be the same for grant applications as they are for academic and clinical institutions; however, to write a successful grant application, the researcher must understand the interests of the funding agency, the extent of available funds, the deadlines for submitting proposals, and the proper format of the application.*

The purpose of this chapter is to discuss the process of developing and writing a research proposal. The exact format of the proposal will depend on the requirements or instructions of the individuals, clinics, faculty or agencies that will review the project.

---

*A reference, such as the Foundation Reporter,[1] can be used to aid in selecting an appropriate agency. This reference provides information about an agency's contact individual, foundation philosophy, typical recipients, application, review procedures and restrictions. Other resources may be found on the Internet, such as Science Careers, sponsored by the AAAS.[2]

TABLE 32.1   **WORKING PLAN FOR DEVELOPING A RESEARCH PROPOSAL**

I. THE RESEARCH PLAN
  A. Title
  B. Abstract
  C. Statement of the research problem
    1. Rationale and justification for the study
    2. Significance of the study
  D. Statement of the purpose of the study
    1. Specific aims or objectives
    2. Research hypotheses or guiding questions
  E. Background of the study
    1. Topics for the review of literature related to:
      a. Theory and supportive rationale
      b. Related studies
      c. Methods
    2. Previous work by the investigator that supports the project
  F. Method
    1. Subjects: characteristics, sampling method and plans for recruitment
    2. Materials: instrumentation, plans to establish reliability and validity
    3. Procedures
      a. Study design
      b. Details of test and treatment administration
      c. Data collection methods
      d. Timetable and organizational chart
    4. Data management and analysis
  G. Literature cited
  H. Documentation of informed consent
II. PLAN FOR ADMINISTRATIVE SUPPORT
  A. Budget: personnel, equipment, facilities and supplies
  B. Resources and environment
  C. Personnel: qualifications, time commitment, job descriptions, consultant

The order of presentation of material may vary, as may the extent of the information required. The following guidelines are meant to reflect the most common elements of a proposal. A research proposal has two basic parts, as shown in Table 32.1. The first part provides details of the research plan, and the other describes the administrative and personnel support required to carry out the project.

COMPONENTS OF THE RESEARCH PLAN

Before writing one word, the researcher spends considerable time thinking, gathering facts, and consulting with individuals who are knowledgeable in the content and methodology of interest. Students should also review guidelines for preparing their proposal with faculty advisors. Researchers who are seeking funding may find it helpful to read other proposals that were submitted to and funded by the agencies that are being considered. As one proceeds with the development of the project and considers its feasibility, it is helpful to follow an organized working plan that focuses the important elements of the project.

Title

The title of a research proposal will be the first thing seen by readers, although it is often easier for the researcher to develop an appropriate title after the study design has been formulated. The title will become the project's introduction to all potential readers. It is the first impression of what the reviewers should expect to read in the subsequent pages. It must be concise and informative. A title such as "Bronchopulmonary Dysplasia" is certainly concise, but the reader is likely to say "what about it?" Expanded, this title could be "Cardiovascular Problems in Bronchopulmonary Dysplasia." This is better, but does not yet suggest a research focus. With a few more words, this title will say much more: "Cardiovascular Effects of Physical Therapy Intervention in Infants with Bronchopulmonary Dysplasia." We now know that this proposed research has an *independent variable* and a *dependent variable* and that the sample will be infants.

Abstract

A summary or **abstract** of the project or program, often limited to one page, is required by most funding agencies and institutional review boards, and may be required for student projects. When a proposed project is to be reviewed by faculty, administrative or foundation committees, all members of these committees will receive the summary, whereas only selected members of such committees may review the full proposal. The abstract should highlight the purpose and importance of the proposed project. A brief description of the method should identify the study subjects, procedures and methods for data analysis. The proposed duration of the study and overall projected costs may be stated. Because the summary is likely to be read before the detailed proposal is read, it must make a positive impression, conveying specifically what is to be done and why the study is important.

Body of the Proposal

The body of the research proposal is the narrative portion that will explain the purpose and importance of the study and describe the design and procedures in detail.

Statement of the Problem

The opening statement of the proposal identifies the subject area to be studied. As an introduction, this statement should convey a clear sense of the importance of the problem in terms of applicability of potential findings to clinical practice and patient care. It may begin as a broad definition but should lead the reader logically toward a definition of the specific delimited topic, which will become the focus of the present project.

As an example, Rudd and co-workers[3] compared a specialist community rehabilitation program with a standard hospital and homecare program for patients with stroke. The statement of the problem, as it might have been written in a proposal, would first establish why the study was needed by defining the problems related to costs of hospitalization and psychosocial aspects of managing these patients. By acknowledging these problems and alternative approaches to rehabilitation, the researchers justify the need to further examine the effectiveness of different treatment settings.

The problem statement, therefore, presents a rationale for the specific question being addressed by the project. In the preceding example, the authors have created a rationale for examining the difference between the structured specialist community program and standard care. No single project can be expected to solve a problem in its entirety. On the other hand, each project should clearly contribute to the solution. Each study expands the evidence that can be used to support the body of knowledge related to the research problem. The content of the opening section of the proposal should clearly demonstrate this contribution.

Purpose, Hypotheses and Specific Aims

In a brief statement, the researcher must state precisely what the project is expected to accomplish. The **purpose** of the study should follow clearly from the justification presented earlier. If the research is to be experimental or correlational, the purpose is translated here into research hypotheses. Research hypotheses are stated in positive terms; they reflect the expectations of outcome. "Null" hypotheses that serve a statistical function do not belong in the text, unless the purpose of the research is specifically to show that no relationship exists between variables. If the research is descriptive in nature, the author will state the characteristics or behaviors that will be documented in this work and what questions the data will answer about the target population.

Many granting agencies require a statement of **specific aims** or **objectives** for a project. For instance, a study's objectives might be to add to the body of knowledge in a certain content area, to test a theoretical proposition, to demonstrate differences between certain treatments to develop more effective and efficient intervention strategies, to document the reliability of an instrument, or to establish the relationship between specific variables as a basis for making treatment planning decisions. These objectives are derived from the research hypotheses or descriptive questions. Objectives help reviewers focus the description of methods and will often help the researcher guide the discussion of results when the study is completed.

Proposals for qualitative research may need to include explanations of the research approach, especially when those who will review the proposal are unfamiliar with naturalistic inquiry. The researcher should include specific reference to the form of qualitative research (for example, ethnography or phenomenology), including assumptions about the nature of knowledge and reality that are relevant to the area of study.[4]

Background

The presentation of background information includes the theoretical rationale for the study and pertinent facts, observations or claims that have led the investigator to the proposed research question. This information is derived from the literature review (see Chapter 7) and from previous or related work done by the investigator. Funding agencies look favorably on projects that are built on previous work by the investigator.

The literature review is difficult to present concisely, and much effort is usually required to integrate published material to make relevant points. While preparing for a project, the researcher will have read and catalogued many references, typically many more than will or should be included in the written proposal. Authors must continually ask, "Is this reference or point of information directly related to this study?" "Does it contribute to the rationale or clarify the basic assumptions that underlie the research question?" If the answer is "No," then the reference should be set aside or discarded. When the references have been selected, they should be organized by topic areas to facilitate organization of the paper.

The presentation of the review of literature includes the main points that serve as the background of the proposed study. A meaningful review of literature provides a clear representation of the author's thought processes in developing the proposed study. It is not simply a series of abstracts of papers on the topic. The author must convey an integration of content that supports the need, importance and rationale for the proposed study. The need and importance of the proposed study are defined in relationship to existing clinical or scientific reports. The first elements of the review may include relevant epidemiological factors, demographics, the impact of the research issue on health care policy or practice and the potential impact on patients. For instance, for the example cited earlier, the investigators might focus on the rising costs of care resulting from the increased incidence of stroke, and the potential psychosocial advantages of the patients' early return to community living.

The major portion of the background focuses on prior research that has been done to address the same or related questions, reflecting current knowledge or lack of knowledge. This includes a synthesis of consistencies and conflicts found in prior reports. The possible reasons for inconsistencies and identifiable limitations of previous studies should be elucidated to provide further evidence that more study is required. The content of this section should show the logic for selecting subjects, selecting the variables to be studied and the methods of measurement. This section should end with a summary of the facts, problems, or controversies found in the literature and the relevant perspectives of the researcher that lead directly back to the specific need and stated purpose of the proposed study.

Method

The method section is probably the most important part of the proposal, and should be both concise and complete. The author should include enough detailed information so that reviewers can judge the soundness of the work, so that members of the institutional review board can determine exactly what the subjects will be asked to do and so that the researcher can determine the feasibility of the study. The opening section identifies the overall study design that will be employed to test the research hypothesis or answer the research question. For example,

> This will be a randomized controlled trial to compare the effects of a specialized community rehabilitation program and a standard hospital-based program on motor abilities, cognition, aphasia, activities of daily living, anxiety and depression in patients who have had a stroke.

The details of the research methods are usually presented in four subsections: Subjects, Materials, Procedures, and Data Analysis.

Subjects.   The description of *subjects* used in human studies is extremely important because of the inherent variability among them and the vast number of extraneous factors that may affect human behavior or performance. The author must describe who the subjects will be in terms of *inclusion* and *exclusion criteria*, how many and from where subjects will be recruited, how they are to be selected, and the method by which they will be assigned to groups for the study. Characteristics such as age, gender, disability, diagnosis and duration of hospitalization should be defined if they are relevant to the study. The author must include all, and only, those factors that could influence the results and the ability to generalize the findings to the target population or to compare findings with other similar studies. Funding agencies and institutional review boards generally require a power analysis to demonstrate the appropriateness of the proposed sample size.

Materials.   *Materials* refer to the equipment, instruments or measuring tools that will be used in the study. Materials should be described according to important characteristics such as brand name and model and should be documented for reliability and validity. If measurement tools are new, relatively unknown, or developed by the researcher, they should be described in sufficient detail and a figure should be included. If the measurement tool is a survey, the entire document may be presented as an appendix to the proposal or a set of sample questions may be included in the narrative.

Procedures.   The *procedures* section describes precisely what is to be done from beginning to end of the investigation, in chronological sequence. Procedures also include how, and by whom data are to be collected. Operational definitions should be provided for independent and dependent variables. If these procedures are extensive and lengthy, they may be briefly described in the text with references to appendixes that will present the details in full. The researcher should include strategies for controlling extraneous variables.

In qualitative study, the proposal should include how the researcher will interact with subjects, describing the kind of data that will be collected (for example, field notes, audio tapes, video tapes, or transcriptions).[4]

A chart or flow sheet, presented in tabular form, will serve to summarize the procedural sequence. Figure 32.1 illustrates the timetable for a hypothetical 2-year study. The study is a pretest-posttest design with subjects randomly assigned to two treatment groups. The intervention period for each subject lasts 6 months. Outcome data will be collected initially, each month for 6 months, and 9 months after the initial evaluation of each patient. The last patients will be admitted to the study in Month 15; their treatment period, lasting 6 months, will end in Month 21, and their follow-up assessment will be made 3 months later, in Month 24. Such a display of the "work schedule" will assist reviewers in evaluating the feasibility of the investigation in terms of time and available funding.

Data Analysis.   The plan for *data analysis* should outline specific procedures for recording, storing, and reducing data and for statistical analysis. Reviewers will examine both descriptive and analytical methods to determine their appropriateness for the

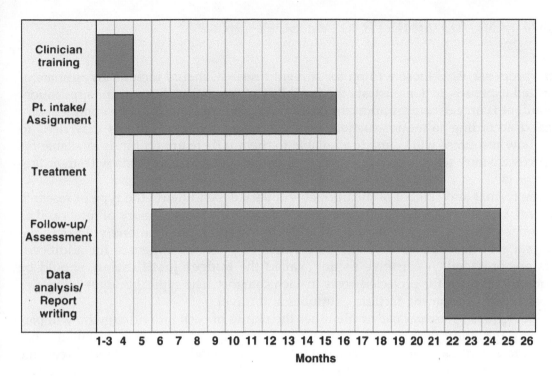

Months

FIGURE 32.1   Graphic display of a hypothetical study time line.

design of the study and the type of measurement. It is often helpful to obtain the services of a statistician to be sure that this section is accurate and complete. The funding agency will probably have a statistician review it.

Proposals for qualitative studies should include descriptions of how notes will be transcribed and reconstructed.[4] The specifics of coding and sorting data may evolve as the project unfolds, but the researcher should discuss the intended format and how the process will be developed. Methods of establishing reliability and validity of data should be included (see Chapter 14).

References.   The final part of the narrative portion of the proposal should be a listing of literature cited in the paper. Some agencies require the use of a specific bibliographic style, but often this is left to the discretion of the researcher.

Documentation of Informed Consent

A copy of the informed consent form must accompany the proposal when subjects will be directly involved in the study. The informed consent form may not be required for secondary analysis studies. Funding agencies and sponsoring institutions may require IRB approval before a proposal is submitted and reviewed. The time delays inherent in obtaining this approval must be built into the timetable for submitting the proposal. Documentation of IRB approval must accompany the proposal. The process and elements of obtaining informed consent are discussed in Chapter 3.

PLAN FOR ADMINISTRATIVE SUPPORT
Budget

Every proposal, even those written for student research, should include an estimate of projected expenses, to demonstrate the feasibility of the project. For a grant application, the budget is an extremely important part of the proposal, and must be complete and detailed according to the instructions of the funding agency. Students may need to show how resources will be made available to them if there are no funds available for the project. Many schools provide small grants that will assist students with their thesis projects.

The format and content of the budget will vary depending on the type of research proposal. Generally, the budget is presented by category as a summary of totals and as an itemized budget. For grants that are expected to run more than one year, only the first year's budget is itemized, and summaries of projected expenses for additional years are provided. A narrative section, called the **budget justification**, should be included to explain the projected costs in each category. The typical budget categories are personnel, equipment, facilities, supplies and travel.

The itemized *personnel budget* identifies the names of each individual who will participate in the study, their proposed title (such as principal investigator, consultant, statistician, research assistant, secretary), the salary for each individual and the percentage of full-time or number of hours that will be devoted to the project. Dollar amounts may be based on percentage of the individual's full-time salary or an hourly wage for a specified number of hours. Some personnel may be asked to participate in the project with no remuneration. These individuals should also be listed, showing no salary request. Associated fringe benefit amounts are listed separately based on the total amount of projected salaries and wages. Reviewers will scrutinize the personnel budget particularly to evaluate the appropriateness of the time commitment of each participant. The budget justification should explain the responsibilities of each participant and should show that the personnel will realistically be able to achieve the desired outcomes.

Equipment costs are given for all equipment that will be purchased with grant funds. Costs should reflect current prices and any charges related to installation, calibration and maintenance. Most granting agencies define a threshold cost for "equipment" as having an extended life expectancy of at least 3 to 5 years. The narrative should provide details of equipment, such as manufacturer, model number and special accessories that are needed for the study. The researcher should indicate if some of the necessary equipment is already available, to show the funding agency that the project can be completed with some contribution by the researcher's institution.

The budget may include a request for funds for *alteration* or *renovations* to facilities. If space must be altered to accommodate equipment or to provide a work area, the contractors' estimates should be confirmed before specifying those costs in the budget. Explanations of all construction costs should be provided in detail, justifying why they are necessary for the study.

The category called *supplies* usually refers to consumable materials as opposed to capital equipment. Specific quantities of these supplies should be given with justification. A category of "other expenses" may also be included to account for miscellaneous items, such as telephone costs and photocopying. Depending on the nature of the project and the regulations of the funding agency, *travel expenses* may be budgeted. Travel to and from the institutional "home base" to collect data is certainly part of conducting a project and is likely to be an acceptable expense. Travel to meetings where data may be presented is more indirectly related to the project, but can often be justified. Travel costs may also be applied to patients who must be transported for purposes of the research.

All of the preceding budget categories are defined as **direct costs. Indirect costs** relate principally to the overhead charged by the sponsoring institution for administrative activities, facility maintenance and any other support services. Funding agencies usually limit the amount of support that may be used for indirect costs based on some defined percentage of the total budget. In cases where the customary institutional charge exceeds the set limit, the budget narrative should specify the manner in which such a discrepancy will be handled. In some cases, granting agencies will negotiate this percentage. The total budget for the project is the sum of all direct and indirect costs.

In every institution where research is conducted, there is an administrative officer responsible for grants and contracts. This individual will be able to assist researchers with the general "anatomy" of a proposal budget and will provide information about fringe benefits, indirect costs and institutional support. Consultation with this individual is essential and should begin early in the process of developing a research proposal budget. The administrative officer must sign off on the proposal before it is submitted, reflecting institutional approval of the proposed project.

Resources and Environment

Many funding agencies and academic or clinical institutions will also ask for information regarding existing resources for carrying out the proposed project. The investigator will be asked to describe available laboratory facilities, equipment, clinical sites, computer capability, office space and so on, to demonstrate that the project is feasible within the institution's environment. The areas in which data collection will take place should be described, as should the areas where equipment will be housed. In addition, administrative support services may need to be described. Documentation of secretarial or technical assistance or the need to acquire such support will be evaluated by reviewers in regard to the feasibility and justification of the applicant's budget request.

Personnel

Identification of the investigators and their qualifications is an important element of a proposal, especially when external funding is being sought. This will probably not be a factor in student research, except where expert assistance is required for carrying out parts of the project. Funding agencies will examine investigators' education, experience, track record of research and prior publications to determine that they have appropriate qualifications. This information is most often provided in the form of biographical summaries for each person working on the project. Some institutions offer a variety of funding programs and the eligibility requirements differ for each program. For example, the Arthritis Foundation offers several programs ranging from postdoctoral fellowships for individuals with 3 to 6 years of research experience to traineeships for supporting the research of individual health professions.[5] Grants through the National Institutes of Health usually require that someone with an MD or PhD and research experience act as primary investigator. Foundations that support new investigators often require that an experienced, competent researcher supervise the proposed work. Because of these kinds of criteria, the inclusion of information about the participants in a proposed study is essential to the process of evaluation by an agency or foundation.

PRESENTATION OF THE PROPOSAL

Style

The research proposal is a forward-looking document. The researcher's thinking begins with the present, acknowledges and draws from the past, but primarily leads to the future. Therefore, the statement of the problem is written in the present tense, the background is written in the past tense, and the method (which is the proposed research) is written in the future tense.

The actual format required for the proposal varies among agencies and schools. The researcher must follow the specific instructions provided by the sponsoring agency. The method of citing references should be consistent throughout, and tables and appendixes should be clearly labeled and cited in the text.

The tone or mood of the document should be positive, persuasive and scholarly. The researcher must convince reviewers that the proposed research is important, that there is a need to conduct the proposed research, and that the research team has the knowledge and ability to accomplish the study objectives. Phrases such as "perhaps the results will contribute" and "we hope to demonstrate" convey hesitation and insecurity. Conversely, the use of superlatives, implying that this work will be the greatest of all, will detract from the substance. A proposal that is sensible, factual and realistic will receive the attention it deserves.

COMMENTARY

Review, Revise, Edit, Revise, Review

Even the most experienced researcher will find writing a proposal challenging. For those with less experience, the empty page may seem like an insurmountable hurdle. The best way to get started is to dive in, with the clear understanding that there will be several drafts and revisions before the proposal is ready for submission.[6] The proposal will not necessarily be written in the order that it will later be read; for example, the abstract is presented at the beginning, but may actually be written last.

Before the "final" version is ready, one final step should be taken: enlisting others to read the whole proposal. Graduate students have "built-in" readers; this is one of the responsibilities of thesis and dissertation advisory committees. Those who are not students should seek three kinds of individuals to review the proposal. One who is knowledgeable about the topic and the relevance of the project should be asked to evaluate the appropriateness, accuracy and thoroughness of the presentation. Another who understands research design and methodology will concentrate on the validity of the research methods relative to the research question and specific aims. The third should be someone who is unfamiliar with the subject matter and who will react to the readability of the paper. All three may notice inconsistencies, instances of unnecessary professional jargon or redundancy. This kind of preliminary review by colleagues is valuable for inspiring the researcher's confidence that the proposal is ready for formal review and subsequent successful implementation.

REFERENCES

1. Foundation Reporter: *Comprehensive Profiles and Guiding Analyses of America's Major Private Foundations*, Ed. 38. Detroit, MI, The Taft Group, 2005.
2. American Association for the Advancement of Science: *Science Careers*. Available at: <http://sciencecareers.sciencemag.org/funding> Accessed June 5, 2006.
3. Rudd AG, Wolfe CDA, Tilling, K and Beech R: Randomised controlled trial to evaluate discharge scheme for patients with stroke. *BMJ* 1997;315:1039–1044.
4. Heath AW. The proposal in qualitative research. *The Qualitative Report* (Online serial). 1997;3(1). Available at: <http://www.nova.edu/ssss/QR/QR3-1/heath.html> Accessed June 11, 2007.
5. Arthritis Foundation. Available at: <http://www.arthritis.org/research/ProposalCentral.asp#chapter> Accessed June 5, 2006.
6. Davitz JR, Davitz LL. *Evaluating Research Proposals: A Guide for the Behavioral Sciences.* Upper Saddle River, NJ. Prentice Hall, 1996.

CHAPTER 33

Reporting the Results of Clinical Research

The culmination of the research process is the communication of results. This final stage may be the most important part of the process in that only shared information can clarify, amplify and expand the professional body of knowledge. Research reports can be developed in a variety of ways. The written article published in a refereed journal provides a permanent record of research that will be available to a large audience. Oral reports and poster presentations at professional meetings serve to disseminate research information in a timely fashion, although the audience is limited and the record of research findings will be found only in abstract form. Students are usually required to document their work in the form of a thesis or dissertation, but may be given the option of writing the paper in the form of a journal article. The purpose of this chapter is to describe the process of preparing manuscripts for publication in scientific journals, poster presentations and oral reports.

THE JOURNAL ARTICLE

Selecting a Journal

The researcher should decide where the manuscript will be submitted before writing the final paper. The expansion of the scope of practice in the health professions has been accompanied by a proliferation of publications serving specialized areas of practice. The choices are numerous and selection of the appropriate one deserves careful thought.

Some journals have a clearly defined focus with priorities explicitly stated. This focus is often stated in a journal's masthead or instructions to authors. For example, the *Journal of Rehabilitation Research and Development* (*JRRD*) has a complete statement that clarifies the kinds of papers that are appropriate, including the priorities:

> *JRRD* responsibly reports the results of rehabilitation research relevant to veterans. Our goal is to publish cutting-edge research that enhances the quality and relevance of Department of Veterans Affairs rehabilitation research and disseminate biomedical and engineering advances. Priority areas are prosthetics, amputations, orthotics, and orthopedics; spinal cord injury and other neurological disorders (with particular interest in traumatic brain injury, multiple sclerosis, and restorative therapies); communication, sensory, and cognitive aids; geriatric rehabilitation; and functional outcome research. *JRRD* accepts national and international submissions.[1]

When a journal's focus is not so obvious, the contents of several issues of that journal should be read to determine if a particular study is consistent with the subject matter and type of research that the journal tends to publish. It is an unfortunate waste of time, effort and perhaps money to make the wrong choice and to have a manuscript returned because it "is not suitable for publication" in a particular journal. This is almost verbatim what the rejection letter will say.

Another consideration in selecting a journal is the readership. The product of research should reach the people who will best be able to use the information. If, for example, a study documents the functional outcome of an orthopedic surgical procedure, the report should be in a journal that orthopedists read. If, on the other hand, the study focuses on the postoperative physical or occupational therapy intervention, journals devoted to these professions will be more appropriate.

Submitting the Article

Every journal publishes **Instructions to Authors** that must be followed in the preparation of a manuscript. Although the general format of a research report is fairly consistent in medical and scientific writing,[2] each journal has its own particular rules about organization and length of a manuscript; preparation of tables, illustrations, or graphs; and method of reference citation. Look carefully at articles published in the journal to follow the format. Failure to follow the instructions may be a reason for rejection; or, at least, the manuscript will be returned for corrections.

Authors must expect delays in responses when their article is being reviewed. Some journal editors are more rigorous about turnaround time than others. Standard policy for scientific journals states that authors should submit an article to only one journal at a time. This protects journals from conflicts in copyright. If an article is rejected, the author can then submit it to a different journal.

The content of this chapter is in keeping with the CONSORT[3] and STARD[4] statements that are designed to assure that papers related to intervention or analysis of diagnostic tools are complete. These statements were described more fully in Chapters 9 and 27 (see Tables 9.3 and 27.3 and Figures 9.1 and 27.4).

Structure and Content of the Written Research Report

The sections of a research report are the abstract, introduction, methods, results, discussion and conclusion, as shown in Table 33.1. The introduction and methods sections serve the same purpose as in the project proposal; that is, they describe the rationale for the study and the specific procedures used to collect the data (see Chapter 32). Although the content of these sections will be similar to the proposal, the author will have to do some serious editing to fit the journal article format. The "forward-looking" statements must be changed to past tense because the project is now completed. The last three sections of the article will be completely new.

Abstract.   Most journals require an **abstract** of the report that the author usually prepares after the manuscript is complete. The abstract summarizes the content of the article including the purpose of the study, the number and type of subjects, the basic procedures used, a summary of the results and the major conclusion. The abstract must

TABLE 33.1 STRUCTURE OF A JOURNAL ARTICLE FOR REPORTING RESEARCH

Section	Should contain
Abstract	• Overview and purpose of the study • General description of methods • Highlights of results • Statement of significance of results • General conclusions
Introduction	• Statement of the problem • Clinical relevance • Review of literature • Rationale and theoretical framework • Specific purpose and hypotheses (or guiding questions)
Methods	• Study design • Criteria for and methods of subject selection • Description and number of subjects • Measurement methods and data collection techniques • Data analysis procedures
Results	• Narrative description of statistical outcomes • Tables and figures that summarize findings • Statements to support or reject hypotheses
Discussion (and Conclusions)	• Interpretation of statistical outcomes • Discussion of clinical significance of outcomes • Importance of the work • Comparison of results with work of others • How results support or conflict with theory • Critique of the study limitations and strengths • Suggestions for further study
References	• List of all references cited in the article

be concise. The prescribed limit may be 150 words, occasionally less. Readers will refer to the abstract first to decide whether to read the complete report. Computerized retrieval systems store author-written abstracts. Therefore, they must be able to stand alone, despite their brevity.

Introduction.   The **introduction** can be drawn from the statement of purpose, the background and specific aims included in the research proposal. As in the proposal, the introduction of an article should provide a description of the research question and the context within which the author intended to answer it. After reading the first one or two paragraphs of the introduction, the reader should have a clear understanding of the problem being studied and why it is important. The literature review should reflect the relevant background that is necessary to support the theoretical rationale for the study, and should provide sufficient information for the reader to understand how the research question will be answered. The introduction should end with a statement of the specific purpose of the study, delineating the variables that were studied and the research hypotheses or guiding questions that have been investigated in the study.

Methods.   The **methods** section should begin by describing the subjects, including how many were studied, what criteria were used to recruit them, how they were selected and how they were assigned to groups. Relevant characteristics of subjects, especially age and sex, should be summarized using means, ranges and frequencies. Most journals require a statement documenting that subjects read and signed an informed consent form and that the appropriate committees approved the project.

The methods section continues with a description of equipment and data collection procedures, presented in chronological order so that the reader can follow the procedural flow of the project. If the measurement or treatment procedures are standardized and well known, they can be described briefly and the author can refer the reader to the original sources for a more detailed description. When manufactured instruments are used, the company name and address should be cited. Operational definitions should be provided for all variables, with the intent that someone could replicate the data collection procedures. Many researchers develop a written protocol that they use as a guide during data collection to be sure that all procedures are followed properly. This protocol can easily serve as an outline for this section of the paper. Diagrams, photographs and tables can clarify and simplify the presentation of methods. For example, demographic information and special characteristics of subjects can be summarized in a table, and photographs of a unique procedural setup may make a lengthy verbal description unnecessary.

The methods section ends with a full description of the procedures used to reduce and analyze the data, including specific statistical procedures. If unique or new statistical methods are used, they should be referenced.

Results.   The **results** section contains *only* a report of results, that is, a narrative description of exactly what happened in order of importance relative to the specific aims or hypotheses of the study. In the course of the study, the researchers may have gained considerable amounts of information, but unless it relates specifically to the stated purpose of the project, such information should not be included in this section. If one simple hypothesis has been proposed, the results section may be stated in a few succinct sentences.

The outcomes of statistical tests must be included to demonstrate or support the statement of results. Although the inclusion of calculated values, degrees of freedom, and the significance level is important, the narrative portion of the results section should emphasize the variables of interest rather than just statistics. For example, in a study of gait comparing elderly and young women, the statement "The differences in step length were significant, $t = -3.13$ ($p < .01$)," is not as meaningful to the reader as "The elderly women demonstrated a significantly shorter step length than the younger group $(t = -3.13, p < .01)$." When detailed statistical or descriptive information related to the study variables is needed in the paper, it is usually easier and often clearer for the reader to refer to tables or graphs that summarize such information.

Two major principles should guide the structure of the results section. One is that tables and figures should not duplicate the narrative; that is, if the author includes values for group means and standard deviations in the body of the text, there is no need to repeat them in a table. The author can refer the reader to the tables and figures for details and should only summarize these details in the text. The reader should be able to understand the results without referring to the tables and should be able to understand the tables without referring to the text. Therefore, the tables and figures should complement but be independent of the text. Second, the author should not discuss results in this section. Statements related to how this information could be applied to practice or interpretation of outcomes should be left to the discussion section.

Discussion.   The **discussion** section is the heart of a research report. It reflects the researcher's interpretation of the results in terms of the purpose of the study and the outside world. This is the part of the paper in which the author can express opinions. The author should comment on the importance of the results, limitations of the study, suggestions for future research and clinical implications.

The commentary about the importance of results should not be a reiteration of the results section, but should focus on alternative explanations of the observed outcomes, emphasizing how they either support or refute previous work or clinical theories. All results should be addressed, including those that were not statistically significant. The author should provide perspectives on the applicability of results to practice or further study.

The limitations of the study, including possible extraneous variables that could have affected the outcomes, should be identified and explained. Some of these factors may have been identified before the study began and others will have become evident during the course of data collection or analysis. These may include small sample size, attrition of subjects or lack of subject adherence to the protocol. The author must consider the relative importance of these limitations to the interpretations of results. It is essential that the author delineate all major extraneous factors so that the reader can examine the results realistically.

Every research endeavor leads to further questions. Sometimes, these questions arise out of the expressed limitations of a study and the need to clarify extraneous factors. In clinical research, alternative methods exist for studying the same or similar research questions and these may need to be examined. Given the results of a study, the author may want to reconsider a particular theory and how it may be applied. Suggestions for future research will develop from these ideas and should be expressed.

Authors should acknowledge the immediate or potential applicability of results to clinical practice. Their perspectives on the clinical relevance of studies are important whether the research focus is primarily on theory, applied science or clinical effectiveness.

Conclusion.   The **conclusion** is a brief restatement of the purpose of the study and its principal findings. It is often written in such a way that the author states the deductions made from the results. Phrases like "the results of this study indicate" and "this study demonstrates" serve to link the summary of results and the meaning of those results.

References.   The style of citing **references** throughout the text and in the listing of references at the end of a manuscript must follow the Instructions to Authors. Many journals use the style suggested by the published "Uniform Requirements."[2] Others may follow the American Psychological Association.[5]

The Internet is an important new source of references. Journals may eventually include instructions for such citations. The Modern Language Association of America (MLA) has published a full array of methods for citing documents that have been obtained from websites.[6]

Tables and Graphs

Tables and graphs should be used in the results section of an article to facilitate explanation of statistical findings and to provide visual explanations. To be effective, the tables and graphs must follow guidelines for the specific journal and general considerations for developing visual materials. The narrative portion of the paper will often present general descriptions of findings, and the tables and figures will present the details.

Tables

The customary table has five components: the title, column headings (horizontally displayed), row headings (vertically displayed), the "field" within which the data are arranged by columns and rows, and footnotes. Journals will format tables according to their style. The well constructed table of research results will present numeric or descriptive data demonstrating the relationships between independent and dependent variables. The title should identify those relationships.

Whether data are oriented vertically or horizontally may depend on the size and format requirement of the journal; however, logically, related numeric data should be presented in the columns, particularly when they will be summarized with totals or means and standard deviations in the last row. The sequence of column headings should progress logically from left to right based on the order of events. In the display of pretest and posttest data, the pretest should come first. The column headings should specify what was measured and the units of measurement, such as "(degrees)." The source of column data must be identified by the row headings, such as subjects by number or code when individual data points are displayed, or with labels, such as "control" and "experimental" when the table represents grouped summaries.

Footnotes may be used to present p-values, to explain abbreviations, or to cite references. A journal's instructions to authors may specify the style for sequentially labeling footnotes. Some may use small italic Arabic letters (a,b,c). Others may use symbolic keys. For example, the Uniform Requirements for Manuscripts Submitted to Biomedical Journals describes a common symbolic sequence: * (asterisk), † (dagger), ‡ (double dagger), § (section mark), || (parallels), ¶ (paragraph symbol), and # (number sign).[2]

Specialized tables are constructed to present statistical test summaries. Many examples are presented in this text. A tabular presentation of a frequency distribution is shown in Table 17.1. A typical analysis of variance table, called a "source table," is shown in Table 20.1.

Graphs

Graphs provide a visual demonstration of research results. Trends, relationships and comparisons may be presented more effectively and more concisely by constructing a graph than by writing a detailed text. Graphs can be drawn in a number of ways. Frequency data are commonly represented using a histogram or a frequency polygon. Figure 17.1 in this text shows examples. In a *histogram* the bars are contiguous, and in a *frequency polygon,* the data points are connected by lines. A *pie chart* graphically can display the proportional distribution of selected characteristics of a whole sample where the percentage of each characteristic is drawn to scale as a piece of the whole pie. A *bar graph,* which is a series of separate bars, may be used to show frequency or magnitude data derived from separate samples, such as control versus experimental group values, or experimental events, such as pretest and posttest values.

In constructing graphs, the author must pay careful attention to the scaling of the units of measurement. Graphs are intended to represent meaningful trends, relationships, or comparisons; therefore scales should be realistic and drawn to illustrate important, true differences in the data. They can, however, be drawn to present a false impression—either exaggerating or diminishing real differences. For example, Figure 33.1 displays shoulder abduction range of motion before and after treatment intervention. The data in both graphs are the same: a mean of 100 degrees for both groups before treatment, 110 degrees for the control group and 120 degrees for the experimental group following treatment. The magnitude of change appears to be greater in Figure 33.1A as compared with Figure 33.1B. Especially considering that normal shoulder abduction range is somewhere between 160 and 180 degrees, Figure 33.1A seems to be an exaggeration of the comparative effectiveness of the treatment intervention.

In deciding what content to present in narrative form or in tables or graphs, the author should consider a general rule that each element of the results section must

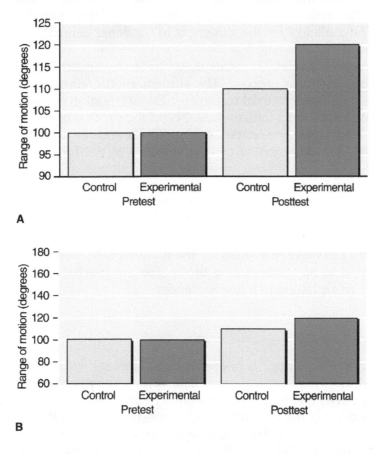

FIGURE 33.1 Two bar graphs showing shoulder abduction range of motion before and after treatment for two groups, illustrating the effect of vertical axis scaling. (**A**) Scale from 90 to 125 degrees; (**B**) Scale from 60 to 180 degrees.

stand alone and each must contribute to the complete and accurate presentation of the research findings.

Unique Elements for Reporting Systematic Reviews

The general principles and procedures for preparing papers for publication apply to reporting systematic reviews. The content of these reports, however, should include descriptions of the special methods that are part of the review process, as described in Chapter 16. The reader is encouraged to look for examples in the Cochrane Database of Systematic Reviews.[7]

Converting Theses and Dissertations for Publication

Most theses and dissertations are written on the basis of a six-chapter format: statement of the problem, review of the literature, methods, results, discussion and conclusion. Journal articles contain the same elements, but are honed carefully by authors to avoid all but the essential content presented succinctly. The full document that is prepared to meet degree requirements is usually too long and over-referenced to be acceptable as a journal article. The challenge for the student is to condense content considerably while retaining substance and meaning.

This is not a simple undertaking; therefore, the student must consider seriously the decision and commitment to proceed. The student should consider whether the outcome of the project will offer journal readers useful information or new insight and perspectives. Only if the answer is affirmative should the process of editing begin.

The review of literature, presentation of methods and results, and discussion will require the most work. The review of the literature in the full document is usually extremely lengthy. The author who writes for publication is obliged to be much more selective, including in the manuscript only those references that provide necessary, contemporary information and explicitly relevant background for the work.

The author of a research paper is also obliged to clearly and explicitly describe the method of study; however, a "blow-by-blow" description is usually unnecessary in a journal article, and can be very tedious for the reader. Often, minute details of the protocol are delineated in appendices of a thesis. For the journal article, the content of appendices must be explained in a few sentences.

Writing Style

The process of scientific writing "is not primarily a `literary' effort, but is an exercise in organization and clarity of expression."[8] The final written report should be strong, reflecting the objectivity and logic of the research project. We have reviewed the customary format and content of the research report to guide the author through the structural elements; however, the readability of the report depends on the author's skill in communicating with precision. Readers often complain that research reports are boring and difficult to follow. These complaints may have nothing to do with the subject but with sentence structure or the flow of ideas—the personal writing style of the author.

We will not present a "style manual" in this text, but will highlight a few common problems and current issues that interfere with clear writing. A selection of useful references for developing and improving writing skills are cited at the end of this chapter. Even the most accomplished author may benefit from consulting such references, especially when the early drafts of a paper seem cumbersome.

People First.   Our patients or clients are indeed people first! It is incumbent on all of us to be sensitive to this basic human issue. We can easily reflect this in the description of subjects who have been studied. In choosing words about people with disabilities, the guiding principle is to refer to the person first, not the disability. In place of saying "the disabled," it is preferable to say "people with disabilities." This way, the emphasis is placed on the person, not the disability. As examples, "stroke patients" are patients who have had a stroke; "learning-disabled children" are children who have learning disabilities. Words like *invalid, suffering,* and *victim* should be avoided. Attention to people-first language demonstrates an underlying respect that should be reflected in our scientific publications.[9]

Active versus Passive Voice.   A sentence written in active voice is powerful and concrete. Passive voice tends to make sentences ponderous and dull. The writer must create sentences that make the intended point most clearly. At times, the choice between active and passive voice is not so obvious. The following sentences illustrate the choices.

Passive: One hour was spent by the raters to observe the patient's movement patterns so that the number of changes in static posture could be documented.

Active: The raters spent one hour observing the patient's movement patterns to document the number of changes in static posture.

The emphasis is different in these two sentences. The amount of time is emphasized in the passive example, whereas the raters and their activity are highlighted in the active example. In addition, the active example is shorter by six words! Consider the following examples as well:

Passive: Increased tension throughout the upper extremity and neck is produced by constant pain in the wrist.

Active: Constant pain in the wrist increases tension throughout the upper extremity and neck.

Note the difference in focus of these sentences. If the author is addressing the potential for dysfunction at sites remote from the pathology, then the first (passive) example may be best. If the author is developing a rationale for eliminating wrist pain, the active example is more appropriate.

Passive voice may be appropriate when the subject of the sentence is unimportant or the object or action should be emphasized. For example, "Patients were randomly assigned..." conveys an important action, and the subject (who assigned) may not be important.

Superfluous passive expressions, such as "it has been suggested..." or "it is thought that..." usually distract the reader because they dilute the strength of the message. Who suggested? Who thought? In citing the work of others, authors should acknowledge the "who," for example, "Jones and Brown suggested...." In discussing present work, the authors might write "Our preliminary results indicate...." Using active voice in such cases is direct and clear.

One special case should be discussed—the use of first-person active voice. For many years, authors went out of their way to avoid using first-person active voice with the notion that to use it detracts from the "scientific," "objective" nature of research reports. Now, the use of first person is acceptable in selected instances. When authors (researchers) are emphasizing their own actions, experiences, assumptions or opinions, their writing may be more readable and indeed more accurate if they say "We think the logical interpretation of this finding is..." or "We found that this technique is...." On the other hand, overuse of "I" and "we" can be intrusive, calling unnecessary attention to the authors, especially when purely scientific information is being conveyed. Presentation of techniques, procedures, and results requires attention to what was done and how, not who. Therefore, it is stronger to say "The subjects were asked to complete the questionnaire," rather than "I asked the subjects to complete the questionnaire."

Simplicity of Language. In conversation, we tend to use expressions and phrases that are spontaneous, but often superfluous to the point we are making. Many such expressions will be found in the early drafts of written work because of the natural effort to "speak" the text. Authors must, however, remain cognizant of the need to be concise in scientific writing. Many of the elements of creative writing that we learned in school, designed to create metaphors and add color to our words, should be discarded for scientific writing. Many authors try to use different words for the same concept to avoid being repetitious; however, where one word will make the point best, it is better to be repetitious than to be unclear or ambiguous. Adjectives and adverbs are especially useless for describing scientific findings. There is no need to say that an outcome is "very practical" or "extremely useful." It would be sufficient to be practical or useful for clinical care.

The use of expressions should also be tempered for scientific reports. Although it is certainly more interesting to read a paper that is written with variations in sentence structure, the purpose of an article is to communicate findings, not to create poetry. Here are a few examples of complex phrases that can usually be avoided:

in light of the fact that	=	because
with the exception of	=	except
in spite of the fact that	=	although
is designed to improve	=	improves
due to the fact that	=	because
was found to have	=	had
immediately prior to	=	before

In early drafts, there may be redundant phrases, such as "exactly identical" and "grouped together," and unnecessary qualifiers, such as "blue in color" and "end result." Correcting these kinds of errors is easy, if the author is looking for them.

THE POSTER PRESENTATION

A poster presentation is a report of research that is displayed on a large board so that it can be read and viewed by groups in an informal atmosphere. Posters afford a special opportunity for researchers and their professional colleagues to exchange ideas in conference settings. Poster sessions are organized so that each poster is available for several hours. Sessions may be somewhat formalized by asking researchers to present a brief oral summary to an assembled group, with a moderator who guides a discussion around each poster in a symposium format. In another format, the open session, posters are displayed in an exhibit hall where interested participants view the posters. In this case, the researcher is available to answer questions or engage in discussion. A major advantage of the poster presentation is that interested members of the audience can study the content and contemplate the implications of a study at a comfortable pace. The researcher has an opportunity to clarify or amplify details of the study. Observers' reactions or questions may be helpful in guiding future work and stimulating new ideas.

Content and Layout

The poster should contain the major elements of the study in a clear, brief series of statements including title, purpose, hypothesis or specific aims, method, results and discussion, and conclusions. The poster should be self-explanatory, but "telegraphic" in style; that is, content should include key words and phrases and not necessarily complete sentences. Tables, graphs or photographs should summarize and illustrate important findings or unique aspects of the method. The most effective posters do not contain so much written material that the observer gets lost, but should be complete enough to allow the observer to understand the full intent of the study.

The conference sponsor will provide guidelines about the size and composition of the board that will be available. The customary size is 4 ft high and 4 to 8 ft wide. The composition is usually cork or particleboard, so that thumbtacks can be used to hang sections of the poster.

In preparing a poster, a scaled template should be drawn, showing the arrangement of text and figures. The content elements can be moved about the template to find the best arrangement for the logical flow of information. Ordinarily, the eye follows from left to right, as in reading. The introductory materials should be placed at the top left and the conclusion at the bottom right. Methods and results should be displayed prominently in the center. Figure 33.2 is an example of a poster with 4' × 6' dimensions.[10]

Materials

Today's posters are typically created using software such as PowerPoint®, allowing the researcher to prepare a colorful and effective presentation. Where posters used to be composed of several mounted documents, they are now output on large printers with many varied formats available.

The effective poster should be legible and uncluttered, with content and graphics presented in sharp contrast to its background. Letters for the title should be 2 inches high, headings should be at least 1 inch high, and text letters should be at least 0.5 inch

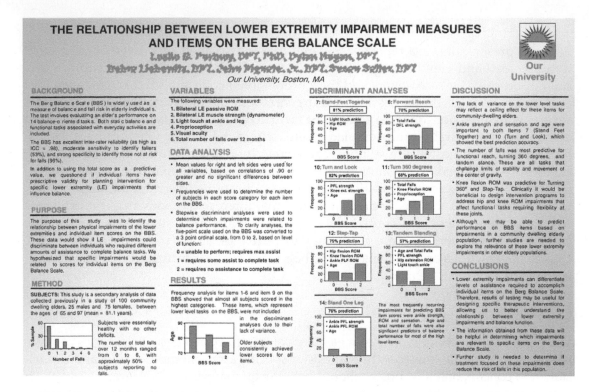

FIGURE 33.2 A sample template for the arrangement of a poster presentation.

high. The size and type of the text should be readable from 4 feet away. The print should be bold with clear, sharp edges. The visual aspect of the poster should remain foremost in its preparation, providing an interesting and attractive presentation for those who will pass by.

THE ORAL PRESENTATION

Oral presentation of research findings in an open forum of colleagues is a time-honored tradition in medicine and science. This avenue of communication offers immediate, timely dissemination of new information. Like the poster presentation, it encourages direct interchange of ideas and stimulates consideration of new directions in research.

The notion of oral reporting is particularly attractive to those who consider writing a difficult task and speaking a much more free, more comfortable, process; however, the oral report of research is not at all the same as conversational speaking. In conversation, ideas are conveyed spontaneously, with facial expressions or gestures for emphasis and opportunities to repeat or reconstruct a thought to clarify a point. In a formal presentation, which usually has a time limit of 15 minutes, language must be chosen carefully to convey the speaker's message correctly. The message is emphasized and illustrated visually with slides. Unlike conversational speaking, the oral presentation of research is highly structured. Thorough planning and preparation including practice are required to ensure success.

Planning and Preparation

Most organizations select individuals to present oral papers on the basis of written abstracts submitted by the researchers. That written abstract can be the skeleton of the presentation because it contains the major elements of the research project.

Because content must be well organized and the presentation will have customary time limits, we suggest that the talk be written. From an initial draft, the speaker can adapt and refine the talk. Key words and phrases can be manipulated to improve precision and emphasis. Logical sequencing and transitions from thought to thought can be refined.

Most organizations require that speakers strictly adhere to the prescribed time limit. Therefore, even at this early stage, the text should be read aloud so the speaker begins to develop a sense of timing. Practice should include using visual materials. The experienced presenter may know that eight pages of double-spaced text including references to slides will be about a 10-minute talk. Each individual must acquire this sense of timing, for which there is no common formula. If the talk is too lengthy, the presenter must abbreviate the content. What can be eliminated? Is the background or introductory material too extensive? Have any extraneous, albeit interesting, sidelights been included? Is the talk complicated by falsely fancy words or jargon?

Editing may continue until the final product is ready, but the major elements must be in place early, so that the slides can be planned and prepared.

Visual Presentation

Visual aids are essential to the success of an oral presentation. Effective slides emphasize and illustrate the content of the presentation and focus the audience's attention to important details. On the other hand, a presentation can be destroyed by poorly constructed, overwhelming, or confusing slides. In this section, we discuss a few important guidelines for planning and preparing slides.

Types of Slides. The type and number of slides to use should be determined by identifying the key points of the written text. The most effective presentations use slides to accompany all parts of the paper, so that the listener is guided through each section of the presentation. Factors of production cost and the time allotted for the presentation may dictate how slides are used. Four types of slides may be presented: words or phrases (text), photographs, graphs and tables. Word slides are customarily used to present the title of the presentation, the statement of the purpose or objectives, important background material, hypotheses, description of subjects and study protocol, summary of results, and conclusions. Photographs can illustrate aspects of the method such as the equipment setup or subject activity. Graphs and tables are used to demonstrate the results.

Limiting Words. Word slides must be legible and should contain no more than six lines of text or 45 characters per line.[11] The choice of font is a matter of preference; however, ornate, italic, uppercase, and open typefaces are usually more difficult to read.

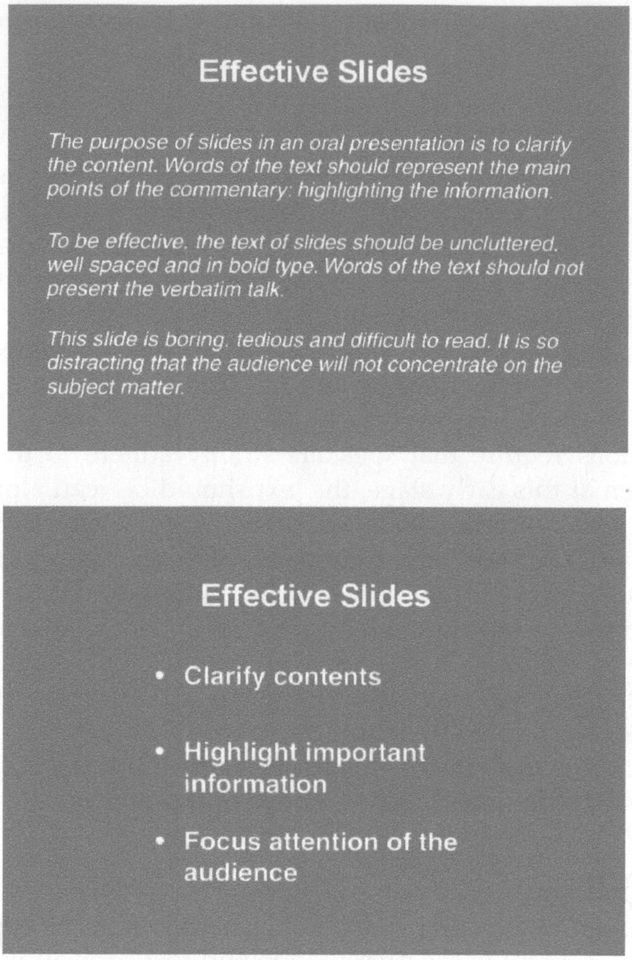

FIGURE 33.3   Illustration of slide content: (**A**) Overcrowded; (**B**) summarized.

Figure 33.3A illustrates a slide that contains too many words to be an effective source of information to a large audience. Figure 33.3B shows how this information can be reduced to present major points, which would then be discussed by the presenter in greater detail. By highlighting each point, the listener can focus on each one as the presenter addresses it. In addition, the text is larger and less cluttered so that the listener can read it quickly and easily without being drawn away from the spoken material. The border of each of these "slides" is based on a template drawn in proportion to a typical PowerPoint® slide.

Content of Slides.   The content of each slide and the accompanying verbal commentary must be synchronized. The listening audience will find it difficult to focus on two separate points at one time. Because many of us are "visual learners," the presenter's remarks will be lost if the slide does not fit the talk. An uncoordinated presentation is distracting and difficult to follow.

Bulleted lists are usually easier to follow than long sentences or descriptions. Presenters should use the slides to essentially outline their talk, allowing the audience to connect the written and spoken word. The number of slides that will be used will depend on how long they stay in view.

Graphics. Graphs and tables must be simple and easily understood. The amount of information included of course depends on how much is needed to present the results adequately. When a study has generated a lot of data, the presenter may have to be selective in what to include in the presentation because listeners cannot absorb mounds of data in such a short time span. Generally, three comparison lines, or six bars on a graph or four rows and columns in a table is a sensible limit. Legends, headings, and numbers should be large enough to be read easily.

Backgrounds and Colors. Presentation programs provide an array of background colors and print styles, as well as designs and patterns that can make slides more attractive. Researchers should be wary of making slides too busy or "glitzy." The background of the slide should not detract from the information it is trying to convey. A variety of slide templates are available, although many are too busy or ornate for scientific presentations.

Rehearsal

After the presentation is written and slides are keyed to the text, rehearsal can begin. First, the presenter should go through the talk incorporating the slide presentation to be sure that the slides are synchronized properly with the verbal commentary and to confirm the length of the talk. Then, presentation to the "home-town" audience is warranted. Not only will staff members, fellow students, and faculty comment on or make suggestions for the presentation, they should be encouraged to ask questions, which may indicate the kind of questions that will come up in discussion following the formal conference presentation. Being well prepared for both the talk and the discussion will inspire confidence and ensure a professional performance.

COMMENTARY

Taking the Final Step

A written report of research findings should provide information that is new, true, important and comprehensible.[11] These criteria can be applied to poster and oral presentations, as well. New treatment or measurement techniques may have been developed and tested. Effectiveness of intervention may have been demonstrated, reaffirmed or refuted. The process of a study may have been valid and objective. The findings may have important implications for clinical practice. But who will know if the report is poorly prepared? Sheen[12] presented the point this way: "As a scientific author, you must write so that you are understood or, perhaps more important, so that you are not misunderstood."

The final step in the research process—to communicate the results—requires time: time to plan, time to write, time to revise. Early drafts of reports and presentations should be put away for a while and then later reread with the intention of editing. The editorial board of a journal and sponsors of a conference establish rules and restrictions for the format and organization, but only the author can make a presentation clear, precise and alive.

REFERENCES

1. Guidelines for Contributors. JRRD. Available at: <http://www.vard.org/guid/guidelns.htm> Accessed June 8, 2006.
2. International Committee of Medical Journal Editors. Uniform requirements for manuscripts submitted to biomedical journals. Available at: <http://www.icmje.org> Accessed June 8, 2006.
3. Moher D, Schulz KF, Altman DG (for the Consort Group). Revised recommendations for improving the quality of reports of parallel group randomized trials 2001. Available at: <http://www.consort-statement.org/statement/revisedstatement.htm> Accessed August 28, 2006.
4. The STARD Statement: Standards for Reporting of Diagnostic Accuracy Studies. Available at: <http://www.stard-statement.org/website%20stard> Accessed October 16, 2006.
5. American Psychological Association. *Publication Manual of the APA* (5th ed.). Washington, DC: APA, 2001.
6. Gibaldi J: *MLA Style Manual and Guide to Scholarly Publishing* (2nd ed.). New York: Modern Language Association of America, 1998.
7. Cochrane Database of Systematic Reviews. Available at: <www.cochrane.org> Accessed April 10, 2007.
8. Staheli LT. *Speaking and Writing for the Physician.* New York: Raven Press, 1986.
9. Guidelines for reporting and writing about people with disabilities. The Life Span Institute. Available at: <http://www.lsi.ku.edu/lsi/internal/guidelines.html> Accessed July 29, 2007.
10. Portney LG, Hogan D, Liebowitz D, Pignato J, Salter S. The relationship between lower extremity impairment measures and items on the Berg Balance Scale. Poster presented at the APTA Combined Sections Meeting, Tampa, FL. *J Geriatr Phys Ther* 2003;25(3):38.
11. DeBakey L: *The Scientific Journal: Editorial Policies and Practices.* St. Louis, MO: CV Mosby, 1976.
12. Sheen AP. *Breathing Life into Medical Writing: A Handbook.* St. Louis, MO: CV Mosby, 1982.

SUGGESTED ADDITIONAL READINGS

Pyrczak F and Bruce RR. *Writing Empirical Research Reports* (5th ed.). Glendale, CA: Pyrczak Publishing, 2005.

Day RA: *How to Write and Publish a Scientific Paper* (5th ed.). Phoenix: Oryx Press, 1998.

Gibaldi J: *MLA Style Manual and Guide to Scholarly Publishing* (2nd ed.). New York: Modern Language Association of America, 1998.

Portney L, Craik R. Sharing your research: Platform and poster presentations. *PT Magazine* 1998;6:72–81.

Strunk W, White EB: *The Elements of Style* (4th ed.). New York: Allyn & Bacon/Longman, 2000.

Zinsser W: *On Writing Well* (3rd ed.). New York: Harper & Row, 1988.

CHAPTER 34
Evaluating Research Reports

The link between research and clinical practice in health professions must be made by those who read reports of completed research. As consumers of research, we have a responsibility to evaluate research reports to determine whether the findings provide sufficient evidence to support the effectiveness of current practices or offer alternatives that will improve patient care. The success of evidence-based practice will depend on how well we incorporate research findings into our clinical judgments and treatment decisions.

For most of us, it is neither practical nor possible to read the plethora of material presented each month in professional journals. Therefore, the first step in effective reading is to select publications and articles that offer the most useful information. When a particular topic is important to practice, readers should begin by searching for systematic reviews that present an analysis of current knowledge on diagnostic methods or treatment effectiveness (see Chapter 16). Readers may also consider textbooks or traditional narrative review articles that provide basic, often in-depth, information on a topic; however, we must realize that the information is second-hand, presented from the perspective of the textbook or review article author. The problem is one of interpretation; the original research may be misrepresented or inadequately described. Therefore, consumers of research must be able to access the first-hand reports of researchers to judge the merits of their work.

Critical analysis of a research report is necessary to determine its validity and, thereby, its applicability for clinical decision making. The structure and content elements of research reports have been described in Chapter 33. The purpose of this chapter is to present a practical approach for critically reading and evaluating published literature, describing the kinds of questions readers should ask. Authors may also use this approach to appraise their own manuscripts before submitting them for publication.* Although this chapter focuses on the written research report, these principles

---

*Through a process of international consensus, specific guidelines have been developed to help authors assess the completeness of their reports of randomized trials and diagnostic accuracy. Known, respectively, as the CONSORT statement (*Consolidated Standards of Reporting Trials*)[1] and the STARD statement (*Standards for Reporting of Diagnostic Accuracy*),[2] these guidelines are composed of checklists and flow diagrams that outline a standard way for researchers to develop their reports. The intent of these statements is to standardize the information that is included in published studies. These standards will also serve to make the research process more transparent, so that readers can determine if flaws are present, and therefore decide if the data are useful for evidence-based decisions. The full checklists and flow diagrams have been presented in Chapters 9 and 27 for clinical trials and diagnostic studies.

apply to the evaluation of oral and poster presentations as well. This evaluative process works for purposes of literature review, answering specific clinical questions for evidence-based practice, or just keeping up with progress in an area of interest.

We will focus this discussion on three areas: trials that test the efficacy of interventions, studies that measure the accuracy of diagnostic/screening tests, and studies that examine the predictive validity of variables for prognosis. Guidelines for evaluating systematic reviews were presented in Chapter 16.

JOURNAL QUALITY

One of the first considerations in evaluating the scientific merit of an article is the reputation of the journal. Scientific journals are generally *refereed*, which means that the articles have been subjected to review by content experts and accepted for publication on the basis of reviewer evaluation. *Instructions to Authors*, provided in most journals, will describe this process. The editors and reviewers of refereed journals follow policies and procedures designed to ensure that published articles meet defined criteria, including importance of the research, originality, appropriateness of design, adequacy of the method, soundness of conclusions and interpretation, relevance of the discussion, and clarity of writing. The manuscript review process is similar, in fact, to the way in which responsible readers will evaluate published articles.

Authors are usually asked to make revisions to improve the quality and clarity of a manuscript before it is accepted for publication. This process does not guarantee, however, that a study is without flaws. It remains the reader's responsibility to evaluate a study's validity and applicability. Important information may be presented in non-refereed journals; however, readers must realize that the contents of those publications have not been scrutinized in the same way as those in refereed journals.

EVALUATING COMPONENTS OF RESEARCH STUDIES

Clinicians and researchers will evaluate literature from three perspectives. First, the assessment will help to determine if the study has validity in terms of design and analysis. Second, the results of the study are examined to determine the importance of the effect of intervention, the accuracy of diagnostic tests, or the risks associated with prognostic variables. Finally, the clinician may consider how effectively the results can be applied to a particular patient's management.

Many useful references are available to guide the process of critical appraisal of published papers.[2-9] Several of these guidelines are also used to assess methodological quality in systematic reviews (see Chapter 16).

What Is the Study About?

Before we can assess the validity of a study, we must first understand its intent. Researchers begin this process at the top, by reading the title and abstract. Titles should be informative, but are often so abbreviated that the reader is unable to learn much about content other than the general topic. If the reader is interested in the topic, then the next step is to read the abstract. Abstracts of research papers will include fairly specific information about the purpose, subjects, method, results, and major conclusions of the presented work. When readers decide that the results and conclusions stated in the abstract could be applied to their practice, they should read the body of the paper.

The **introduction** to an article tells us about the purpose of the study and how the authors developed the research question. It informs readers by providing a review of literature that frames the theoretical foundation for the study. The following questions help to focus the content of the introduction:

- What is the problem being investigated? Has it been clearly stated? Why is it important?
- How has the author used the literature to form a sound and logical rationale?
- What is the theoretical context for the study?
- Are references appropriate and comprehensive?
- What type of research does the study represent?
- What is the specific purpose of the study?
- What are hypotheses or guiding questions that form the basis of the study?

In the opening sentences of an article, the author should establish the problem being investigated. The background material should demonstrate that the researchers have thoughtfully and thoroughly synthesized the literature and related theoretical models. This synthesis should provide a rationale for pursuing this line of research. Readers should be convinced that the study was needed.

By the end of the introduction, the specific purpose or aims of the study should have been clearly stated and the research question should be evident. The authors of an intervention study should have explicitly stated the hypotheses that were to be tested. If not, however, readers should be able to determine what the researchers expected to find. For a diagnostic accuracy study, it should be clear if the intent is to compare two tests, to estimate the accuracy of one test, or to examine a test's utility across participant groups. Studies of prognosis should document the relevance of predictive variables and validity of outcomes.

Are the Results of the Study Valid?

The foundation of a research report is the method section, providing the details of the study. This is where we learn enough to decide if the results and conclusions of the study are meaningful. Flaws or omissions detected in the methods section affect the usefulness of interpretations derived from the study. Table 34.1 shows the questions that should be asked to assess the validity of an intervention study. Questions relevant to diagnostic accuracy and prognosis are shown in Tables 34.2 and 34.3.

Subjects

Readers must know who the subjects were in order to interpret the validity of a study's conclusions and to understand the extent to which the findings can be generalized or applied to specific patients. We can ask questions to determine whether sampling bias might have existed and to identify potentially confounding factors. Age, gender, diagnosis, comorbidities and level of function of the subjects are among the many factors that may affect the validity of findings. Inclusion and exclusion criteria should be specified so that the target population for the study is clearly identified.

TABLE 34.1 QUESTIONS TO DETERMINE VALIDITY OF AN INTERVENTION STUDY

Are the Results of the Study Valid?

Subjects	• How were subjects selected? • Can results be generalized based on the accessible population? • Was a power analysis done to determine sample size? • What were the specific inclusion and exclusion criteria used?
Design	• Was random assignment used to form study groups? • Were the intervention and control groups similar at the start of the trial? • Were data standardized and collected at specific intervals according to a pre-planned protocol? • Were measurements taken at reasonable time intervals, and were subjects followed for a sufficient time period? • Was the study internally valid? (Were other factors present that could have affected the outcome?) • Was everyone involved in the study (subjects, investigators, and testers) "blind" to treatment?
Procedures	• Did the authors provide a rationale for the interventions and measurements used? • Were the groups treated equally (aside from the intervention)? • Were measurements reliable and valid? • Were operational definitions provided for independent and dependent variables, such that they could be replicated?
Data Analysis	• Are all participants who entered the trial properly accounted for at its conclusion? • Were subjects analyzed in the groups to which they were initially assigned (intention-to-treat analysis)? • Were appropriate statistical analyses utilized?

Are the Results Meaningful?

- Are the results clinically as well as statistically significant?
- Were outcomes addressed in terms of a minimally important clinical change?
- Are the authors' conclusions valid based on findings?
- If a negative outcome, was a power analysis done?

Will the Results Help in Caring for My Patient?

- Are the subjects similar to my patient?
- Is the intervention feasible in my setting?
- Is the intervention consistent with my patient's preferences?
- Are the treatment benefits worth the potential harm or cost?

The number of subjects in a study is a consideration when interpreting the results of the statistical analysis. Specifically, failure to demonstrate statistically significant effects should not be assumed to mean that no effect truly exists. The authors should present the results of a power analysis to determine the possibility of a Type II error resulting from an inadequate sample size.

For intervention studies, the description of subjects should include information about the accessible population and whether a probability or nonprobability sampling process was used. This information provides a foundation for deciding how well the findings can be generalized.

In diagnostic studies, the sample should reflect an appropriate spectrum of patients for whom the test would be applied. A diagnostic test is useful only to the extent it can identify those with varied degrees of the target disorder.[10]

TABLE 34.2 QUESTIONS TO DETERMINE VALIDITY OF A DIAGNOSTIC ACCURACY STUDY

Are the Results of the Study Valid?

Subjects	• How were subjects selected?
	• What were the relevant inclusion and exclusion criteria?
	• Was the diagnostic test evaluated in an appropriate spectrum of patients (like those for whom we would use it in practice)?
Design	• Was there an independent comparison with a reference standard of diagnosis (i.e., how was the true diagnosis determined)?
	• Was the reference standard used regardless of the diagnostic test result?
	• Were those performing the test blind to the patients' true diagnosis?
Procedures	• Were the methods for performing the test described sufficiently to allow replication?
	• Did the investigators repeat the test on a second group of subjects?
Data Analysis	• Were measures of diagnostic accuracy performed, including sensitivity, specificity, and likelihood ratios?

Are the Results Meaningful?

- Were data provided to allow calculations of diagnostic accuracy?
- What were the sensitivity, specificity and likelihood ratios?

Will the Results Help in Caring for My Patient?

- Are the subjects similar to my patient?
- Can the test be reproduced in my setting?
- Are the results applicable to my patient?
- Will the results of the test change the management of my patient?
- Will my patient benefit from the results of the test?

TABLE 34.3 QUESTIONS TO DETERMINE VALIDITY OF A PROGNOSIS STUDY

Are the Results of the Study Valid?

Subjects	• From what accessible population were subjects chosen?
	• Was the sample composed of a representative group of subjects at a similar point in their disease?
Design	• Was follow-up sufficiently long and complete?
	• Were the individuals collecting data blinded to the subjects' prognostic status?
	• Were objective and unbiased outcome measures used?
Procedures	• Were operational definitions provided for prognostic and outcome measures?
Data Analysis	• Were subgroups of subjects examined for differences in prognostic estimates?
	• Were appropriate prognostic estimates performed?

Are the Results Meaningful?

- How likely are the outcomes within a given period of time?
- How precise are the prognostic estimates (based on confidence intervals)?

Will the Results Help in Caring for My Patient?

- Are the subjects similar to my patient?
- Will results lead to selecting or avoiding certain intervention approaches?
- Will results affect what I tell my patient?

For prognostic studies, authors should provide a complete description of the duration of the disease or disorder at the time patients entered the study.[11] Patients should be at a similar stage of disease to demonstrate consistency of outcomes.

Design

Based on the stated purpose of the project, readers should be able to judge the appropriateness of the design choices that were made. For studies of interventions, randomized designs are important for the control of internal validity, although quasi-experimental studies may still provide useful findings with sufficient description and controls. In diagnostic and prognostic studies, cohort designs are most useful for following subjects over time. Levels of evidence that are appropriate for these studies have been summarized in Chapter 16 (Table 16.1). It is important, however, to take these recommendations as guidelines only, understanding that the quality of the study must be examined to determine its applicability as evidence for clinical practice.

Information on study design will allow the reader to determine if the study is free from bias. As much as possible, researchers should incorporate **blinding** of subjects, testers, and investigators to protect against such bias. For intervention studies with two or more comparison groups, blinding provides some assurance that responses are not distorted because of inconsistent application of procedures or measurements. For diagnostic studies, those who administer and score tests should be blinded to the subject's true diagnosis. In prognostic studies, those who measure outcomes should be blinded to the subject's prior status.

The design will also provide a framework for understanding points of data collection, and the extent to which subjects are followed over time. For intervention studies, this has implications for understanding differences in trends and changes across groups. For prognosis studies, where the presence of a prognostic factor can precede outcomes by long periods, follow-up is most important to be sure that the study duration is long enough to detect the outcomes of interest.

The balance between efficacy and effectiveness should also be considered. When true experimental designs are employed, with the strict control inherent in these designs, readers should consider how to relate the findings to their "real world." In the "experimental" setting, where confounding factors and internal validity are rigorously controlled, the effects of manipulating or imposing the independent variable can be accepted with a high degree of confidence. But have these controls created such an "artificial" situation that it would be unrealistic to expect the same outcome when methods or procedures are implemented in clinical practice?

On the other hand, if quasi-experimental designs or descriptive methods are employed, readers must be alert to the possibility that extraneous variables have interfered with the interpretation of the results. The validity of an experimental or quasi-experimental study will depend in large part on how subjects are assigned to groups and whether or not a control group was included in the design. For example, when intact groups are used as in case-control designs, the author should specify the basis on which the subjects were selected.

Procedures

Readers should know what specific instruments or tools were used for measurements. If these are standard and commercially available, the model numbers and names and addresses of manufacturers should be included. If standardized questionnaires or survey instruments are used, references must be cited. When appropriate, reliability of measurements should be documented. Such documentation may be referenced from previous studies, or the researcher may establish reliability within the context of the study being reported.

The description of procedures should report the sequence of events from beginning to end. Description of data collection methods should include who performed the measurements, what the subjects were asked to do, what the data collectors did, and when and how often measurements were taken. All of these activities must be described in sufficient detail so that readers could, in a similar setting with similar subjects, replicate the study procedures. Studies of interventions typically involve comparison of groups or conditions, and the author should document the extent to which these groups were treated equally, except for the experimental treatment.

Data Analysis

Both descriptive and inferential statistical analyses should be identified. If inferential statistics were used, the acceptable significance level, such as $\alpha = .05$, should have been established by the researchers and reported. The statistical tests should be described not merely by name, but by specifying to which data the analyses were applied. This information is necessary for readers to evaluate the appropriateness of the analyses. The use or misuse of statistics should be judged on the basis of two major factors: the nature of measurements (scale, reliability, linearity, and so on) and the study design (the number of groups or variables and frequency of measurement). Discrepancies in the proper application of statistical tests interfere with the statistical conclusion validity of the study and detract from the interpretation of the data.

Authors should report the degree of follow-up that was achieved and if attrition was present in the study sample. Reasons for attrition should be provided, to help determine if bias was present. In intervention studies, the author should specify if an intention to treat analysis was done, and how missing data were handled. The degree of follow-up is especially important for prognostic studies, to assure that outcomes are representative of the sample.

Are the Results Meaningful?

The results section of a research report should contain the findings of the study without interpretation or commentary. Readers should find a narrative description of results, typically including test statistic values, such as t or F, odds ratios, or likelihood ratios.

It is rarely sufficient to simply determine that values are "significant," however. The usefulness of a study's results lies in the size of the effect that was demonstrated. **Effect size** tells us about the strength of the observed relationships. As we strive for greater application of evidence in clinical practice, we must understand just how much change we should expect from an intervention, how accurate a diagnostic will be, or how likely prognostic outcomes will occur. Statistics such as risk ratios, likelihood ratios, and number needed to treat will help us understand these effects. The precision of these estimates should be reflected in confidence intervals.

The narrative description of findings may be illustrated with or complemented by figures and tables to clarify and summarize the characteristics of the data. Readers should study graphs and tables carefully. The effect size indices are often presented in tabular fashion, rather than in the text. It is a useful exercise to compare data from tables with information found in the text, to be sure that the discussion of results follows what was actually reported.

What Does It All Mean?

A research report ends with the authors' discussion and conclusions, putting the results of the study in context. The discussion section of an article should address each of the research questions, and should show how relevant literature helps to support the author's conclusions. Some useful questions to focus this part of the review include:

- How does the author interpret results?
- Did the author clarify if hypotheses were rejected or accepted?
- What alternative explanations does the author consider for the obtained findings?
- How are the findings related to prior reports?
- What limitations are described? Are there limitations that are not addressed?
- If results are not significant, does the author consider the possibility of Type II error?
- Regardless of the statistical outcome, are the results clinically important?
- Does the author discuss how the results apply to practice?
- Does the author present suggestions for further study?
- Do the stated conclusions flow logically from the obtained results?

Readers should find a clear statement of the authors' major conclusions based on their interpretation of the results and research hypotheses. The authors should compare and contrast results with other related work, to offer support for existing clinical theory or propose an alternative theory or explanation. The authors should acknowledge factors about the subjects, materials, or methods that could have complicated the interpretation of the results. As the authors discuss these limitations, they should share their ideas for approaching the research question differently. On the other hand, if the authors expressed confidence in the design and execution of the study and, therefore, have confidence in the results, they should suggest a direction that future studies might take. Finally, and perhaps most importantly, the authors should discuss the impact of the results on clinical practice. Is their evidence strong enough to suggest a need to change some aspect of treatment intervention or practice models? As critical consumers of the products of clinical research, readers should study the discussion and conclusion sections of the research report to decide whether the authors' answers to these kinds of questions are true, appropriate, and justified.

CRITICALLY APPRAISED TOPICS (CATs)

As we search for information to apply to our clinical decision making, we all benefit from applying literature to patient cases. A systematic review is one approach to critically understanding the quality of evidence on a topic (see Chapter 16). The systematic review, however, is based on an overview of the topic, not its application to a specific patient. An alternative format, called a **critically appraised topic (CAT),** has become popular to provide a brief summary of a search and critical appraisal of literature related to a focused clinical question.[12–16]

A CAT provides a standardized format to present a critique of one or more articles and a statement of the clinical relevance of the results. A CAT is typically initiated by a patient encounter that reveals a knowledge gap.[17] The author of a CAT searches for and appraises "current best evidence" from the literature, summarizes the evidence, integrates it with clinical expertise, and finally suggests how the information can be applied to a patient scenario.[18] The critique will address internal, external, and statistical conclusion validity. Table 34.4 shows a sample CAT of an intervention study.

Format of a CAT

The format of a CAT can vary, although the essential elements remain fairly constant. It is generally a brief document, typically one to two pages in length. Information is intended to be concise. Table 34.4 shows one common layout. At minimum, a CAT should contain the following information:

- **Title:**   A concise statement that will be used to catalogue the CAT.
- **Author and Date:**   The author of the CAT should be specified, as well as the date the search was executed. A revision date should be proposed.
- **Clinical Scenario:**   A concise description of the patient case that prompted the question.
- **Clinical Question:**   This is the question that was developed from the patient case. It includes the elements of PICO (see Chapter 1): The patient/population, the intervention that is being considered (diagnostic test or prognostic variables), a comparison (if relevant), and the outcome of interest. This structure helps to refine the question and identifies key elements of an efficient database search.
- **Clinical Bottom Line:**   A concise summary of how the results can be applied; a description of how results will affect clinical decisions or actions.
- **Search History:**   Description of the search strategy used to obtain the studies that are being appraised (see Chapter 31). This includes databases used and terms entered at each step. Relevant studies are selected, often based on achieving highest levels of evidence (see Chapter 16).
- **Citations:**   Full bibliographic citations of studies selected for review.
- **Summary of the Study:**   Is the evidence in this study valid? This section should provide a description of the study based on the questions shown in Tables 34.1 through 34.3, including the type of study, subjects, procedures, and design elements.

TABLE 34.4	FORMAT FOR A CRITICALLY APPRAISED TOPIC (CAT) ON INTERVENTION

Title: Community-based occupational therapy improves functioning in older adults with dementia.

Appraiser: Leslie Portney

Date of Appraisal: August 2007
Review Date: August 2009

Clinical Scenario: AR is an 85-year-old female who experiences mild Alzheimer's dementia. She lives with her daughter and her daughter's family (husband and two teen-age children). AR is able to function with supervision, but has exhibited increasing problems with activities of daily living. She has also exhibited some agitation in her interactions with the family. Her daughter works from home, and is able to supervise her mother around the house. Her daughter has expressed concern for her own ability to handle her mother's functional limitations. She has asked if community occupational therapy services would be beneficial for improving her mother's function.

Clinical Question:

Patient/Problem: Community-dwelling elders with mild to moderate dementia
Intervention: Community-based occupational therapy
Comparison: No treatment
Outcomes: Functional performance

In older patients with dementia, does community-based occupational therapy improve daily functioning?

Clinical Bottom Line: Community-based occupational therapy improves daily functioning in older adults with dementia and increases caregivers' feelings of competence.

Search History:
Databases: CINAHL, MEDLINE
Search Terms (MeSH): Occupational therapy/
                     Dementia/
                     Community.mp[a]

Citation: Graff MJ, Vernooij-Dassen MJ, Thijssen M, et al. Community based occupational therapy for patients with dementia and their care givers: Randomized controlled trial. *BMJ* 2006;333:1196–1201.

Summary of Study:

Design: Randomized controlled trial.

Sample: Patients recruited from memory clinics and day clinics of a geriatrics department in one region of the Netherlands. 135 patients $\geq$ 65 years of age who had mild-to-moderate dementia were living in the community and were visited by caregivers at least once weekly. Exclusion criteria included depression, severe behavioral symptoms, severe illness and < 3 months of treatment with same dose of a cholinesterase inhibitor or memantine.

Intervention: Patients randomly assigned to 10 one-hour sessions of OT at home over 5 weeks (n = 68) or no OT (n = 67), stratified by mild or moderate dementia. Assessors were blind to group allocation. First 4 sessions focused on evaluation of options and goal setting. In remaining sessions, patients were taught to optimize strategies to improve ADLs, and caregivers were trained in supervisory, problem solving and coping strategies. OTs were experienced in the use of client-centered guidelines for patients with dementia.

Outcome Measures: Patients assessed for motor and process skills and deterioration of ADLs; caregivers assessed for sense of competence. All measurements utilized standardized tools. Assessments made at baseline, 6 weeks and 12 weeks.

Data Analysis: Intention to treat analysis applied at 12 weeks (78% retention), with last observation carried forward. Analysis of covariance applied with age, sex, and baseline scores as covariates.

The Evidence

At 6 and 12 weeks, patients in the OT group had better motor and process skills and less deterioration in ADL, and caregivers in the OT group had higher competence scores than the non-OT group.

	Process		Performance		Competence	
	6 wks	12 wks	6 wks	12 wks	6 wks	12 wks
% Improved						
OT Group	84%	75%	78%	82%	58%	48%
Control Group	9%	9%	12%	10%	18%	24%
NNT	1.3	1.5	1.5	1.4	2.5	4.2
(95% CI)	(1.2 to 1.4)	(1.4 to 1.6)	(1.4 to 1.6)	(1.3 to 1.5)	(1.3 to 2.7)	(4.0 to 4.4)

Comments

- Randomized block design provided good control over bias, including assessor blinding.
- Sample may have limited generalizability because of recruitment from specific outpatient clinics, eliminating general practice and other institutions.
- Outcomes were based on selected tasks and goals developed with OT. We do not know if these tasks were similar to those in baseline measurements, which could have inflated the beneficial effects of intervention. However, targeting goals that are personalized and important to the patient and caregiver makes the difference in effect sizes more meaningful.
- Inclusion of caregiver perceptions of confidence provide an important context for evaluating the success of the program.
- Results can only be generalized to patients who are already stable on cholinesterase inhibitors at the outset. The benefits of intervention are, therefore, in addition to those of the medication. We don't know how these strategies will work in the absence of such medication.
- NNTs are quite low with narrow confidence intervals.
- OTs trained in providing community-based support can effectively improve function of those with dementia and confidence of their caregivers following a 10-week program.

[a]MeSH abbreviation .mp = keyword search in title, abstract or MeSH heading

References:
Hirsch C. Community-based occupational therapy improved daily functioning in older patients with dementia. Comment in *ACP Journal Club* March/April 2007;146(2); Golden J., Lawlor B. Treatment of dementia in the community [Editorial]. *BMJ* 2006;333:1184–1185.

- **Summary of the Evidence:**   The results of the study should be summarized in narrative and/or tabular format. Specific effect size estimates should be provided as appropriate, such as means and mean differences, confidence intervals, odds ratios, likelihood ratios, sensitivity and specificity, and number needed to treat. If these estimates are not included in the research report, the CAT author may be able to calculate them if sufficient data are provided in the study.
- **Additional Comments:**   Provide critical comments on the study, including issues related to the sampling, methods, data analysis, quality of discussion, and interpretation of results. This is where you should comment on the internal, external, and statistical validity of the study. Comment on positive and negative aspects of the study.

A CAT has two important distinguishing features for evidence-based practice. First, it is based on a specific clinical question, prompted by a clinician's need to clarify an aspect of patient care related to intervention, diagnosis, prognosis, or harm.[13] This question is developed using the PICO format, as shown in Table 34.4. The clinician searches the literature explicitly to provide an answer to this question, with the intent of influencing management of the patient.

The second unique feature of a CAT is the inclusion of a *clinical bottom line,* or conclusion by the CAT author as to the value of the findings. The usefulness of the bottom line depends on the ability of the CAT author to accurately assess the validity of the literature and to grasp the relevance of findings for a particular patient's management.[18] This information is then useful to others who may encounter similar patients, who can take advantage of the summary for efficient decision making.

Using CATs for Clinical Decision Making

The utility of CATs will depend on the clinician's ability to readily access the information within the clinical setting. Wyer[14] suggests that CATs may serve to make the results of journal clubs or case conferences available to clinical staff to improve the care of subsequent patients. He offers the perspective that building such bridges and making them available at the point of care should be an essential part of evidence-based practice. Many institutions have established online "CAT Banks" that provide ready access to summaries of articles on specific topics.[12,19-24]

CATs do have limitations as a source of clinical data. They have a short shelf life as new evidence becomes available, which is why revision dates are included. Clinicians must recognize that CATs do not represent a rigorous search of the literature, as in a systematic review. CATs are often based on only one or two references and may not represent the full scope of literature on a topic. Their usefulness is conditional on the critical appraisal skills and accuracy of the author. It is, therefore, the clinician's responsibility to determine the relevance of the clinical question, the logic of the search strategy, and the application of validity criteria in the review.[25] It is also important to assess the strength of the CAT author's conclusions in relation to the evidence provided. Notwithstanding these limitations, however, in the hands of discerning clinicians, CATs provide a practical method for disseminating evidence from the literature to inform clinical decisions.

COMMENTARY

The Reader's View

The final published report of research does not end the story. Readers have an opportunity to comment in the journal that published the report by submitting a letter to the editor or by being invited by the editor to present a formal commentary that will accompany the report at the time of publication. The purpose of responding or reacting to reports through the journal is to offer points of view that may differ from those of the researchers or to raise questions about some aspect of the research design, methods, or interpretation of results. Comments should never be confrontational or degrading, but should provide constructive criticisms or offer evidence to support the published findings. Written dialogue between researchers and respondents may stimulate new ideas for keeping the line of research alive. Readers should look for and evaluate letters or commentaries with the same kind of scrutiny that they applied to the evaluation of the original report.

Critical appraisal of research reports is a skill that must be developed and practiced. We offer one caveat. As one develops this ability, there is a tendency to be overly critical, finding many flaws, major and minor, real and potential. Because of the nature of clinical research, there will always be some aspects of the design that could have been tighter or cleaner. The important element is whether the limitations in the design are so great that the findings are useless. In refereed journals these flaws are not likely to be "fatal"; that is, the articles that make it to the publication stage have been screened. Regardless of the imperfections that exist in the clinical research process, we must remember to find the merits of each project and accept them in the context of the entire endeavor. With careful attention to the details of all research reports we choose to read, we should expect to learn something valuable from each one.

REFERENCES

1. CONSORT website. Available at: <http://www.consort-statement.org/> Accessed August 19, 2005.
2. The STARD Statement: Standards for reporting of diagnostic accuracy studies. Available at: <http://www.stard-statement.org/website%20stard> Accessed on October 16, 2006.
3. Physiotherapy Evidence Database (PEDro). Available at: <http://www.pedro.fhs.usyd.edu.au/index.html> Accessed on June 26, 2006.
4. Critical Appraisal Skills Programme (CASP). Critical Appraisal Tools. Available at: <http://www.phru.nhs.uk/casp/critical_appraisal_tools.htm> Accessed August 28, 2006.
5. Critical Appraisal and Using the Literature. Available at: <http://www.shef.ac.uk/scharr/ir/units/critapp/introduction.htm> Accessed August 28, 2006.
6. Bhogal SK, Teasell RW, Foley NC, Speechly MR. The PEDro scale provides a more comprehensive measure of methodological quality than the Jadad scale in stroke rehabilitation literature. *J Clin Epidemiol* 2005;58:668–673.
7. Moher D, Schultz KF, Altman DG (for the Consort Group). Revised recommendations for improving the quality of reports of parallel group randomized trials. 2001. Available

at: <http://www.consort–statement.org/statement/revisedstatement.htm> Accessed August 28, 2006.

8. MacDermid JC. An introduction to evidence-based practice for hand therapists. *J Hand Ther* 2004;17:105–117.

9. Hopayian K. The need for caution in interpreting high quality systematic reviews. *BMJ* 2001;323:681–684.

10. Jaeschke R, Guyatt G, Sackett DL. Users' guides to the medical literature. III. How to use an article about a diagnostic test. A. Are the results of the study valid? Evidence-Based Medicine Working Group. *JAMA* 1994;271:389–391.

11. Laupacis A, Wells G, Richardson WS, Tugwell P. Users' guides to the medical literature. V. How to use an article about prognosis. Evidence-Based Medicine Working Group. *JAMA* 1994;272:234–237.

12. Critically Appraised Topics in Rehabilitation Therapy. Available at: <http://www.rehab.queensu.ca/cats/> Accessed August 3, 2007.

13. Straus SE, Richardson WS, Glasziou P, Haynes RB. *Evidence-based Medicine: How to Practice and Teach EBM.* 3rd ed. Edinburgh: Churchill Livingstone, 2005.

14. Wyer PC. The critically appraised topic: Closing the evidence-transfer gap. *Ann Emerg Med* 1997;30:639–640.

15. Sauve S, Lee HN, Meade MD, et al. The critically appraised topic: A practical approach to learning critical appraisal. *Ann Roy Coll Phys Surg Canada* 1995;28:396–398.

16. Johnson CJ. Getting started in evidence-based practice for childhood speech-language disorders. *Am J Speech Lang Pathol* 2006;15:20–35.

17. Wingerchuk DM, Demaerschalk BM. Critically appraised topics: The evidence-based neurologist. *Neurologist* 2007;13(1):1.

18. Fetters L, Figueiredo EM, Keane-Miller D, McSweeney DJ, Tsao C. Critically appraised topics. *Pediatr Phys Ther* 2004;16:19–21.

19. Sample scenarios, searches, completed worksheets and CATs for Evidence-based Physiotherapy Practice. Available at: <http://www.cebm.utoronto.ca/syllabi/physio/samples.htm> Accessed August 3, 2007.

20. UNC-CH School of Medicine. Index of CAT sheets by subject. Available at: <http://www.med.unc.edu/medicine/edursrc/!catlist.htm> Accessed August 3, 2007.

21. Evidence-Based Pediatrics Web Site. University of Michigan. Available at: <http://www.med.umich.edu/pediatrics/ebm/Cat.htm> Accessed August 3, 2007.

22. Occupational Therapy Critically Appraised Topics. Available at: <http://www.otcats.com/> Accessed August 3, 2007.

23. University of British Columbia. Critically Appraised Topics (Cats). Available at: <http://www.mrsc.ubc.ca/site_page.asp?pageid=98> Accessed August 3, 2007.

24. South African Medical Research Council. CATbank. Available at: <http://www.mrc.ac.za/cochrane/catbank.htm> Accessed August 5, 2007.

25. Dawes M. Critically appraised topics and evidence-based medicine journals. *Singapore Med J* 2005;46(9):442–449.

APPENDIX A
Statistical Tables

TABLE A.1   AREAS UNDER THE NORMAL CURVE (z)

z	Area between 0 and z	Area above z	z	Area between 0 and z	Area above z	z	Area between 0 and z	Area above z
0.00	.0000	.5000	0.40	.1554	.3446	0.80	.2881	.2119
0.01	.0040	.4960	0.41	.1591	.3409	0.81	.2910	.2090
0.02	.0080	.4920	0.42	.1628	.3372	0.82	.2939	.2061
0.03	.0120	.4880	0.43	.1664	.3336	0.83	.2967	.2033
0.04	.0160	.4840	0.44	.1700	.3300	0.84	.2995	.2005
0.05	.0199	.4801	0.45	.1736	.3264	0.85	.3023	.1977
0.06	.0239	.4761	0.46	.1772	.3228	0.86	.3051	.1949
0.07	.0279	.4721	0.47	.1808	.3192	0.87	.3078	.1922
0.08	.0319	.4681	0.48	.1844	.3156	0.88	.3106	.1894
0.09	.0359	.4641	0.49	.1879	.3121	0.89	.3133	.1867
0.10	.0398	.4602	0.50	.1915	.3085	0.90	.3159	.1841
0.11	.0438	.4562	0.51	.1950	.3050	0.91	.3186	.1814
0.12	.0478	.4522	0.52	.1985	.3015	0.92	.3212	.1788
0.13	.0517	.4483	0.53	.2019	.2981	0.93	.3238	.1762
0.14	.0557	.4443	0.54	.2054	.2946	0.94	.3264	.1736
0.15	.0596	.4404	0.55	.2088	.2912	0.95	.3289	.1711
0.16	.0636	.4364	0.56	.2123	.2877	0.96	.3315	.1685
0.17	.0675	.4325	0.57	.2157	.2843	0.97	.3340	.1660
0.18	.0714	.4286	0.58	.2190	.2810	0.98	.3365	.1635
0.19	.0753	.4247	0.59	.2224	.2776	0.99	.3389	.1611
0.20	.0793	.4207	0.60	.2257	.2743	1.00	.3413	.1587
0.21	.0832	.4168	0.61	.2291	.2709	1.01	.3438	.1562
0.22	.0871	.4129	0.62	.2324	.2676	1.02	.3461	.1539
0.23	.0910	.4090	0.63	.2357	.2643	1.03	.3485	.1515
0.24	.0948	.4052	0.64	.2389	.2611	1.04	.3508	.1492
0.25	.0987	.4013	0.65	.2422	.2578	1.05	.3531	.1469
0.26	.1026	.3974	0.66	.2454	.2546	1.06	.3554	.1446
0.27	.1064	.3936	0.67	.2486	.2514	1.07	.3577	.1423
0.28	.1103	.3897	0.68	.2517	.2483	1.08	.3599	.1401
0.29	.1141	.3859	0.69	.2549	.2451	1.09	.3621	.1379
0.30	.1179	.3821	0.70	.2580	.2420	1.10	.3643	.1357
0.31	.1217	.3783	0.71	.2611	.2389	1.11	.3665	.1335
0.32	.1255	.3745	0.72	.2642	.2358	1.12	.3686	.1314
0.33	.1293	.3707	0.73	.2673	.2327	1.13	.3708	.1292
0.34	.1331	.3669	0.74	.2704	.2296	1.14	.3729	.1271
0.35	.1368	.3632	0.75	.2734	.2266	1.15	.3749	.1251
0.36	.1406	.3594	0.76	.2764	.2236	1.16	.3770	.1230
0.37	.1443	.3557	0.77	.2794	.2206	1.17	.3790	.1210
0.38	.1480	.3520	0.78	.2823	.2177	1.18	.3810	.1190
0.39	.1517	.3483	0.79	.2852	.2148	1.19	.3830	.1170

TABLE A.1   AREAS UNDER THE NORMAL CURVE (z)

z	Area between 0 and z	Area above z	z	Area between 0 and z	Area above z	z	Area between 0 and z	Area above z
1.20	.3849	.1151	1.55	.4394	.0606	1.90	.4713	.0287
1.21	.3869	.1131	1.56	.4406	.0594	1.91	.4719	.0281
1.22	.3888	.1112	1.57	.4418	.0582	1.92	.4726	.0274
1.23	.3907	.1093	1.58	.4429	.0571	1.93	.4732	.0268
1.24	.3925	.1075	1.59	.4441	.0559	1.94	.4738	.0262
1.25	.3944	.1056	1.60	.4452	.0548	1.95	.4744	.0256
1.26	.3962	.1038	1.61	.4463	.0537	**1.96**	**.4750**	**.0250**
1.27	.3980	.1020	1.62	.4474	.0526	1.97	.4756	.0244
1.28	.3997	.1003	1.63	.4484	.0516	1.98	.4761	.0239
1.29	.4015	.0985	1.64	.4495	.0505	1.99	.4767	.0233
			1.645	**.4500**	**.0500**			
1.30	.4032	.0968	1.65	.4505	.0495	2.00	.4772	.0228
1.31	.4049	.0951	1.66	.4515	.0485	2.01	.4778	.0222
1.32	.4066	.0934	1.67	.4525	.0475	2.02	.4783	.0217
1.33	.4082	.0918	1.68	.4535	.0465	2.03	.4788	.0212
1.34	.4099	.0901	1.69	.4545	.0455	2.04	.4793	.0207
1.35	.4115	.0885	1.70	.4554	.0446	2.05	.4798	.0202
1.36	.4131	.0869	1.71	.4564	.0436	**2.054**	**.4800**	**.0200**
1.37	.4147	.0853	1.72	.4573	.0427	2.06	.4803	.0197
1.38	.4162	.0838	1.73	.4582	.0418	2.07	.4808	.0192
1.39	.4177	.0823	1.74	.4591	.0409	2.08	.4812	.0188
						2.09	.4817	.0183
1.40	.4192	.0808	1.75	.4599	.0401	2.10	.4821	.0179
1.41	.4207	.0793	**1.751**	**.4600**	**.0400**	2.11	.4826	.0174
1.42	.4222	.0778	1.76	.4608	.0392	2.12	.4830	.0170
1.43	.4236	.0764	1.77	.4616	.0384	2.13	.4834	.0166
1.44	.4251	.0749	1.78	.4625	.0375	2.14	.4838	.0162
			1.79	.4633	.0367			
1.45	.4265	.0735	1.80	.4641	.0359	2.15	.4842	.0158
1.46	.4279	.0721	1.81	.4649	.0351	2.16	.4846	.0154
1.47	.4292	.0708	1.82	.4656	.0344	2.17	.4850	.0150
1.48	.4306	.0694	1.83	.4664	.0336	2.18	.4854	.0146
1.49	.4319	.0681	1.84	.4671	.0329	2.19	.4857	.0143
1.50	.4332	.0668	1.85	.4678	.0322	2.20	.4861	.0139
1.51	.4345	.0655	1.86	.4686	.0314	2.21	.4864	.0136
1.52	.4357	.0643	1.87	.4693	.0307	2.22	.4868	.0132
1.53	.4370	.0630	1.88	.4699	.0301	2.23	.4871	.0129
1.54	.4382	.0618	**1.881**	**.4700**	**.0300**	2.24	.4875	.0125
			1.89	.4706	.0294			

TABLE A.1   AREAS UNDER THE NORMAL CURVE (z)

z	Area between 0 and z	Area above z	z	Area between 0 and z	Area above z	z	Area between 0 and z	Area above z
2.25	.4878	.0122	2.60	.4953	.0047	2.95	.4984	.0016
2.26	.4881	.0119	2.61	.4955	.0045	2.96	.4985	.0015
2.27	.4884	.0116	2.62	.4956	.0044	2.97	.4985	.0015
2.28	.4887	.0113	2.63	.4957	.0043	2.98	.4986	.0014
2.29	.4890	.0110	2.64	.4959	.0041	2.99	.4986	.0014
2.30	.4893	.0107	**2.65**	**.4960**	**.0040**	3.00	.4987	.0013
2.31	.4896	.0104	2.66	.4961	.0039	3.01	.4987	.0013
2.32	.4898	.0102	2.67	.4962	.0038	3.02	.4987	.0013
2.326	**.4900**	**.0100**	2.68	.4963	.0037	3.03	.4988	.0012
2.33	.4901	.0099	2.69	.4964	.0036	3.04	.4998	.0012
2.34	.4904	.0096						
2.35	.4906	.0094	2.70	.4965	.0035	3.05	.49886	.00114
2.36	.4909	.0091	2.71	.4966	.0034	3.06	.49889	.00111
2.37	.4911	.0089	2.72	.4967	.0033	3.07	.49893	.00107
2.38	.4913	.0087	2.73	.4968	.0032	3.08	.49896	.00104
2.39	.4916	.0084	2.74	.4969	.0031	**3.09**	**.49900**	**.00100**
2.40	.4918	.0082	**2.75**	**.4970**	**.0030**	3.10	.49903	.00097
2.41	.4920	.0080	2.76	.4971	.0029	3.11	.49906	.00094
2.42	.4922	.0078	2.77	.4972	.0028	3.12	.49910	.00090
2.43	.4925	.0075	2.78	.4973	.0027	3.13	.49913	.00087
2.44	.4927	.0073	2.79	.4974	.0026	3.14	.49916	.00084
2.45	.4929	.0071	2.80	.4974	.0026	3.15	.49918	.00082
2.46	.4931	.0069	2.81	.4975	.0025	3.16	.49921	.00079
2.47	.4932	.0068	2.82	.4976	.0024	3.17	.49924	.00076
2.48	.4934	.0066	2.83	.4977	.0023	3.18	.49926	.00074
2.49	.4936	.0064	2.84	.4977	.0023	3.19	.49929	.00071
2.50	.4938	.0062	2.85	.4978	.0022	3.20	.49931	.00069
2.51	.4940	.0060	2.86	.4979	.0021	3.21	.49934	.00066
2.52	.4941	.0059	2.87	.4979	.0021	3.22	.49936	.00064
2.53	.4943	.0057	**2.88**	**.4980**	**.0020**	3.23	.49938	.00062
2.54	.4945	.0055	2.89	.4981	.0019	3.24	.49940	.00060
2.55	.4946	.0054	2.90	.4981	.0019	3.25	.49942	.00058
2.56	.4948	.0052	2.91	.4982	.0018	3.26	.49944	.00056
2.57	.4949	.0051	2.92	.4982	.0018	3.27	.49946	.00054
2.576	**.4950**	**.0050**	2.93	.4983	.0017	3.28	.49948	.00052
2.58	.4951	.0049	2.94	.4984	.0016	**3.29**	**.49950**	**.00050**
2.59	.4952	.0048						

TABLE A.1 AREAS UNDER THE NORMAL CURVE (z)

z	Area between 0 and z	Area above z	z	Area between 0 and z	Area above z	z	Area between 0 and z	Area above z
3.30	.49951	.00048	3.35	.49960	.00040	3.40	.49966	.00034
3.31	.49953	.00047	3.36	.49961	.00039	3.45	.49972	.00028
3.32	.49955	.00045	3.37	.49962	.00038	3.50	.49977	.00023
3.33	.49957	.00043	3.38	.49964	.00036	3.60	.49984	.00016
3.34	.49958	.00042	3.39	.49965	.00035	3.70	.49989	.00011
						3.80	.49993	.00007
						3.90	.49995	.00005
						4.00	.49997	.00003

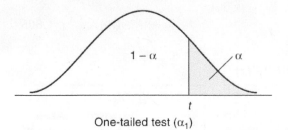

One-tailed test (α_1)

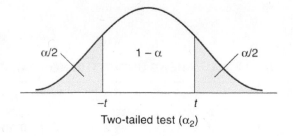

Two-tailed test (α_2)

TABLE A.2 CRITICAL VALUES OF t

df	α_1	.10	.05	.025	.01	.005	.0005
	α_2	.20	.10	.05	.02	.01	.001
1		3.078	6.314	12.706	31.821	63.657	636.619
2		1.886	2.920	4.303	6.965	9.925	31.598
3		1.638	2.353	3.182	4.541	5.841	12.924
4		1.533	2.132	2.776	3.747	4.604	8.610
5		1.476	2.015	2.571	3.365	4.032	6.859
6		1.440	1.943	2.447	3.143	3.707	5.959
7		1.415	1.895	2.365	2.998	3.499	5.405
8		1.397	1.860	2.306	2.896	3.355	5.041
9		1.383	1.833	2.262	2.821	3.250	4.781
10		1.372	1.812	2.228	2.764	3.169	4.587
11		1.363	1.796	2.201	2.718	3.106	4.437
12		1.356	1.782	2.179	2.681	3.055	4.318
13		1.350	1.771	2.160	2.650	3.012	4.221
14		1.345	1.761	2.145	2.624	2.977	4.140
15		1.341	1.753	2.131	2.602	2.947	4.073
16		1.337	1.746	2.120	2.583	2.921	4.015
17		1.333	1.740	2.110	2.457	2.898	3.965
18		1.330	1.734	2.101	2.552	2.878	3.922
19		1.328	1.729	2.093	2.539	2.861	3.883
20		1.325	1.725	2.086	2.528	2.845	3.850
21		1.323	1.721	2.080	2.518	2.831	3.819
22		1.321	1.717	2.074	2.508	2.819	3.792
23		1.319	1.714	2.069	2.500	2.807	3.767
24		1.318	1.711	2.064	2.492	2.797	3.745
25		1.316	1.708	2.060	2.485	2.787	3.725
26		1.315	1.706	2.056	2.479	2.779	3.707
27		1.314	1.703	2.052	2.473	2.771	3.690
28		1.313	1.701	2.048	2.467	2.763	3.674
29		1.311	1.699	2.045	2.462	2.756	3.659
30		1.310	1.694	2.042	2.457	2.750	3.646
40		1.303	1.684	2.021	2.423	2.704	3.551
60		1.296	1.671	2.000	2.390	2.660	3.460
120		1.289	1.658	1.980	2.358	2.617	3.373
∞		1.282	1.645	1.960	2.326	2.576	3.291

For unpaired t-test $df = (n_1 - 1) + (n_2 - 1)$. For paired t-test, $df = n - 1$. Test statistic must be greater than or equal to critical value to reject H_b.

TABLE A.3 **CRITICAL VALUES OF F, $\alpha = .05$**

df_e for denominator	df_b for numerator															
	1	2	3	4	5	6	7	8	9	10	12	15	20	30	60	∞
1	161.4	199.5	215.7	224.6	230.2	234.0	236.8	238.9	240.5	241.9	243.9	245.9	248.0	250.1	252.2	254.3
2	18.51	19.00	19.16	19.25	19.30	19.33	19.35	19.37	19.38	19.40	19.41	19.43	19.45	19.46	19.48	19.50
3	10.13	9.55	9.28	9.12	9.01	8.64	8.89	8.85	8.81	8.79	8.74	8.70	8.66	8.62	8.57	8.53
4	7.71	6.94	6.59	6.39	6.26	6.16	6.09	6.04	6.00	5.96	5.91	5.86	5.80	5.75	5.69	5.63
5	6.61	5.79	5.41	5.19	5.05	4.95	4.88	4.82	4.77	4.74	4.68	4.62	4.56	4.50	4.43	4.36
6	5.99	5.14	4.76	4.53	4.39	4.28	4.21	4.15	4.10	4.06	4.00	3.94	3.87	3.81	3.74	3.67
7	5.59	4.74	4.35	4.12	3.97	3.87	3.79	3.73	3.68	3.64	3.57	3.51	3.44	3.38	3.30	3.23
8	5.32	4.46	4.07	3.84	3.69	3.58	3.50	3.44	3.39	3.35	3.28	3.22	3.15	3.08	3.01	2.93
9	5.12	4.26	3.86	3.63	3.48	3.37	3.29	3.23	3.18	3.14	3.07	3.01	2.94	2.86	2.79	2.71
10	4.96	4.10	3.71	3.48	3.33	3.22	3.14	3.07	3.02	2.98	2.91	2.85	2.77	2.70	2.62	2.54
11	4.84	3.98	3.59	3.36	3.20	3.09	3.01	2.95	2.90	2.85	2.79	2.72	2.65	2.57	2.49	2.40
12	4.75	3.89	3.49	3.26	3.11	3.00	2.91	2.85	2.80	2.75	2.69	2.62	2.54	2.47	2.38	2.30
13	4.67	3.81	3.41	3.18	3.03	2.92	2.83	2.77	2.71	2.67	2.60	2.53	2.46	2.38	2.30	2.21
14	4.60	3.74	3.34	3.11	2.96	2.85	2.76	2.70	2.65	2.60	2.53	2.46	2.39	2.31	2.22	2.13
15	4.54	3.68	3.29	3.06	2.90	2.79	2.71	2.64	2.59	2.54	2.48	2.40	2.33	2.25	2.16	2.07

TABLE A.3 CRITICAL VALUES OF F, $\alpha = .05$

df_e for denominator									df_b for numerator							
	1	**2**	**3**	**4**	**5**	**6**	**7**	**8**	**9**	**10**	**12**	**15**	**20**	**30**	**60**	**∞**
16	4.49	3.63	3.24	3.01	2.85	2.74	2.66	2.59	2.54	2.49	2.42	2.35	2.28	2.19	2.11	2.01
17	4.45	3.59	3.20	2.96	2.81	2.70	2.61	2.55	2.49	2.45	2.38	2.31	2.23	2.15	2.06	1.96
18	4.41	3.55	3.16	2.93	2.77	2.66	2.58	2.51	2.46	2.41	2.34	2.27	2.19	2.11	2.02	1.92
19	4.38	3.52	3.13	2.90	2.74	2.63	2.54	2.48	2.42	2.38	2.31	2.23	2.16	2.07	1.98	1.88
20	4.35	3.49	3.10	2.87	2.71	2.60	2.51	2.45	2.39	2.35	2.28	2.20	2.12	2.04	1.95	1.84
21	4.32	3.47	3.07	2.84	2.68	2.57	2.49	2.42	2.37	2.32	2.25	2.18	2.10	2.01	1.92	1.81
22	4.30	3.44	3.05	2.82	2.66	2.55	2.46	2.40	2.34	2.30	2.23	2.15	2.07	1.98	1.89	1.78
23	4.28	3.42	3.03	2.80	2.64	2.53	2.44	2.37	2.32	2.27	2.20	2.13	2.05	1.96	1.86	1.76
24	4.26	3.40	3.01	2.78	2.62	2.51	2.42	2.36	2.30	2.25	2.18	2.11	2.03	1.94	1.84	1.73
25	4.24	3.39	2.99	2.76	2.60	2.49	2.40	2.34	2.28	2.24	2.16	2.09	2.01	1.92	1.82	1.71
26	4.23	3.37	2.98	2.74	2.59	2.47	2.39	2.32	2.27	2.22	2.15	2.07	1.99	1.90	1.80	1.69
27	4.21	3.35	2.96	2.73	2.57	2.46	2.37	2.31	2.25	2.20	2.13	2.06	1.97	1.88	1.79	1.67
28	4.20	3.34	2.95	2.71	2.56	2.45	3.26	2.29	2.24	2.19	2.12	2.04	1.96	1.87	1.77	1.65
29	4.18	3.33	2.93	2.79	2.55	2.43	2.35	2.28	2.l22	2.18	2.10	2.03	1.94	1.85	1.75	1.64
30	4.17	3.32	2.92	2.69	2.53	2.42	2.33	2.27	2.21	2.16	2.09	2.01	1.93	1.84	1.74	1.62
40	4.08	3.23	2.84	2.61	2.45	2.34	2.25	2.18	2.12	2.08	2.00	1.92	1.84	1.74	1.64	1.51
60	4.00	3.15	2.76	2.53	2.37	2.25	2.17	2.10	2.04	1.99	1.92	1.84	1.75	1.65	1.53	1.39
120	3.92	3.07	2.68	2.45	2.29	2.17	2.09	2.02	1.96	1.91	1.83	1.75	1.66	1.55	1.43	1.25
∞	3.84	3.00	2.60	2.37	2.21	2.10	2.01	1.94	1.88	1.83	1.75	1.67	1.57	1.46	1.32	1.00

df_b = between-groups degrees of freedom.
df_e = error (within-groups) degrees of freedom.
Test statistic must be greater than or equal to critical value to reject H_0.

TABLE A.4   CRITICAL VALUES OF r

df	α_1 α_2	.05 .10	.025 .05	.01 .02	.005 .01	.0005 .001
1		.988	.997	.9995	.9999	.9999
2		.900	.950	.980	.990	.999
3		.805	.878	.934	.959	.991
4		.729	.811	.882	.917	.974
5		.669	.755	.833	.875	.951
6		.622	.707	.789	.834	.925
7		.582	.666	.750	.798	.898
8		.549	.632	.716	.765	.872
9		.521	.602	.685	.735	.847
10		.497	.576	.658	.708	.823
11		.476	.553	.634	.684	.801
12		.458	.532	.612	.661	.780
13		.441	.514	.592	.641	.760
14		.426	.497	.574	.623	.742
15		.412	.482	.558	.606	.725
16		.400	.468	.543	.590	.708
17		.389	.456	.529	.575	.693
18		.378	.444	.516	.561	.679
19		.369	.433	.503	.549	.665
20		.360	.423	.492	.537	.652
25		.323	.381	.445	.487	.597
30		.296	.349	.409	.449	.554
35		.275	.325	.381	.418	.519
40		.257	.304	.358	.393	.490
45		.243	.288	.338	.372	.465
50		.231	.273	.322	.354	.443
60		.211	.250	.295	.325	.408
70		.195	.232	.274	.302	.380
80		.183	.217	.257	.283	.357
90		.173	.205	.242	.267	.338
100		.164	.195	.230	.254	.321

$df = n - 2.$

Test statistic must be greater than or equal to critical value to reject H_0.

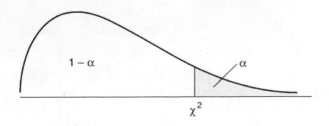

TABLE A.5 CRITICAL VALUES OF CHI-SQUARE, χ^2

df	α	.05	.02	.01	.005	.001
1		3.84	5.02	6.64	7.88	10.83
2		5.99	7.38	9.21	10.60	13.82
3		7.82	9.35	11.35	12.84	16.27
4		9.49	11.14	13.28	14.86	18.47
5		11.07	12.83	15.09	16.75	20.52
6		12.59	14.45	16.81	18.55	22.46
7		14.07	16.01	18.48	20.28	24.32
8		15.51	17.53	20.09	21.96	26.13
9		16.92	19.03	21.67	23.59	27.88
10		18.31	20.48	23.21	25.19	29.59
11		19.68	21.92	24.73	26.76	31.26
12		21.03	23.34	26.22	28.30	32.91
13		22.36	24.74	27.69	29.82	34.53
14		23.69	26.12	29.14	31.32	36.12
15		25.00	27.49	30.58	32.80	37.70
16		26.30	28.85	32.00	34.27	39.25
17		27.59	30.19	33.41	35.72	40.79
18		28.87	31.53	34.81	37.16	42.31
19		30.14	32.85	36.19	38.58	43.82
20		31.41	34.17	37.57	40.00	45.32
21		32.67	35.48	38.93	41.40	46.80
22		33.92	36.78	40.29	42.80	48.27
23		35.17	38.06	41.64	44.18	49.73
24		36.42	39.36	42.98	45.56	51.18
25		37.65	40.65	44.31	46.93	52.62
26		38.89	41.92	45.64	48.29	54.05
27		40.11	43.19	46.96	49.65	55.47
28		41.34	44.46	48.28	50.99	56.89
29		42.56	45.72	49.59	52.34	58.30
30		43.77	46.98	50.89	53.67	59.70
40		55.76	59.34	63.69	66.77	73.40
50		67.51	71.42	76.15	79.49	86.66
60		79.08	83.30	88.38	91.95	99.61
70		90.53	95.02	100.43	104.22	112.32
80		101.88	106.63	112.33	116.32	124.84
90		113.15	118.14	124.12	128.30	137.21
100		124.34	129.56	135.81	140.47	149.45

For one-sample test, $df = k - 1$. For two-sample test, $df = (R - 1)(C - 1)$. Test statistic must be greater than or equal to critical value to reject H_0.

TABLE A.6 **CRITICAL VALUES OF THE STUDENTIZED RANGE STATISTIC, q, FOR TUKEY'S HONESTLY SIGNIFICANT DIFFERENCE (HSD) AND NEWMAN-KEULS (NK) COMPARISONS**

df_e	α	r = number of means (HSD) or size of comparison interval (NK)										
		2	**3**	**4**	**5**	**6**	**7**	**8**	**9**	**10**	**11**	**12**
5	.05	3.64	4.60	5.22	5.67	6.03	6.33	6.58	6.80	6.99	7.17	7.32
	.01	5.70	6.98	7.80	8.42	8.91	9.32	9.67	9.97	10.24	10.48	10.70
6	.05	3.46	4.34	4.90	5.30	5.63	5.90	6.12	6.32	6.49	6.65	6.79
	.01	5.24	6.33	7.03	7.56	7.97	8.32	8.61	8.87	9.10	9.30	9.48
7	.05	3.34	4.16	4.68	5.06	5.36	5.61	5.82	6.00	6.16	6.30	6.43
	.01	4.95	5.92	6.54	7.01	7.37	7.68	7.94	8.17	8.37	8.55	8.71
8	.05	3.26	4.04	4.53	4.89	5.17	5.40	5.60	5.77	5.92	6.05	6.18
	.01	4.75	5.64	6.20	6.62	6.96	7.24	7.47	7.68	7.86	8.03	8.18
9	.05	3.20	3.95	4.41	4.76	5.02	5.24	5.43	5.59	5.74	5.87	5.98
	.01	4.60	5.43	5.96	6.35	6.66	6.91	7.13	7.33	7.49	7.65	7.78
10	.05	3.15	3.88	4.33	4.65	4.91	5.12	5.30	5.46	5.60	5.72	5.83
	.01	4.48	5.27	5.77	6.14	6.43	6.67	6.87	7.05	7.21	7.36	7.49
11	.05	3.11	3.82	4.26	4.57	4.82	5.03	5.20	5.35	5.49	5.61	5.71
	.01	4.39	5.15	5.62	5.97	6.25	6.48	6.67	6.84	6.99	7.13	7.25
12	.05	3.08	3.77	4.20	4.51	4.75	4.95	5.12	5.27	5.39	5.51	5.61
	.01	4.32	5.05	5.50	5.84	6.10	6.32	6.51	6.67	6.81	6.94	7.06
13	.05	3.06	3.73	4.15	4.45	4.69	4.88	5.05	5.19	5.32	5.43	5.53
	.01	4.26	4.96	5.40	5.73	5.98	6.19	6.37	6.53	6.67	6.79	6.90
14	.05	3.03	3.70	4.11	4.41	4.64	4.83	4.99	5.13	5.25	5.36	5.46
	.01	4.21	4.89	5.32	5.63	5.88	6.08	6.26	6.41	6.54	6.66	6.77
15	.05	3.01	3.67	4.08	4.37	4.59	4.78	4.94	5.08	5.20	5.31	5.40
	.01	4.17	4.84	5.25	5.56	5.80	5.99	6.16	6.31	6.44	6.55	6.66
16	.05	3.00	3.65	4.05	4.33	4.56	4.74	4.90	5.03	5.15	5.26	5.35
	.01	4.13	4.79	5.19	5.49	5.72	5.92	6.08	6.22	6.35	6.46	6.56
17	.05	2.98	3.63	4.02	4.30	4.52	4.70	4.86	4.99	5.11	5.21	5.31
	.01	4.10	4.74	5.14	5.43	5.66	5.85	6.01	6.15	6.27	6.38	6.48
18	.05	2.97	3.61	4.00	4.28	4.49	4.67	4.82	4.96	5.07	5.17	5.27
	.01	4.07	4.70	5.09	5.38	5.60	5.79	5.94	6.08	6.20	6.31	6.41
19	.05	2.96	3.59	3.98	4.25	4.47	4.65	4.79	4.92	5.04	5.14	5.23
	.01	4.05	4.67	5.05	5.33	5.55	5.73	5.89	6.02	6.14	6.25	6.34
20	.05	2.95	3.58	3.96	4.23	4.45	4.62	4.77	4.90	5.01	5.11	5.20
	.01	4.02	4.64	5.02	5.29	5.51	5.69	5.84	5.97	6.09	6.19	6.28

TABLE A.6 **CRITICAL VALUES OF THE STUDENTIZED RANGE STATISTIC, q, FOR TUKEY'S HONESTLY SIGNIFICANT DIFFERENCE (HSD) AND NEWMAN-KEULS (NK) COMPARISONS**

24	.05	2.92	3.53	3.90	4.17	4.37	4.54	4.68	4.81	4.92	5.01	5.10
	.01	3.96	4.55	4.91	5.17	5.37	5.54	5.69	5.81	5.92	6.02	6.11
30	.05	2.89	3.49	3.85	4.10	4.30	4.46	4.60	4.72	4.82	4.92	5.00
	.01	3.89	4.45	4.80	5.05	5.24	5.40	5.54	5.65	5.76	5.85	5.93
40	.05	2.86	3.44	3.79	4.04	4.23	4.39	4.52	4.63	4.73	4.82	4.90
	.01	3.82	4.37	4.70	4.93	5.11	5.26	5.39	5.50	5.60	5.69	5.76
60	.05	2.83	3.40	3.74	3.98	4.16	4.31	4.44	4.55	4.65	4.73	4.81
	.01	3.76	4.28	4.59	4.82	4.99	5.13	5.25	5.36	5.45	5.53	5.60
120	.05	2.80	3.36	3.68	3.92	4.10	4.24	4.36	4.47	4.56	4.64	4.71
	.01	3.70	4.20	4.50	4.71	4.87	5.01	5.12	5.21	5.30	5.37	5.44
∞	.05	2.77	3.31	3.63	3.86	4.03	4.17	4.29	4.39	4.47	4.55	4.62
	.01	3.64	4.12	4.40	4.60	4.76	4.88	4.99	5.08	5.16	5.23	5.29

TABLE A.7   CRITICAL VALUES OF $t(B)$ FOR BONFERRONI'S MULTIPLE COMPARISON TEST

df_e	α_2	Number of comparisons (c)								
		2	3	4	5	6	7	8	9	10
2	.10	4.243	5.243	6.081	6.816	7.480	8.090	8.656	9.188	9.691
	.05	6.164	7.582	8.774	9.823	10.769	11.639	12.449	13.208	13.927
	.01	14.071	17.248	19.925	22.282	24.413	26.372	28.196	29.908	31.528
3	.10	3.149	3.690	4.115	4.471	4.780	5.055	5.304	5.532	5.744
	.05	4.156	4.826	5.355	5.799	6.185	6.529	6.842	7.128	7.394
	.01	7.447	8.565	9.453	10.201	10.853	11.436	11.966	12.453	12.904
4	.10	2.751	3.150	3.452	3.669	3.909	4.093	4.257	4.406	4.542
	.05	3.481	3.941	4.290	4.577	4.822	5.036	5.228	5.402	5.562
	.01	5.594	6.248	6.751	7.166	7.520	7.832	8.112	8.367	8.600
5	.10	2.549	2.882	3.129	3.327	3.493	3.638	3.765	3.880	3.985
	.05	3.152	3.518	3.791	4.012	4.197	4.358	4.501	4.630	4.747
	.01	4.771	5.243	5.599	5.888	6.133	6.346	6.535	6.706	6.862
6	.10	2.428	2.723	2.939	3.110	3.253	3.376	3.484	3.580	3.668
	.05	2.959	3.274	3.505	3.690	3.845	3.978	4.095	4.200	4.296
	.01	4.315	4.695	4.977	5.203	5.394	5.559	5.704	5.835	5.954
7	.10	2.347	2.618	2.814	2.969	3.097	3.206	3.302	3.388	3.465
	.05	2.832	3.115	3.321	3.484	3.620	3.736	3.838	3.929	4.011
	.01	4.027	4.353	4.591	4.782	4.941	5.078	5.198	5.306	5.404
8	.10	2.289	2.544	2.726	2.869	2.987	3.088	3.176	3.254	3.324
	.05	2.743	3.005	3.193	3.342	3.464	3.569	3.661	3.743	3.816
	.01	3.831	4.120	4.331	4.498	4.637	4.756	4.860	4.953	5.038
9	.10	2.246	2.488	2.661	2.796	2.907	3.001	3.083	3.155	3.221
	.05	2.677	2.923	3.099	3.237	3.351	3.448	3.532	3.607	3.675
	.01	3.688	3.952	4.143	4.294	4.419	4.526	4.619	4.703	4.778
10	.10	2.213	2.446	2.611	2.739	2.845	2.934	3.012	3.080	3.142
	.05	2.626	2.860	3.027	3.157	3.264	3.355	3.434	3.505	3.568
	.01	3.580	3.825	4.002	4.141	2.256	4.354	4.439	4.515	4.584
11	.10	2.186	2.412	2.571	2.695	2.796	2.881	2.955	3.021	3.079
	.05	2.586	2.811	2.970	3.094	3.196	3.283	3.358	3.424	3.484
	.01	3.495	3.726	3.892	4.022	4.129	4.221	4.300	4.371	4.434
12	.10	2.164	2.384	2.539	2.658	2.756	2.838	2.910	2.973	3.029
	.05	2.553	2.770	2.924	3.044	3.141	3.224	3.296	3.359	3.416
	.01	3.427	3.647	3.804	3.927	4.029	4.114	4.189	4.356	4.315

TABLE A.7   **CRITICAL VALUES OF $t(B)$ FOR BONFERRONI'S
MULTIPLE COMPARISON TEST (continued)**

df_e	α_2	Number of comparisons (c)								
		2	**3**	**4**	**5**	**6**	**7**	**8**	**9**	**10**
13	.10	2.146	2.361	2.512	2.628	2.723	2.803	2.872	2.933	2.988
	.05	2.526	2.737	2.886	3.002	3.096	3.176	3.245	3.306	3.361
	.01	3.371	3.582	3.733	3.850	3.946	4.028	4.099	4.162	4.218
14	.10	2.131	2.342	2.489	2.603	2.696	2.774	2.841	2.900	2.953
	.05	2.503	2.709	2.854	2.967	3.058	3.135	3.202	3.261	3.314
	.01	3.324	3.528	3.673	3.785	3.878	3.956	4.024	4.084	4.138
15	.10	2.118	2.325	2.470	2.582	2.672	2.748	2.814	2.872	2.924
	.05	2.483	2.685	2.827	2.937	3.026	3.101	3.166	3.224	3.275
	.01	3.285	3.482	3.622	3.731	3.820	3.895	3.961	4.019	4.071
16	.10	2.106	2.311	2.453	2.563	2.652	2.726	2.791	2.848	2.898
	.05	2.467	2.665	2.804	2.911	2.998	3.072	3.135	3.191	3.241
	.01	3.251	3.443	3.579	3.684	3.771	3.844	3.907	3.963	4.013
18	.10	2.088	2.287	2.426	2.532	2.619	2.691	2.753	2.808	2.857
	.05	2.439	2.631	2.766	2.869	2.953	3.024	3.085	3.138	3.186
	.01	3.195	3.379	3.508	3.609	3.691	3.760	3.820	3.872	3.920
20	.10	2.073	2.269	2.405	2.508	2.593	2.663	2.724	2.777	2.824
	.05	2.417	2.605	2.736	2.836	2.918	2.986	3.045	3.097	3.143
	.01	3.152	3.329	3.454	3.550	3.629	3.695	3.752	3.802	3.848
25	.10	2.047	2.236	2.367	2.466	2.547	2.614	2.672	2.722	2.767
	.05	2.379	2.558	2.683	2.779	2.856	2.921	2.976	3.025	3.069
	.01	3.077	3.243	3.359	3.449	3.521	3.583	3.635	3.682	3.723
30	.10	2.030	2.215	2.342	2.439	2.517	2.582	2.638	2.687	2.731
	.05	2.354	2.528	2.649	2.742	2.816	2.878	2.932	2.979	3.021
	.01	3.029	3.188	3.298	3.384	3.453	3.511	2.561	3.605	3.644

df_e	α_2	Number of comparisons (c)												
		2	**3**	**4**	**5**	**6**	**7**	**8**	**9**	**10**	**15**	**20**	**25**	**30**
40	.10	2.009	2.189	2.312	2.406	2.481	2.544	2.597	2.644	2.686	2.843	2.952	3.036	3.103
	.05	2.323	2.492	2.608	2.696	2.768	2.827	2.878	2.923	2.963	3.113	3.218	3.298	3.363
	.01	2.970	3.121	3.225	3.305	3.370	3.425	3.472	3.513	3.549	3.689	3.787	3.862	3.923
60	.10	1.989	2.163	2.283	2.373	2.446	2.506	2.558	2.603	2.643	2.793	2.897	2.976	3.040
	.05	2.294	2.456	2.568	2.653	2.721	2.777	2.826	2.869	2.906	3.049	3.148	3.223	3.284
	.01	2.914	3.056	3.155	3.230	3.291	3.342	3.386	3.425	3.459	3.589	3.679	3.749	3.805
120	.10	1.968	2.138	2.254	2.342	2.411	2.469	2.519	2.562	2.600	2.744	2.843	2.918	2.978
	.05	2.265	2.422	2.529	2.610	2.675	2.729	2.776	2.816	2.852	2.987	3.081	3.152	3.209
	.01	2.859	2.994	3.087	3.158	3.215	3.263	3.304	3.340	3.372	3.493	3.577	3.641	3.693
∞	.10	1.949	2.114	2.226	2.311	2.378	2.434	2.482	2.523	2.560	2.697	2.791	2.862	2.920
	.05	2.237	2.388	2.491	2.569	2.631	2.683	2.727	2.766	2.300	2.928	3.016	3.083	3.137
	.01	2.806	2.934	3.022	3.089	3.143	3.186	3.226	3.260	3.289	3.402	3.480	3.539	3.587

TABLE A.8 CRITICAL VALUES FOR THE MANN-WHITNEY U-TEST

n_1	α_1	α_2	3	4	5	6	7	8	9	10	11	12	13	14	15	16	17	18	19	20	21	22	23	24	25
																n_2 (larger sample size)								
3	.005	.01	—	—	—	—	—	—	0	0	0	1	1	1	2	2	2	2	3	3	3	4	4	4	5
	.01	.02	—	—	—	—	0	0	1	1	1	2	2	2	3	3	4	4	4	5	5	6	6	6	7
	.025	.05	—	—	0	1	1	2	2	3	3	4	4	5	5	6	6	7	7	8	8	9	9	10	10
	.05	.10	0	0	1	2	2	3	4	4	5	5	6	7	7	8	9	9	10	11	11	12	13	13	14
4	.005	.01	—	—	—	0	0	1	1	2	2	3	3	4	5	5	6	6	7	8	8	9	9	10	10
	.01	.02	—	—	0	1	1	2	3	3	4	5	5	6	7	7	8	9	9	10	11	11	12	13	13
	.025	.05	—	0	1	2	3	4	4	5	6	7	8	9	10	11	11	12	13	14	15	16	17	17	18
	.05	.10	0	1	2	3	4	5	6	7	8	9	10	11	12	14	15	16	17	18	19	20	21	22	23
5	.005	.01	—	—	0	1	1	2	3	4	5	6	7	7	8	9	10	11	12	13	14	14	15	16	17
	.01	.02	—	—	1	2	3	4	5	6	7	8	9	10	11	12	13	14	15	16	17	18	19	20	21
	.025	.05	—	—	2	3	5	6	7	8	9	11	12	13	14	15	17	18	19	20	22	23	24	25	27
	.05	.10	—	—	4	5	6	8	9	11	12	13	15	16	18	19	20	22	23	25	26	28	29	30	32
6	.005	.01	—	—	—	2	3	4	5	6	7	9	10	11	12	13	15	16	17	18	19	21	22	23	24
	.01	.02	—	—	—	3	4	6	7	8	9	11	12	13	15	16	18	19	20	22	23	24	26	27	29
	.025	.05	—	—	—	5	6	8	10	11	13	14	16	17	19	21	22	24	25	27	29	30	32	33	35
	.05	.10	—	—	—	7	8	10	12	14	16	17	19	21	23	25	26	28	30	32	34	36	37	39	41
7	.005	.01	—	—	—	—	4	6	7	9	10	12	13	15	16	18	19	21	22	24	25	27	29	30	32
	.01	.02	—	—	—	—	6	7	9	11	12	14	16	17	19	21	23	24	26	28	30	31	33	35	36
	.025	.05	—	—	—	—	8	10	12	14	16	18	20	22	24	26	28	30	32	34	36	38	40	42	44
	.05	.10	—	—	—	—	11	13	15	17	19	21	24	26	28	30	33	35	37	39	41	44	46	48	50
8	.005	.01	—	—	—	—	—	7	9	11	13	15	17	18	20	22	24	26	28	30	32	34	35	37	39
	.01	.02	—	—	—	—	—	9	11	13	15	17	20	22	24	26	28	30	32	34	36	38	40	42	45
	.025	.05	—	—	—	—	—	13	15	17	19	22	24	26	29	31	34	36	38	41	43	45	48	50	53
	.05	.10	—	—	—	—	—	15	18	20	23	26	28	31	33	36	39	41	44	47	49	52	54	57	60

TABLE A.8 CRITICAL VALUES FOR THE MANN-WHITNEY U-TEST

n_1	α_1	α_2	9	10	11	12	13	14	15	16	17	18	19	20	21	22	23	24	25
									n_2 (larger sample size)										
9	.005	.01	11	13	16	18	20	22	24	27	29	31	33	36	38	40	43	45	47
	.01	.02	14	16	18	21	23	26	28	31	33	36	38	40	43	45	48	50	53
	.025	.05	17	20	23	26	28	31	34	37	39	42	45	48	50	53	56	59	62
	.05	.10	21	24	27	30	33	36	39	42	45	48	51	54	57	60	63	66	69
10	.005	.01	—	16	18	21	24	26	29	31	34	37	39	42	44	47	50	52	55
	.01	.02	—	19	22	24	27	30	33	36	38	41	44	47	50	53	55	58	61
	.025	.05	—	23	26	29	33	36	39	42	45	48	52	55	58	61	64	67	71
	.05	.10	—	27	31	34	37	41	44	48	51	55	58	62	65	68	72	75	79
11	.005	.01	—	—	21	24	27	30	33	36	39	42	45	48	51	54	57	60	63
	.01	.02	—	—	25	28	31	34	37	41	44	47	50	53	57	60	63	66	70
	.025	.05	—	—	30	33	37	40	44	47	51	55	58	62	65	69	73	76	80
	.05	.10	—	—	34	38	42	46	50	54	57	61	65	69	73	77	81	85	89
12	.005	.01	—	—	—	27	31	34	37	41	44	47	51	54	58	61	64	68	71
	.01	.02	—	—	—	31	35	38	42	46	49	53	56	60	64	67	71	75	78
	.025	.05	—	—	—	37	41	45	49	53	57	61	65	69	73	77	81	85	89
	.05	.10	—	—	—	42	47	51	55	60	64	68	72	77	81	85	90	95	99
13	.005	.01	—	—	—	—	34	38	42	45	49	53	57	60	64	68	72	75	79
	.01	.02	—	—	—	—	39	43	47	51	55	59	63	67	71	75	79	83	87
	.025	.05	—	—	—	—	45	50	54	59	63	67	72	76	80	85	89	94	98
	.05	.10	—	—	—	—	51	56	61	65	70	75	80	84	89	94	98	103	108
14	.005	.01	—	—	—	—	—	42	46	50	54	58	63	67	71	75	79	83	87
	.01	.02	—	—	—	—	—	47	51	56	60	65	69	73	78	82	87	91	95
	.025	.05	—	—	—	—	—	55	59	64	69	74	78	83	88	93	98	102	107
	.05	.10	—	—	—	—	—	61	66	71	77	82	87	92	97	102	107	113	118
15	.005	.01	—	—	—	—	—	—	51	55	60	64	69	73	78	82	87	91	96
	.01	.02	—	—	—	—	—	—	56	61	66	70	75	80	85	90	94	99	104
	.025	.05	—	—	—	—	—	—	64	70	75	80	85	90	96	101	106	111	117
	.05	.10	—	—	—	—	—	—	72	77	83	88	94	100	105	111	116	122	128
16	.005	.01	—	—	—	—	—	—	—	60	65	70	74	79	84	89	94	99	104
	.01	.02	—	—	—	—	—	—	—	66	71	76	82	87	92	97	102	108	113
	.025	.05	—	—	—	—	—	—	—	75	81	86	92	98	103	109	115	120	126
	.05	.10	—	—	—	—	—	—	—	83	89	95	101	107	113	119	125	131	137

(continued)

TABLE A.8   **CRITICAL VALUES FOR THE MANN-WHITNEY *U*-TEST (continued)**

n_1	α_1	α_2	n_2 (larger sample size)								
			17	18	19	20	21	22	23	24	25
17	.005	.01	70	75	81	86	91	96	102	107	112
	.01	.02	77	82	88	93	99	105	120	126	132
	.025	.05	87	93	99	105	111	117	123	129	135
	.05	.10	96	102	109	115	121	128	134	141	147
18	.005	.01	—	81	87	92	98	104	109	115	121
	.01	.02	—	88	94	100	106	112	118	124	130
	.025	.05	—	99	106	112	119	125	132	138	145
	.05	.10	—	109	116	123	130	136	143	150	157
19	.005	.01	—	—	93	99	105	111	117	123	129
	.01	.02	—	—	101	107	113	120	126	133	139
	.025	.05	—	—	113	119	126	133	140	147	154
	.05	.10	—	—	123	130	138	145	152	160	167
20	.005	.01	—	—	—	105	112	118	125	131	138
	.01	.02	—	—	—	114	121	127	134	141	148
	.025	.05	—	—	—	127	134	141	149	156	163
	.05	.10	—	—	—	138	146	154	161	169	177
21	.005	.01	—	—	—	—	118	125	132	139	146
	.01	.02	—	—	—	—	128	135	142	150	157
	.025	.05	—	—	—	—	142	150	157	165	173
	.05	.10	—	—	—	—	154	162	170	179	187
22	.005	.01	—	—	—	—	—	133	140	147	155
	.01	.02	—	—	—	—	—	143	150	158	166
	.025	.05	—	—	—	—	—	158	166	174	182
	.05	.10	—	—	—	—	—	171	179	188	197
23	.005	.01	—	—	—	—	—	—	148	155	163
	.01	.02	—	—	—	—	—	—	158	167	175
	.025	.05	—	—	—	—	—	—	175	183	192
	.05	.10	—	—	—	—	—	—	189	198	207
24	.005	.01	—	—	—	—	—	—	—	167	172
	.01	.02	—	—	—	—	—	—	—	175	184
	.025	.05	—	—	—	—	—	—	—	192	201
	.05	.10	—	—	—	—	—	—	—	207	217
25	.005	.01	—	—	—	—	—	—	—	—	180
	.01	.02	—	—	—	—	—	—	—	—	192
	.025	.05	—	—	—	—	—	—	—	—	211
	.05	.10	—	—	—	—	—	—	—	—	227

The test statistic must be equal to or less than the critical value to reject H_0.

When groups are of unequal size, n_1 is the smaller group.

Adapted from Table 1 in Verdooren LR. Extended tables of critical values for Wilcoxon's test statistic. *Biometrika* 1963;50(1 and 2):177, with the permission of the Biometrika Trustees.

TABLE A.9 PROBABILITIES* ASSOCIATED WITH VALUES OF x IN THE BINOMIAL TEST

									x								
n	0	1	2	3	4	5	6	7	8	9	10	11	12	13	14	15	16
4	.062	.312	.688	.938	—	—	—	—	—	—	—	—	—	—	—	—	—
5	.031	.188	.500	.812	.969	—	—	—	—	—	—	—	—	—	—	—	—
6	.016	.109	.344	.656	.891	.984	—	—	—	—	—	—	—	—	—	—	—
7	.008	.062	.227	.500	.773	.938	.992	—	—	—	—	—	—	—	—	—	—
8	.004	.035	.145	.363	.637	.855	.965	.996	—	—	—	—	—	—	—	—	—
9	.002	.020	.090	.254	.500	.746	.910	.980	.998	—	—	—	—	—	—	—	—
10	.001	.011	.055	.172	.377	.623	.828	.945	.989	.999	—	—	—	—	—	—	—
11	—	.006	.033	.113	.274	.500	.726	.887	.967	.994	—	—	—	—	—	—	—
12	—	.003	.019	.073	.194	.387	.613	.806	.927	.981	.997	—	—	—	—	—	—
13	—	.002	.011	.046	.133	.291	.500	.709	.867	.954	.989	.998	—	—	—	—	—
14	—	.001	.006	.029	.090	.212	.395	.605	.788	.910	.971	.994	.999	—	—	—	—
15	—	—	.004	.018	.059	.151	.304	.500	.696	.849	.941	.982	.996	—	—	—	—
16	—	—	.002	.011	.038	.105	.227	.402	.598	.773	.895	.962	.989	.998	—	—	—
17	—	—	.001	.006	.025	.072	.166	.315	.500	.685	.834	.928	.975	.994	.999	—	—
18	—	—	.001	.004	.015	.048	.119	.240	.407	.593	.760	.881	.952	.985	.996	.999	—
19	—	—	—	.002	.010	.032	.084	.180	.324	.500	.676	.850	.916	.968	.990	.998	—
20	—	—	—	.001	.006	.021	.058	.132	.252	.412	.588	.748	.868	.942	.979	.994	.999
21	—	—	—	.001	.004	.013	.039	.095	.192	.332	.500	.668	.808	.902	.961	.987	.996
22	—	—	—	—	.002	.008	.026	.067	.143	.262	.416	.584	.738	.857	.933	.974	.992
23	—	—	—	—	.001	.005	.017	.047	.105	.202	.339	.500	.661	.798	.895	.953	.983
24	—	—	—	—	.001	.003	.011	.032	.076	.154	.271	.419	.581	.729	.846	.924	.968
25	—	—	—	—	—	.002	.007	.022	.054	.115	.212	.345	.500	.655	.788	.885	.946
26	—	—	—	—	—	.001	.005	.014	.038	.084	.163	.279	.423	.577	.721	.837	.916
27	—	—	—	—	—	.001	.003	.010	.026	.061	.124	.221	.351	.500	.649	.779	.876
28	—	—	—	—	—	—	.002	.006	.018	.044	.092	.172	.286	.425	.575	.714	.828
29	—	—	—	—	—	—	.001	.004	.012	.031	.068	.132	.229	.356	.500	.644	.771
30	—	—	—	—	—	—	.001	.003	.008	.021	.049	.100	.181	.292	.428	.572	.708

*Tabled probabilities are for one-tailed tests. Double values in table for a two-tailed test.

TABLE A.10 CRITICAL VALUES OF T FOR THE WILCOXON SIGNED-RANKS TEST

N	α_1 α_2	.025 .05	.01 .02	.005 .01
6		0	—	—
7		2	0	—
8		4	2	0
9		6	3	2
10		8	5	3
11		11	7	5
12		14	10	7
13		17	13	10
14		21	16	13
15		25	20	16
16		30	24	20
17		35	28	23
18		40	33	28
19		46	38	32
20		52	43	38
21		59	49	43
22		66	56	49
23		73	62	55
24		81	69	61
25		89	77	68

The test statistic must be equal to or less than the critical value to reject H_0.

TABLE A.11   CRITICAL VALUES OF SPEARMAN'S RANK CORRELATION COEFFICIENT, r_s

n	α_2 0.10 α_1 0.05	0.05 0.025	0.02 0.01	0.01 0.005	0.005 0.0025	0.002 0.001	0.001 0.0005
4	1.000						
5	0.900	1.000	1.000				
6	0.829	0.886	0.943	1.000	1.000		
7	0.714	0.786	0.893	0.929	0.964	1.000	1.000
8	0.643	0.738	0.833	0.881	0.905	0.952	0.976
9	0.600	0.700	0.783	0.833	0.867	0.917	0.933
10	0.564	0.648	0.745	0.794	0.830	0.879	0.903
11	0.536	0.618	0.709	0.755	0.800	0.845	0.873
12	0.503	0.587	0.671	0.727	0.776	0.825	0.860
13	0.484	0.560	0.648	0.703	0.747	0.802	0.835
14	0.464	0.538	0.622	0.675	0.723	0.776	0.811
15	0.443	0.521	0.604	0.654	0.700	0.754	0.786
16	0.429	0.503	0.582	0.635	0.679	0.732	0.765
17	0.414	0.485	0.566	0.615	0.662	0.713	0.748
18	0.401	0.472	0.550	0.600	0.643	0.695	0.728
19	0.391	0.460	0.535	0.584	0.628	0.677	0.712
20	0.380	0.447	0.520	0.570	0.612	0.662	0.696
21	0.370	0.435	0.508	0.556	0.599	0.648	0.681
22	0.361	0.425	0.496	0.544	0.586	0.634	0.667
23	0.353	0.415	0.486	0.532	0.573	0.622	0.654
24	0.344	0.406	0.476	0.521	0.562	0.610	0.642
25	0.337	0.398	0.466	0.511	0.551	0.598	0.630
26	0.331	0.390	0.457	0.501	0.541	0.587	0.619
27	0.324	0.382	0.448	0.491	0.531	0.577	0.608
28	0.317	0.375	0.440	0.483	0.522	0.567	0.598
29	0.312	0.368	0.433	0.475	0.513	0.558	0.589
30	0.306	0.362	0.425	0.467	0.504	0.549	0.580
31	0.301	0.356	0.418	0.459	0.496	0.541	0.571
32	0.296	0.350	0.412	0.452	0.489	0.533	0.563
33	0.291	0.345	0.405	0.446	0.482	0.525	0.554
34	0.287	0.340	0.399	0.439	0.475	0.517	0.547
35	0.283	0.335	0.394	0.433	0.468	0.510	0.539
36	0.279	0.330	0.388	0.427	0.462	0.504	0.533
37	0.275	0.325	0.383	0.421	0.456	0.497	0.526
38	0.271	0.321	0.378	0.415	0.450	0.491	0.519
39	0.267	0.317	0.373	0.410	0.444	0.485	0.513
40	0.264	0.313	0.368	0.405	0.439	0.479	0.507
41	0.261	0.309	0.364	0.400	0.433	0.473	0.501
42	0.257	0.305	0.359	0.395	0.428	0.468	0.495
43	0.254	0.301	0.355	0.391	0.423	0.463	0.490
44	0.251	0.298	0.351	0.386	0.419	0.458	0.484
45	0.248	0.294	0.347	0.382	0.414	0.453	0.479

TABLE A.11 CRITICAL VALUES OF SPEARMAN'S RANK CORRELATION COEFFICIENT, r_s (continued)

n	α_2 α_1	0.10 0.05	0.05 0.025	0.02 0.01	0.01 0.005	0.005 0.0025	0.002 0.001	0.001 0.0005
46		0.246	0.291	0.343	0.378	0.410	0.448	0.474
47		0.243	0.288	0.340	0.374	0.405	0.443	0.469
48		0.240	0.285	0.336	0.370	0.401	0.439	0.465
49		0.238	0.282	0.333	0.366	0.397	0.434	0.460
50		0.235	0.279	0.329	0.363	0.393	0.430	0.456
60		0.214	0.255	0.300	0.331	0.360	0.394	0.418
70		0.198	0.235	0.278	0.307	0.333	0.365	0.388
80		0.185	0.220	0.260	0.287	0.312	0.342	0.363
90		0.174	0.207	0.245	0.271	0.294	0.323	0.343
100		0.165	0.197	0.233	0.257	0.279	0.307	0.326

APPENDIX B

Relating the Research Question to the Choice of Statistical Test

Research Question	Refer to Chart
Is there a difference between means (or medians)?	
1 independent variable, 2 levels	B1
1 independent variable, $\geq$ 3 levels	B2
2 or more independent variables	B3
Is there a difference in proportions?	B4
Is there an association between variables?	B5
Is there a predictive relationship between variables?	B6
Are measurements reliable?	B7

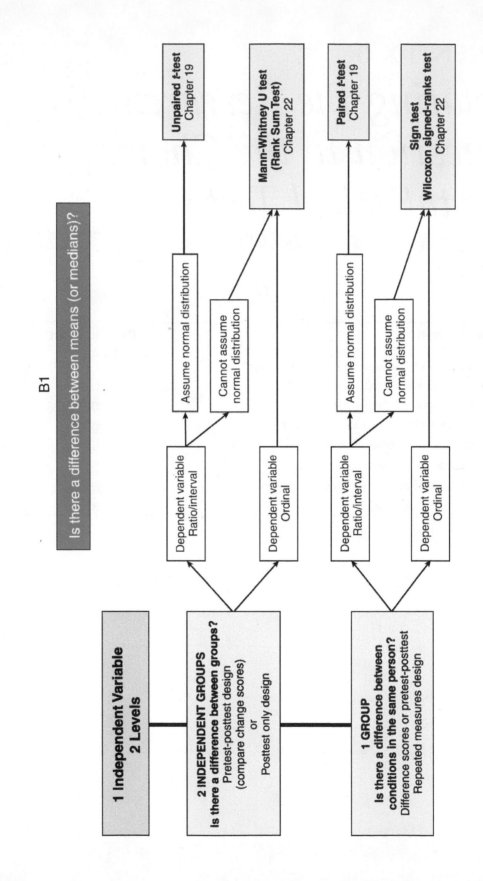

B1

Is there a difference between means (or medians)?

1 Independent Variable 2 Levels

2 INDEPENDENT GROUPS
Is there a difference between groups?
Pretest-posttest design
(compare change scores)
or
Posttest only design

Dependent variable
Ratio/interval

Assume normal distribution

→ **Unpaired *t*-test**
Chapter 19

Cannot assume
normal distribution

Dependent variable
Ordinal

→ **Mann-Whitney U test
(Rank Sum Test)**
Chapter 22

1 GROUP
**Is there a difference between
conditions in the same person?**
Difference scores or pretest-posttest
Repeated measures design

Dependent variable
Ratio/interval

Assume normal distribution

→ **Paired *t*-test**
Chapter 19

Cannot assume
normal distribution

Dependent variable
Ordinal

→ **Sign test
Wilcoxon signed-ranks test**
Chapter 22

B2

Is there a difference between means (or medians)?

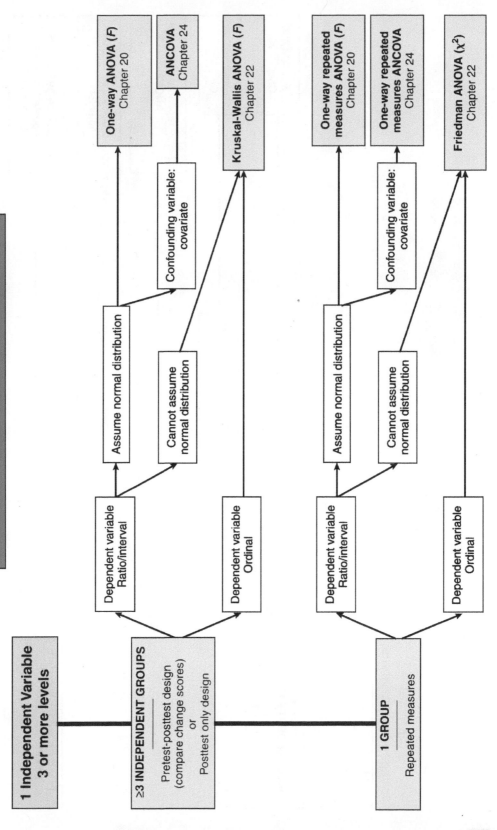

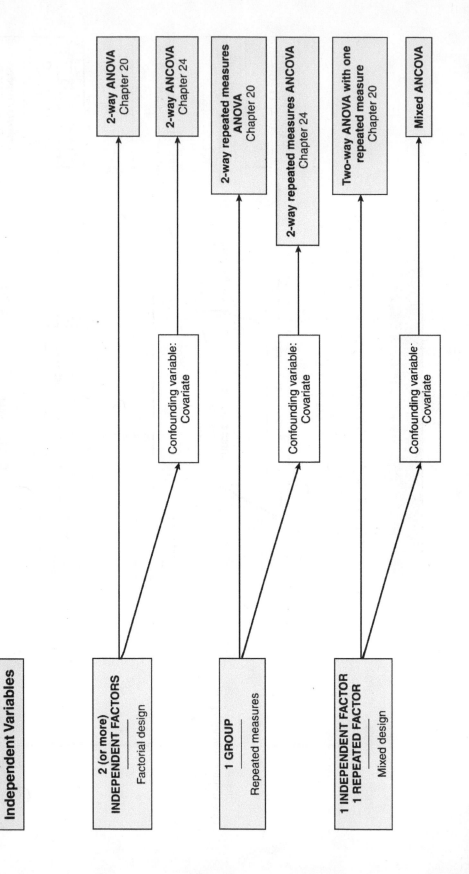

B3

Is there a difference between means (or medians)?

2 (or more) Independent Variables

2 (or more) INDEPENDENT FACTORS
Factorial design

1 GROUP
Repeated measures

1 INDEPENDENT FACTOR 1 REPEATED FACTOR
Mixed design

Confounding variable: Covariate

Confounding variable: Covariate

Confounding variable: Covariate

2-way ANOVA
Chapter 20

2-way ANCOVA
Chapter 24

2-way repeated measures ANOVA
Chapter 20

2-way repeated measures ANCOVA
Chapter 24

Two-way ANOVA with one repeated measure
Chapter 20

Mixed ANCOVA

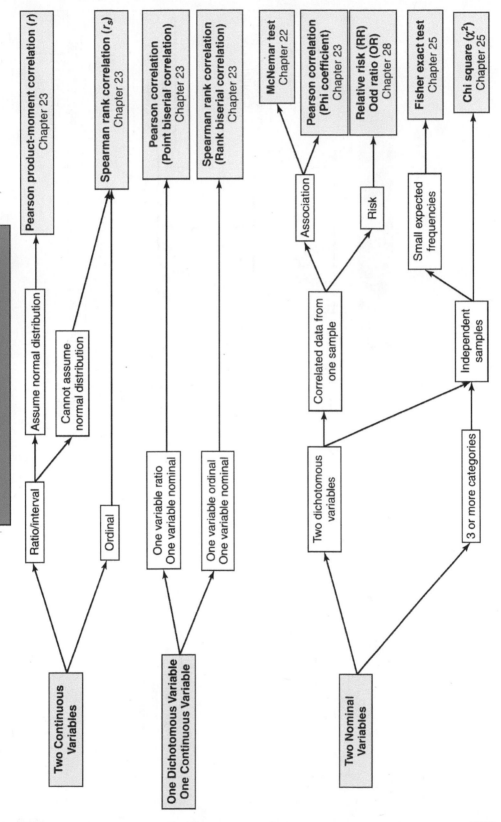

B4

Is there an association between variables?

Two Continuous Variables → Ratio/interval

Ratio/interval → Assume normal distribution → **Pearson product-moment correlation (r)** Chapter 23

Ratio/interval → Cannot assume normal distribution → **Spearman rank correlation (r_s)** Chapter 23

Two Continuous Variables → Ordinal → **Spearman rank correlation (r_s)** Chapter 23

One Dichotomous Variable One Continuous Variable → One variable ratio One variable nominal → **Pearson correlation (Point biserial correlation)** Chapter 23

One Dichotomous Variable One Continuous Variable → One variable ordinal One variable nominal → **Spearman rank correlation (Rank biserial correlation)** Chapter 23

Two Nominal Variables → Two dichotomous variables → Correlated data from one sample → Association → **McNemar test** Chapter 22

Correlated data from one sample → Association → **Pearson correlation (Phi coefficient)** Chapter 23

Two dichotomous variables → Risk → **Relative risk (RR) Odd ratio (OR)** Chapter 28

Two Nominal Variables → Independent samples → Small expected frequencies → **Fisher exact test** Chapter 25

Independent samples → 3 or more categories → **Chi square (χ^2)** Chapter 25

B5

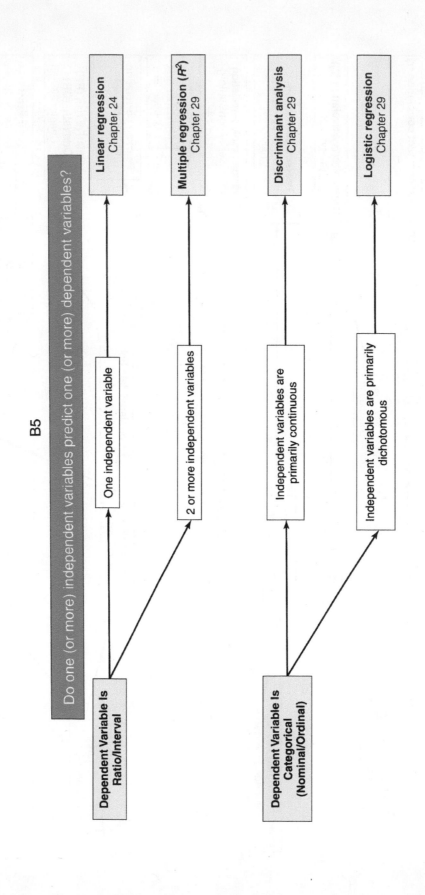

B6

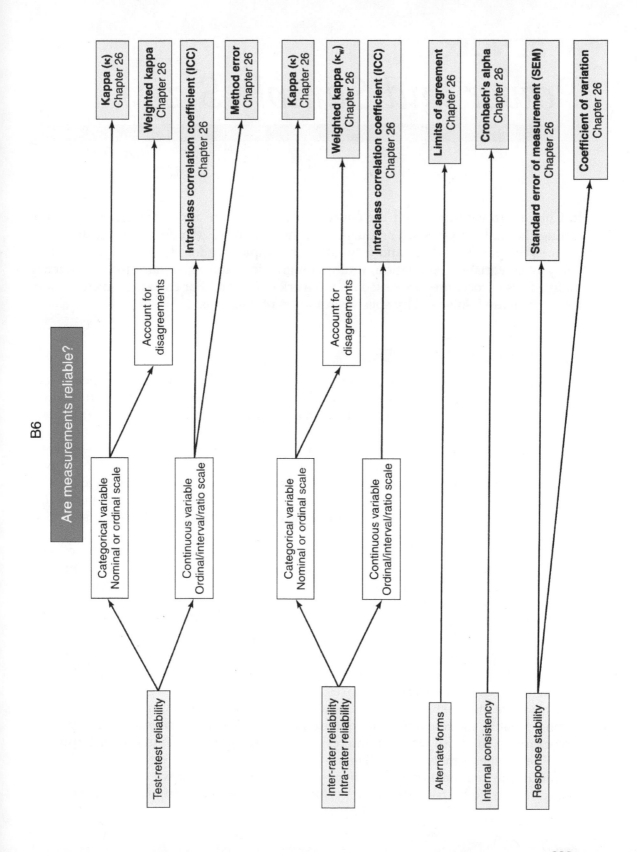

APPENDIX C
Power and Sample Size

In Chapter 18 we introduced the concept of power as an important consideration in testing the null hypothesis. The purpose of this appendix is to describe statistical procedures for power analysis and estimation of sample size for studies using the *t*-test, analysis of variance, correlation, multiple regression, and chi-square for contingency tables. These procedures are based on the work of Cohen.[1] For each procedure, formulas are provided, followed by specific examples of their use.

THE EFFECT SIZE INDEX

In power analysis we are concerned with five statistical elements: the significance criterion (α), the sample size (n), sample variance (s^2), effect size (ES), and power ($1 - \beta$). These elements are related in such a way that given any four, the fifth is readily determined.

Effect size is a measure of the magnitude of difference or correlation. The larger the observed effect, the more likely it will result in a significant statistical test (given a specific alpha level). An *effect size index* is a statistic that represents effect size using a standardized value that is universally applicable for all units of data, just as *t*, *F* and *r* are unit free. A different form of effect size index is used for each statistical procedure.

It is a simple process to calculate a sample effect size index following completion of a study. We know the sample size, and we can calculate the actual variance, means, correlations, or proportions in the data. This information can then be used to determine the degree of power achieved.

During planning stages of a study we use effect size to determine how many subjects will be needed. But because data are not yet available, the researcher must make an educated guess as to the expected effect size. This hypothesis is often based on previous research or pilot data, where studies can provide reasonable estimates for mean differences, correlations and variances. When such data are not available, the effect size estimate may be based on the researcher's opinion of a clinically meaningful difference; that is, the researcher can determine how large an effect would be important. For example, suppose we were interested in studying two treatments for improving shoulder range of motion in patients with adhesive capsulitis. We might say that the results of the treatments should differ by at least 20 degrees, or we would not consider the difference to be meaningful. Therefore, if we observed a difference this large, we would want it to be significant. This would be the effect size we would propose. Similarly, for a correlational study we could propose that a correlation of at least .60 would be important. These types of clinical judgments can then be used to guide the estimation of sample size.

Conventional Effect Sizes

When the researcher wants to establish the required sample size prior to data collection, and no clinical judgment or previous data provide a reasonable guide, Cohen proposes the use of conventional values, which are based on operational definitions for "small," "medium," and "large" effect sizes.[1] Although these definitions are purely relative and somewhat intuitive, Cohen suggests that they represent reasonable estimates for planning purposes. Specific values for small, medium and large effects are proposed for each statistical procedure. Cohen emphasizes, however, that these descriptions are necessarily relative, and must be operationalized for a given research situation. A small effect size for tests of movement may be quite different from a small effect for psychological phenomena.

As a starting point then, a *small effect size* is considered small enough so that changes are not perceptible to the human eye, but not so small as to be minute. In new areas of inquiry, effect sizes are likely to be small because the phenomenon under study is typically not well understood and perhaps not under good experimental control. Many behavioral effects are likely to fall into this category, because of the influence of extraneous variables and the subtleties of human performance.

A *medium effect size* is conceived as large enough to be visible to the naked eye, so that one would be aware of the change in the course of normal observation.

A *large effect size* represents a great degree of separation, so that there is very little overlap between population distributions. Differences should be grossly observable. Large effect sizes are often seen in sociology, economics, and physiology, fields characterized by studies with large samples and good experimental control.

One way to conceptualize these definitions is to think of effect size in terms of variance. Using a simple framework involving two group means, the difference between means would be considered small if it is 20% of one standard deviation (assuming both groups have the same standard deviation). A medium effect would be equivalent to half a standard deviation, and a large effect would be 80% of a standard deviation. It is useful to think of effect size, then, as a ratio of the variance between groups relative to the variance within groups.

Estimating Sample Size

So what happens if the estimate of effect size is incorrect? What happens if we predict a large effect size and choose the appropriate sample, but the actual scores reveal a small effect, which turns out to be nonsignificant? Well, then we go back and determine the probability of a Type II error, and what level of power was actually achieved. This information can then be used for interpreting the study's results and in planning future studies. It is usually more prudent to be conservative in effect size estimates, so that a large enough sample will be recruited. If several analyses are planned for a given set of data (such as several regression equations or multiple analyses of variance), the sample size must be large enough to support the smallest hypothesized effect for the most complex analysis.[2]

Tables

Tables are provided for power and sample size estimates at the end of this appendix. Power can be determined by knowing effect size and sample size, and sample size can be determined by knowing the expected effect size and the desired level of power. Tables are included for $\alpha = .05$, for one- and two-tailed test where appropriate. Each statistical procedure requires its own set of tables. We have limited these tables to basic configurations for the t-test, analysis of variance, correlation, regression, and chi-square. The reader is referred to Cohen for additional tables.[1]

POWER ANALYSIS FOR THE t-TEST

Power analysis for the t-test is based on the effect size index, d, which expresses the difference between the two sample means in standard deviation units.

Unpaired t-Test: Equal Variances

For the unpaired t-test with equal variances, the effect size index is calculated according to:

$$d = \frac{\overline{X}_1 - \overline{X}_2}{s} \tag{C.1}$$

where $\overline{X}_1$ and $\overline{X}_2$ are the group means, and s is their common standard deviation. Assuming equality of variance, s can be the standard deviation from either group, or it can be their arithmetic average, the square root of the pooled variance, $\sqrt{s_p^2}$ (see Equation 19.2).

If used after data analysis, the d index can also be computed using the calculated value of t:

$$d = t\sqrt{\frac{n_1 + n_2}{n_1 n_2}} \tag{C.2}$$

With a nondirectional alternative hypothesis, only the absolute value of d is considered. With a directional hypothesis, the sign of d must correspond to the predicted direction.

Unpaired *t*-Test: Unequal Variances

When the assumption of homogeneity of variance is not met, the calculation of d is based on the *root mean square* (s') of s_1 and s_2 as follows:

$$s' = \sqrt{\frac{s_1^2 + s_2^2}{2}} \qquad \text{(C.3)}$$

The value of s' is used in the denominator of Equation C.1.

Paired *t*-Test

When data are collected in a repeated measures design, calculation of d is based on paired scores. In this case, we first calculate d' using the means for the two test conditions and a common standard deviation:

$$d' = \frac{\overline{X}_1 - \overline{X}_2}{s} \qquad \text{(C.4)}$$

We account for the fact that these values are correlated by adjusting d as follows:

$$d = \frac{d'}{\sqrt{1 - r}} \qquad \text{(C.5)}$$

where r is the correlation coefficient for the paired data.
    When no estimate of r can be made, we can substitute the formula

$$d' = \frac{\overline{d}}{s_d} \qquad \text{(C.6)}$$

where $\overline{d}$ is the mean of the difference scores, and s_d is the standard deviation of the difference scores. The value of d to be used in the power tables is then determined by

$$d = d'\sqrt{2} \qquad \text{(C.7)}$$

Conventional Effect Sizes

When d cannot be computed directly, the following conventions can be used to assign value to the effect size index: small $d = .20$, medium $d = .50$, and large $d = .80$.

Power and Sample Size Tables

To determine the power achieved for a given sample size and effect size, we use Tables C.1.1 and C.1.2, found at the end of this appendix, for estimates at α_1 and $\alpha_2 = .05$. Along the top of the table we locate the appropriate value of d, and down the side, the known sample size, n. For the unpaired test, sample size refers to the number of subjects in *each group* (assuming equal groups), not both groups combined. For the paired *t*-test, this is the number of subjects in the study. Power levels, in percentages, are given in the body of the table.

Unequal Samples

When sample sizes are different for the two groups being compared, the *harmonic mean* of the two sample sizes, n', is computed:

$$n' = \frac{2n_1 n_2}{n_1 + n_2} \qquad (C.8)$$

The value of n' is then used to locate n in the power table.

Table C.2 is used to determine the sample size needed for the t-test to achieve a desired level of power for one- and two-tailed tests at $\alpha = .05$ and .01. For each sub-table, the value of d is located across the top, and the desired power is given at the left. Power levels are listed for .70, .80, and .90. The sample sizes found in the body of the table represent the number of subjects required *in each group*, or the total number of subjects for paired observations.

When the exact value of d is not provided in the table, an adequate approximation of n can be given by

$$n = \frac{n_{.10}}{100d^2} + 1 \qquad (C.9)$$

where $n_{.10}$ is the sample size given for $d = .10$ in Table C.2, and d is the exact calculated value of the effect size index.*

Examples

Unpaired t-Test: Equal Variances

Consider the data from Table 19.1 in Chapter 19. In that hypothetical study, we measured change in pinch strength in two groups, with $\overline{X}_1 = 10.11$, $\overline{X}_2 = 5.45$, and $s_p^2 = 14.695$. A directional hypothesis was proposed. Therefore, using Equation C.1,

$$s = \sqrt{s_p^2} = \sqrt{14.695} = 3.83 \qquad d = \frac{10.11 - 5.45}{3.83} = 1.22$$

Alternatively, $t = 2.718$, with $n = 10$ per group. Therefore, using Equation C.2,

$$d = 2.718\sqrt{\frac{10 + 10}{(10)(10)}} = 2.718\sqrt{.20} = 1.22$$

To determine the power achieved with this test, we refer to Table C.1.1 for $\alpha_1 = .05$ and $n = 10$. With $d = 1.2$, we achieve 83% power. If we use these values to determine sample size for 80% power, we refer to Table C.2 for $\alpha_1 = .05$, where we find that we would need 9 subjects per group.

---

*When using an average value for n the power estimates will be underestimates; that is, the power value in the table will be slightly lower than the true power. This underestimate will be trivial when $n' > 25$. Note that when sample sizes and variances are both unequal, the estimates of power using these tables may be inaccurate.[1]

Now suppose we are planning this study. We state a nondirectional hypothesis and propose that a difference of 5 pounds would be important. We guess that a standard deviation of 8.0 would be expected. Therefore, we estimate that $d = 5/8 = .625$. Referring to Table C.2 for $\alpha_1 = .05$ and $d = .60$, we would estimate that we will need 35 subjects *per group* (a total of 70) to achieve 80% power. If once the study is completed, we obtain an effect size index of 1.2 with $n = 35$, we would then have achieved more than 99% power (Table C.1.1).

Unpaired t-Test: Unequal Variances

Consider the data in Table 19.2 in Chapter 19 for change in pinch strength, where $\overline{X}_1 = 10.80$, $\overline{X}_2 = 5.65$ and $s_1^2 = 25.17$, $s_2^2 = 4.89$. Therefore, using Equations C.3 and C.1,

$$s' = \sqrt{\frac{25.17 + 4.89}{2}} = 3.88 \qquad d = \frac{10.80 - 5.65}{3.88} = 1.33$$

Because the samples are of unequal size, we compute the harmonic mean to determine n' using Equation C.8. With $n_1 = 10$ and $n_2 = 15$:

$$n' = \frac{2n_1n_2}{n_1 + n_2} = \frac{2(10)(15)}{10 + 15} = \frac{300}{25} = 12$$

Using $n = 12$ in Table C.1.1, we find for $d = 1.2$ power is 89%, and for $d = 1.4$ power is 96%. We can, therefore, estimate that power is approximately 93% for $d = 1.3$.

To determine sample size requirements with $d = 1.3$ we can use Table C.2. For 80% power with $\alpha_1 = .05$, we would need between 9 and 7 subjects (between $d = 1.2$ and 1.4). To calculate the exact sample size for $d = 1.3$, we use Equation C.9:

$$n = \frac{n_{.10}}{100d^2} + 1 = \frac{1237}{100(1.3)^2} + 1 = 7.32 + 1 = 8.32$$

These results should always be rounded up to the nearest whole number. We would need 9 subjects per group to achieve 80% power with this effect size.

Paired t-Test

Consider the data in Table 19.3 in Chapter 19 for paired data. We examined the angle of the pelvis with and without a lumbar pillow in a sample of 8 subjects. For the paired *t*-test, we found that $\overline{X}_1 = 102.38$, $\overline{X}_2 = 99.00$ and $s_1 = 7.41$, $s_2 = 8.64$. A nondirectional hypothesis was proposed. The analysis also showed that $r = .86$ for the paired scores. Therefore, we use Equations C.4 and C.5:

$$s = \frac{7.41 + 8.64}{2} = 8.025 \qquad d' = \frac{102.38 - 99.00}{8.025} = 0.42 \qquad d = \frac{0.42}{\sqrt{1 - .71}} = 0.78$$

Alternatively, using $\overline{d} = -3.375$ and $s_d = 6.232$, with Equations C.6 and C.7:

$$d' = \frac{-3.375}{6.232} = 0.54 \qquad d = 0.54\sqrt{2} = 0.76$$

Note that the minus sign is ignored.

To determine power at $\alpha_2 = .05$, we use Table C.1.2. For $n = 8$ and $d = .80$ (rounded) we can see that we achieve 31% power. This study had a good effect size, but the sample size was quite small, resulting in low power. Using Table C.2, we find we would have needed 26 subjects to achieve 80% power.

POWER ANALYSIS FOR THE ANALYSIS OF VARIANCE

For the analysis of variance (ANOVA) the effect size index, f, is defined by

$$f = \sqrt{\frac{SS_b}{SS_e}} \tag{C.10}$$

where SS_e is the error sum of squares from the ANOVA summary table.[†] For a one-way ANOVA, SS_b is the between-groups sum of squares. For a two-way ANOVA, SS_b can represent either an individual main effect or the interaction effect; that is, a separate effect size index can be computed for each effect.[‡] This index can be applied to independent samples and repeated measures designs.

If we do not have access to the ANOVA summary, we can also calculate f using the following formula:

$$f = \frac{s_m}{s} \tag{C.11}$$

where s_m is the standard deviation of the group means around the grand mean, and s is the common standard deviation for each group. For planning purposes, to estimate f, researchers may be able to hypothesize values for group means and their common standard deviation, based on theory and previous research. With equal sample sizes, s_m is obtained by

$$s_m = \sqrt{\frac{\Sigma(\overline{X}_i - \overline{X}_G)^2}{k}} \tag{C.12}$$

where $(\overline{X}_i - \overline{X}_G)$ represents the deviation of each individual group mean $(\overline{X}_i)$ from the grand mean $(\overline{X}_G)$ and k is the number of groups.[§] Equation C.12 will work for the between-groups effect in a one-way ANOVA and for the main effects in a factorial design.

[†]Some statistical programs report this effect size index as eta squared (η^2):[3] $\eta^2 = \dfrac{SS_b}{SS_b + SS_e}$

These indices are related:[1] $f = \sqrt{\dfrac{\eta^2}{1 - \eta^2}}$ and $\eta^2 = \dfrac{f^2}{1 + f^2}$

[‡]Alternatively, an effect size index can also be computed for the overall two-way ANOVA model, combining all between-groups effects. The term SS_b would then be the sum of all between-groups sums of squares (i.e., SS_A, SS_B, and $SS_{A \times B}$).

[§]If groups are not of equal size, the difference between each group mean and the grand mean must be weighted by the sample size, using $s_m = \sqrt{\dfrac{\Sigma n_i(\overline{X}_i - \overline{X}_G)^2}{N}}$ where n_i is the number of subjects in each group and N is the total sample size for all groups combined.

For two-way interactions, the f index must account for the variability among the interaction means with reference to the main effects (A and B) and the grand mean as follows:

$$s_{m(AB)} = \sqrt{\frac{\Sigma(\overline{X}_{AB} - \overline{X}_A - \overline{X}_B + \overline{X}_G)^2}{df_{AB} + 1}} \tag{C.13}$$

where $\overline{X}_{AB}$ is the individual cell mean, $\overline{X}_A$ is the marginal mean for variable A and $\overline{X}_B$ is the marginal mean for variable B for that cell, and $\overline{X}_G$ is the grand mean for the sample. The term df_{AB} represents the degrees of freedom associated with the interaction term $(A - 1)(B - 1)$.

Conventional Effect Sizes

When effect sizes cannot be estimated from existing data, conventional values are as follows: small $f = .10$, medium $f = .25$, large $f = .40$.[11]

Power and Sample Size Tables

Power tables for the analysis of variance are arranged according to the degrees of freedom associated with each F-test (df_b). In a one-way ANOVA, this is the between-groups effect. In a two-way ANOVA (or larger) these effects will include each main effect and an interaction effect. Tables C.3.1 through C.3.4 give power estimates for different values of the effect size index, f, at $df_b = 1, 2, 3,$ and 4 at $\alpha = .05$. See Cohen for additional tables.[1]

Sample sizes can be found using Table C.4 for various levels of α and df_b. These tables are used in the same way as the tables for the t-test.

To find n for a value of f that is not tabled, we use

$$n = \frac{n_{.05}}{400f^2} + 1 \tag{C.14}$$

where $n_{.05}$ is the sample size for $f = .05$ at the desired level of power and f is the exact value of the effect size index.

Examples

One-Way Analysis of Variance

Consider the data for a one-way analysis of variance presented in Table 20.1 in Chapter 20. In this study we examined the effect of different modalities on ROM in 44 patients with elbow tendinitis. Four groups were compared ($k = 4$). Using data from the ANOVA output summary table, we found that $SS_b = 3158.09$ and $SS_e = 3541.64$. Therefore, using Equation C.10,

$$f = \sqrt{\frac{SS_b}{SS_e}} = \sqrt{\frac{3158.09}{3541.64}} = \sqrt{0.892} = 0.944$$

---

[11]Using η^2 these conventional effect sizes are equivalent to small $\eta^2 = .01$, medium $\eta^2 = .06$, large $\eta^2 = .14$.

Given conventional effect sizes for f, this is a large effect.

To determine the power achieved with this test, we refer to Table C.3.3 for $df_b = 3$. The sample size used in the table refers to the number of subjects *in each group,* in this case $n = 11$. In this example, the f index is larger than .80, which is the highest value listed in the table. If we look across the row for $n = 11$, for $f = .80$ the power is 99%. Therefore, we can expect that power for $f = 0.94$ is 100%. Note that we actually would not do a power analysis for this study, as it resulted in a significant F-test. We use it here for illustration only.

Suppose we did not know these results, but we wanted to plan this study to determine the needed sample size. We hypothesize that ROM change will be greatest for those using ice, slightly less for those using ultrasound, less for those using massage, and much less for those with no intervention. As an estimate, based on our experience, we guess that the means will be 50, 40, 30, and 20, respectively. Using the literature as a guide, we also estimate that the standard deviation will be 8.0. With these values, we estimate a grand mean of $(50 + 40 + 30 + 20)/4 = 35$. Therefore, we can estimate f using Equations C.12 and C.11 as follows:

$$s_m = \sqrt{\frac{\Sigma(\overline{X}_i - \overline{X}_G)}{k}} = \sqrt{\frac{(50 - 8)^2 + (40 - 8)^2 + (30 - 8)^2 + (20 - 8)^2}{4}} = 58.45$$

$$f = \frac{s_m}{s} = \frac{58.45}{8} = 7.31$$

We turn to Table C.4 ($df_b = 3$) to determine the sample size needed to achieve 80% power with this estimated effect size. Using $f = .80$ (the largest value), we find that we would need 5 subjects per group, or a total sample of 20 subjects. Based on conventional effect sizes, this is considered a large effect, achieving high power even with a relatively small sample.

Two-Way Analysis of Variance

In a two-way ANOVA, power can be determined for each of the main effects and interaction effects. Consider the data presented in Table 20.3 in Chapter 20, for a study comparing the effect of three types of stretch (A) in two knee positions (B) for increasing ankle range of motion. A total of 60 subjects were assigned to six unique treatment groups. This analysis resulted in a significant interaction as well as a significant main effect for Stretch, but no significant effect for Position.

Main Effect.   To look at the main effect of Position (variable B), we estimate effect size using Equation C.10 as follows:

$$f_B = \sqrt{\frac{SS_B}{SS_e}} = \sqrt{\frac{2.02}{697.36}} = \sqrt{.003} = .0548$$

where SS_B is the sum of squares associated with Position (variable B).[#] Based on conventional values, this would be considered an extremely small effect. To determine the

---

[#]For these examples, please do not confuse subscripts A and B, which represent values associated with factors A and B, and subscript b which indicates the between-groups effect.

power of this test with two levels, we use Table C.3.1 for $df_B = 1$. Each level of Position includes 30 subjects. This test achieves 6% power. Therefore, we have a 94% chance that we committed a Type II error. However, we must also consider the fact that the difference between main effect means for the two positions was 0.36 degrees (see Figure 20.6); that is, the observed effect size was extremely small. Given that we are measuring range of motion, such an effect would not be considered important. Therefore, it is unlikely that we have truly committed a Type II error. It is more likely that these positions are not different.

How many subjects would we have needed to achieve 80% power with this effect? We use Table C.4 for $df_b = 1$. For $f = .05$ at 80% power, we would need 1,571 subjects *per group*. As this is surely unreasonable, we might reconsider the inclusion of this variable in our research hypothesis.

Interaction Effect.   To determine power for the interaction effect (an illustration, as this effect was significant), we use Equation C.10 as follows:

$$f_{AB} = \sqrt{\frac{SS_{AB}}{SS_e}} = \sqrt{\frac{707.72}{697.36}} = \sqrt{1.02} = 1.01$$

We refer to Table C.3.2 for $df_b = 2$ (the degrees of freedom associated with the interaction effect). The effect size values do not go as high as 1.00, but for $n = 10$ at $f = .80$, power is 97%. Therefore, we know that we have achieved maximal power for this effect.

In planning this study, suppose we hypothesized that prolonged stretch would be most effective, and that the control group would not change. We also believe that greater ankle range of motion will be achieved when stretch is given with the knee extended. We project the following means:

Stretch		Knee Position		Marginal Means
		Flexion B$_1$	Extension B$_2$	
Prolonged	A$_1$	15	20	$\overline{X}_{A_1} = 17.5$
Quick	A$_2$	10	10	$\overline{X}_{A_2} = 10$
Control	A$_3$	0	0	$\overline{X}_{A_3} = 0$
Marginal Means		$\overline{X}_{B_1} = 8.3$	$\overline{X}_{B_2} = 10$	$\overline{X}_G = 9.15$

From the literature we estimate that the standard deviation in our data will be 5.0. Using these values, we compute $s_{m(AB)}$ using Equation C.13 as follows:

$$s_{m(AB)} = \sqrt{\frac{(15 - 17.5 - 8.3 + 9.15)^2 + (20 - 17.5 - 10 + 9.15)^2 + \cdots + (0 - 0 - 10 - 9.15)^2}{2 + 1}} = \sqrt{2.78} = 1.67$$

Therefore, according to Equation C.10,

$$f_{AB} = \frac{1.67}{5.0} = .33$$

To determine sample size, we look at Table C.4 for $df_b = 2$, power = 80%, and $f = .30$. We would need 36 subjects *per group*, or a total of 72 subjects. If we were doing this type of planning for a two-way design, we would project sample sizes for each main effect and interaction, and use the largest sample size as our guideline.

POWER ANALYSIS FOR CORRELATION

Power analysis for correlations is based on the magnitude of association, or the correlation coefficient. Because the correlation coefficient is a unit-free index, the effect size index does not need to be adjusted, and is simply the value of r.

Conventional Effect Sizes

Cohen addresses the dilemma that often surfaces when interpreting values of r; that is, even small correlations are often considered meaningful.[1] This is especially common in the behavioral and clinical sciences, where significant correlations will often be less than .60. Therefore, how does one conceptualize a "large" or "small" effect? This must be a relative frame of reference, based on knowledge of the literature and clinical hypotheses; that is, how much of the variance in clinical phenomena can we truly expect to predict?

Based on this understanding, Cohen hesitates to offer conventional effect sizes for r, but does suggest the following may be used when no other statistical rationale is obvious: small $r = 1.0$, medium $r = .30$, large $r = .50$.

Power and Sample Size Tables

Tables C.5.1 and C.5.2 can be used to estimate power for the Pearson and Spearman correlations for one- and two-tailed tests at $\alpha = .05$. Table C.6 provides estimated sample sizes required to achieve various levels of power for the same significance levels. The values of n in the tables represent the number of paired observations.

Example

Refer to Table 23.2 in Chapter 23, showing the correlation of proximal and distal behaviors in a sample of 12 normal infants, with a resulting correlation of $r = .37$, which was not significant at $\alpha_1 = .05$. To determine the level of power achieved, we refer to Table C.5.1. With $r = .40$ and 12 subjects, we attained 38% power; that is, there is a 62% chance we committed a Type II error. To find how many subjects we needed for 80% power, we use Table C.6 ($\alpha_1 = .05$). We should have recruited a sample of 37 subjects. In planning a study, we simply hypothesize a meaningful value for r and use this value in Table C.6.

POWER ANALYSIS FOR REGRESSION

In regression analysis, a quantitative dependent variable (Y) is correlated with a set of independent variables (X_1, X_2, through X_k). As with correlation, the degree of association within the regression equation represents the effect size, in this case R^2. The independent variables may represent quantitative or categorical variables (see Chapters 24 and 27).

In determining power, however, we must convert R^2 to another index that will account for both the number of subjects and the number of independent variables in the regression. This index, called lambda (λ)** is calculated as follows:

$$\lambda = \frac{R^2}{1 - R^2}(N)$$
(C.15)

Power and Sample Size Tables

Table C.7 is used to determine the power of the regression for $\alpha = .05$. To use this table we must know three elements: (1) the number of independent variables, k, in the left-most column, (2) the number of residual degrees of freedom, df_{res}, in the analysis of variance of regression (equal to $N - k - 1$), in the second column, and (3) the value for λ, along the top. For values of λ that fall between the values in the table, power can be determined by linear interpolation. Four values for df_{res} are given: 20, 60, 120, and ∞. Although not strictly linear, for degrees of freedom that fall between these values, power can be estimated with reasonable accuracy.

To determine sample size, we specify a level of power, the number of independent variables, and a projected R^2. We then use Table C.8 to determine a value for lambda and substitute that value in the formula:

$$N = \frac{\lambda(1 - R^2)}{R^2}$$
(C.16)

The obvious dilemma in this process is that finding a value for lambda requires estimating df_{res}, which is a function of sample size, which we are trying to determine! Therefore, the process becomes one of limited trial and error. We start with one value for lambda, determine the associated sample size, and then calculate df_{res} for that sample ($df_{res} = N - k - 1$). If the numbers do not correspond, we go back and choose a different value for df_{res} and try again. One choice in the table will provide a reasonable estimate.

Example

To illustrate power analysis for multiple regression, consider a hypothetical study involving five independent variables ($k = 5$) as predictors of hospital length of stay (LOS). Suppose our sample consists of 30 patients, and results show that $R^2 = .20$ ($p = .176$). Because this is not significant, we want to determine the power of

---

**Lambda is the *noncentrality parameter* of the F-test. Some statistical programs, such as SPSS, will generate a value for the noncentrality parameter as part of a power analysis for an analysis of variance. This value by itself is not used to represent power, but is needed to obtain power estimates.

the test. First we calculate lambda for $k = 5$, $R^2 = .20$, $df_{res} = 24$, and $N = 30$, using Equation C.15:

$$\lambda = \frac{R^2}{1 - R^2}(N) = \frac{.20}{1 - .20}(30) = 7.5$$

We refer to Table C.7. Using the closest values for $df_{res} = 20$, $k = 5$, and $\lambda = 8$, we find that our test achieved approximately 44% power, indicating a 56% probability of committing a Type II error.

Table C.7 also shows us how the number of independent variables included in the regression will influence the number of subjects needed. As k increases, we can see that power decreases for a given value of λ. Just to illustrate, look at $k = 3$ for $\lambda = 14$ at $df_{res} = 20$. Power is 82%. If we double the number of independent variables, $k = 6$, power decreases to 66%. With 10 independent variables, we are down to 51%. Researchers will often use stepwise regression or factor analysis to decrease the number of independent variables in a regression analysis, which clearly will have the effect of improving power.

Now let us suppose we are planning this study and we want to determine how many subjects would be needed to achieve 80% power in the analysis with five independent variables. A literature search suggests that the hypothesized effect will be $R^2 = .40$. We start by referring to Table C.8 to determine the value for lambda. Since we do not know how many subjects we need, we must first choose a trial value for df_{res}. Cohen suggests that, as the values of lambda do not vary greatly among the four choices for residual degrees of freedom, using a trial value for $df_{res} = 120$ will generally yield an N of sufficient accuracy.[1] Starting there, for $k = 5$ at 80% power, we find $\lambda = 13.3$. Using Equation C.16, we determine N as follows:

$$N = \frac{\lambda(1 - R^2)}{R^2} = \frac{13.3(1 - .40)}{.40} = 19.95$$

This projection tells us we would need 20 subjects to achieve 80% power.[tt] If we use this estimate, the residual degrees of freedom would then be $N - k - 1 = 20 - 5 - 1 = 14$. Obviously, a great disparity exists between this value and $df_{res} = 120$, which we used to calculate N. This is the trial and error part. Now we return to Table C.8 and find $\lambda = 16.7$ for $k = 5$ and 80% power at $df_{res} = 20$, which we guess will be closer to our required N. This time we find

$$N = \frac{\lambda(1 - R^2)}{R^2} = \frac{16.7(1 - .40)}{.40} = 25.05$$

[tt]We can demonstrate that using 120 degrees of freedom for the calculation will yield a value for N that is not much different from those that would be calculated using the other values. For instance, for $df_{res} = 60$, $\lambda = 11.5$, which would yield $N = 36.42$. For $df_{res} = 20$, $\lambda = 13.2$, which would yield $N = 41.8$. We can generally expect these sample sizes to vary by no more than 10 subjects. Cohen does provide a formula for obtaining a more exact value of N using an adjusted value for λ.[1]

If we use a sample of 25 subjects, df_{res} will be $25 - 5 - 1 = 19$, which corresponds with the tabled values, so we can be comfortable with the outcome. Note that in planning this study, we hypothesized a value for R^2 that is much higher than the value we actually obtained, and therefore, the sample size estimate would not have been adequate for finding a significant effect. Projections of sample size are only as good as the projected effect size.

POWER ANALYSIS FOR CHI-SQUARE

We can establish power for the chi-square test for goodness of fit tests as well as contingency tables. The effect size index is given the symbol w.

For a 2×2 contingency table,[‡‡]

$$w = \sqrt{\frac{\chi^2}{N}} \tag{C.17}$$

For a contingency table with more than two rows or columns,[§§]

$$w = \sqrt{\frac{\chi^2}{N(q-1)}} (\sqrt{q}-1) \tag{C.18}$$

where q is the number of rows or columns, *whichever is smaller.*

Conventional Effect Sizes

Cohen offers values for conventional effect sizes: small $w = .10$, medium $w = .30$, large $w = .50$. He suggests, however, that these values be used with caution, as the value of w will vary with the number of rows, columns, and degrees of freedom in a set of data, even when the true degree of association is the same.

Power and Sample Size Tables

Tables C.9.1 through C.9.4 provide power estimates for $\alpha = .05$ for degrees of freedom $= 1, 2, 3,$ and 4 associated with chi-square $[(R-1)(C-1)]$. To use the tables, we must specify the overall sample size (N) and the value of w. Table C.10 provides sample size estimates, based on a given α level and degrees of freedom. If the value for w is not given in the table, we can determine an exact N according to:

$$N = \frac{N_{.10}}{100w^2} \tag{C.19}$$

[‡‡]Note that this value is identical to the phi coefficient, described in Chapters 23 and 25.
[§§]Note that this value is related to Cramer's V, described in Chapter 25.

where N_{10} is the required sample size for $w = .10$ for the desired power and degrees of freedom.

Example

To illustrate this application for a 2×2 contingency table, refer to the study described in Chapter 25, Table 25.3. This study examined the frequency of diabetic wound healing with a total contact cast (TCC) and a removable cast walker (RCW) (a 2×2 design). For these data, $\chi^2 = 5.24$ and $N = 50$. This study did result in a significant chi-square test, but we will illustrate the process using this data. We can apply these data to determine the probability of committing a Type II error using Equation C.17:

$$w = \sqrt{\frac{5.24}{50}} = \sqrt{.105} = 0.324$$

Using Table C.9.1, for 1 degree of freedom, this study achieves 56% power (at $w = .30$). We can estimate an associated probability of Type II error of 44%.

To determine how many subjects we would need to achieve 80% power, we refer to Table C.10. For $w = .30$, we need 87 subjects (substantially more than the original study used).

REFERENCES

1. Cohen J. *Statistical Power Analysis for the Behavioral Sciences.* 2d ed. Hillsdale, NJ: Lawrence Erlbaum Associates, 1988.
2. Knapp TR. The overemphasis on power analysis. *Nurs Res* 1996;45:379–380.
3. Green SB, Salkind NJ, Akey TM. *Using SPSS for Windows: Analyzing and Understanding Data* (4th ed.). Upper Saddle River, NJ: Prentice-Hall, 2004.

TABLE C.1.1 POWER OF THE *t*-TEST FOR $\alpha_1 = .05$

n	.10	.20	.30	.40	.50	.60	.70	.80	1.00	1.20	1.40
8	07	10	13	19	25	31	38	46	61	74	85
9	07	11	15	20	27	34	41	50	66	79	88
10	08	11	16	22	29	36	45	53	70	83	91
11	08	12	17	23	31	39	48	57	74	86	94
12	08	12	18	25	33	41	51	60	77	89	96
13	08	13	18	26	34	44	54	63	80	91	97
14	08	13	19	27	36	46	57	66	83	93	98
15	08	13	20	28	38	48	59	69	85	94	98
16	09	14	21	30	40	51	62	72	87	95	99
17	09	14	22	31	42	53	64	74	89	96	99
18	09	15	22	32	43	55	66	76	90	97	99
19	09	15	23	33	45	57	68	78	92	98	
20	09	15	24	34	46	59	70	80	93	98	
30	10	19	31	46	61	74	85	92	99		
40	11	22	38	55	72	84	93	97			
50	12	26	44	63	80	91	97	99			
100	17	41	68	88	97						
200	26	64	91	99							

TABLE C.1.2 POWER OF THE *t*-TEST FOR $\alpha_2 = .05$

n	.10	.20	.30	.40	.50	.60	.70	.80	1.00	1.20	1.40
8	05	07	09	11	15	20	25	31	46	60	73
9	05	07	09	12	16	22	28	35	51	65	79
10	06	07	10	13	18	24	31	39	56	71	84
11	06	07	10	14	20	26	34	43	61	76	87
12	06	08	11	15	21	28	37	46	65	80	90
13	06	08	11	16	23	31	40	50	69	83	93
14	06	08	12	17	25	33	43	53	72	86	94
15	06	08	12	18	26	35	45	56	75	88	96
16	06	08	13	19	28	37	48	59	78	90	97
17	06	09	13	20	29	39	51	62	80	92	98
18	06	09	14	21	31	41	53	64	83	94	98
19	06	09	15	22	32	43	55	67	85	95	99
20	06	09	15	23	33	45	58	69	87	96	99
30	07	12	21	33	47	63	76	86	97		
40	07	14	26	42	60	75	87	94	99		
50	08	17	32	50	70	84	93	98			
100	11	29	56	80	94	99					
200	17	51	85	98							

Adapted from Tables 2.3.2 and 2.3.5 in Cohen J. *Statistical Power Analysis for the Behavioral Sciences*, ed 2. Hillsdale, NJ: Lawrence Erlbaum Associates, 1988. Used with permission of the publisher and author.

TABLE C.2 SAMPLE SIZES NEEDED FOR THE *t*-TEST

Power	.10	.20	.30	.40	.50	.60	.70	.80	1.00	1.20	1.40
$\alpha_1 = .05$											
.70	942	236	105	60	38	27	20	15	10	7	6
.80	1237	310	138	78	50	35	26	20	13	9	7
.90	1713	429	191	108	69	48	36	27	18	13	10
$\alpha_2 = .05$											
.70	1235	310	138	78	50	35	26	20	13	10	7
.80	1571	393	175	99	64	45	33	26	17	12	9
.90	2102	526	234	132	85	59	44	34	22	16	12

Adapted from Table 2.4.1 in Cohen J. *Statistical Power Analysis for the Behavioral Sciences*, ed 2. Hillsdale, NJ: Lawrence Erlbaum Associates, 1988. Used with permission of the publisher and author.

TABLE C.3.1 POWER OF THE F-TEST IN ANALYSIS OF VARIANCE FOR $\alpha = .05$ AND $df_b = 1$

n	.05	.10	.15	.20	.25	.30	.35	.40	.50	.60	.70	.80
5	05	06	07	08	11	13	16	20	38	29	50	61
6	05	06	07	09	12	15	20	34	35	47	60	71
7	05	06	08	10	14	18	23	28	41	55	68	79
8	05	06	08	11	15	20	26	32	47	62	75	85
9	05	07	09	12	17	22	29	36	52	68	80	89
10	05	07	09	13	18	25	32	40	57	73	85	93
11	05	07	10	14	20	27	35	44	62	77	88	95
12	05	07	10	15	22	29	38	47	66	81	91	97
13	05	07	11	16	23	32	41	51	70	84	93	98
14	05	08	11	17	25	34	44	54	73	87	95	98
15	06	08	12	18	26	36	47	57	76	89	96	99
16	06	08	12	19	28	38	49	60	79	91	97	99
17	06	08	13	20	30	40	52	63	82	93	98	
18	06	08	14	21	31	42	54	66	84	94	98	
19	06	09	14	22	33	44	57	68	86	95	99	
20	06	09	15	23	34	46	59	70	88	96	99	
30	06	11	21	34	49	64	77	87	97			
40	07	14	27	43	61	77	88	95	99			
50	07	16	32	52	71	85	94	98				
60	08	19	38	60	79	94	97	99				
80	09	24	48	72	89	97	99					
100	10	29	57	81	94	99						
120	11	34	65	88	94							
140	13	39	72	92	99							
160	14	44	77	95	99							
180	15	48	82	97								
200	16	52	86	98								

TABLE C.3.2 POWER OF THE F-TEST IN ANALYSIS OF VARIANCE FOR $\alpha = .05$ AND $df_b = 2$

n	.05	.10	.15	.20	.25	.30	.35	.40	.50	.60	.70	.80
5	05	06	07	09	11	14	17	22	32	44	56	69
6	05	06	07	10	13	16	21	26	39	53	67	79
7	05	06	08	11	14	19	25	31	46	62	76	87
8	05	06	08	12	16	22	28	36	53	69	83	92
9	05	07	09	13	18	24	32	40	59	75	88	95
10	05	07	10	14	20	27	35	45	64	81	91	97
11	05	07	10	15	21	30	39	49	69	85	94	98
12	06	07	11	16	23	32	42	53	74	88	96	99
13	06	08	11	17	25	35	46	57	77	91	97	99
14	06	08	12	18	27	38	49	61	81	93	98	
15	06	08	13	20	29	40	52	64	84	95	99	
16	06	08	13	21	31	43	55	94	86	96	99	
17	06	09	14	22	33	45	58	70	89	97	99	
18	06	09	14	23	34	48	61	73	90	98		
19	06	09	15	24	36	50	64	76	92	99		
20	06	09	16	26	38	52	66	78	93	99		
30	06	12	22	37	55	71	85	93	99			
40	07	15	29	48	68	84	94	98				
50	08	18	36	58	79	92	98	99				
60	08	21	42	67	86	96	99					
80	09	27	54	80	94	99						
100	11	32	64	88	98							
120	12	38	73	94	99							
140	14	44	79	97								
160	15	49	85	98								
180	16	54	89	99								
200	18	59	92									

TABLE C.3.3 POWER OF THE F-TEST IN ANALYSIS OF VARIANCE FOR $\alpha = .05$ AND $df_b = 3$

n	.05	.10	.15	.20	.25	.30	.35	.40	.50	.60	.70	.80
5	05	06	07	09	12	15	19	24	36	50	64	76
6	05	06	08	10	13	18	23	29	44	60	75	86
7	05	06	08	11	15	21	27	35	52	69	83	92
8	05	07	09	12	17	24	31	40	59	77	89	96
9	05	07	09	14	19	27	36	46	66	82	93	98
10	05	07	10	15	21	30	40	51	71	87	96	99
11	06	07	11	16	24	33	44	55	76	91	97	99
12	06	08	11	17	26	36	48	60	81	93	98	
13	06	08	12	19	28	39	52	64	84	95	99	
14	06	08	13	20	30	42	55	68	87	97	99	
15	06	08	13	21	32	45	59	71	90	98		
16	06	09	14	23	34	48	62	75	92	98		
17	06	09	15	24	37	51	65	78	94	99		
18	06	09	16	26	39	53	68	80	95	99		
19	06	09	16	27	41	56	71	83	96	99		
20	06	10	17	28	43	59	73	85	97			
30	07	13	25	42	61	79	90	96	99			
40	07	16	32	54	76	90	97	99				
50	08	19	40	65	85	96	99					
60	09	22	47	74	91	98						
80	10	29	61	86	97							
100	11	36	71	93	99							
120	13	43	80	97								
140	14	49	86	99								
160	16	55	94	99								
180	18	61	94									
200	19	66	96									

TABLE C.3.4 **POWER OF THE F-TEST IN ANALYSIS OF VARIANCE FOR $\alpha = .05$ AND $df_b = 4$**

n	.05	.10	.15	.20	.25	.30	.35	.40	.50	.60	.70	.80
5	05	06	07	09	12	16	21	26	40	55	70	83
6	05	06	08	10	14	19	25	32	49	66	81	91
7	05	06	09	12	16	22	30	39	58	79	88	96
8	05	07	09	13	19	26	35	45	65	83	93	98
9	05	07	10	14	21	29	40	51	72	88	96	99
10	06	07	10	16	23	33	44	56	78	92	98	
11	06	08	11	17	26	37	49	61	82	94	99	
12	06	08	12	19	28	40	53	66	86	96	99	
13	06	08	13	20	31	43	57	70	89	98		
14	06	08	13	22	33	47	61	74	92	98		
15	06	09	14	23	36	50	65	78	94	99		
16	06	09	15	25	38	53	68	81	95	99		
17	06	09	16	26	40	56	71	83	96			
18	06	09	17	28	43	59	74	86	97			
19	06	10	17	30	45	62	77	88	98			
20	06	10	18	31	47	65	79	90	99			
30	07	13	27	46	67	84	94	98				
40	07	17	36	60	81	94	99					
50	08	21	44	81	90	98						
60	09	24	52	80	95	99						
80	10	32	66	91	99							
100	12	40	77	96								
120	13	47	85	99								
140	15	54	91	99								
160	17	61	94									
180	18	67	97									
200	20	72	98									

Adapted from Tables 8.3.12 to 8.3.15 in Cohen, J. *Statistical Power Analysis for the Behavioral Sciences*, ed 2. Hillsdale, NJ: Lawrence Erlbaum Associates, 1988. Used with permission of the publisher and author.

TABLE C.4   SAMPLE SIZES NEEDED FOR THE ANALYSIS OF VARIANCE FOR $\alpha = .05$

Power	.05	.10	.15	.20	.25	.30	.35	.40	.50	.60	.70	.80
$df_b = 1$												
.70	1235	310	138	78	50	35	26	20	13	10	7	6
.80	1571	393	175	99	64	45	33	26	17	12	9	7
.90	2102	526	234	132	85	59	44	34	22	16	12	9
$df_b = 2$												
.70	1028	258	115	65	42	29	22	17	11	8	6	5
.80	1286	322	144	81	52	36	27	21	14	10	8	6
.90	1682	421	188	106	68	48	35	27	18	13	10	8
$df_b = 3$												
.70	881	221	99	56	36	25	19	15	10	7	6	5
.80	1096	274	123	69	45	31	23	18	12	9	7	5
.90	1415	354	158	89	58	40	30	23	15	11	8	7
$df_b = 4$												
.70	776	195	87	49	32	22	17	13	9	6	5	4
.80	956	240	107	61	39	27	20	16	10	8	6	5
.90	1231	309	138	78	50	35	26	20	13	10	7	6
$df_b = 5$												
.70	698	175	78	44	29	20	15	12	8	6	5	4
.80	856	215	96	54	35	25	18	14	9	7	5	4
.90	1098	275	123	69	45	31	23	18	12	9	7	5
$df_b = 6$												
.70	638	160	72	41	26	18	14	11	7	5	4	4
.80	780	195	87	50	32	22	17	13	9	6	5	4
.90	995	250	112	63	41	29	21	16	11	8	6	5
$df_b = 8$												
.70	548	138	61	35	23	16	12	9	6	5	4	3
.80	669	168	75	42	27	19	14	11	8	6	4	4
.90	848	213	95	54	35	24	18	14	9	7	5	4
$df_b = 10$												
.70	488	123	55	31	20	14	11	8	6	4	3	3
.80	591	148	66	38	24	17	13	10	7	5	4	3
.90	747	187	84	48	31	22	16	13	8	6	5	4

Adapted from Tables 8.4.4 and 8.4.5 in Cohen J. *Statistical Power Analysis for the Behavioral Sciences,* ed 2. Hillsdale, NJ: Lawrence Erlbaum Associates, 1988. Used with permission of the publisher and author.

TABLE C.5.1 **POWER OF THE CORRELATION COEFFICIENT, $r(\alpha_1 = .05)$**

n	.10	.20	.30	.40	.50	.60	.70	.80	.90
8	08	12	18	26	37	52	68	85	97
9	08	13	20	29	42	57	74	90	99
10	08	14	22	32	46	62	79	93	99
11	09	15	23	35	50	67	83	95	
12	09	15	25	38	54	71	87	97	
13	09	16	26	40	57	74	89	98	
14	10	17	28	43	60	78	91	98	
15	10	18	30	45	63	81	93	99	
20	11	22	37	56	75	90	98		
30	13	28	50	72	90	98			
40	15	35	60	83	96				
50	17	41	69	90	98				
60	19	45	76	94	99				
80	22	45	86	98					
100	26	64	82	99					
200	41	89							
500	72								
1000	94								

TABLE C.5.2 **POWER OF THE CORRELATION COEFFICIENT, $r(\alpha_2 = .05)$**

n	.10	.20	.30	.40	.50	.60	.70	.80	.90
8	06	07	11	16	25	37	54	75	94
9	06	08	12	19	29	43	62	82	97
10	06	08	13	21	33	49	68	87	98
11	06	09	14	23	36	54	73	91	99
12	06	09	16	26	40	58	78	93	99
13	06	10	17	28	44	63	82	95	
14	06	10	18	30	47	66	85	96	
15	06	11	19	32	50	70	88	98	
20	07	14	25	43	64	83	96		
30	08	19	37	61	83	95			
40	09	24	48	74	92	99			
50	11	29	57	83	97				
60	12	34	65	90	99				
80	14	43	78	96					
100	17	52	86	99					
200	29	81	99						
500	61	99							
1000	89								

Adapted from Tables 3.3.2 and 3.3.5 in Cohen, J. *Statistical Power Analysis for the Behavioral Sciences*, ed 2. Hillsdale, NJ: Lawrence Erlbaum Associates, 1988. Used with permission of the publisher and author.

TABLE C.6 **SAMPLE SIZES NEEDED FOR THE CORRELATION COEFFICIENT, r**

Power	.10	.20	.30	.40	.50	.60	.70	.80	.90
$\alpha_1 = .05$									
.70	470	117	52	28	18	12	8	6	4
.80	617	153	68	37	22	15	10	7	5
.90	854	211	92	50	31	20	13	9	6
$\alpha_2 = .05$									
.70	616	153	67	37	23	15	10	7	5
.80	783	194	85	46	28	18	12	9	6
.90	1047	259	113	62	37	24	16	11	7

Adapted from Table 3.4 1 in Cohen, J. *Statistical Power Analysis for the Behavioral Sciences*, ed 2. Hillsdale, NJ: Lawrence Erlbaum Associates, 1988. Used with permission of the publisher and author.

TABLE C.7 POWER OF THE F-TEST FOR REGRESSION ANALYSIS AT $\alpha = .05$

k	df_{res}	2	4	6	8	10	12	14	16	18	20	24	28	32	36	40
1	20	27	48	64	77	85	91	95	97	98	99					
	60	29	50	67	79	88	92	96	98	99	99					
	120	29	51	68	80	88	93	96	98	99	99					
	∞	29	52	69	81	89	93	96	98	99	99					
2	20	20	36	52	65	75	83	88	92	95	97	99				
	60	22	40	56	69	79	87	91	95	97	98					
	120	22	41	57	71	80	87	92	95	97	98					
	∞	23	42	58	72	82	88	93	96	97	99					
3	20	17	30	44	56	67	75	82	87	91	94	97	99			
	60	19	34	49	62	73	81	87	92	95	97	98				
	120	19	35	50	64	75	83	89	93	95	97	99				
	∞	19	36	52	65	76	84	90	93	96	98	99				
4	20	15	26	38	49	60	69	76	83	87	91	95	98	99		
	60	17	30	44	57	68	77	83	89	92	95	98	99			
	120	17	31	46	58	70	78	85	90	93	96	98	99			
	∞	17	32	47	60	72	80	87	91	94	96	99				
5	20	13	23	34	44	54	63	71	78	83	87	93	96	98	99	
	60	15	27	40	52	63	72	80	86	90	93	97	99			
	120	16	29	41	54	65	75	82	87	91	94	98	99			
	∞	16	29	43	56	68	77	84	89	93	95	98	99			
10	20	09	16	23	30	37	44	51	58	64	70	79	86	91	94	96
	60	10	20	30	39	48	56	65	72	78	83	90	95	97	99	99
	120	11	21	31	42	51	60	69	75	81	86	93	96	98	99	
	∞	12	21	32	43	54	64	72	79	85	89	94	98	99		
15	20	08	12	17	22	27	33	39	44	50	55	65	74	81	86	90
	60	09	15	22	30	38	46	54	61	67	73	83	89	94	96	98
	120	10	16	24	33	42	51	59	66	73	78	87	92	96	98	99
	∞	10	18	27	37	47	56	64	72	78	83	91	95	97	99	99
20	20	08	11	14	18	22	26	31	36	40	45	54	63	70	77	82
	60	08	13	19	25	31	38	45	52	58	64	75	83	89	93	96
	120	09	14	21	28	36	43	51	58	65	71	81	88	93	96	98
	∞	09	16	24	32	41	50	58	65	72	78	87	92	96	98	99

λ

Adapted from Table 9.3.2 in Cohen, J. *Statistical Power Analysis for the Behavioral Sciences*, ed 2. Hillsdale, NJ: Lawrence Erlbaum Associates, 1988. Used with the permission of the publisher and author.

TABLE C.8 VALUES OF LAMBDA (λ) USED TO DETERMINE SAMPLE SIZE FOR THE F-TEST FOR REGRESSION ANALYSIS (α = .05)

k	df_{res}	Power										
		.25	.50	.60	.67	.70	.75	.80	.85	.90	.95	.99
1	20	1.9	4.1	5.3	6.2	6.7	7.5	8.5	9.7	11.4	14.1	20.1
	60	1.7	3.9	4.9	5.8	6.2	7.0	7.9	9.1	10.6	13.2	18.7
	120	1.7	3.8	4.9	5.7	6.2	6.9	7.8	9.0	10.5	13.0	18.4
	∞	1.6	3.8	4.9	5.7	6.2	6.9	7.8	9.0	10.5	13.0	18.4
2	20	2.6	5.7	7.1	8.2	8.9	9.9	11.1	12.6	14.6	17.9	24.9
	60	2.3	5.1	6.4	7.4	8.0	8.9	10.0	11.3	13.2	16.1	22.4
	120	2.3	5.0	6.3	7.2	7.8	8.7	9.7	11.1	12.8	15.7	21.8
	∞	2.2	5.0	6.2	7.2	7.7	8.6	9.6	10.9	12.7	15.4	21.4
3	20	3.2	6.9	8.6	9.9	10.6	11.8	13.2	14.9	17.2	20.9	28.7
	60	2.8	6.0	7.5	8.6	9.3	10.3	11.5	13.0	15.0	18.3	25.1
	120	2.7	5.8	7.3	8.4	9.0	10.0	11.1	12.6	14.5	17.7	24.3
	∞	2.7	5.8	7.2	8.2	8.8	9.8	10.9	12.3	14.2	17.2	23.5
4	20	3.8	8.0	9.9	11.4	12.2	13.5	15.0	16.9	19.5	23.5	32.1
	60	3.3	6.8	8.5	9.7	10.4	11.5	12.8	14.4	16.6	20.1	27.4
	120	3.1	6.6	8.1	9.3	10.0	11.0	12.3	13.9	16.0	19.3	26.3
	∞	3.1	6.4	7.9	9.1	9.7	10.7	11.9	13.4	15.4	18.6	25.2
5	20	4.4	9.0	11.1	12.7	13.6	15.0	16.7	18.8	21.6	26.0	35.2
	60	3.7	7.5	9.3	10.6	11.3	12.6	14.0	15.7	18.0	21.7	29.4
	120	3.5	7.2	8.9	10.1	10.8	12.0	13.3	15.0	17.2	20.7	28.1
	∞	3.4	7.0	8.6	9.8	10.5	11.6	12.8	14.4	16.5	19.8	26.7
10	20	6.9	13.7	16.7	18.9	20.1	22.1	24.4	27.3	31.0	37.0	49.2
	60	5.3	10.5	12.8	14.5	15.4	17.0	18.7	20.9	23.8	28.3	37.7
	120	5.0	9.8	11.9	13.5	14.3	15.8	17.4	19.5	22.1	26.4	35.2
	∞	4.4	9.2	11.2	12.6	13.4	14.7	16.8	18.1	20.5	24.4	32.4
15	20	9.2	18.0	21.8	24.6	26.1	28.7	31.6	35.1	39.8	47.1	62.2
	60	6.7	13.1	15.8	17.8	18.9	20.7	22.8	25.3	28.7	33.9	44.7
	120	6.1	11.9	14.3	16.2	17.2	18.8	20.7	23.1	26.1	30.9	40.8
	∞	5.6	10.9	13.1	14.7	15.6	17.1	18.8	20.9	23.6	27.8	36.6
20	20	11.4	22.2	26.8	30.1	32.0	35.0	38.5	42.7	48.3	57.0	74.8
	60	8.1	15.4	18.5	20.8	22.1	24.1	26.5	29.4	33.2	39.1	51.2
	120	7.2	13.7	16.5	18.6	19.7	21.6	23.7	26.3	29.6	34.9	45.8
	∞	6.4	12.3	14.7	16.5	17.5	19.1	21.0	23.2	26.1	30.7	40.1

Adapted from Table 9.4.2 in Cohen, J. *Statistical Power Analysis for the Behavioral Sciences*, ed 2. Hillsdale, NJ: Lawrence Erlbaum Associates, 1988. Used with permission of the publisher and the author.

TABLE C.9.1   POWER OF THE χ^2 TEST AT $\alpha = .05$ FOR $df = 1$

| | | | | | w | | | | |
N	.10	.20	.30	.40	.50	.60	.70	.80	.90
25	08	17	32	52	70	85	94	98	99
30	08	19	38	59	78	91	97	99	
35	09	22	43	66	84	94	99		
40	10	24	47	71	89	97	99		
45	10	27	52	76	92	98			
50	11	29	56	81	94	99			
60	12	34	64	87	97				
70	13	39	71	92	99				
80	15	43	76	95	99				
90	16	47	81	97					
100	17	52	85	98					
120	19	59	91	99					
140	22	66	94						
160	24	71	97						
180	27	76	98						
200	29	81	99						
300	41	93							
500	61	99							
600	69								
700	75								
800	81								
900	85								
1000	89								

TABLE C.9.2   POWER OF THE χ^2 TEST AT $\alpha = .05$ FOR $df = 2$

| | | | | | w | | | | |
N	.10	.20	.30	.40	.50	.60	.70	.80	.90
25	07	13	25	42	60	77	89	96	99
30	07	15	29	49	69	85	94	98	
35	08	17	34	55	76	90	97	99	
40	08	19	38	61	82	93	98		
45	09	21	42	67	86	96	99		
50	09	23	46	72	90	97			
60	10	26	54	80	94	99			
70	11	30	61	86	97				
80	12	34	67	90	99				
90	12	38	72	93	99				
100	13	42	77	96					
120	15	49	85	98					
140	17	55	90	99					
160	19	61	93						
180	21	67	96						
200	23	72	97						
300	32	88							
500	50	99							
600	58								
700	66								
800	72								
900	77								
1000	82								

TABLE C.9.3   POWER OF THE χ^2 TEST AT $\alpha = .05$ FOR $df = 3$

N	.10	.20	.30	.40	.50	.60	.70	.80	.90
25	07	12	21	36	54	71	85	93	98
30	07	13	25	42	62	80	90	97	99
35	07	15	29	49	70	86	95	99	
40	07	16	32	55	76	90	97	99	
45	08	18	36	60	81	94	99		
50	08	19	40	65	86	96	99		
60	09	22	47	74	92	98			
70	09	26	54	81	95	99			
80	10	29	60	86	98				
90	11	32	66	90	99				
100	12	36	71	93	99				
120	13	42	80	97					
140	15	49	86	99					
160	16	55	90	99					
180	18	60	94						
200	19	65	96						
300	27	84							
500	44	98							
600	52	99							
700	59								
800	65								
900	71								
1000	76								

TABLE C.9.4   POWER OF THE χ^2 TEST AT $\alpha = .05$ FOR $df = 4$

N	.10	.20	.30	.40	.50	.60	.70	.80	.90
25	06	11	19	32	50	66	81	91	97
30	07	12	22	38	57	75	88	96	99
35	07	13	26	44	65	82	93	98	
40	07	14	29	50	72	88	96	99	
45	07	16	32	55	77	92	98		
50	08	17	36	60	82	94	99		
60	08	20	43	70	89	98			
70	09	23	49	77	94	99			
80	09	26	55	83	96				
90	10	29	61	88	98				
100	11	32	66	91	99				
120	12	38	75	96					
140	13	44	82	98					
160	14	50	88	99					
180	16	55	92						
200	17	60	94						
300	24	80	99						
500	40	96							
600	47	99							
700	54								
800	60								
900	66								
1000	72								

Adapted from Tables 7.3.15 to 7.3.18 in Cohen, J. *Statistical Power Analysis for the Behavioral Sciences*, ed 2. Hillsdale, NJ: Lawrence Erlbaum Associates, 1988. Used with permission of the publisher and author.

TABLE C.10   SAMPLE SIZES NEEDED FOR χ^2 FOR $\alpha = .05$

Power	.10	.20	.30	.40	.50	.60	.70	.80	.90
$df = 1$									
.70	617	154	69	39	25	17	13	10	8
.80	785	196	87	49	31	22	16	12	10
.90	1051	263	117	66	42	29	21	16	13
$df = 2$									
.70	770	193	86	48	31	21	16	12	10
.80	964	241	107	60	39	27	20	15	12
.90	1265	316	141	79	51	35	26	20	16
$df = 3$									
.70	879	220	98	55	35	24	18	14	11
.80	1090	273	121	68	44	30	22	17	13
.90	1417	354	157	89	57	39	29	22	17
$df = 4$									
.70	968	242	108	61	39	27	20	15	12
.80	1194	298	133	75	48	33	24	19	15
.90	1540	385	171	96	62	43	31	24	19
$df = 6$									
.70	1114	279	124	70	45	31	23	17	14
.80	1362	341	151	85	54	38	28	21	17
.90	1742	435	194	109	70	48	36	27	22
$df = 8$									
.70	1235	309	137	77	49	34	25	19	15
.80	1502	376	167	94	60	42	31	23	19
.90	1908	477	212	119	76	53	39	30	24
$df = 9$									
.70	1289	322	143	81	52	36	26	20	16
.80	1565	391	174	98	63	43	32	24	19
.90	1983	496	220	124	79	55	40	31	24
$df = 12$									
.70	1435	359	159	90	57	40	29	22	18
.80	1734	433	193	108	69	48	35	27	21
.90	2183	546	243	136	87	61	45	34	27

Adapted from Tables 7.4.6 to 7.4.9 in Cohen, J. *Statistical Power Analysis for the Behavioral Sciences,* ed 2. Hillsdale, NJ, Lawrence Erlbaum Associates, 1988. Used with the permission of the publisher and author.

APPENDIX D
Transformation of Data

Many statistical procedures, like the *t*-test, analysis of variance and linear regression are based on assumptions about homogeneity of variance and normality that should be met to ensure the validity of the test. Although most parametric statistical procedures are considered robust to moderate violations of these assumptions, some modification to the analysis is usually necessary with striking departures. When this occurs, the researcher can choose one of two approaches to accommodate the analysis. The analytic procedure can be modified, by using nonparametric statistics or nonlinear regression, or the dependent variable, X, can be transformed to a new variable, X', which more closely satisfies the necessary assumptions. The new variable is created by changing the scale of measurement for X. In this appendix we introduce five approaches to *data transformation*.

The three most common reasons for using data transformation are to satisfy the assumption of homogeneity of variance, to conform data to a normal distribution, and to create a more linear distribution that will fit the linear regression model. Fortunately, the same transformation will often accomplish more than one of these goals.[1]

The most commonly used transformations are the square root transformation, the square transformation, the log transformation, the reciprocal transformation, and the arc sine transformation. The choice of which method to use will depend on characteristics of the data. Before we describe the guidelines for using each of these approaches, it may be helpful to illustrate the transformation process using the square root transformation.

The *square root transformation* $(X' = \sqrt{X})$ replaces each score in a distribution with its square root. This method is most appropriate when variances are roughly proportional to group means, that is, when $s^2/\overline{X}$ is similar for all samples. The square root transformation will typically have the effect of equalizing variances.

Suppose we were given two sample distributions shown on the left panel in Table D.1. These variances, $s_A^2 = 8.5$ and $s_B^2 = 26.5$, are obviously quite different from one another. We determine the applicability of the square root transformation by demonstrating that $s^2/\overline{X}$ is similar for both distributions: $s_A^2/\overline{X}_A = 2.15$ and $s_B^2/\overline{X}_B = 2.65$.

Each score in both distributions is transformed to its square root on the right in Table D.1. As we can see, the effect of this transformation is a reduction in the discrepancy between the two variances; now $s_A^2 = .56$ and $s_B^2 = .61$. These transformed values can now be used in a statistical analysis.

When data contain many small numbers (equal or close to zero), the square root transformation is more valid using $X' = \sqrt{X + .5}$ as the converted score.

The *square transformation* $(X' = X^2)$ is used primarily in regression analysis when the relationship between X and Y is curvilinear downward; that is, slope steadily decreases

TABLE D.1   EFFECT OF SQUARE ROOT TRANSFORMATION

	Original Data (X)		Transformed Data ($\sqrt{X}$)	
	A	B	A	B
	1	8	1.00	2.83
	3	7	1.73	2.65
	8	12	2.83	3.46
	6	5	2.45	2.24
	2	18	1.41	4.24
Σ	20	50	9.42	15.42
$\overline{X}$	4	10	1.88	3.08
s^2	8.5	26.5	.56	.61
$s^2/\overline{X}$	2.125	2.65		

as the value of the independent variable increases.[1] This transformation will cause the relationship to appear more linear. It will also have the effect of stabilizing variances and will normalize the dependent variable when the residuals are negatively skewed.

The *log transformation* ($X' = \log X$) is most appropriately used when the standard deviations of the original data are proportional to the mean; that is, the ratio $s/\overline{X}$ (the coefficient of variation) will be roughly constant across distributions. In addition to equalizing variances, the log transformation is used most often to normalize a skewed distribution. In regression analyses, the log transformation can also be used to create a more linear relationship between X and Y when the regression model shows a consistently increasing slope.[1] When data are numerically small, the transformation should be made on the basis of $X' = \log X + 1$.[2] The effect of log transformation can be easily demonstrated by plotting scores on logarithmic or semilogarithmic graph paper.

The *reciprocal transformation* ($X' = 1/X$) is used when the standard deviations of the original data are proportional to the square of the mean $s/\overline{X}^2$.[3] It is effective for attaining homogeneity of variance or normality. Use of this approach will minimize the skewing effect of large values of X, which will be close to zero in their reciprocal form. With numeric data close to zero, this transformation should be obtained by using $X' = 1/X + 1$.

The *arc sine transformation* ($X' = \arcsin \sqrt{X}$) is also called angular transformation. It is used when data are collected in the form of proportions or percentages, such as the proportion of successful responses in a given number of trials. The relationship $s^2 = \overline{X}(1 - \overline{X})$ should be constant for all samples. This transformation is based on an angular scale, whereby each proportion, p, is replaced by the angle whose sine is $\sqrt{p}$. Angles are usually given in radians. Tables for arc sine transformations are provided in Fisher and Yates[4] and Snedecor and Cochran.[5]

CHOOSING THE BEST TRANSFORMATION

Selecting the best transformation may be a less than obvious task. Many researchers use trial and error to determine the transformation that is most successful at reorienting the data. Kirk has suggested a method that may be helpful in facilitating this decision.[3] He uses each transformation to convert the largest and smallest scores in each distribution. The difference between the largest and smallest score, or the range of the distribution, is calculated using the transformed values. The ratio of the larger to the smaller range is then calculated for each transformation. The transformation that produces the smallest ratio is selected. This process is illustrated in Table D.2.

Data are obtained from two treatment groups. For this example, the largest and smallest raw scores in each distribution are transformed using the square root, log, and reciprocal transformations. The differences between the transformed values of the smallest and largest scores is calculated. For example, the difference between the square roots of 18 and 10 (the largest and smallest scores in Distribution 1) is 1.08. The difference between the square roots of 40 and 20 (Distribution 2) is 1.85. For the square root transformation, the ratio of the larger to the smaller range is $1.85/1.08 = 1.71$. A similar ratio is calculated for each of the other transformations, as shown in Table D.2. The log transformation would be selected because it results in the smallest ratio.

When more than two distributions are compared, the ratio is calculated using the largest and smallest ranges for each transformation. For instance, suppose we added a third group to the data, and the differences between the square roots of the largest and smallest values were 1.08, 1.85, and 1.13. The ratio for this transformation would be formed using only 1.85 and 1.08, as these are the largest and smallest ranges for this transformation.

Once data are analyzed using transformed data, all further interpretations of data must be made using the transformed values. For example, epidemiologists have shown that the distribution of incubation periods of communicable diseases tends to be normally distributed on a logarithmic scale.[6] Therefore, further analyses of these data have used the log incubation period as the unit of measurement.[7]

There are situations where data will be of sufficient variability that no transformation will be successful at smoothing the data. When this occurs, the researcher may consider choosing a different response measure as the dependent variable, one that would be more evenly distributed. Alternatively, nonparametric statistics can be applied. These tests, discussed in Chapter 22, do not require normality or equal variances.

Tables are provided in many statistics texts to facilitate log, square, and square root transformations.[4,8] In addition, most computer programs provide a mechanism for data transformation prior to analysis.

TABLE D.2   TRANSFORMATION BASED ON LARGEST AND SMALLEST SCORES IN TWO DISTRIBUTIONS

	Treatment group		$\sqrt{X}$		log X		$1/X$	
	1	2	1	2	1	2	1	2
Largest	18	40	4.24	6.32	1.26	1.60	.06	.02
Smallest	10	20	3.16	4.47	1.00	1.30	.10	.05
Range	8	20	1.08	1.85	.26	.30	.04	.03
Ratio	$\dfrac{\text{range}_{largest}}{\text{range}_{smallest}}$		$\dfrac{1.85}{1.08} = 1.71$		$\dfrac{.30}{.26} = 1.15$		$\dfrac{.04}{.03} = 1.33$	

REFERENCES

1. Kleinbaum DG, Kupper LL: *Applied Regression Analysis and Other Multivariable Techniques.* North Scituate, MA, Duxbury Press, 1978.
2. Winer BJ: *Statistical Principles in Experimental Design,* ed 2. New York, McGraw-Hill, 1971.
3. Kirk RE: *Experimental Design: Procedures for the Behavioral Sciences,* ed 2. Belmont, CA, Brooks/Cole, 1982.
4. Fisher RA, Yates F: *Statistical Tables for Biological, Agricultural and Medical Research,* ed 6. London, Longman, 1963.
5. Snedecor GW, Cochran WG: *Statistical Methods,* ed 6. Ames, Iowa University Press, 1967.
6. Sartwell PE: The distribution of incubation periods of infectious disease. *Am J Hyg* 51:310, 1950.
7. Colton T: *Statistics in Medicine.* Boston, Little, Brown, 1974.
8. Dixon WJ, Massey FJ: *Introduction to Statistical Analysis,* ed 3. New York, McGraw-Hill, 1969.

Sample Informed Consent Form

University Research Consent Form

Title: The Effect of a Tai Chi Program on Falling in the Elderly
Principal Investigator: Joe Smith, Ph. D.

About this form:

This form gives you important information about a research study. Please read it carefully. One of our staff members will be with you to answer any questions you may have about the study and what you will be asked to do. If you decide to be a participant (called a "subject"), you will have to sign this form. We will give you a copy of it to keep.

Why is this research being done?

The purpose of this research is to find out if special exercises (Tai Chi) are helpful in preventing falls and helping people to be more confident in doing daily activities. We are inviting you to join the study because you have told your doctor that you have fallen down a few times this year. We would like about 100 people to take part in this study.

How long will I take part in this study?

You will spend 10 weeks from the beginning to the end of the study. During this time, we will teach you activities that you will do at home every other day and you will come to this clinic for learning the activities and for testing.

What will happen in this research study?

If you agree to be in this study, you will be assigned by chance (like flipping a coin) to receive one of two activity programs. One of these is called Tai Chi Chuan that includes gentle stretching, standing and balancing. The other group will be instructed in a daily activity program.

Before your program begins, you will perform a walking test. You will walk down the corridor as fast as you can. A tester will time how fast you go. You will also do a few balance tests, like standing on one leg, standing with your feet one in front of the other, standing with eyes closed and turning around. We will also ask you to complete a questionnaire about how confident you are about doing certain daily activities like reaching overhead or going shopping.

If you are in the Tai Chi group, you will come to the clinic and will learn a series of special exercises. You will be given pictures and descriptions of what to do at home. Once a week, one of us will come to your home to review the exercises with you.

If you are in the activity program group, you will come to the clinic and will review your daily activities with one of us. We will give you a list of activities that you should be sure to do every other day.

We will give you a calendar chart for marking each time you do your planned exercise or activity program and to make a note if you have a fall at any time.

You will return to the clinic to repeat the tests and the questionnaire during the tenth week.

What are the risks and possible discomforts from being in this research study?

During the testing and during your activities program, it is possible that you could fall. We will help you to figure out ways to keep this from happening at home and while you are in the clinic, someone will be right beside you. You may feel tired at the end of the testing or activities period. If this happens, a short rest period would be a good idea.

What are the possible benefits from being in this study?

You may feel more active and may be more comfortable doing your daily household and outdoor activities.

Every institution that has an IRB will have several additional "boilerplate" sections. These will include:
- **Description of alternative treatments (if they exist)**
- **Assurance that nonparticipation will not affect routine medical care**
- **Financial compensation (if relevant)**
- **Injury statement, indicating the patient's responsibility for cost of care if needed**

- **Contact individual including phone number**
- **Privacy and HIPAA authorization, explaining what information will be taken and how it will be used**
- **Right to withdraw from the study at any time without prejudice or bias**

Statement of Subject or Person Giving Consent/Assent

- I have read this consent form.
- This research study has been explained to me, including risks and possible benefits (if any), other options for treatments or procedures, and other important things about the study.
- I have had the opportunity to ask questions.

If you understand the information we have given you, and would like to take part in this research study, and also agree to allow your health information to be used and shared as described above, then please sign below.

Signature of Subject:

_____   _____
Adults or minors ages 14--17   Date/Time

Signature of Witness:

_____   _____
Witness (when required)   Date/Time

Statement of Individual Obtaining Consent:

- I have explained the research to the study subject, and
- I have answered all questions about this research study to the best of my ability.

_____   _____
Investigator or Person Obtaining Consent   Date/Time

The question format of this sample form is taken from the standard Informed Consent Form of Partners Human Research Committee, Partners HealthCare System, Boston, 2007.

Glossary

Numbers in parentheses indicate the chapter in which the term is introduced.

A–B design.   A single-case design with two phases: A represents the baseline phase, and B represents the intervention phase. (12)

A–B–A design.   A single-case withdrawal design in which a second baseline phase is introduced. (12)

absolute risk increase (ARI).   The increase in risk associated with an intervention as compared to risk without the intervention (or control condition); the absolute difference between the control event rate (CER) and the experimental event rate (EER). (28)

absolute risk reduction (ARR).   The reduction in risk associated with an intervention as compared to the risk without the intervention (or the control condition); the absolute difference between the experimental event rate (EER) and the control event rate (CER). (28)

accessible population.   The actual population of subjects available to be chosen for a study. This group is usually a nonrandom subset of the target population. (8)

active variable.   An independent variable with levels that can be manipulated and assigned by the researcher. (9)

adjusted means.   Means that have been adjusted based on the value of a covariate in an analysis of covariance. (24)

agreement.   (See *percent agreement*.)

alpha coefficient.   (See *Cronbach's alpha*.)

alpha level (α).   Level of statistical significance, or risk of Type I error; maximum probability level that can be achieved in a statistical test to reject the null hypothesis. Symbols α_1 and α_2 are used to denote level of significance for one- and two-tailed tests, respectively. (18)

alphanumeric data.   In data processing, the entry of values that contain symbols or letters. (30)

alternate forms reliability.   Reliability of two equivalent forms of a measuring instrument. (5, 26)

alternating treatment design.   A single-case design in which two (or more) treatments are compared by alternating them within a session (or in alternate sessions). (12)

alternative hypothesis (H_1).   Hypothesis stating the expected relationship between independent and dependent variables; considered the negation of the null hypothesis. The alternative hypothesis is accepted when the null hypothesis is rejected. (18)

analysis of covariance (ANCOVA).   Statistical procedure used to compare two or more treatment groups while controlling for the effect of one or more confounding variables (called covariates). (24)

analysis of variance (ANOVA).   Statistical procedure appropriate for comparison of three or more treatment groups or conditions, or the simultaneous manipulation of two or more independent variables; based on the F statistic. (20)

a priori comparisons.   (See *planned comparisons*.)

area probability sample.   A form of cluster sampling in which geographic areas serve as the units of analysis. (8)

ARIMA (autoregressive integrated moving average). Statistical technique for analysis of data from time-series studies. (11)

attribute variable. An independent variable with levels that cannot be manipulated or assigned by the researcher, but that represent subject characteristics (such as age and sex). (9)

attrition (experimental mortality). A threat to internal validity, referring to the differential loss of participants during the course of data collection, potentially introducing bias by changing the composition of the sample. (9)

audit trail. Comprehensive process of documenting interpretation of qualitative data. (14)

autocorrelation. Correlation of consecutive data points in a time series design. (12)

backward selection. A process used in stepwise multiple regression that enters all independent variables into the equation, and then removes nonsignificant variables in successive steps, until all remaining variables are significant. (29)

Bayes' theorem. The calculation of the probability of one event based on the probability of another event; used to estimate posterior (posttest) probabilities based on prior (pretest) probabilities of a diagnostic outcome. (27)

beta (β). Probability of making a Type II error. (18)

beta weight. In a multiple regression equation, the standardized weight for each independent variable. (29)

between-groups variance. That portion of the total variance in a set of scores that is attributed to the difference between groups. (19, 20)

between subjects design. An experimental design that is based on comparison between independent groups. (10)

between subjects factor. An independent variable for which levels are applied to independent groups. (20)

bimodal distribution. A distribution having two modes. (17)

binomial variable. (See *dichotomy*.)

bivariate statistics. Statistics involving the analysis of two variables for the purpose of determining the relationship between them, for example, correlation. (23)

blinding. Techniques to reduce experimental bias by keeping the subjects and/or investigators ignorant of group assignments and research hypotheses. (9)

block. Level of an attribute variable in which subjects are homogeneous on a particular characteristic. (9, 10)

Bonferroni's adjustment (correction). A correction often used when multiple *t*-tests are performed, to reduce Type I error. The desired level of significance (α) is divided by the number of comparisons. The resulting value is then used as the level of signficance for each comparison to reject the null hypothesis. (21)

Bonferroni *t*. A post hoc method to compare means following an analysis of variance; based on planned comparisons; also called the Dunn multiple comparison procedure. (21)

Boolean logic. In literature searches, the terms AND, NOT and OR used to expand or narrow search terms. (31)

box plot. Also called box and whisker plot. A graphic display of a distribution, showing the median, 25th and 75th percentiles, and highest and lowest scores. (17)

canonical correlation. A multivariate correlation procedure, whereby two sets of variables are correlated. (29)

case–control study. A design in analytic epidemiology in which the investigator selects subjects on the basis of their having or not having a particular disease and then determines their previous exposure. (13)

ceiling effect. A measurement limitation of an instrument whereby the scale cannot determine increased performance beyond a certain level. (6)

celeration line. In single-case research, a line that divides the data points within a phase into two equal halves, indicating the trend of the data within that phase. (12)

censored observation. An observation whose value is unknown because the subject has not been in the study long enough for the outcome to have occurred; used to estimate survival curves. (29)

central tendency. Descriptive statistics that represent "averages" or scores that are representative of a distribution; includes mean, median, and mode. (17)

centroid. A point determined from the intersection of two means of two dependent variables (X, Y), used in multivariate analysis. (29)

change score. Difference between two measurements taken at different times, typically between pretest and posttest or followup. Also called a gain score. (6, 27)

chi square test (χ^2). A nonparametric test applied to nominal data, comparing observed frequencies within categories to frequencies expected by chance. (25)

clinical prediction rule. A statistical tool that quantifies the relative contribution of examination and history findings to determine a diagnosis, prognosis, or likely response to intervention. (27)

cluster analysis. A multivariate statistical procedure that classifies subjects into homogeneous subsets. (29)

cluster sampling. A form of probability sampling in which large subgroups (clusters) are randomly selected first, and then smaller units from these clusters are successively chosen; also called multistage sampling. (8)

coefficient of determination (r^2). Coefficient representing the amount of variance in one variable (Y) that can be explained (accounted for) by a second variable (X). (24)

coefficient of variation (CV). A measure of relative variation; based on the standard deviation divided by the mean, expressed as a percentage. (17, 26)

cohort study. An observational study design in which a specific group is followed over time. Subjects are classified according to whether they do or do not have a particular risk factor or exposure and followed to determine disease outcomes. (13)

common cause variation. Fluctuation in response resulting in random and expected variation in performance. (12)

completer analysis. Analysis of data in a clinical trial only for those subjects who complete the study. (9)

concurrent validity. A type of measurement validity; a form of criterion-related validity; the degree to which the outcomes of one test correlate with outcomes on a criterion test, when both tests are given at relatively the same time. (6)

confidence interval (CI). The range of values within which a population parameter is estimated to fall, with a specific level of confidence. (18, 19)

confounding. The contaminating effect of extraneous variables on interpretation of the relationship between independent and dependent variables. (9, 28)

confounding variable. A variable that is more likely to be present in one group of subjects than another, and that is related to the outcome of interest, thereby potentially "confounding" interpretation of the outcome. (28)

consecutive sampling. A form of nonprobability sampling, where subjects are recruited as they become available. (8)

constant comparative method. Inductive process in qualitative research that calls for continual testing of a theory as data are examined. (14)

construct validity. 1. A type of measurement validity; the degree to which a theoretical construct is measured by an instrument. (6) 2. Design validity related to operational definitions of independent and dependent variables. (9)

content analysis. A procedure for analyzing and coding narrative data in a systematic way. (13)

content validity. A type of measurement validity; the degree to which the items in an instrument adequately reflect the content domain being measured. (6)

contingency table. A two-dimensional table displaying frequencies or counts, with rows (R) and columns (C) representing categories of nominal or ordinal variables; also referred to as cross-tabulation. (25)

continuous variable. A quantitative variable that can theoretically take on values along a continuum. (4)

control event rate (CER). The number of subjects in the control group who develop the outcome of interest. (28)

convenience sampling. A nonprobability sampling procedure, involving selection of the most available subjects for a study. (8)

convergent validity. An approach in construct validation, assessing the degree to which two different instruments or methods are able to measure the same construct. (6)

correlation. The tendency for variation in one variable to be related to variation in a second variable; those statistical procedures used to assess the degree of covariation between two variables. (23)

correlational research. A descriptive research approach that explores the relationship among variables without active manipulation of variables by the researcher. (13)

counterbalancing. Systematic alternation of the order of treatment conditions, to avoid order effects in a repeated measures design. (10)

covariate. An extraneous variable that is statistically controlled in an analysis of covariance, so that the relationship between the independent and dependent variables is analyzed with the effect of the extraneous factor removed. (24)

Cox's proportional hazards regression. A regression procedure used when the outcome has not yet occurred (a censored variable). Used in survival analysis. (29)

criterion-related validity. A type of measurement validity; the degree to which the outcomes of one test correlate with outcomes on a criterion test; can be assessed as concurrent validity or predictive validity. (6)

criterion-referencing. Interpretation of a score based on its actual value. (6)

critical value. The value of a test statistic that must be exceeded for the null hypothesis to be rejected; the value of a statistic that separates the critical region; the value that defines a statistically significant result at the set alpha level. (18)

Cronbach's alpha. Reliability index of internal consistency, on a scale of 0.00 to 1.00. (5, 26)

crossover design. A repeated measures design used to control order effects when comparing two treatments, where half of the sample receives treatment A first followed by treatment B, and the other half receives treatment B first followed by treatment A. (10)

cross-sectional study. A study based on observations of different age or developmental groups at one point in time, providing the basis for inferring trends over time. (13)

cross-tabulation. (See *contingency table*.)

crude rate. A rate for a population that is not adjusted for any subset of the population. (28)

cumulative incidence (CI). The number of new cases of a disease during a specified time period divided by the total number of people at risk; the proportion of new cases of a disease in a population. (28)

cumulative scale. A scale designed so that agreement with higher-level responses assumes agreement with all lower-level responses. (15)

curvilinear relationship. The relationship between two variables that does not follow a linear proportional relationship. (23)

cut-off score. Score used as the demarcation of a positive or negative test outcome. (27)

deductive reasoning. The logical process of developing specific hypotheses based on general principles. (1)

degrees of freedom (*df*).   Statistical concept indicating the number of values within a distribution that are free to vary, given restrictions on the data set; usually $n - 1$. (18) For analysis of variance, df_e = error degrees of freedom; df_b = between groups degrees of freedom; df_t = total degrees of freedom. (20)

Delphi survey.   Survey method whereby decisions on items are based on consensus of a panel. (14)

dependent variable.   A response variable that is assumed to depend on or be caused by another (independent) variable. (7)

developmental research.   A descriptive research approach designed to document how certain groups change over time on specific variables. (14)

deviation score ($X - \overline{X}$).   The distance of a single data point from the mean of the distribution. The sum of the deviation scores for a given distribution will always equal zero. (17)

dichotomy (dichotomous variable).   A nominal variable having only two categories, such as yes/no and male/female; a binomial variable. (7)

difference score (*d*).   The difference between two scores taken on the same individual. (19)

directional hypothesis.   A research hypothesis (or alternative hypothesis) that predicts the direction of a relationship between two variables. (7, 18)

discrete variable.   A variable that can only be measured in separate units and that cannot be measured in intervals of less than 1. (4)

discriminant analysis.   A multivariate statistical technique used to determine if a set of variables can predict group membership. (29)

discriminant validity.   An approach in construct validation assessing the degree to which an instrument yields different results when measuring two different constructs; that is, the ability to discriminate between the constructs. (6)

double-blind study.   An experiment in which both the investigator and the subject are kept ignorant of group assignment. (9)

dummy variable (coding).   In regression procedures, the assignment of codes to a nominal variable, reflecting the presence or absence of certain traits. (29)

effect size.   A statistical expression of the magnitude of the difference between two treatments or the magnitude of a relationship between two variables, based on the proportional relationship of the difference to the variance. (18, 27, Appendix C)

effectiveness.   Benefits of an intervention as tested under "real world" conditions, often using quasi-experimental methods. (10)

efficacy.   Benefit of an intervention as tested under controlled experimental conditions, usually with a control group in a randomized controlled trial. (10)

eigenvalue.   A measure of the proportion of the total variance accounted for by a factor in a factor analysis. (29)

epidemiology.   Study of the distribution of disease in relation to person, place and time, and measures of risk associated with exposures to disease. (28)

error variance.   That portion of the total variance in a data set that cannot be attributed to treatment effects, but that is due to differences between subjects. (19)

ethnography.   An approach to qualitative research in which the experiences of a specific cultural group are studied. (14)

event rate.   The proportion of subjects in a group in whom a specific event or outcome is observed. (See *control event rate [CER]* and *experimental event rate [EER]*.) (28)

evidence-based practice.   The application of clinical decision making for patient management based on research evidence, clinical expertise, patient values and preferences and clinical circumstances. (1)

exempt review.   Exemption from review of a proposal by an Institutional Review Board for projects that do not involve direct contact with subjects, presenting no risk. (3)

expedited review.   Accelerated review of a proposal by an Institutional Review Board, based on minimal risk. (3)

expected frequencies.   In a contingency table, the frequencies that would be expected if the null hypothesis is true; frequencies that are expected just by chance. (25)

experimental event rate (EER).   The number of subjects in the experimental or treatment group who develop the outcome of interest. (28)

experimenter effects (experimenter bias).   Biases that are present in research data because of behaviors, expectations, or attitudes of those collecting the data. (9)

explained variance.   Between-groups variance; that portion of the total variance in a data set that can be attributed to the differences between groups or treatment conditions. (19)

exploratory research.   Research that has as its purpose the exploration of data to determine relationships among variables. (13)

external validity.   The degree to which results of a study can be generalized to persons or settings outside the experimental situation. (9)

extraneous variable.   A variable that confounds the relationship between the independent and dependent variables. (9)

facets.   In generalizability theory, specific conditions under which reliability of a measurement can be generalized. (5, 26)

face validity.   The assumption of validity of a measuring instrument based on its appearance as a reasonable measure of a given variable. (6)

factor.   1. A variable. (7) 2. A set of interrelated variables in a factor analysis. (29)

factor analysis.   An exploratory multivariate statistical technique used to examine the structure within a large set of variables and to determine the underlying dimensions that exist within that set of variables. (6, 29)

factorial design.   An experimental design involving two or more independent variables, allowing for the interpretation of main effects and interaction effects. (10)

false negative.   A test result that is negative in a person who has the disease or condition of interest. (27)

false positive.   A test result that is positive in a person who does not have the disease or condition of interest. (27)

Fisher's exact test.   A nonparametric procedure applied to nominal data in a 2×2 contingency table, comparing observed frequencies within categories to frequencies expected by chance. Used when samples are too small to use the chi-square test. (25)

floor effect.   A measurement limitation of an instrument whereby the scale cannot determine decreased performance beyond a certain level. (6)

forward selection.   A process used in stepwise multiple regression that enters variables one at a time into the equation based on the strength of their association with the outcome variable, until all statistically significant variables are included. (29)

frequency distribution.   A list of values that occur in a distribution, with a count of the number of times each value occurs. (17)

Friedman two-way analysis of variance by ranks (χ^2_r).   A nonparametric statistical procedure for repeated measures, comparing more than two treatment conditions of one independent variable; analogous to the one-way repeated measures analysis of variance. (22)

gain score.   (See *change score*.)

Gaussian distribution.   (See *normal distribution*.)

generalizability.   1. The quality of research that justifies inference of outcomes to groups or situations other than those directly involved in the investigation. (9) 2. The concept of reliability theory in which measurement error is viewed as multidimensional and must be interpreted under specific measurement conditions. (5, 26)

gold standard. A measurement that defines the true value of a variable. In criterion-related validity, an instrument that is considered a valid measure and that can be used as the standard for assessing validity of other instruments. (6) In diagnostic testing, a procedure that accurately identifies the true disease condition (negative or positive) of the subject. (27)

goodness of fit test. Use of chi square to determine if an observed distribution of categorical variables fits a given theoretical distribution. (25)

grand mean. The mean of all scores across groups in an analysis of variance. (20)

grounded theory. An approach to collecting and analyzing data in qualitative research, with the goal of developing theories to explain observations and experience. (14)

Guttman scale. (See *cumulative scale.*)

Hawthorne effect. The effect of subjects' knowledge that they are part of a study on their performance. (9)

hazard function. The probability that a subject will achieve a specific outcome in a certain time interval. (29)

histogram. A bar graph of a frequency distribution. (17)

historical controls. Subjects from previous research studies that serve as controls for experimental subjects in a subsequent study. (11)

historical research. Research that seeks to examine relationships and facts based on documentation of past events. (13)

history effect. A threat to internal validity, referring to the occurrence of extraneous events prior to a posttest that can affect the dependent variable. (9)

homogeneity of variance. An underlying assumption in parametric statistics that variances of samples are not significantly different. (18, 19)

hypothesis. A statement of the expected relationship between variables. (7)

incidence. The proportion of people who develop a given disease or condition within a specified time period. (28)

independent factor. An independent variable in which the levels represent independent groups of subjects. (7)

independent variable. The variable that is presumed to cause, explain or influence a dependent variable; a variable that is manipulated or controlled by the researcher, who sets its "values" or levels. (7)

inductive reasoning. The logical process of developing generalizations based on specific observations or facts. (1)

inferential statistics. That branch of statistics concerned with testing hypotheses and using sample data to make generalizations concerning populations. (18)

informed consent. An ethical principle that requires obtaining the consent of the individual to participate in a study based on full prior disclosure of risks and benefits. (3)

instrumentation effect. A threat to internal validity in which bias is introduced by an unreliable or inaccurate measurement system. (9)

intention-to-treat. Principle whereby data are analyzed according to group assignments, regardless of how subjects actually completed the study. (9)

interaction effect. The combined effect of two or more independent variables on a dependent variable. (10, 20)

intercorrelations. A set of bivariate correlations for several variables within a sample. (23)

internal consistency. A form of reliability, assessing the degree to which a set of items in an instrument all measure the same trait. Typically measured using Cronbach's alpha. (5, 26)

internal validity. The degree to which the relationship between the independent and dependent variables is free from the effects of extraneous factors. (9)

interquartile range.   The difference between the first and third quartiles in a distribution, often expressed graphically in a boxplot. (17)

interrater reliability.   The degree to which two or more raters can obtain the same ratings for a given variable. (5, 26)

interrupted time-series design.   A design involving a series of measurements over time, interrupted by one or more treatment occasions. (10)

interval scale.   Level of measurement in which values have equal intervals, but no true zero point. (4)

intraclass correlation coefficient (ICC).   A reliability coefficient based on an analysis of variance; a generalizability coefficient. (26)

intrarater reliability.   The degree to which one rater can obtain the same rating on multiple occasions of measuring the same variable. (5, 26)

item-to-total correlation.   Correlation of individual items in a scale with the total scale score; an indication of internal consistency. (5, 26)

Kaplan-Meier Estimate.   A common method of determining survival time which generates a step function, changing the survival estimate each time a patient dies (or reaches the terminal event). (29)

kappa (κ).   A correction factor for percent agreement measures of reliability, accounting for the potential effect of chance agreements. (26)

known groups method.   A technique for construct validation, in which validity is determined by the degree to which an instrument can demonstrate different scores for groups known to vary on the variable being measured. (6)

Kruskal–Wallis one-way analysis of variance by ranks (H).   A nonparametric statistical procedure for comparing more than two independent groups representing levels of one independent variable; analogous to the one-way analysis of variance. (22)

Latin square.   A matrix of columns and rows used to assign sequences of treatments to control for order effects. (10)

Least squares method.   A method of fitting a regression line to a set of bivariate data so as to minimize the sum of the squared vertical deviations of Y values around that line. (24)

level.   1. The "value" or classification of an independent variable. (7) 2. In single-case research, the magnitude of the target behavior; changes in level are associated with differences in magnitude between the end of one phase and the beginning of the following phase. (12)

level of measurement.   The precision of a scale based on how a characteristic is measured; nominal, ordinal, interval and ratio levels. (4)

level of significance (α).   The probability that an observed effect could be attributed to chance; the standard for rejecting the null hypothesis; traditionally set at a = .05. (18)

Levene's test.   A test of the equality of variances, used with the independent t test and the analysis of variance. (19)

Likert scale.   A summative scale based on responses to a set of statements for which respondents are asked to rate their degree of agreement or disagreement. (15)

likelihood ratio.   In diagnostic testing, the ratio indicating the usefulness of the test for ruling in or ruling out a condition. (See *negative likelihood ratio* and *positive likelihood ratio*.) (27)

limits of agreement.   Index of reliability between alternate forms of an instrument. (26)

linear regression.   The process of determining a regression equation to predict values of Y based on a linear relationship with values of X. (24)

line of best fit.   The regression line, representing the relationship between two variables, usually plotted on a scatter diagram. (24)

logistic regression.   Multiple regression procedure where the dependent variable is a dichotomous outcome; predicts odds associated with presence or absence of the dependent variable based on the independent variables. (29)

logrank test. A statistical procedure for comparing two survival curves when censored observations are present. (29)

longitudinal study. A study designed to collect data over time, usually for the purpose of describing developmental changes in a particular group. (13)

main effect. The separate effect of one independent variable in a multifactor design. (10, 20)

Mann-Whitney U test. A nonparametric statistical test for comparing two independent groups; analogous to the unpaired t-test. (22)

MANOVA. (See *multivariate analysis of variance*.)

maturation effect. A threat to internal validity, in which changes occur in the dependent variable as a result of the passing of time. (9)

McNemar test. A nonparametric statistical test for nominal level measures, for correlated samples; a form of the chi square test. (25)

mean ($\overline{X}$). A measure of central tendency, computed by summing the values of several observations and dividing by the number of observations. (17)

mean square (MS). In an analysis of variance, that value representing the variance; calculated by dividing the sum of squares for a particular effect by the degrees of freedom for that effect. The symbol MS_e = error mean square; MS_b = between groups mean square. (20)

measurement error. The difference between an observed value for a measurement and the theoretical true score; may be the result of systematic or random effects. (5, 26)

median. A measure of central tendency representing the 50th percentile in a ranked distribution of scores; that is, that point at which 50 percent of the scores fall below and 50 percent fall above. (17)

meta-analysis. Use of statistical techniques in a systematic review to integrate the results of included studies to determine overall outcome, usually based on effect size. (16)

method error (ME). A form of reliability testing for assessing response stability based on the discrepancy between two sets of repeated scores. (26)

methodological research. Research designed to develop or refine procedures or instruments for measuring variables, generally focusing on reliability and validity. (13)

minimal clinically important difference (MCID). The smallest difference in a measured variable that signifies an important rather than trivial difference in the patient's condition. The smallest difference a patient or clinician would perceive as beneficial, and that would result in a change in the management of the patient. Also called minimal clinically important change (MCIC) or minimally important change (MIC). (6, 27)

minimal detectable difference (MDD). That amount of change in a variable that must be achieved to reflect a true difference; the smallest amount of change that passes the threshold of error. Also called minimal detectable change (MDC). (5, 26)

mixed design. A design that incorporates independent variables that are independent (between-subjects) and repeated (within-subjects) factors. Also called a split-plot design. (10)

mode. A measure of central tendency representing the most commonly occurring score. (17)

μ (mu). Mean of a population. (17)

multicolinearity. The correlation between independent variables in a multiple regression equation, causing them to provide redundant information. (29)

multiple baseline design. In single-case research, a design for collecting data for more than one subject, behavior, or treatment condition. Baseline phases are staggered to provide control. (12)

multiple comparison test. A test of differences between individual means following analysis of variance, used to control for Type I error. (21)

multiple regression. A multivariate statistical technique for establishing the predictive relationship between one dependent variable (Y) and a set of independent variables ($X_1, X_2, \ldots$). (29)

multistage sampling. (See *cluster sampling*.)

multivariate analysis. A set of statistical procedures designed to analyze the relationship among three or more variables; includes techniques such as multiple regression, discriminant analysis, factor analysis and multivariate analysis of variance. (29)

multivariate analysis of variance (MANOVA). An advanced multivariate procedure that provides a global test of significance for multiple dependent variables using an analysis of variance. (29)

natural history. Longitudinal study of a disease or disorder, demonstrating the typical progress of the condition. (14)

naturalistic inquiry. Qualitative observation and interaction with subjects in their own natural environment. (14)

negative likelihood ratio (LR−). A ratio that indicates how much the odds of a disease are decreased if a diagnostic test is negative. Equals specificity/1 − sensitivity. (27)

negative predictive value (PV−). In diagnostic testing, the proportion of subjects who are correctly identified as not having the condition of interest. (27)

nested design. A multifactor design in which one variable is not crossed with other variables. (10)

Newman-Keuls (NK) multiple comparison test. A multiple comparison procedure, used following a significant analysis of variance. Also called the Student-Newman-Keuls (SNK) test. (21)

nominal scale. Level of measurement for classification variables; assignment of "values" based on mutually exclusive and exhaustive categories with no inherent rank order. (4)

nondirectional hypothesis. A research hypothesis (or alternative hypothesis) that does not indicate the expected direction of the relationship between variables. (7,18)

nonequivalent control group. A control group (or comparison group) that was not created by random assignment. (11)

nonparametric statistics. A set of statistical procedures that are not based on assumptions about population parameters, or the shape of the underlying population distribution; most often used when data are measured on the nominal or ordinal scales. (22)

nonprobability sample. A sample that was not selected using random selection. (8)

normal distribution (curve). A symmetrical bell-shaped theoretical distribution that has defined properties; also called a Gaussian distribution. (17, 18)

normative research. A descriptive research approach designed to determine normal values for specific variables within a population. (14)

norm referencing. Interpretation of a score based on its value relative to a standard or "normal" score. (6)

null hypothesis (H_0). A statement of no difference or no relationship between variables; the statistical hypothesis. (7, 18)

number needed to harm (NNH). The number of patients that need to be treated to observe one adverse outcome. (28)

number needed to treat (NNT). The number of patients that need to be treated to prevent one adverse outcome or achieve one successful outcome; the reciprocal of absolute risk reduction (ARR). (28)

observational study. A study that does not involve an intervention or manipulation of an independent variable. (13)

odds ratio (OR). Estimate of relative risk in a case-control study. (28)

one-tailed test. A statistical test based on a directional alternative hypothesis, in which critical values are obtained for only one tail of a distribution. (18)

one-way analysis of variance. An analysis of variance with one independent variable. (20)

one-way design. An experimental or quasi-experimental design that involves one independent variable. (10)

on-protocol analysis.   Analysis of data in an experiment based only on subjects who completed the study according to assigned groups. Also called completer analysis or on-treatment analysis. (9)

open-ended question.   A question on a survey (interview or questionnaire) that does not restrict the respondent to specific choices, but allows for a free response. (15)

operational definition.   Definition of a variable based on how it will be used in a particular study; how a dependent variable will be measured, how an independent variable will be manipulated. (7)

order effects.   The sequential effect of one subject being exposed to several treatments in the same order; potentially manifested as carryover or practice effects. (10)

ordinal scale.   Level of measurement in which scores are ranks. (4)

outlier.   Numeric value that does not fall within the range of most scores in a distribution. (24)

paired _t_-test.   A parametric test for comparing two means for correlated samples or repeated measures; also called a correlated _t_-test. (19)

paradigm.   A set of assumptions, concepts or values that constitute a way of viewing reality within an intellectual community. (1)

parameter.   A measured characteristic of a population. (17)

parametric statistics.   Statistical procedures for estimating population parameters and for testing hypotheses based on population parameters, with assumptions about the distribution of variables, and for use with interval or ratio measures. (18)

partial correlation.   A statistical technique for establishing the correlation between two variables, with the effect of a third variable removed; also called a first-order correlation. (29)

participant observation.   A method of data collection in qualitative research in which the researcher becomes a participant in the group that is being observed. (14)

Pearson product-moment coefficient of correlation (r).   A parametric statistical technique for determining the relationship between two variables. (23)

percent agreement.   A reliability test for categorical variables, estimating the ability of researchers to agree on category ratings. (26)

percentile.   The percentage of a distribution that is below a specified value. Data are divided into 99 equal ranks, or percentiles, with 1 percent of the scores in each rank. (17)

person-years.   The total number of years that a set of subjects have participated in a study, typically used when subjects begin and end their participation at different times. (28)

phenomenology.   An approach to qualitative research involving the study of complex human experience as it is actually lived. (14)

phi coefficient (r_Φ).   A nonparametric correlation statistic for estimating the relationship between two dichotomous variables. (23,25)

point biserial correlation (r_{pb}).   A correlation statistic for estimating the relationship between a dichotomy and a continuous variable on the interval or ratio scale. (23)

point estimate.   A single sample statistic that serves as an estimate of a population parameter. (18)

polynomial regression.   Regression procedure for nonlinear data. (24)

pooled variance estimate (s_p^2).   Estimate of population variance based on the weighted average of sample variances; used in the unpaired _t_-test when group variances are not significantly different (under conditions of homogeneity of variance). (19)

population.   The entire set of individuals or units to which data will be generalized. (8)

positive likelihood ratio (LR +).   A ratio that indicates how much the odds of a disease are increased if a diagnostic test is positive. Equals sensitivity/1 − specificity. (27)

positive predictive value (PV +).   Estimate of the likelihood that a person who tests positive actually has the disease. (27)

posterior probability.   (See _posttest probability_.)

post hoc comparisons.   Multiple comparison tests that follow an analysis of variance. (21)

posttest-only design.   An experimental design in which only one measurement is taken following treatment. (10)

posttest probability.   The probability of a condition existing after performing a diagnostic test; predictive value of a diagnostic test. Also called posterior probability. Depends on the pretest probability, and the test's sensitivity and specificity. (27)

power $(1 - \beta)$.   The ability of a statistical test to find a significant difference that really does exist; the probability that a test will lead to rejection of the null hypothesis. (18, Appendix C)

predictive validity.   A form of measurement validity in which an instrument is used to predict some future performance. (6)

predictive value (PV).   (see *negative predictive value* and *positive predictive value*)

preference.   In sequential clinical trials, the expression of which treatment is considered better within a sequential pair. (10)

pretest probability.   The probability that a condition exists prior to performing a diagnostic test. Equal to the prevalence of the condition in a specified group of subjects. Also called prior probability. (27)

pretest-posttest design.   An experimental design involving a pretest prior to intervention and a posttest following intervention. (10)

prevalence.   The number of existing cases of a disease or condition at a given point in time, expressed as a proportion of the total population at risk. (27, 28)

primary source.   Reference source that represents the original document by the original author. (7)

prior probability.   (See *pretest probability*.)

probability sample.   A sample chosen using randomized methods. (8)

proportional hazards model.   (See *Cox's regression*.)

prospective study.   A study designed to collect data following development of the research question. (13)

publication bias.   Tendency for researchers and editors to treat positive experimental results (finding an effect) differently from negative or inconclusive results (finding no effect), often with a preference for publication of positive findings. (16)

purposive sample.   A nonprobability sample in which subjects are specifically selected by the researcher on the basis of subjective judgment that they will be the most representative. (8)

q.   Studentized range statistic, used in multiple comparison tests. (21)

Q-sort.   An analytic technique used to characterize attitudes, opinions, or judgments of individuals through a process of comparative rank ordering. (15)

quadratic trend.   A nonlinear trend, with one turn in direction. (21, 24)

quartile (Q).   Three quartiles divide a distribution of ranked data into four equal groups, each containing 25 percent of the scores. (17)

quasi-experimental research.   Comparative research approach in which subjects cannot be randomly assigned to groups or control groups are not used. (11)

quota sampling.   Nonprobability sampling method in which stratification is used to obtain representative proportions of specific subgroups. (8)

R^2 (R squared).   Multiple correlation coefficient squared; represents the proportion of variance in Y explained by several independent variables in a multiple regression equation. (29)

random assignment.   Assignment of subjects to groups using probability methods, where every subject has an equal chance of being assigned to each group. (9)

random sampling.   Probability method of selecting subjects for a sample, where every subject in the population has an equal chance of being chosen. (8)

random selection.   (See *random sampling*.)

randomized block design. An experimental design in which one independent variable is an attribute variable, creating homogeneous blocks of subjects who are then randomly assigned to levels of the other independent variable. (10)

randomized controlled trial (RCT). An experimental study in which a clinical treatment is compared with a control condition, where subjects are randomly assigned to groups. Also called a randomized clinical trial. (10)

rank sum test. A nonparametric statistical procedure, used to compare two independent samples; equivalent to the Mann-Whitney U test. Analogous to the unpaired t-test. (22)

Rasch analysis. Transformation of items on an ordinal scale to an interval scale, demonstrating the unidimensional nature of a scale. (15)

ratio scale. The highest level of measurement, in which there are equal intervals between score units and a true zero point. (4)

reactive measurement. A measurement that distorts the variable being measured, either by the subject's awareness of being measured or by influence of the measurement process. (9)

recall bias. The possible inaccuracy of recalling medical history or previous exposures; of particular concern in retrospective studies. (28)

receiver operating characteristic (ROC) curve. In diagnostic testing, a plot of the true positives (sensitivity) against false positives (1 − specificity) at several cutoff points for defining a positive test. (27)

refereed journal. Journals that utilize a peer review process to evaluate manuscript submissions as a basis for choosing which ones will be published. (33)

reference standard. A value used as a standard against which to judge a criterion; may or may not be a gold standard. Used to judge criterion-related validity or diagnostic accuracy. (6, 27)

regression analysis. A statistical procedure for examining the predictive relationship between a dependent (criterion) variable and an independent (predictor) variable. (24, 29)

regression coefficient. In a regression equation, the weight (b) assigned to the independent variable; the slope of the regression line. (24, 29)

regression line. The straight line that is drawn on a scatter plot for bivariate data from the regression equation, summarizing the relationship between variables. (24)

regression toward the mean. A statistical phenomenon in which scores on a pretest are likely to move toward the group mean on a posttest because of inherent positive or negative measurement error; also called statistical regression. (5, 9)

relative risk (RR). Estimate of the magnitude of the association between an exposure and disease, indicating the likelihood that the exposed group will develop the disease relative to those who are not exposed. (28)

relative risk reduction (RRR). The reduction in risk associated with an intervention relative to the risk without the intervention (control); the absolute difference between the experimental event rate and the control event rate divided by the control event rate. (28)

reliability. The degree of consistency with which an instrument or rater measures a variable. (5, 26)

repeated measure (repeated factor). An independent variable for which subjects act as their own control; that is, all subjects are exposed to all levels of the variable. Also called a within-subjects factor. (7, 10)

research hypothesis. A statement of the researcher's expectations about the relationship between variables under study. (7)

residual ($Y - \hat{Y}$). In regression analysis, the difference between the value of the dependent variable predicted by the regression equation and the actual value. (24)

responsiveness. The ability of a test to demonstrate change. (6, 27)

retrospective study. A study that analyzes observations that were collected in the past. (13)

ρ (rho). Correlation coefficient for a population. (23)

risk-benefit ratio.   An ethical principle that is an element of informed consent, in which the risks of a research study to the participant are evaluated in relation to the potential benefits of the study's outcomes. (3)

risk factor.   A characteristic or exposure that potentially increases the likelihood of having a disease or condition. (28)

ROC curve.   (See *receiver operating characteristic curve*.)

sampling bias.   Bias that occurs when individuals who are selected for a sample overrepresent or underrepresent the underlying population characteristics. (8)

sampling distribution.   A theoretical frequency distribution of a statistic, based on the value of the statistic over an infinite number of samples. (18)

sampling error.   The difference between an observed statistic from a sample and the population parameter. (18)

scale of measurement.   (See *level of measurement*.)

scatter plot.   A graphic representation of the relationship between two variables. (23)

Scheffé's multiple comparison test.   A multiple comparison procedure for comparing means following a significant analysis of variance. Considered the most conservative of the multiple comparison methods. (21)

secondary analysis.   An approach to research involving the use of data that were collected for another purpose, usually for the purpose of testing new hypotheses. (13)

secondary source.   Reference source that represents a review or report of another's work. (7)

selection bias.   A threat to internal validity in which bias is introduced by initial differences between groups, when these differences are not random. (9)

semantic differential.   A technique used to measure attitudes by asking respondents to rate concepts on a 7-point scale which represents a continuum across two extremes. (15)

sensitivity.   A measure of validity of a screening procedure, based on the probability that someone with a disease will test positive. (27)

sensitivity analysis.   A procedure in decision making to determine how decisions change as values are systematically varied. (16)

sequential clinical trial.   Experimental research design that allows consecutive entrance to a clinical trial and continuous analysis of data, permitting stopping of the trial when data are sufficient to show a significant effect. (10)

serial dependency.   Correlation in a set of data collected over time, in which one observation can be predicted based on previous observations. (12)

σ (sigma).   Standard deviation of a population. σ^2 is the population variance. (17)

Σ (sigma, uppercase).   Read as: "the sum of." (17)

sign test.   A nonparametric statistical procedure for comparing two correlated samples, based on comparison of positive or negative outcomes; analogous to the paired t-test. (22)

significance level (α).   (See *alpha level*.)

single-blind study.   An experiment in which either the investigator or the subject is kept ignorant of group assignment, but not both. (9)

single-factor design.   An experimental design involving one independent variable. (10)

single-subject design.   An experimental design based on time-series data from one or more subjects, with data compared across baseline and intervention phases. Also called single-case designs. (12)

skewed distribution.   A distribution of scores that is asymmetrical, with more scores to one extreme. (17)

slope.   1. In regression analysis, the rate of change in values of Y for one unit of change in X. (24) 2. In single-case research, the rate of change in the magnitude of the target behavior over time. (12)

SnNout.   When a test has high sensitivity, a negative test rules out the diagnosis. (27)

snowball sampling.   A nonprobability sampling method in which subjects are successively recruited by referrals from other subjects. (8)

Spearman-Brown formula.   The statistical procedure used to analyze split-half reliability; also called the Spearman-Brown prophecy formula. (5)

Spearman's rank correlation coefficient (r_s).   A nonparametric correlation procedure for ordinal data. Also called Spearman's rho. (23)

special cause variation.   Fluctuation in response caused by known factors that results in non-random and unexpected performance.

specificity.   A measure of validity of a screening procedure, based on the probability that someone who does not have a disease will test negative. (27)

split-half reliability.   A reliability measure of internal consistency based on dividing the items on an instrument into two halves and correlating the results. (5)

split middle line.   In single-case research, a line used to separate data points within one phase into two equal halves, reflecting the trend of the data within that phase. (See *celeration line.*) (12)

split-plot design.   (See *mixed design.*)

SpPin.   When a test has high specificity, a positive test rules in the diagnosis. (27)

standard deviation (s).   A descriptive statistic reflecting the variability or dispersion of scores around the mean. (17)

standard error of measurement (SEM).   A reliability measure of response stability, estimating the standard error in a set of repeated scores. (26)

standard error of the estimate (SEE).   In regression analysis, an estimate of prediction accuracy; a measure of the spread of scores around the regression line. (24)

standard error of the mean ($s_{\overline{x}}$).   The standard deviation of a distribution of sample means; an estimate of the population standard deviation. (18)

standardized residual.   In a chi square test, the contribution of each cell to the overall statistic. (25)

standardized response mean (SRM).   One approach to evaluating effect size with change scores. Calculated as the difference between pretest and posttest scores, divided by the standard deviation of the change scores. (27)

standardized score.   (See *z-score.*)

statistic.   A measured characteristic of a sample. (12)

statistical conclusion validity.   The validity of conclusions drawn from statistical analyses, based on the proper application of statistical tests and principles. (9)

statistical hypothesis.   (See *null hypothesis.*)

statistical process control (SPC).   A method of charting production outcomes over time to identify and monitor variances; can be used as a method of analysis for single-subject designs. (12)

statistical regression.   (See *regression toward the mean.*)

statistical significance.   The term indicating that the results of an analysis are unlikely to be the result of chance at a specified probability level; rejection of the null hypothesis. (18)

stem-and-leaf plot.   A graphic display for numerical data in a frequency distribution showing each value in the distribution. (17)

stepwise regression.   An approach to multiple regression that involves a sequential process of selecting variables for inclusion in the prediction equation. (29)

stopping rule.   In a sequential clinical trial, the threshold for stopping a study based on crossing a boundary that indicates a difference or no difference between treatments. (10)

stratification.   The grouping of individuals in a population into homogeneous groups on some characteristic prior to sampling. (8)

sum of squares (SS).   A measure of variability in a set of data, equal to the sum of squared deviation scores for a distribution ($\Sigma(X - \overline{X})^2$; the numerator in the formula for variance. (17)

Used in analysis of variance as the basis for partitioning between-groups (SS_b) and within-groups error (SS_e) variance components. (20)

survival analysis.   Multivariate analysis to estimate survival time, or time to a defined outcome, based on probabilities that an individual will achieve the outcome. (29)

systematic error.   A form of measurement error, where error is constant across trials. (5)

systematic review.   Review of a clearly formulated question that uses systematic and explicit methods to identify, select and critically appraise relevant research. (16)

systematic sample.   A probability sampling method where subjects are chosen from lists of population members using specified intervals, such as every 10th person. (8)

***t*-test.**   A parametric test for comparing two means; also called Student's *t*-test. (See paired *t*-test and unpaired *t*-test.) (19)

target population.   The larger population to which results of a study will be generalized. (8)

testing effect.   The effect that occurs when a test itself is responsible for observed changes in the measured variable. (5, 9)

test-retest reliability.   The degree to which an instrument is stable, based on repeated administrations of the test to the same individuals over a specified time interval. (5)

time-series design.   A quasi-experimental design in which performance changes are assessed over time, prior to and following the administration of treatment. (11)

transformation.   Mathematical conversion of a distribution to a different scale by a constant (such as square root or log) to change the shape or variance characteristics of the distribution. (Appendix D)

translational research.   Clinical investigation with human subjects in which knowledge obtained from basic research is translated into diagnostic or therapeutic interventions that can be applied to treatment or prevention. (1)

treatment arm.   Another term for each independent group in a clinical trial. (10)

treatment threshold.   In clinical decision making, the point at which a decision is reached to treat the patient without first performing a diagnostic test. (27)

treatment-received analysis.   Analysis of subject data in an experiment according to the treatment subjects actually did receive, regardless of their original group assignment. (9)

trend.   1. The shape of a distribution of scores taken over time, reflecting the distribution's linearity or lack of linearity. (21) 2. In single-case research, the direction of change in the target behavior within a phase or across phases. (12)

trend analysis.   Part of an analysis of variance, used to assess trend within data taken over ordered intervals; can express data as linear, quadratic, cubic, and so on, reflecting the number of changes in direction in the data over time. (21)

triangulation.   The use of multiple methods to document phenomena. (14)

true negative.   A test result that is negative for those who do not have the disease or condition of interest. (27)

true positive.   A test result that is positive for those who do have the disease or condition of interest. (27)

Tukey's honestly significant difference (HSD).   A multiple comparison test for comparing multiple means following a significant analysis of variance. (21)

Two standard deviation band method.   A method of data analysis in single-subject research. (12)

two-tailed test.   A statistical test based on a nondirectional alternative hypothesis, in which critical values represent both positive and negative tails of a distribution. (18)

two-way analysis of variance.   An analysis of variance with two independent variables. (20)

two-way design.   An experimental or quasi-experimental study that involves two independent variables. (10)

Type I error.   An incorrect decision to reject the null hypothesis, concluding that a relationship exists when in fact it does not. (18)

Type II error.   An incorrect decision to accept the null hypothesis, concluding that no relationship exists when in fact it does. (18)

univariate analysis.   Statistical procedures for analyzing one dependent variable. (29)

unpaired *t*-test.   A parametric test for comparing two means for independent samples; also called an independent *t*-test. (19)

validity.   1. The degree to which an instrument measures what it is intended to measure. (6) 2. The degree to which a research design allows for reasonable interpretations from the data, based on controls (internal validity), appropriate definitions (construct validity), appropriate analysis procedures (statistical conclusion validity), and generalizability (external validity). (9)

variable.   A characteristic that can be manipulated or observed and that can take on different values, either quantitatively or qualitatively. (2, 7)

variance (s^2).   A measure of variablity in a distribution, equal to the square of the standard deviation. (17)

vital statistics.   Mortality and morbidity rates. (28)

washout period.   In a crossover design, that period of time between administration of the two treatments, allowing effects of the experimental treatment to dissipate. (10)

weighted kappa (κ_w).   An estimate of percentage agreement, corrected for chance, based on weights reflecting levels of seriousness of disagreements. (26)

Wilcoxon rank-sum test.   (See *Mann Whitney U test*.)

Wilcoxon signed-ranks test (*T*).   A nonparametric statistical procedure, comparing two correlated samples (repeated measures); analogous to the paired *t*-test. (22)

withdrawal design.   In single-case research, a design that involves withdrawal of the intervention. (12)

within-groups variance.   (See *error variance*.)

within-subjects design.   A research design that incorporates only repeated measures. (10)

within-subjects factor.   (See *repeated measure*.)

$\overline{X}$.   Mean of a sample. (17)

Yates' correction for continuity.   In the chi square test, a correction factor applied when expected frequencies are too small, effectively reducing the chi square statistic. (25)

z distribution.   The standardized normal distribution, with a mean of 0 and a standard deviation of 1. (17)

z-score   The number of standard deviations that a given value is above or below the mean of the distribution; also called a standardized score. (17)

zero-order correlation.   A bivariate correlation. (29)

Index